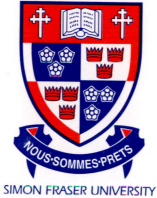

INTEGRATIVE ONCOLOGY

Principles and practice

Dedication

This book is dedicated to all whose lives are touched by cancer – that you may have the courage, knowledge and resources to heal

INTEGRATIVE ONCOLOGY

Principles and practice

Edited by

Matthew P Mumber MD
Harbin Clinic Radiation Oncology Center
Rome, Georgia, USA

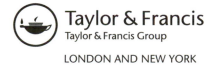

Taylor & Francis
Taylor & Francis Group

LONDON AND NEW YORK

© 2006 Taylor & Francis, an imprint of the Taylor & Francis Group

First published in the United Kingdom in 2006
by Taylor & Francis,
an imprint of the Taylor & Francis Group,
2 Park Square, Milton Park
Abingdon, Oxon OX14 4RN, UK

Tel.:   +44 (0) 20 7017 6000
Fax.:   +44 (0) 20 7017 6699
E-mail: info.medicine@tandf.co.uk
Website: http://www.tandf.co.uk/medicine

Although every effort has been made to ensure that all owners of copyright material have been acknowledged in this publication, we would be glad to acknowledge in subsequent reprints or editions any omissions brought to our attention.

British Library Cataloguing in Publication Data
Data available on application

Library of Congress Cataloging-in-Publication Data
Data available on application

ISBN10 0-41537-415-4
ISBN13 9-78-0-41537-415-6

Distributed in North and South America by

Taylor & Francis
2000 NW Corporate Blvd
Boca Raton, FL 33431, USA
Within Continental USA
Tel.: 800 272 7737; Fax.: 800 374 3401
Outside Continental USA
Tel.: 561 994 0555; Fax.: 561 361 6018
E-mail: orders@crcpress.com

Distributed in the rest of the world by
Thomson Publishing Services
Cheriton House
North Way
Andover, Hampshire SP10 5BE, UK
Tel.: +44 (0) 1264 332424
E-mail: salesorder.tandf@thomsonpublishingservices.co.uk

Composition by Parthenon Publishing
Printed and bound by Antony Rowe Ltd, Chippenham, Wiltshire, UK

Cover graphic design by Jeremy Clewell

Contents

Contributing authors   xi

Foreword   xiii

Introduction   xv

Acknowledgments   xix

Section I: Principles   1

1. Principles of integrative oncology   3
    Matthew P. Mumber

2. Clinical research and evidence   17
    Nancy Stark, Suzanne Hess and Edward Shaw

3. Physician training in integrative medicine   43
    Patrick B. Massey

4. The health of the healer: physician/health-care provider wellness   57
    Danna M. Park

5. Models of care   77
    Judith Boyce

6. Legal issues   101
    Michael H. Cohen and David Rosenthal

7. Business assessment   121
    Joan Kines

Section II. Practice   141

  8. Clinical decision analysis   145
      Matthew P. Mumber

  9. Stages of change   165
      Robert B. Lutz

 10. Modalities – overview   169
     a. Physical activity   171
        Robert B. Lutz
     b. Nutrition   177
        Cynthia Thomson and Mara Vitolins
     c. Mind–body interventions   183
        Linda E. Carlson and Shauna L. Shapiro
     d. Botanicals   191
        Lise Alschuler
     e. Manual therapy   197
        J. Michael Menke
     f. Energy medicine   203
        Suzanne Clewell
     g. Spirituality   221
        Howard Silverman and Toby Schneider
     h. Alternative medical systems   243
        Lawrence Berk

 11. Modalities – cancer prevention   255
     a. Physical activity   257
        Robert B. Lutz
     b. Nutrition   263
        Cynthia Thomson and Mara Vitolins
     c. Mind–body interventions   281
        Linda E. Carlson and Shauna L. Shapiro
     d. Botanicals   287
        Lise Alschuler
     e. Energy medicine   295
        Suzanne Clewell

 12. Modalities – supportive care   301
     a. Physical activity   303
        Robert B. Lutz
     b. Nutrition   307
        Mara Vitolins and Cynthia Thomson
     c. Mind–body interventions   319
        Linda E. Carlson and Shauna L. Shapiro

d. Botanicals   331
    Lise Alschuler

e. Manual therapy   339
    J. Michael Menke

f. Energy medicine   341
    Suzanne Clewell

g. Alternative medical systems   367
    Lawrence Berk

13. Modalities – antineoplastic therapy   377

a. Nutrition   379
    Mara Vitolins and Cynthia Thomson

b. Mind–body interventions   381
    Linda E. Carlson and Shauna L. Shapiro

c. Botanicals   383
    Lise Alschuler

d. Energy medicine   393
    Suzanne Clewell

14. Tobacco, alcohol and integrative oncology   397
    Dennett Gordon

15. Specific malignancies

a. Breast cancer   409
    Matthew P. Mumber

    Physical activity   412
    Robert B. Lutz

    Nutrition   418
    Cynthia Thomson and Mara Vitolins

    Mind–body interventions   419
    Linda E. Carlson and Shauna L. Shapiro

    Botanicals   420
    Lise Alschuler

    Energy medicine   425
    Suzanne Clewell

b. Prostate cancer   429
    Matthew P. Mumber

    Physical activity   432
    Robert B. Lutz

    Nutrition   438
    Mara Vitolins and Cynthia Thomson

    Mind–body interventions   439
    Linda E. Carlson and Shauna L. Shapuro

Botanicals   440
Lise Alschuler

Energy medicine   443
Suzanne Clewell

c.   Lung cancer   445
Matthew P. Mumber

Physical activity   447
Robert B. Lutz

Nutrition   452
Mara Vitolins and Cynthia Thomson

Mind–body interventions   453
Linda E. Carlson and Shauna L. Shapiro

Botanicals   454
Lise Alschuler

Energy medicine   455
Suzanne Clewell

d.   Colorectal cancer   457
Matthew P. Mumber

Physical activity   460
Robert B. Lutz

Nutrition   466
Mara Vitolins and Cynthia Thomson

Mind–body interventions   467
Linda E. Carlson and Shauna L. Shapiro

Botanicals   468
Lise Alschuler

Energy medicine   469
Suzanne Clewell

e.   Skin cancer   471
Matthew P. Mumber

Physical activity   473
Robert B. Lutz

Nutrition   477
Cynthia Thomson and Mara Vitolins

Mind–body interventions   478
Linda E. Carlson and Shauna L. Shapiro

Botanicals   479
Lise Alschuler

Energy medicine   480
Suzanne Clewell

f. Other cancers   483
    Matthew P. Mumber
        Physical activity   484
        Robert B. Lutz
        Botanicals   485
        Lise Alschuler
        Energy medicine   490
        Suzanne Clewell

g. Palliative and end-of-life care   495
    Matthew P. Mumber

Index   503

Contributing authors

Lise N Alschuler ND
Naturopathic Medicine Department
Midwestern Regional Medical Center
2520 Elisha Avenue
Zion, IL 60099
USA

Lawrence B Berk MD PhD
Central Ohio Radiation Oncology
115 McMillen Drive
Newark, OH 43055
USA

Judith M Boyce MD
Floyd Center for Health and Healing
420 East 2nd Avenue
Rome, GA 30161
USA

Linda E Carlson PhD CPsych
Department of Psychosocial Resources
Tom Baker Cancer Centre – Holy Cross Site
2202 2nd Street SW
Calgary
Alberta T2S 3C1
Canada

Suzanne Clewell RN BSN HNC
Harbin Clinic Radiation Oncology Center
321 West 5th Street
Rome, GA 30165
USA

Michael H Cohen JD
Harvard Medical School Osher Institute
401 Park Drive, 22-W
Boston, MA 02215
USA

Dennett Gordon PhD
111 Greenview Road
Rome, GA 30165
USA

Suzanne M Hess PhD
Department of Radiation Oncology
Wake Forest University School of Medicine
Medical Center Boulevard
Winston-Salem, NC 27157
USA

Joan Kines
Harbin Clinic Radiation Oncology Center
321 West 5th Street
Rome, GA 30165
USA

Robert B Lutz MD MPH
College of Medicine and Public Health
University of Arizona
Tucson, AZ 85721
USA

Patrick B Massey MD PhD
Complementary and Alternative Medicine
Alexian Brothers Hospital
1544 Nerge Road
Elk Grove Village, IL 60007
USA

J Michael Menke MA DC
1836 Bryant Street
Palo Alto, CA 94301
USA

Matthew P Mumber MD
Harbin Clinic Radiation Oncology Center
321 West 5th Street
Rome, GA 30165
USA

Danna M Park MD
Program in Integrative Medicine
University of Arizona
PO Box 245153
Tucson, AZ 85724-5153
USA

David Rosenthal MD
Leonard P Zakim Center for Integrated
  Therapies
Dana-Farber Cancer Institute
44 Binney Street
Boston, MA 02215
USA

Toby Schneider
11345 Kallgren Road
Bainbridge Island, WA 98110
USA

Shauna L Shapiro PhD
Department of Psychology
Santa Clara University
500 El Camino
Santa Clara, CA 95053-0201
USA

Edward G Shaw MD
Division of Radiation Oncology
Wake Forest University School of Medicine
Medical Center Boulevard
Winston-Salem, NC 27157
USA

Howard D Silverman MD MS
Program in Integrative Medicine
College of Medicine
University of Arizona
PO Box 245153
Tucson, AZ 85724-5153
USA

Nancy Stark RN PhD
Section of Hematology and Oncology
Wake Forest University Health Sciences
Medical Center Boulevard
Winston-Salem, NC 27157
USA

Cynthia A Thomson PhD RD
Department of Nutritional Sciences
University of Arizona
Shantz Building 328
1177 East 4th Street
Tucson, AZ 85721-0038
USA

Mara Z Vitolins DrPH MPH RD
Department of Public Health Sciences
Wake Forest University Health Sciences
Piedmont Plaza II, Suite 512
2000 West First Street
Winston-Salem, NC 27104
USA

Foreword

Integrative Oncology: Principles and Practice is a text whose time has come. For 25 years, people with cancer have been asking their oncologists, and providers like my colleagues and myself, two urgent questions about integrative care: 'What else can I do aside from conventional cancer treatment?' and 'Where can I go to find a professional who can help me to do it?'

These questions cover a great deal of territory: Where can I find an integrative oncologist who will offer a second opinion? What can I do in addition to conventional care to improve my chances for living longer and better? How can I use those therapies that are called 'complementary' together with conventional care? Are there alternatives to conventional approaches that I should be aware of, particularly if conventional care has no further answers for me? And, where can I go to find these services? And, inevitably, why doesn't my oncologist know more about this? In the mid-1990s, 70% of *all* queries to the NIH Office of Alternative Medicine were about complementary and alternative medicine (CAM) therapies for cancer.

For these past 25 years, as a clinician in private practice, as the Founder and Director of the non-profit Center for Mind–Body Medicine (CMBM), and as an advisor to the National Institutes of Health and the National Cancer Institute, I've been helping people find these answers, and, indeed, helping to develop programs of integrative care.

In 1998, the CMBM created the first international Comprehensive Cancer Care Conference to bring leading clinicians and researchers in conventional cancer care together with those doing the most thoughtful and promising work in CAM therapies and integrative approaches. A number of contributors to *Integrative Oncology* participated in these meetings.

More recently, we've been working to train oncology and other health professionals to be CancerGuides®. CancerGuides are professionals who supply the answers to the questions I've listed above, and who are willing to be there – intellectually, emotionally, spiritually – for people with cancer and their families, from the moment of diagnosis, through and beyond treatment.

Now, Matt Mumber and his colleagues have responded to many of the questions oncology professionals and their patients are asking. They have created a text for us to use as an educational resource.

Integrative Oncology: Principles and Practice brings together, in one place, some of the most progressive and important thinking in the field. There are thoughtful descriptions of models of integrative care and of the perspectives and practices of alternative systems of healing; discussions of the spirit of transformation that the cancer experience may bring; clear summaries of research considerations and legal issues; reviews of the contributions of complementary therapies to palliative care and to dealing with the side-effects of conventional care; and comprehensive references to help all of us learn more.

Integrative Oncology: Principles and Practice offers a thoughtful and generous perspective on integrative care, an outstanding overview of the exciting work that is now being done and a guide to the new territories that all of us – physicians and patients, oncologists and CAM practitioners – need to explore and understand. I'm deeply grateful for this book for myself and for the Cancer Guides we are training, and I fully expect that you and your patients will be as well.

James S Gordon MD
Founder and Director of the Center for
Mind–Body Medicine
Author of *Comprehensive Cancer Care:*
Integrating Alternative, Complementary and
Conventional Therapies
jgordon@cmbm.org

Introduction

INTEGRATIVE ONCOLOGY: AN EVOLVING DISCIPLINE

What is integrative oncology? Why is this the right time to develop the field and to publish a book on its principles and practice? Complementary and alternative medicine (CAM), as this evolving field is currently known, has had a dramatic history over the past several decades as to nomenclature and utilization. The terminology itself, 'complementary and alternative medicine', as a descriptor, has created significant difficulties in scientific acceptance by physicians and other health professionals in oncology settings. Historians of this discipline would describe how far the field has come in the past 30 years, when the scientific community often referred to such interventions as 'quackery'. Since then, descriptive terms have shown a gradual trend toward acceptance from a Western medical perspective, while retaining a commitment to hold these therapies up to scientific scrutiny, e.g. from 'questionable methods of therapy' to 'unproven methods' to 'complementary and alternative methods of therapy' and now to 'integrative therapies'. In the USA, CAM has become a multibillion dollar unregulated industry, with the costs – and the potential risks of unsupervised use – incurred almost totally by the patients. Cancer patients are high utilizers of CAM therapies for a variety of reasons, including symptom management, improved quality of life and, in some cases, the hope of improving the disease process. CAM practices have increasingly gained the attention of the biomedical research community. The major governmental biomedical research agency, the National Institutes of Health (NIH), has two centers dedicated to cancer research in CAM: the National Center for Complementary and Alternative Medicine (NCCAM) and the Office of Cancer Complementary and Alternative Medicine (OCCAM), a division of the National Cancer Institute (NCI). Having sources of federally funded, peer-reviewed research in CAM has expanded medical professionals' knowledge and education about these modalities. Furthermore, it has helped to establish the legitimacy of CAM as the subject of scientific inquiry, moving the field forward through greater co-operation between clinical investigators and CAM practitioners.

Why the name-change from CAM to integrative oncology (IO)? IO emphasizes the incorporation of complementary therapies (e.g. acupuncture, meditation, music therapy) with conventional cancer treatment. CAM was initially patient driven and, as is known from the literature, patients often have not disclosed their self-care or self-directed care to their treating oncologist. This is true whether it involves the use of over-the-counter vitamin supplements, antioxidants, herbs or other approaches or technologies. At the same time, physicians often do not ask patients pertinent CAM-related questions. This lack of communication occurs despite the high interest and use of complementary therapies by cancer patients. These therapies need to be part of a patient–physician dialogue, because they may positively or negatively impact on treatment decisions, medical issues, or a patient's overall sense of well-being. In the new discipline of integrative oncology, emerging questions need to be addressed by the oncologist. What are some of the CAM practices utilized in the community to address cancer prevention, to lessen side-effects during cancer treatment and/or to support patients during rehabilitation and beyond? Are there legal and ethical issues that clinicians need to be aware of when patients consume herbs that may alleviate some cancer symptoms, but also may contain constituent chemicals within the product which have unknown intrinsic effects or side-effects due to contaminants? How can we be reassured about the consistency of a product or the standardization of the amount of product on a lot-to-lot basis? In addition to the well-recognized problem of drug–drug interactions, what are other interactions that could interfere with treatment effectiveness, such as interactions between drugs and herbs, and between antioxidants and chemotherapy or radiation therapy? These are some of the issues that need to be addressed in order to provide optimal, comprehensive cancer care.

Integration also means that patients, their clinicians and CAM providers are working closely together. In most cases, the oncologist is the primary co-ordinator and conductor of the patient's care and needs to be aware of all the care that the patient receives. When complementary therapies are effectively combined with conventional therapies in order to address the whole being and experience of the patient, the primary care oncologist is helping to meet the total needs of the cancer patient. Examples of this assimilation of therapies involve the recognition of evidence-based treatment options of complementary therapies, with the assurance that they are safe and efficacious, and that they could satisfy a risk–benefit analysis. Both the patient and the oncologist need to agree that integrative therapies are providing preventive and supportive care and are not being used for a 'cure' or as an alternative to conventional therapies. As one patient expressed, 'Integrative oncology is like building bridges between patients and their physicians.' The judicious use of complementary therapies alongside conventional therapies within a therapeutic and empathic doctor–patient relationship helps to ensure that the patient is treated as a whole person, rather than just as a cancer subject.

In establishing integrative oncology centers, whether in a hospital, ambulatory setting, or in a group practice, there are many principles that should be observed. Most important, however, are the clinical data behind complementary therapies and their role in oncology practice. How are treatment decisions made? How are complementary therapies initiated? When should complementary therapies be recommended to our patients? To advise their patients, the primary care oncologists need knowledge about which complementary therapies can be recommended, accepted, or discouraged. Research in CAM/IO is essential for physician acceptance.

A new society was formed to address scientifically the many questions raised. The Society for Integrative Oncology (SIO) provides such a forum. Although IO is in its infancy, the first international conference of the SIO, held in November 2004, included over 600 participants from four continents. The goal of the conference was to 'educate oncology professionals and other health care stakeholders about state of the art integrative therapies'. The conference addressed the data behind complementary therapies and their efficacy in oncology practice, essentially emphasizing evidence-based practices. Attendees at the conference learned about important work that is being done internationally in developing Integrative Cancer Centers. Plenary sessions and research studies covered areas such as acupuncture for cancer symptoms, as well as the use of botanicals, phytoestrogens and antioxidants in the treatment of cancer. Participants also learned about the importance of Phase I and II trials of CAM therapies and how to navigate the investigational new drug (IND) submissions of these agents to the Food and Drug Administration (FDA). Although models of integrative medicine in disciplines other than oncology are being formulated, 'integrative oncology' may serve as a model for other specialties.

The SIO will serve as a forum for the presentation of scientific data on complementary therapies, while emphasizing the importance of developing an infrastructure that promotes the principles and practices of IO. The ultimate goal is to develop multidisciplinary expertise, as well as therapeutic synergy, between conventional and complementary therapies.

We look forward to this initial edition of *Integrative Oncology: Principles and Practice* as a reference to be updated periodically as this dynamic field continues on a new trajectory as part of 21st century medicine.

David S Rosenthal MD
President of the Society of Integrative Oncology
Professor of Medicine, Harvard Medical School
Medical Director of the Zakim Center for
Integrated Therapies at DFCI

Henry K Oliver Professor of Hygiene and
Director of Harvard University Health Services,
Cambridge, MA

Acknowledgments

There are many individuals and organizations that have influenced the development of this text. None of this would be possible without the patience and diligence of all of the contributing authors and medical editors, especially Kath Burrow and Martin Lister, who remained focused during the dynamic and creative process that brought this text to life.

From a personal perspective, I would like, first and foremost, to thank my wife, Laura, for her unwavering support, unconditional love and steady guidance. My sons, J.T., Samson and Marcus remind me of the reason why I went into medicine in the first place, and give meaning to every part of my life, including the production of this text. I thank my mentors – Dr Lewis Barnett (Dr B.), Dr Bernie Siegel – all of the instructors and fellow classmates from the University of Arizona Program in Integrative Medicine Associate Fellowship, my patients with cancer, their families and care providers, the staff at Regional Radiation Oncology Center at Rome, and all board members, volunteers and providers associated with Many Streams Healing Systems, Incorporated. I would also like to thank my friends and family, and all those who helped in review, including Judy Boyce MD, Michael Cohen JD, Melissa Dillmon MD, J. Chris Eastman BA, Denny Gordon PhD, Joan Kines, Suzanne Hess, David Rosenthal MD, and Thomas Wolfe.

A portion of the after tax sales proceeds from this text will be donated to the Georgia Cancer Coalition.

Section I

Principles

1

Principles of integrative oncology

Matthew P. Mumber

'As we acquire more knowledge, things do not become more comprehensible, but more mysterious.'
– Albert Schweitzer

OVERVIEW

Integrative oncology (IO) is the next step in the evolution of cancer care. It addresses the limitations of the current system, while retaining its successful features. It includes the use of evidence-based tools that translate into definable outcomes in the fields of preventive, supportive and antineoplastic care. These tools have their origin both in Western, conventional medicine and in complementary and alternative medicine (CAM) traditions. IO addresses all participants in a sustainable process of cancer care, at all levels of their being and experience. Along with tools that translate into definable outcomes, it also includes methods that can transform the health of individual participants and the entire medical system.

INTRODUCTION

IO has developed as a specialized field within integrative medicine (IM) that is focused on oncology. IM is an evolving field, with broad and varied definitions[1,2]. In general, IM has grown out of the realization that an exclusive application of the tools and philosophy of conventional, allopathic medicine may result in a practice that is unsustainable and restrictive. IM proponents want to address health care needs fully with all available evidence-based types of intervention, regardless of the origin or goals of a specific application. The purpose of IM is eventually to eliminate the terms CAM and conventional, and arrive at a form of medicine that delivers 'what works'[3–7].

'What works' has typically been defined by analyzing the levels of evidence available for a specific intervention. The section on Research and Evidence focuses on this crucial aspect of evidence-based implementation. Therapies that differ in intent and outcomes have different levels of evidence requirements for recommendation. The study of both CAM and conventional modalities is tending toward a more individualized approach to patient care. In conventional medicine, this is seen in microassays and genetic profiling for resistance to therapy. In CAM, this can be seen in innovative approaches to research design that respect a systems-based approach, rather than trying to reduce a complex set of interventions to a single substance or therapeutic approach. It is important to remember that both individualized patient care and scientific reproducibility of results are necessary for a sustainable integrative approach to oncology. Once 'what works' has been clearly demonstrated, education of the main gatekeepers of medicine – physicians – can begin. Many methods are under way to address instruction in IM, as addressed in Chapter 3. One of the central messages that IM brings is an appropriate concern for the health of physician providers, addressed in Chapter 4. Since IM is an evolving field, there are multiple methods currently in use in a variety of settings; many are covered in Chapter 3. There are significant non-medical challenges involved in starting up this new method of health-care service, and these are outlined in Chapters 6 and 7.

This text does not include a discussion of conventional medicine approaches that are generally used to treat cancer: namely chemotherapy, radiation therapy and surgery. These fields are adequately and thoroughly defined in specialized medical texts[8–10]. This text also does not include the entire range of options from the CAM world that have been applied to cancer. Other texts provide comprehensive information covering this broad spectrum of approaches[11–13]. In keeping with the intent to provide a practical guide to the state of the art and science of IO, only modalities with a significant foundation of evidence are presented. An attempt is also made to build upon previous efforts at clinical decision guidelines[14,15].

DEFINITIONS

The words 'conventional', 'complementary' and 'alternative' have different meanings in various medical systems throughout the world. This is based on the fact that each culture thinks of its own traditional system as being 'conventional'. For the purposes of this text, the following definitions will apply:

Conventional medicine: Therapies that are part of the standard of care in biomedicine, with demonstrated safety and efficacy for cancer treatment in humans. This usually includes Western allopathic medicine, which is based on the scientific method, technology and formulation.

Complementary medicine: Modalities that provide beneficial additions to conventional approaches, yet are not widely utilized or considered a part of standard care.

Alternative medicine: Options that have no clinical, scientific basis of efficacy or safety in treating cancer in humans.

Integrative oncology: A comprehensive, evidence-based approach to cancer care that addresses all participants at all levels of their being and experience.

An integrative approach to oncology expands the level of care possible for all of the participants involved in the process through several important mechanisms:

(1) Inclusion of all participants involved at all levels of their being: their experience of body, mind, soul and spirit within the self, and within the specific culture and the natural world;

(2) A renewed focus on the guiding principles of medicine;

(3) An expansion of the goals of interventions to include the general categories of translational and transformational approaches and specific categories of preventive, supportive and antineoplastic care;

(4) A focus on variable levels of evidence required for recommendations based upon the goals of a therapy and an individualized risk–benefit analysis. This includes judicious use of the Precautionary Principle.

The remainder of this chapter will discuss these points in detail.

WHY INTEGRATIVE ONCOLOGY?

Biomedicine has resulted in significant successes; the rates of cancer deaths have decreased significantly over the past 20 years[16]. According to figures from the American Cancer Society (ACS), approximately two-thirds of cancer patients diagnosed today will experience 5-year survival. There are multiple reasons for this reduction in death rates, including improved screening, technology and conventional therapeutic advances[16]. Rates of disease control have improved dramatically in some malignancies in the USA, including stomach and uterine cancer, while they have improved very little in others, such as lung cancer[17].

Unfortunately, these advances have come at the cost of a breakdown in the therapeutic relationship, with both patients and physicians expressing dissatisfaction with the system[18]. At the same time, a medical malpractice crisis exists in the face of skyrocketing costs and increasing cancer incidence rates[19]. The National Institutes of Health (NIH) estimate the overall cost for cancer in the year 2003 at 189.5 billion dollars –

64.2 billion for direct medical costs, 16.3 billion for indirect morbidity costs and 109 billion for indirect mortality costs. It is estimated that the current lifetime risk of developing cancer in the USA is 1 in 2 for men and 1 in 3 for women[17]. In addition, there are now over 10 million cancer survivors who are often ill-equipped to handle their special needs. These needs include medical, psychosocial and lifestyle issues[20].

Cancer patients increasingly turn to practitioners of CAM, while remaining high users of conventional approaches as well. They spend billions of dollars per year out of their own pockets on various CAM therapies. There has been a trend away from use of CAM by specific subgroups, such as highly educated females, to a more diverse user group[21]. It is obvious that, despite significant biomedical advances, patients seek a more holistic approach[3]. The literature documents both a 'push' away from conventional medicine and a 'pull' toward CAM[22–32] (Table 1.1). Physicians have scant formal education in CAM approaches and can offer little advice concerning these modalities. The result is a double-edged sword: beneficial CAM therapies are under-utilized in the realms of prevention and supportive care; dangerous interactions can exist between some CAM and conventional treatments; and delays in beginning conventional

Table 1.1 'Push and pull' driving patients toward complementary and alternative medicine (CAM)

Push away from conventional medicine	Pull toward CAM
More focused on the doctor and treatment than on the individual	Individual needs are addressed in a caring manner with few time constraints
Treatment too costly or toxic	Non-toxic, 'natural' treatments
Focus on disease	Focus on the whole person
Frightening technology	Hands-on approach
Emphasis on 'fixing' as an external action	Emphasis on self-care; increase in control; possible improved outcomes
Lack of attention to emotional and spiritual dimensions	Addresses mind, body and spirit

Table 1.2 Integrative medicine: positive and negative attributes	
Positive	**Negative**
Addresses all participants involved, at all levels of their being and experience	Limited data on outcomes; untested hypotheses are common
Includes prevention, supportive care and disease treatment, as well as interventions that have transformational intent	Cost may be prohibitive to implement and sustain
Focus on healing as opposed to curing	No well-defined decision trees for patient care Lack of communication and trust between conventional and CAM providers Limited standardization, which complicates reproducibility and research

treatment can result in cancer dissemination and death[14].

INTEGRATIVE ONCOLOGY: THE NEXT STEP?

The philosopher Ken Wilber has published extensively on the evolution of integrative systems. Wilbur states that evolution occurs through a combination of transcendence and inclusion[33]. In this context, integrative oncology must include the positive aspects of biomedicine while going beyond its limitations. An integrative approach also has significant positive and negative attributes (Table 1.2); these must be recognized in order to move forward with implementation[34,35].

EXPANDED DOMAIN

A truly comprehensive integrative approach will address all participants at all levels of their being and experience[33]. It will address all of the individuals involved – patient, family, providers, community and society – at all levels of their being (mind, body, soul and spirit) in all levels of their experience, including the self, their role in a specific culture, and the effects of and on the natural environment (Figure 1.1).

In order to meet the needs of this diverse group of individuals, a team approach to care will be necessary. That team will require an appropriate co-ordinator. In the field of cancer care, conventionally trained oncologists would appear to be the best candidates to serve as 'conductor of the orchestra' because their knowledge of conventional therapy is key to a safe and efficacious integrative approach. It would certainly seem to be more efficient to educate conventional physicians concerning referral to appropriate CAM providers, rather than vice versa. This is mainly due to the extent of biomedical information that must be digested in order to fully understand, recommend and treat individuals with conventional approaches.

RENEWED FOCUS ON GUIDING PRINCIPLES OF MEDICINE

One of the main features that will guide the evolution of biomedicine into an integrative approach is a return to the basic philosophic principles upon which medicine was founded[36]. A renewed focus on these principles will eliminate much of the 'push and pull' phenomenon

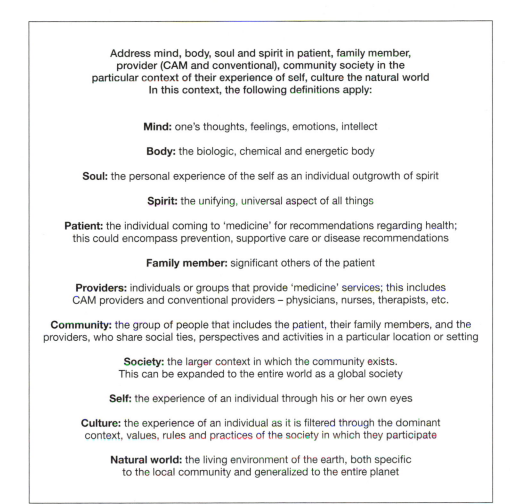

Address mind, body, soul and spirit in patient, family member, provider (CAM and conventional), community society in the particular context of their experience of self, culture the natural world
In this context, the following definitions apply:

Mind: one's thoughts, feelings, emotions, intellect

Body: the biologic, chemical and energetic body

Soul: the personal experience of the self as an individual outgrowth of spirit

Spirit: the unifying, universal aspect of all things

Patient: the individual coming to 'medicine' for recommendations regarding health; this could encompass prevention, supportive care or disease recommendations

Family member: significant others of the patient

Providers: individuals or groups that provide 'medicine' services; this includes CAM providers and conventional providers – physicians, nurses, therapists, etc.

Community: the group of people that includes the patient, their family members, and the providers, who share social ties, perspectives and activities in a particular location or setting

Society: the larger context in which the community exists. This can be expanded to the entire world as a global society

Self: the experience of an individual through his or her own eyes

Culture: the experience of an individual as it is filtered through the dominant context, values, rules and practices of the society in which they participate

Natural world: the living environment of the earth, both specific to the local community and generalized to the entire planet

Figure 1.1   Definition of a comprehensive integrative approach

that has resulted in patients moving away from conventional approaches and towards CAM practitioners (see Table 1.1). In addition, there are some distinct, clear principles of IO/IM:

(1)   Relationship centered;

(2)   Cultural sensitivity;

(3)   Individualized care based on mind, body and spirit;

(4)   Patient as active partner;

(5)   Focus on prevention and health maintenance;

(6)   Providers as educators and role models, i.e. self-care;

(7)   Evidence-based approach from multiple sources of information to integrate the best therapy for the individual – conventional or CAM;

(8)   Seeks and removes barriers to innate healing:

(9) Sees compassion as always helpful;

(10) Works collaboratively with patient and a team of providers;

(11) Maintains that healing is always possible even when curing is not;

(12) Agrees that the physician's job is, paraphrasing Hippocrates: to cure sometimes, heal often and support always[37].

Much can be learned about creating a sustainable model of medicine from the philosophy of many CAM approaches, and their foundation in medicine's guiding principles. In Energy Medicine (see Chapter 10f for definition), for example, the *intention to do only good* is actively approached by the provider *serving as a conduit of healing, not as the source*. The providers open themselves to the passing of energy in such a way that their own energy is not depleted. In order to be a conduit of energy for another, one must receive that energy as well. The care of the self is seen as paramount to being able to deliver sustainable care to others. This philosophy lies in stark contrast to conventional medicine, where self-care is routinely ignored during the medical education process through long work hours in emotionally demanding settings, information overload and constant performance evaluation.

The guiding principles of integrative oncology include:

• Harmlessness/beneficence;

• Service among equals;

• Compassion;

• Focus on healing.

Harmlessness is the foundation of modern medicine: 'first do no harm'. Unfortunately, when carried to its logical extreme, this could result in complete inaction. *Beneficence*, or 'doing good', will accomplish the same edict of harmlessness, while allowing for the fact that benefits can often occur despite negative side-effects. Reconnection with the principles of harmlessness and beneficence must take into account that 'doing harm or good' is a potential part of any interaction; one could not exist without the other. This concept is represented by the theory of Yin and Yang in traditional Chinese medicine. There is always a degree of Yin included in Yang – one can never be totally without the presence of the other.

One of the most difficult aspects of the cancer experience, whether as a physician, cancer patient or family member, is living with the uncertainty of outcomes. Unrealistic expectations of outcomes can result in significant harm, and this can have an end result of patient dissatisfaction, physician burnout and malpractice suits. Embracing this uncertainty can lead one into a state of *being comfortable with the presence of paradox*, in everyday life and in the practice of medicine. Regardless of how tightly we control the variables associated with health care – the level of perfection of our technology; personal care practices; and/or adherence to protocol or intellectual abilities – the outcomes of our actions are ultimately beyond our control. No matter what we do, we cannot eliminate the possibility of doing harm from the intention of doing good. Coming to grips with this fact, and living in peace with the presence of paradox (one can do everything 'right' and still have events turn out 'wrong') may be an important aspect in our development of integrative oncology. This allows mystery and awe back into the practice of medicine to the degree that we open ourselves up to the fact that we are not ultimately in control of who lives and who dies.

Michael Lerner, founder of Commonweal, an organization that offers residential retreats for cancer patients and physicians, provides an interesting perspective on outcomes: 'Peace of mind is never a function of success – it is the result of knowing that no matter what the outcome, we have chosen to live our lives dedicated to what matters.'

Service among equals implies that an important element of the relationship between doctor and patient is their common humanity. It is tempting to try to 'fix something that is broken' or 'help someone who is weaker', but true service can only take place among equals.

There is generally a large difference in knowledge base concerning specific therapeutic options. The common experience of being human, however, can allow care providers to be open to the experience of *compassion*. An experience of compassion realizes that 'there but for the grace of God, go I'. Patients desire that their physicians relate to their suffering in a compassionate way[38].

A focus on *healing* as opposed to *curing* brings back the mystery, meaning and awe that technology and time constraints have snuffed out in the practice of biomedicine. The word 'healing' is often mentioned as a descriptive, purely positive term, almost as a panacea, as in: 'heal the world' or 'healing substances'. This use of the word belies the depth and breadth of the actual process of healing.

Stephen Levine is a noted author who works with patients through the death and dying experience. In order to deepen his practice of service to others in this situation, Levine was intrigued by the question of what it would be like for him personally to have only 1 year to live. How would he use that time? How could he live mindfully in the process? Where would his priorities lie? He set a date in which he would die in exactly 1 year, and went about living mindfully through this process. Following this experience he wrote the book *A Year to Live*[39]. Levine reflected afterwards, 'If there is a single definition of healing, it is to look with mercy and awareness on those pains, both mental and physical, which we have dismissed in judgment and despair.' Far from being a panacea, healing is difficult work, and the outcomes are not always what we would think that they would be. For example, a relationship may be healed during end-of-life care in a patient with advanced malignancy. Healing can take place in people and situations in which curing is not possible (Table 1.3).

A focus on healing has the potential for the entire system of medicine and everyone involved in it, to look upon those pains with mercy and awareness that have been too quickly judged in the past. Addressing the following and other questions may help to create a sustainable health-care system in the future. Why do we educate our physicians in a manner that places their own health and well-being at risk? Why is it considered inappropriate for a physician to share their emotions with patients? Why does the medical education system encourage competition instead of co-operation among colleagues?

Table 1.3   Characteristics of healing versus curing

Healing	*Curing*
A process, often difficult and mysterious	A definable event or result of a set of events
Involves all levels of the person	Occurs on a physical level only
Involves some action, either conscious or unconscious, of the person being healed. Cannot be forced upon another	Is done by one person to another. Does not involve active cooperation or effort from the person being cured
Outcome is often unknown	Well-defined outcome
The person undergoing healing is the expert	The person delivering the cure is the expert

Why is there such a wide gap between reimbursement for procedure-oriented health care and prevention-oriented primary care?

FUNCTIONAL ASPECTS OF INTEGRATIVE ONCOLOGY

Adherence to the guiding principles of medicine provides the foundation for some of the specific functional aspects which further differentiate integrative oncology from a purely conventional biomedical approach (Table 1.4).

TRANSLATION VERSUS TRANSFORMATION

The addition of CAM methods to a physician's complement of tools is quickly becoming a reality as more positive research on the benefits of these tools becomes available. Nevertheless, the addition of new tools through research and clinical application, regardless of whether they are CAM or conventional, will do little to differentiate integrative oncology from biomedicine. It will merely add new options to an already bulging tool box.

However, most CAM therapies are rooted in systems that can provide an entirely new viewpoint. This dual nature can be thought of as the translational and transformational aspects of CAM approaches. *Translation* is defined as that aspect of an intervention that translates directly into a specific desired outcome. For example, one proven translation of a yoga practice might be increased flexibility and improved sleep. *Transformation* is defined as that aspect of an intervention which opens up the possibility of seeing the world from a new frame of reference, to 'see the world with new eyes'[40,41]. An example of transformation: a yoga practice may bring about a new sense of mastery, a physical, emotional, mental and spiritual opening, allowing an individual to forgive old grievances and to develop comprehensive healthy lifestyle changes.

There are significant differences between the translational and transformational aspects of care (Table 1.5). There are also shared features, namely that both aspects are experiential and contextual. They are both experienced on multiple levels – physically, mentally, emotionally and spiritually. They are also contextual on multiple levels – as they relate to the self, the individual's culture and the surrounding natural environment.

One method of incorporating CAM is to develop logical guidelines to assist in clinical decision making. The translational tool aspect of CAM must be judged using appropriate levels of evidence, similar to those used for the majority of conventional translational approaches. When the goal of CAM is primarily transformational as a part of supportive care, clinical decision guidelines based in part on efficacy and safety are not as applicable. This is because of the rather nebulous outcomes that are intrinsically a part of a transformational experience. Outcomes are distinctly individualized and difficult to define, predict or measure, except through a qualitative, testimonial type of feedback. Therefore, the primary concern for transformational interventions

Table 1.4 Defining functional aspects of integrative oncology
Tools may have transformational and translational intent
Inclusion of preventive, supportive and antineoplastic goals
Use of the Precautionary Principle for situations with limited data

Table 1.5 Differentiating characteristics of interventions with translational and transformational intent

Translational	Transformational
A specific tool, technique or instrument designed to deliver a specific measurable outcome	A highly individualized experience which involves a profound perspective shift of the essence of one's true nature, bringing a larger sense of purpose, meaning and/or fulfillment
Outcome is measurable quantitatively	Outcome is qualitative and difficult to define or measure
External locus of control	Internal locus of control
Reductionistic; can be broken into parts	Irreducible; whole
Definable, discrete, deliverable and replicable	Ultimately mysterious; can set up condition but cannot force
Understandable on a rational level	Frequently indescribable
Has levels of effect	All or nothing

is that they are demonstrated to be safe. Safety is measured in this context with regard to cost, applicability at a specific time in the patient's care, methods used, provider experience and skills. This represents a significant difference with regards to level of evidence requirements for tools with specific outcomes that must meet both safety and efficacy requirements.

For example, in order to recommend yoga as an intervention to help improve sleep, one would need evidence concerning safety and efficacy. If a patient were to desire to enter into a practice that could improve self understanding, the recommendation of yoga would be based primarily on its safety, taking into account the patient's situation.

This also brings up the important concept of a 'match' in advising CAM therapies as a part of integrative care. Owing to the heavy dependence upon the interpersonal relationship, the characteristics of a CAM provider's personality and practice may have a significant effect upon the type of individual who will fit best with their service[42,43]. Again using yoga as an example, there are a variety of types of yoga practice and significant variation among teachers. Some yoga is very physically demanding, akin to aerobic

exercise, while other yoga is more meditative and rejuvenating in nature. Different patients with specific scenarios would potentially benefit from one or the other approach. As the conductor of an orchestrated approach, the conventional oncologist would need to devise a method for appropriate discussion of cases and refer to a 'matched' CAM provider.

PREVENTIVE, SUPPORTIVE AND ANTINEOPLASTIC CARE

The addition of preventive and supportive care as a part of an integrative oncology program may result in several beneficial outcomes: reduction in the lifetime risk for developing cancer; lowering of cancer recurrence rates in survivors; and improvement in the therapeutic ratio.

It is estimated that one-third of cancers may be prevented through dietary changes alone[17]. Providing education at an early age concerning healthy eating and lifestyle patterns could greatly reduce lifetime risk. Families of cancer patients represent a significant population with a vested interest in primary prevention.

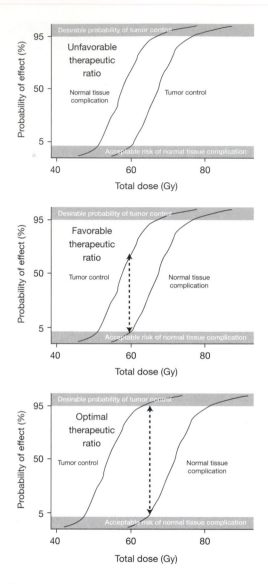

Figure 1.2 The concept of therapeutic ratio under conditions in which the relationship between the normal tissue tolerance and tumor control dose–response curves is unfavorable (upper panel), favorable (middle panel) and optimal (lower panel). Reproduced from reference 44, with permission

Prevention of cancer recurrence may likewise be lowered in cancer survivors through a variety of lifestyle changes. Survivors can be educated concerning healthy lifestyles and then trained to become lay health advisors in the community.

The therapeutic ratio is basically a risk–benefit analysis whereby clinicians attempt to limit toxicity to normal tissue and function, while maximizing tumor control. This is best described graphically, as in Figure 1.2[44]. Treatments that will eliminate cancer from the body may be so toxic as to be intolerable for patients. Improvements in the therapeutic ratio can therefore come through increasing patient tolerance to therapy, or by increasing the effectiveness of antineoplastic treatments. CAM therapies have significant potential as supportive care options that improve patient tolerance and compliance. There are also CAM options that are worthy of further research with regard to potential improvements in antineoplastic care[11].

THE PRECAUTIONARY PRINCIPLE

The development of clinical guidelines requires that providers make appropriate recommendations, even in situations where there are limited data. Categorizing treatment intent as translational versus transformational in nature demonstrates one example of differing levels of evidence required in order to make a recommendation. Another method is through the use of the Precautionary Principle.

The Precautionary Principle was originally formulated as a way of making environmental policy in situations where data were limited. The Rio Declaration defined it as a precautionary approach that is used to protect the environment when there are threats of serious or irreversible damage, and scientific uncertainty should not be used to postpone cost-effective measures[45–49].

This principle was developed in order to address situations in which the collection of data that would absolutely prove efficacy and safety was prohibitive. As an extreme example, it is not practical to carry out a randomized trial of dumping sewage into the water supply in order to measure health effects. The Precautionary Principle (among other things) would tell us that this would have significant health hazards and be inadvisable based on the limited data that are available. A more subtle example exists in the difficulty of prospectively measuring the health effects of xenoestrogens from pesticides used on foods meant for humans. The Precautionary Principle would tell us to avoid them, if possible, until further data are available[50].

This principle has been expanded for use in health-care situations, specifically for breast cancer prevention[51]. It can be applied to preventive and supportive interventions, in which the usual tools of biomedical research are impractical. Using the Precautionary Principle should not be seen as an excuse to advance one's hypotheses without evidence, but can allow physicians and other providers to act in situations where limited data are available, if that action is almost certainly safe and deemed necessary.

Another aspect of the Precautionary Principle deems that significant risk of adverse outcomes be absent in order to justify going forward with limited data. This is inherently a judgment call, and may be difficult to quantify, especially in the supportive and preventive care realms. For example, the use of antioxidant vitamins during radiation has been debated for years. Proponents say that it may lessen side-effects, while detractors say that it could protect the tumor from being destroyed by treatments. The Precautionary Principle in this situation could result in recommending against use of antioxidant supplements during treatments, because of the possibility that it might protect tumor cells from lethal damage and thereby affect disease control – a significant and irreversible risk. Following treatment, patients may be interested in taking antioxidants for general supportive care and prevention of recurrence, despite the fact that there are limited data for either. In this situation, the Precautionary Principle may lead one to recommend supplementation, owing to the significant risk of recurrence, persistent fatigue, etc. In this case, the risk of adverse outcomes and the presence of preliminary data on safety and efficacy could tip the scales in favor of recommendation. These types of decision are not to be taken lightly. A significant caveat of the Precautionary Principle is that future data may show that we have made a mistake and recommended something that was detrimental. Therefore, an analysis of the entire clinical situation, with appropriate informed consent, is always necessary.

CONCLUSIONS

Integrative oncology has the potential to transform both individuals and the system of cancer care. In the process, a more sustainable approach to health care can emerge, grounded in the guiding principles of medicine, and focusing on all participants at all levels of their experience. Integrative oncology also has the potential to improve outcomes with regard to prevention, supportive care and antineoplastic approaches.

We are at a critical juncture in the evolution of health care. In order to be successful in developing an integrative approach to oncology, the efforts of researchers, clinicians, patient advocate groups, corporate health-care workers and policy makers will need to be combined. This will allow for rational planning, development and implementation in the setting of diminishing resources.

References

1. Boon H, Verhoef M, O'Hara D, et al. Integrative healthcare: arriving at a working definition. Altern Ther Health Med 2004; 10: 48–56

2. Caspi O, Sechrest L, Pitluk HC, et al. On the definition of complementary, alternative, and integrative medicine: societal mega-stereotypes vs. the patients' perspectives. Altern Ther Health Med 2003; 9: 58–62

3. Barrett B, Marchand L, Scheder J, et al. Themes of holism, empowerment, access, and legitimacy define complementary, alternative, and integrative medicine in relation to conventional biomedicine. J Altern Complement Med 2003; 9: 937–47

4. Dalen JE. Is integrative medicine the medicine of the future? A debate between Arnold S. Relman, MD, and Andrew Weil, MD. Arch Intern Med 1999; 159: 2122–6

5. Kligler B, Maizes V, Schachter S, et al. Core competencies in integrative medicine for medical school curricula: a proposal. Acad Med 2004; 79: 521–31

6. Markman M. Interactions between academic oncology and alternative/complementary/integrative medicine: complex but necessary. J Clin Oncol 2001; 19(Suppl 18): 52S–3S

7. Oumeish OY. The philosophical, cultural, and historical aspects of complementary, alternative, unconventional, and integrative medicine in the Old World. Arch Dermatol 1998;134:1373–86

8. DeVita VT, Hellman S, Rosenberg S. Cancer: Principles and Practice of Oncology. 6th edn. Philadelphia: Lippincott, Williams and Wilkins, 2001

9. Leibel S, Phillips T. Textbook of Radiation Oncology. Philadelphia: WB Saunders, 1998

10. Perez C, Brady L, Halperin EC, Schmidt-Ullrich RK. Principles and Practice of Radiation Oncology. Philadelphia: Lippincott, Williams & Wilkins, 2004

11. American Cancer Society's Guide to Complementary and Alternative Cancer Methods. Atlanta: American Cancer Society, 2000

12. Low Dog T, Micozzi M. Women's Health in Complementary and Integrative Medicine. St Louis, MO: Elsevier Churchill Livingstone, 2005

13. Freeman LW. Mosby's Complementary & Alternative Medicine: A Research-Based Approach, 2nd edn. St Louis, MO: Mosby, 2004

14. Weiger WA, Smith M, Boon H, et al. Advising patients who seek complementary and alternative medical therapies for cancer. Ann Intern Med 2002; 137: 889–903

15. Adams KE, Cohen MH, Eisenberg D, Jonsen AR. Ethical considerations of complementary and alternative medical therapies in conventional medical settings. Ann Intern Med 2002; 137: 660–4

16. Jemal A, Clegg LX, Ward E, et al. Annual report to the nation on the status of cancer, 1975–2001, with a special feature regarding survival. Cancer 2004; 101: 3–27

17. Cancer Facts and Figures 2004. Atalanta: American Cancer Society, 2004

18. Maizes V, Schneider C, Bell I, Weil A. Integrative medical education: development and implementation of a comprehensive curriculum at the University of Arizona. Acad Med 2002; 77: 851–60

19. Borges W. Living in fear. Physicians face mounting liability insurance crisis. Tex Med 2002; 98: 34–40

20. President's Cancer Panel. Living Beyond Cancer: Finding a New Balance. Bethesda, MD: NIH, 2004

21. Kessler RC, Davis RB, Foster DF, et al. Long-term trends in the use of complementary and alternative medical therapies in the United States. Ann Intern Med 2001; 135: 262–8

22. Balneaves LG, Kristjanson LJ, Tataryn D. Beyond convention: describing complementary therapy use by women living with breast cancer. Patient Educ Couns 1999; 38: 143–53

23. Boon H, Brown JB, Gavin A, Westlake K. Men with prostate cancer: making decisions about complementary/alternative medicine. Med Decis Making 2003; 23: 471–9

24. Boon H, Brown JB, Gavin A, et al. Breast cancer survivors' perceptions of complementary/alternative medicine (CAM): making the decision to use or not to use. Qual Health Res 1999; 9: 639–53

25. Eng J, Ramsum D, Verhoef M, et al. A population-based survey of complementary and alternative medicine use in men recently diagnosed with prostate cancer. Integr Cancer Ther 2003; 2: 212–16

26. Hall JD, Bissonette EA, Boyd JC, Theodorescu D. Motivations and influences on the use of complementary medicine in patients with localized prostate cancer treated with curative intent: results of a pilot study. Br J Urol Int 2003; 91: 603–7

27. Herbert CP, Verhoef M, White M, et al. Complementary therapy and cancer: decision making by patients and their physicians setting a research agenda. Patient Educ Couns 1999; 38: 87–92

28. Kimby CK, Launso L, Henningsen I, Langgaard H. Choice of unconventional treatment by patients with cancer. J Altern Complement Med 2003; 9: 549–61

29. Shumay DM, Maskarinec G, Kakai H, Gotay CC. Why some cancer patients choose complementary and alternative medicine instead of conventional treatment. J Fam Pract 2001; 50: 1067

30. Truant T, Bottorff JL. Decision making related to complementary therapies: a process of regaining control. Patient Educ Couns 1999; 38: 131–42

31. Truant T. Complementary therapies: the decision-making process of women with breast cancer. Can Oncol Nurs J 1997; 7: 119

32. Verhoef MJ, White MA. Factors in making the decision to forgo conventional cancer treatment. Cancer Pract 2002; 10: 201–7

33. Wilber K. A Brief History of Everything. Boston: Shambhala, 2000

34. Lynoe N. Ethical and professional aspects of the practice of alternative medicine. Scand J Soc Med 1992; 20: 217–25

35. Truant T, McKenzie M. Discussing complementary therapies: there's more than efficacy to consider. CMAJ 1999; 160: 351–2

36. Marketos SG, Skiadas PK. The modern hippocratic tradition. Some messages for contemporary medicine. Spine 1999; 24: 1159–63

37. Rakel D. Integrative Medicine. Philadelphia, PA: Saunders, 2003

38. Stevenson AC. Compassion and patient centred care. Aust Fam Physician 2002; 31: 1103–6

39. Levine S. A Year to Live. New York: Bell Tower, 1997

40. Jobst KA, Shostak D, Whitehouse PJ. Diseases of meaning, manifestations of health, and metaphor. J Altern Complement Med 1999; 5: 495–502

41. Kirmayer LJ. The cultural diversity of healing: meaning, metaphor and mechanism. Br Med Bull 2004; 69: 33–48

42. Caspi O, Bell IR. One size does not fit all: aptitude chi treatment interaction (ATI) as a conceptual framework for complementary and alternative medicine outcome research. Part II – research designs and their applications. J Altern Complement Med 2004; 10: 698–705

43. Caspi O, Bell IR. One size does not fit all: aptitude χ treatment interaction (ATI) as a conceptual framework for complementary and alternative medicine outcome research. Part 1 – what is ATI research? J Altern Complement Med 2004; 10: 580–6

44. Gunderson LL, Tepper JE. Clinical Radiation Oncology. Philadelphia: Churchill Livingstone, 2003: 1–3

45. Davis DL, Axelrod D, Bailey L, et al. Rethinking breast cancer risk and the environment: the case for the precautionary principle. Environ Health Perspect 1998; 106: 523–9

46. De BC, Lagasse R. [The precautionary principle applied to lung cancer risk caused by residential radon]. Rev Epidemiol Sante Publique 2002; 50: 147–57

47. Hardell L. From phenoxyacetic acids to cellular telephones: is there historical evidence for the precautionary principle in cancer prevention? Int J Health Serv 2004; 34: 25–37

48. Jamieson D, Wartenberg D. The precautionary principle and electric and magnetic fields. Am J Public Health 2001; 91: 1355–8

49. Richter ED, Laster R. The Precautionary Principle, epidemiology and the ethics of delay. Int J Occup Med Environ Health 2004; 17: 9–16

50. Ringvold S, Rottingen JA. [Environmental pollutants with hormonal effects. Is estrogen theory a good model?]. Tidsskr Nor Laegeforen 1997; 117: 66–70

51. Davis DL, Axelrod D, Bailey L, et al. Rethinking breast cancer risk and the environment: the case for the precautionary principle. Environ Health Perspect 1998; 106: 523–9

2

Clinical research and evidence

Nancy Stark, Suzanne Hess and Edward Shaw

'We shall not cease from exploration. And the end of all our exploring. Will be to arrive where we started. And know the place for the first time. Through the unknown, remembered gate. When the last of earth left to discover. Is that which was the beginning...' – T.S. Eliot

INTRODUCTION

An integrative approach to oncology cannot be founded upon the indiscriminate addition of new methods, tools and providers to our biomedical system. An integrative approach must involve a critical appraisal of modalities that may enhance the response to biomedical therapies or, at a minimum, improve the quality of life for cancer patients, their families and providers of care. Complementary and alternative medicine (CAM) modalities are increasingly popular among cancer patients, with the majority either using or inquiring about the use of CAM for cancer treatment, prevention and symptom management[1]. For oncologists and medical providers caring for cancer patients, the growing interest in CAM therapies raises concerns about efficacy and safety, and appropriate ways to counsel patients about CAM use. The deaths of prostate cancer patients taking PC-SPES reinforce the importance of assuring that therapies are safe, in addition to efficacious. It is necessary not only to assure the safety of a therapy taken as a single agent, but also to know the potential adverse effects if it is combined with other medications or therapeutic regimens.

The concern is of particular importance in cancer treatment, where patients may be receiving multiple concurrent or continuous forms of therapy for extended periods. Oncologists and other practitioners treating or counseling cancer patients concerning treatment options face significant challenges in deciding how to counsel patients on the use of CAM therapies and to determine the value of incorporating CAM therapies into clinical practice. The ability to understand research findings on CAM therapies and the applicability of findings to practice are essential.

The purpose of this chapter is to provide clinicians with a framework within which to make decisions about recommending or incorporating CAM therapies into clinical practice. To that end, we review research methods and types of research used in evidence-based medicine and safety issues, and provide a rationale for decision making in the use of CAM.

CAM CLASSIFICATIONS

There is a need for rigorous testing of CAM therapies as they are employed in the prevention, supportive care and treatment related to cancer. Testing is complicated by a lack of standardization inherent to many of the forms of complementary and alternative therapies. CAM therapies are also often difficult to categorize, owing to lack of appropriate controls, inability to measure the actual modality, interpractitioner skill differences, and the individualization of treatment that is the hallmark of many CAM approaches. In order to research CAM treatments systematically, a classification scheme for the variety of therapies is needed. The National Center for Complementary and Alternative Medicine (NCCAM)[2] classifies the major types of CAM medicine into five domains: alternative medical systems; mind–body interventions; biologically based therapies; manipulative and body-based methods; and energy therapies (Table 2.1). A key feature of this scheme is the delineation of certain alternative medical systems as a domain of CAM.

Another classification scheme, developed by Kemper[3], is useful in understanding the range of CAM therapies in cancer care. The Kemper model defines four categories of complementary therapy: biomechanical, bioenergetic, biochemical and lifestyle (Table 2.2). Kemper classifies therapies based on the action alone, thus she does not recognize medical systems as a discreet domain. Rather, the Kemper scheme incorporates various medical system therapies across domains based on the source of therapeutic action.

Biochemical therapies, for example, share a common biochemical mechanism of action, whether herbal, nutritional, or manufactured medicines. Bioenergetic therapies, on the other hand, are rooted in the principle of an 'energy' or 'spirit' that surrounds, flows through, or gives life to the body. Biomechanical therapies involve those affecting larger organs and tissues by movement, stimulation, realignment or removal. Massage, spinal manipulation and surgery are included in this classification. Lifestyle therapies include exercise and nutrition, and extend to environmental adjustments such as the use of air filters, phototherapy and the like. There are areas of possible overlap in this system, however, as

Table 2.1 NCCAM classification of complementary and alternative medicines	
Classification of therapy	*Definition and examples*
Alternative medical systems	Complete systems of medical theory and practice: homeopathic, traditional Chinese, ayurvedic medicine
Mind–body	Interventions or therapies that build the mind's capacity to affect health or bodily function: prayer, meditation, art, music or dance as therapy
Biologically based	Substances found in nature used for health purposes: herbs, vitamins, shark cartilage
Manipulative and body-based	Manipulation or movement of one or more parts of the body: chiropractic therapy, massage therapy
Energy-based	Manipulation of energy fields surrounding the body: Qi Gong, Reiki, Healing Touch, Therapeutic Touch

Table 2.2 Kemper classification of complementary and alternative therapy and optimal research design to result in the highest possible level of evidence

Biochemical	Bioenergetic	Biomechanical	Lifestyle
Randomized double-blinded controlled trial	*Randomized controlled trial*	*Randomized controlled trial*	*Randomized controlled trial*
Medications	Acupuncture*	Massage	Nutritional
Herbal remedies	Therapeutic touch*	Spinal manipulation	Exercise
Nutritional supplements	Healing touch*		Environmental
	Prayer*		Mind–body
	Homeopathy**		

*Single-blinded possible; **double-blinded possible

acupuncture may have both biochemical and bioenergetic effects.

This schema can be used to determine the most suitable types of research for each classification. For instance, biochemical, herbal and nutritional supplement interventions should ultimately be tested using double-blinded, randomized controlled trials. While double blinding may be possible, it may not be feasible. A major challenge to conducting a double-blinded controlled trial to test nutritional or herbal supplements is obtaining the look-alike placebo. Overencapsulation is a method used to create look-alike placebo and intervention drugs. However, the process can affect the chemical compound under study, rendering a double-blinded study impossible. Similarly, the cost of overencapsulation may be prohibitive, making the design less feasible.

Lifestyle therapies such as exercise or dietary interventions may be tested in randomized trials, but not blinded. Bioenergetic therapy trials testing modalities such as healing touch or reiki may randomize participants, and potentially blind participants, if sham practitioners are incorporated into the control group. The advantage of using a sham practitioner is to account for the potential confounding variable of what has been described as a caring presence, or an individual who interacts with the participant as a therapist figure. However, feasibility can again be an issue; clinical settings may not have the space, resources or funding to identify and train individuals to perform as sham practitioners.

KEY FEATURES OF RESEARCH

It is important to have an understanding of research design in order to lay the groundwork for determining levels of evidence with regards to efficacy and safety. A first step in establishing a framework for evaluating CAM therapy is an insight into key features of clinical research. Two issues of importance are: levels of evidence that certain types of clinical trials provide; and hypothesis-driven research.

Levels of evidence

Reviewing the research on a particular CAM therapy requires an understanding of the weight of the findings. A scheme that ranks the importance of research is the concept of 'levels of evidence', which is based on the study design and sample size. Two organizations, the National Cancer Institute (NCI) and the US Agency for Health Care Policy and Research (AHCPR), have developed ranking criteria for levels of evidence[4,5]. The NCI developed a classification scheme for ranking cancer treatment studies according to strength of outcome or endpoints, and study design[4]. The classification system has been adapted for CAM clinical trials reporting a therapeutic outcome such as tumor response, improved survival, or quality of life. The scheme consists of the following categories ranked from 1 to 4, with a rank of 1 representing the highest level of evidence, and a rank of 4 the lowest.

Level 1 evidence: randomized controlled clinical trials

Participants are assigned by chance to separate groups for treatment comparison:

(1) Double-blinded: neither researcher nor patient knows the participant's group assignment (in single-blinded studies, participant only is blinded).

(2) Non-blinded: researcher and participant know the group assignment.

Level 2 evidence: non-randomized controlled clinical trial

Participants are assigned to a treatment group based on certain criteria, e.g. date of birth, medical record number, etc. There is less confidence about comparability of those assigned to a treatment group versus the control group as compared to using a purely randomized assignment.

Level 3 evidence: case series

This type of research describes the results of a group or series of patients who all received the treatment being investigated. There is no control or comparison group. There are three types of case series. In order of descending level of evidence, these are:

(1) Population-based, consecutive case series. Analyzes a representative sample of a well-defined population; patients received treatment as they were identified.

(2) Consecutive case series. Involves a less well-defined population; patients also received treatment in order of identification by researchers.

(3) Non-consecutive case series. Participants were not limited to a specific population, nor did they consecutively receive treatment in order of identification by researchers.

Level 4 evidence: best case series

This represents a subset of cases that actually benefited from the treatment in question.

In addition to ranking types of research in order of strength of evidence, the NCI scheme ranks endpoints or outcome measures. The strongest endpoint, ranked as 'A', is the most objective and easily defined: total mortality. Total mortality is also referred to as death rate, or the proportion of the study population that died, and is often reported as overall survival (OS). Endpoint 'B' is cause-specific mortality, or death in the study population from a specified cause. This is less objective than total mortality. Carefully assessed quality of life (QOL), endpoint C, is more subjective and dependent upon the use of validated instruments. The weakest endpoint, D, is a set of measures referred to as indirect surrogates. These measures include the following in order of decreasing strength: disease-free survival (DFS) – length of time the patient was cancer free following the studied treatment; progression-free survival (PFS) – length of time disease did not progress after the treatment, and tumor response rate – a complete response (CR) or partial response (PR) – the percentage of patients whose tumors decreased in size or the extent to which the tumors responded to therapy.

According to the NCI system, the most influential data would have a classification of 1A, while the least compelling would be classified as 4D. However, when considering the evidence necessary to recommend (or not discourage) a CAM therapy, it may be possible that 4D level of evidence is satisfactory, particularly if the intervention is essentially free of risk. The main strength of this system is its ease of use with regards to analyzing the weight of data supporting the efficacy of a certain treatment. Its main weakness is that it lowers the weight of data focused on quality of life, in favor of measuring mortality. As the Kemper classification notes, some modalities cannot be measured using tests that would result in level 1A data. This should not be interpreted as a lack of strong data to support recommendation of a therapy, but rather, as inherent to the type of treatment itself. While it is certainly true that overall survival is the most accurate and easily identifiable endpoint, the majority of CAM methods do not focus on antineoplastic approaches. Owing to the very nature of some CAM approaches, arriving at level 1 data through a randomized trial may also be difficult, because the absence of a control arm would make such an investigation impossible or impractical to conduct. The NCI system does not mention how to make clinical decisions based on the level of evidence needed to recommend a therapy. This decision is based on several factors, including the therapeutic goal – preventive, supportive or antineoplastic – and a risk/benefit ratio based on reports of both safety and efficacy.

The AHCPR classification system is less detailed than the NCI scheme[5]. The AHCPR levels of evidence are defined as follows:

- Ia. Evidence is from a meta-analysis of randomized controlled trials.

- Ib. Evidence is from at least one well-designed randomized controlled trial.

- IIa. Evidence is based on well-designed controlled trials without randomization.

- IIb. Evidence comes from at least one other well-designed, quasi-experimental study, such as a cohort or case–control analytic study.

- III. Evidence is based on well-designed, descriptive studies.

- IV. Evidence is based upon reports, opinions or clinical experience of respected authorities or expert committees.

The AHCPR system does not prioritize endpoints such as quality of life, or overall survival, as being of greater or lesser weight. It also allows for a level of evidence based upon the opinion of individuals or committees – something that most researchers would term as 'anecdotal experience'. The fact that this scale was developed by an agency focusing on prevention may be significant. Again, level I data may be impossible to obtain for some modalities, and should not be misconstrued as a lack of significant enough data to justify a recommendation for use. Owing to the less restrictive nature of this system, as well as its relative simplicity, a modified AHCPR system will be used throughout this text when analyzing modalities and their levels of evidence (Table 2.3). Level IV will represent preclinical evidence through *in vitro* and *in vivo* (animal) studies. Level II data will be considered as one group, rather than as subgroups. It is important to remember that both safety and efficacy of the agent must be analyzed with regards to level of evidence.

The second key feature in understanding clinical research is the necessity for hypothesis-driven research.

Hypothesis-driven research: what is the study question?

Scientific rigor demands that all clinical trials test a hypothesis. A hypothesis is defined as a specific study question that helps to define the components of a study. These components include the study sample, design, independent variables, and dependent, or outcome, variables[6]. A good hypothesis is simple and specific, and is stated at the outset of the study in order to keep the

Table 2.3 Levels of evidence: integrative oncology	
Level I:	Well-designed, randomized, controlled clinical trial(s)
Level II:	Prospective and retrospective non-randomized clinical trials and analyses
Level III:	Opinions of expert committees, best case series
Level IV:	Preclinical *in vitro* and *in vivo* studies, and traditional uses

research focused on the primary issue of inquiry. Hypothesis testing is not limited to clinical trial research, but is essential to *in vitro* and animal research.

Pre-clinical trials: in vitro and animal research and traditional uses – does it work in the test tube or in animals?

Preclinical studies are essential to determine which agents/modalities may prove to be beneficial for cancer patients. While not all domains of CAM therapies may be tested with *in vitro* and animal studies, i.e. body–mind approaches or body-manipulation therapies, other domains are appropriate for this type of experimental approach. For example, few *in vitro* or animal studies involving energy medicine have been published in peer-reviewed journals in the USA; however, this area of research is growing. Most *in vitro* data involving CAM has been generated in the area of biological and natural agents, such as St John's wort, or ginger.

In vitro studies provide key information necessary prior to testing in humans. Preclinical research may address questions of the efficacy of a whole agent or active metabolites in solid tumor versus non-solid tumor cell lines, the specificity of an agent in one cancer type versus another, or the efficacy of single agent versus combination therapies or mechanisms of action. In addition, there is no placebo effect and the cost of conducting these studies is relatively low compared to clinical trials. The primary disadvantage of using an *in vitro* system is that it is not the whole system. The bioavailability of either

single or multiple agents will be altered once inside an animal. Detoxification by phase I and II enzymes also occurs and differences exist in the P450 systems between species. While some safety and efficacy issues can be measured in an animal model, such as a nude mouse model system which typically is used for conventional cancer assessments, not all positive animal studies translate into efficacy in the clinical studies. Other facts to note about CAM *in vitro* studies are what endpoints will be used, the use of proper controls, the use of reproducible and high-quality agents, the time points used for assessment and, in some cases such as energy medicine studies, the skills of the practitioner performing the intervention, as well as the choice of sham practitioner.

Additionally, it should be noted that the model of integrative/CAM studies has differed somewhat from the Western model of conducting conventional research. While a Western model focuses on the generation of *in vitro* and animal data to determine which agents to pursue in clinical trials, an integrative model has relied more heavily on observing what has seemed to be effective as traditional uses in the general population, then trying to pursue early-phase clinical trials with these agents, and finally to pursue laboratory and animal models. *In vivo* and *in vitro* trials then may confirm what has been observed in the population, and also add to the existing knowledge about that agent. A case in point is epidemiological studies suggesting that consumption of green tea may decrease cancer risk[7–10]. *In vitro* and *in vivo* studies with polyphenolic compounds have shown evidence for protection against specific cancers including skin, lung, mammary gland and gastrointestinal cancers[11–16]. Additional studies with one major component of green tea, epigallocatechin gallate, or EGCG, have reported that this compound is a chemopreventative agent that inhibits tumor invasion and angiogenesis. Phase I studies have been performed[17] and phase II are in progress[18].

Additional preclinical laboratory and animal studies in the area of CAM have led to a variety of outcomes. Some examples are given below. Negative results from laboratory and animal studies with some proposed treatments for cancer patients have led to studies not being deemed worthy of clinical trials. Two such examples of this are the use of Cancell/Entelev (also known as Sheridan's Formula, Jim's Juice, Crocinic Acid, JS-114, JS-101, 126-F and Canctron), and 714-X. Cancell/Entelev is a liquid composed of at least 12 different chemical compounds including inositol, nitric acid, sodium sulfite, potassium hydroxide, sulfuric acid and catechol. In 1978 and 1980, the NCI conducted animal studies on Cancell, and in vitro studies followed in the Anticancer Drug Discovery Program in 1990 and 1991. Both studies confirmed that Cancell lacked anticancer activity and the IND number was pulled for this drug, because of lack of in vitro, animal and human data published in peer-reviewed journals[19]. Another compound, 714-X, a naturally derived camphor, was proposed to protect and stabilize the immune system to help destroy cancer cells. To date, there have been no laboratory and animal studies conducted with 714-X; however, a few studies that have been conducted with camphor also did not lead to peer-reviewed publications[20].

Some published preclinical studies can have conflicting data, as in the case of ginseng extracts and their effects on the growth of breast cancer cells[21–23]. This may be due to the presence of various phytoestrogens present in some preparations of ginseng and their contribution to estrogenic effects and the cell growth effects observed. This example addresses a critical point of analyzing data from an agent that lacks proper purity and quality control, i.e. using an adulterated or mixed CAM agent for in vitro testing.

Purity of the agent being tested is not only critical in terms of assessing efficacy, but in determining safety as well. PC-SPES, described in detail later, is a primary example of this. PC-SPES is an oral supplement composed of eight herbs that has been shown to demonstrate estrogenic effects in vitro[24–28], in rodents[29,30], and in humans[31,32]. PC-SPES can inhibit the growth of both androgen-sensitive and androgen-insensitive cancer cells. While antitumorigenic activity has been shown with some phytochemicals of PC-SPES, mixed results have been observed in androgen-insensitive prostate cells. While PC-SPES has been shown to decrease levels of prostate-specific antigen (PSA)[31–35], improve metastatic disease[33], pain and quality of life[35], contamination of PC-SPES with conventional medications such as diethylstilbestrol (DES), warfarin and indomethacin has led to a recall of PC-SPES and a halt in clinical studies[36]. This documents a case where clinical observation of safety and efficacy led to further preclinical study which determined the presence of contaminants.

Because of the need to prioritize CAM-based research according to the amount of research that still needs to be performed and the amount of grant dollars to perform these studies, both in vitro and animal studies will continue to play a major role in helping to determine those agents that should be further pursued in clinical trials.

PHASE I–PHASE IV CLINICAL TRIALS: SAFETY AND EFFICACY IN HUMANS?

CAM therapies used in cancer treatment, prevention or supportive care must be tested using the most scientifically rigorous methodologies possible. However, the Kemper classification suggests that the optimal study design will vary according to type of therapy: herbal, energy based, or lifestyle related. Similarly, the study hypothesis or question will also determine the optimal study design. For instance, a trial designed to identify whether a therapy has any efficacy will be likely to be an open label study with a small sample and no control group. A trial designed to compare the efficacy and safety of the proposed therapy relative to the standard of care will involve a randomized and, if possible, a blinded trial, with a much larger sample.

Well-designed research ultimately addresses questions of efficacy, safety, dosage, etc. These are the same questions that are addressed in strictly biomedical cancer clinical trials. These questions are studied in phases. Clinical trials are divided into four phases (I–IV) depending on the type of question addressed. Each trial phase targets a specific question with regards to a therapy, e.g. safety, efficacy, improvement over current treatment options, and optimal administration. Generally, trials are conducted in stepwise fashion – beginning with phase I and culminating in a phase IV study (Figure 2.1).

Phase I cancer clinical trials address the question of treatment *safety*, and are conducted to determine the highest dose of a therapy that may safely be administered. The outcome measure for a phase I study is treatment toxicity. This is measured by patient-reported or clinically evident symptoms, blood or other laboratory tests. Phase I trials are the first studies that involve human subjects. Significant basic science research performed on the proposed therapy nearly always precedes testing in humans. Usually, the Food and Drug Administration (FDA) will demand a designation as an Investigational New Drug (IND) in order to begin further testing. The sample size for a phase I trial is usually small, around 15–40 subjects, and may include patients with different types of cancer. The dose or exposure of a substance or modality being tested in a phase I

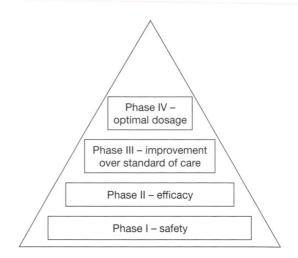

Figure 2.1   Clinical trial classification scheme

trial may be increased during the course of the study, if initial lower doses or exposures are tolerated by study participants. Phase I trials may be particularly difficult to design for CAM therapies that are not classified as biochemical in nature. For example, how could one design a phase I trial testing prayer as an intervention? However, one glaring weakness in CAM research is the lack of phase I data concerning those modalities that do lend themselves to this type of format, including any ingestible forms of therapy – homeopathics, botanicals, nutraceuticals – as well as some lifestyle measures, such as exercise and meditation. Many CAM studies will take traditional uses of a modality as the evidence that a particular dose or exposure is the most effective; this places data gathered by further studies at risk, in that one may never know whether the modality is either ineffective due to too low a dose or exposure, or not maximally effective. It also brings up questions of whether safety may exist at lower than traditional doses. Whenever possible, phase I trials should be an important first step in building the pyramid of evidence.

Phase II studies address the question of *efficacy*, and determine whether the therapy actually results in a measurable clinical improvement.

These studies have a larger sample size, 25–100 participants, and comprise individuals with a particular type of cancer, or clinical situation. All participants receive the same dose or exposure, previously determined in the phase I trial to be the maximally tolerated amount. Outcome measures are dependent upon the hypothesis being tested and may include such measures as reduced tumor size, increase in the length of time to recurrence, or improved pain scores. These are usually reported as occurring in a certain percentage of study subjects. Although placebos are not used, some phase II trials do involve randomizing participants into one of two treatment groups. Participants are still monitored for side-effects.

Once a treatment has gone through preliminary safety and efficacy testing with positive results, it is then ready to be compared to the current standard of care for its specific goal, whether that be tumor control, overall survival, or improved quality of life.

Phase III trials address the question of whether the treatment represents an improvement over currently available treatments in both safety and efficacy. These studies involve larger numbers of participants (several hundred). Patients are randomized and the study is double-blinded or single-blinded when possible, meaning that either the patient (single-blinded) or both the researcher and patient (double-blinded) are not aware of which treatment the participant receives. Placebos are used in phase III trials when possible. In fact the double-blind, placebo-controlled trial is considered the 'gold standard' of testing for a treatment and is discussed further in the next section. Randomization reduces the chance for one group to be different from the other, as differences could bias the study findings. Blinding ensures that participants are not treated differently by study personnel because of their treatment arm, as well as reducing the chance of participants exhibiting a placebo effect. Substances successfully tested in phase III clinical trials may be submitted for FDA approval.

Phase IV cancer clinical trials are conducted to determine the optimal way to use an approved therapy, e.g. the optimal length of time to give therapy, or the most effective frequency. Attempts to identify rare side-effects of the intervention are also made. Drugs used in phase IV trials are FDA approved and available for use in standard care.

The description of phases of clinical trials is based on drug treatment, not surprisingly. However, various therapies, with possible modification in methods, may be tested within this framework, such as surgical techniques, behavioral interventions, devices, etc. CAM therapies that involve bioenergetic therapies, lifestyle or biomechanical therapies, all may be tested through clinical trial research. Whereas blinding researchers and/or participants may be impossible, randomization of participants for any therapy is feasible. Whenever possible, however, CAM therapies should be tested keeping in mind the highest level of evidence possible for that modality.

THE GOLD STANDARD IN CAM: RANDOMIZED DOUBLE-BLIND PLACEBO-CONTROLLED CLINICAL TRIALS?

There has been intense debate as to whether randomized controlled trials are also the gold standard when it comes to assessing the efficacy of complementary and alternative therapies[37–46]. Recently a panel was assembled to discuss the use of clinical trials for evaluating integrative or CAM therapies for cancer patients[47]. To date, a consensus protocol has not been established for the use of standardized integrative therapies in cancer patient populations. Part of the reason for this may be the complex nature of cancer and the frequent individualization of patient treatment by oncologists. It is interesting to note that only 20–50% of conventional medical decisions appear to be based on data generated from clinical trials[48].

Several challenges to testing CAM therapies by randomized control-trials have been identified:

(1) The lack of participation of oncologists due to strict adherence to protocol and lack of individualization for the patients' needs[49];

(2) Low rates of participation in randomized controlled trials in general (3–4%) combined with the potential for randomization to an unproven therapy;

(3) The role of non-specific effects such as the physician–patient relationship;

(4) Failure to measure endpoints important to cancer patients or CAM practitioners, such as relaxation;

(5) Conducting single versus multiple modality trials;

(6) The use of proper controls;

(7) Standardization of CAM therapy;

(8) Quality control of the CAM agent and/or practitioners;

(9) The cost of conducting clinical trials;

(10) Accurate time points for assessing outcomes;

(11) Complexity of the nature of the disease (metastatic disease);

(12) Complexity of some of the interventions (traditional Chinese medicine).

Several of these concerns may be addressed with well-designed, correctly powered, randomized controlled trials that may be prioritized based on relevance in the cancer field. The field may need to reassess or shift the paradigm of what clinical trial endpoints are the most relevant for CAM trials. New quality of life questionnaires may need to be developed that address the needs of cancer patients and focus on outcomes such as feeling 'less blocked', or 'more centered'. More individualization, such as dose escalation, may need to be built into different treatment arms associated with randomized controlled trials so that a more accurate assessment may be made as to whether a particular therapy is beneficial, as well as possibly to convince conventional oncologists that their patient's treatment is not being compromised and it is worthwhile for them to participate in the trial.

The randomized controlled trial and the placebo effect

Keeping the above caveats in mind, the phase III placebo-controlled randomized double-blinded trial is the most rigorous study design and provides the highest level of evidence in clinical trial research. However, even the randomized controlled trial can have confounding variables, such as the placebo effect. As an illustration of this research approach we will discuss a trial reported in the *Journal of the American Medical Association*, 'Effect of *Hypericum perforatum* (St John's wort) in major depressive disorder: a randomized controlled trial', April 10, 2002[50].

St John's wort is a herbal treatment available over the counter and used by many in the USA and Europe to relieve depression. Several trials had indicated that St John's wort is well tolerated (see reference 51 for a review). Phase II trials had suggested that moderately severe depression would respond to St John's wort. Phase III trials had shown that *Hypericum* was superior to placebo for mild to moderate depression. Another phase III study had demonstrated that the herbal pill was comparable to active controls such as fluoxetine and amitryptyline. However, questions were raised about the types of study reporting positive results. The issues include: the lack of placebo-controlled trials that include a selective serotonin reuptake inhibitor arm (a phase IV trial); little information about the use of St John's wort in clinically defined major depression; the lack of controlled data for continued treatment; and concerns about adverse interaction of St John's wort with certain drugs[52]. The study reported in the *Journal of the American Medical Association*[50] had been conducted as a result of issues raised about previous studies specifically to address the issue of efficacy of St John's wort as a treatment for clinically defined major depression. The majority of trials investigating St John's wort had focused on mild to moderate depression. Below is a summary of the objectives, methods and outcomes as published.

The objective of the study was to test the efficacy and safety of a known form of St John's wort (LI-160) in major depressive disorder. The study, a double-blind, randomized, placebo-controlled trial was conducted in 12 academic and community psychiatric research clinics in the USA. A total of 340 adults diagnosed with major depression (as defined by the *Diagnostic and Statistical Manual of Mental Disorders*, 4th edition or DSM-IV), using the modified Structured Clinical Interview for Axis I DSM-IV, were recruited to be randomly assigned to one of three arms: placebo, sertraline 50 mg/day, or *Hypericum* 900 mg/day for 8 weeks, following a 1-week run-in period of taking a placebo. Those who responded could continue blinded treatment for an additional 18 weeks.

Eligible patients for the study had to be at least 18 years old, and have scored a minimum of 20 on a 17-item Hamilton Depression (HAM-D) scale and maximum of 60 on the Global Assessment of Functioning (GAF) at screening, and at baseline, following a 1-week, single-blinded placebo run-in. Participants were excluded if they scored above 2 on the HAM-D suicide item, or if they had attempted suicide in the past year, or if they were a current suicide or homicide risk. Other exclusion criteria included

pregnancy, breast feeding, not using medically accepted form of birth control for reproductive-aged women, clinically significant liver disease, or liver enzyme values to at least twice normal levels, any serious unstable medical condition, history of seizure disorder, severe combined immune deficiency (SCID), diagnosis of alcohol or substance abuse disorder, and certain other psychiatric disorders.

The St John's wort (LI-160), sertraline and placebo used in the study had been procured from established, well-known pharmaceutical companies in Germany and the USA. The LI-160 drug extract had been standardized, and had come from a single batch. The study was conducted under an investigational new drug application filed by the manufacturer.

The dosage given during the study could be increased after 3–4 weeks and again if the participant scored ≥ 4 on the CGI-scale at week 3, or ≥ 3 at weeks 4 or 6. After week 8, the dose of those still eligible for the study could be increased a final time. Medications were dispensed in 'double dummy' blister packs. Medications could be held or reduced if side-effects occurred, and those who reported insomnia could receive zolpidem 5–10 mg up to twice weekly during weeks 1 and 2, and up to a total of six times during the study.

Outcome measures

The primary measure for efficacy was a change in the HAM-D total score from baseline to week 8 and the incidence of full response at week 8, or early study termination. Full response was defined as a Clinical Global Impressions (CGI-I) score of 1–2 and a HAM-D total score of " 8. Partial response was defined as a CGI-I score of 1–2 and a decrease of $\geq 50\%$ in the HAM-D score from baseline, and a total raw score of 9–12. Suicidal ideation or the development of psychosis were criteria for withdrawal from the study. Secondary outcome measures were also taken and included scores on the GAF,

CGI-I, Beck Depression Inventory (BDI) and Self-rating Depression Scale (SDS). Safety assessments were obtained by the physician interviewing participants about adverse effects and documenting them, and having the patient complete a 44-item symptom checklist. Compliance was defined as taking at least 80% of the medication as measured by pill counts at each follow-up visit.

Results

A total of 428 patients consented to participate and undergo the run-in period, and 340 were randomized. No differences were seen between the placebo, sertraline and *Hypericum* groups at week 8 as measured by the HAM-D, although the sertraline group showed better scores on the secondary measure, CGI-I. Side-effects for sertraline were consistent with those reported for the drug, whereas the group assigned to take St John's wort reported more frequent anorgasmia, swelling and urination. The placebo group had a complete response rate of 37% in contrast to the *Hypericum* and sertraline groups, in which only 27% had a complete response.

It is important to point out several key issues of interest in this study. First, in addition to the randomized double-blind, placebo-controlled design, the study had clearly defined eligibility criteria for entering and remaining in the study. The outcome measures were well defined and accepted tests used to measure depression. The level of data generated by this study would be NCI level 1C and could contribute to Pennsylvania Trauma Systems Foundation (PTSF) level I data, and level I data as defined through this text. The intervention contained three arms, so that *Hypericum* was compared not only to a control but also to a standard, prescribed antidepressant. The study design allowed for increased dosage over time, in order to account for the possibility that a higher dose might lead to a response.

The results showed that neither St John's wort nor sertraline were more effective than placebo in treating major depression as measured and treated in this study. The results pointed out a common occurrence in research – the placebo effect. In this study, the placebo group had the highest complete response rate of the three arms, and overall participants randomized to the placebo arm did better than those in the arm receiving St John's wort and the standard drug. The placebo effect is often seen as a confounding variable in clinical research. In this case, the complete response to an inert substance, or placebo, was greater than the response to the study and standard drug.

Even though this was a well-designed clinical trial generating a reasonable level of evidence, the results can still be held in doubt, owing to the superiority of an inert substance over both the test drug and a standard, accepted medication. How does one deal with the effect of placebo in clinical research?

The placebo effect as a confounding factor in clinical research

The term 'placebo', derived from the Latin 'to please', is defined as a pill, injection, procedure or even surgery that is inert, or has no value for a given condition[52,53]. Shapiro and Shapiro[54] define the 'placebo effect' as a non-specific psychologic or psychophysiologic therapeutic effect produced by a placebo.

Generally, placebo effects will occur in 21–58% of study participants[54]. In studies of depression, the range is 30–50%. The placebo response is lowest in double-blind controlled studies, and highest in uncontrolled studies involving therapies believed to be effective but later demonstrated to be ineffective. Several reports[54–56] have suggested that the placebo effect is greater in conditions characterized by symptom fluctuation or spontaneous remission. Cancer may be subject to the placebo effect[54]; however, the effect may be limited to symptom relief rather than disease remission[57].

The limitations of evaluating the literature on reported placebo effects include the absence of a systematic method of measuring the placebo effect, no way to replicate studies, and lack of a method to draw general conclusions. The placebo reaction involves three components: expectancy, conditioning and meaning[58,59].

Expectancy is tied to motivation, i.e. those who are encouraged to have a positive response to a treatment[60]. A study of placebo and antidepressants[61], found that 50% of the response was explained by expectancy. Belief in treatment efficacy is only one part of the belief constellation, however. The patient's faith in a higher power[62,63], or the clinician/physician–patient interaction[58], have been suggested to stimulate the placebo effect. Kirsch[64] refers to beliefs that mediate the placebo effect as response expectancies (anticipating responses such as vomiting or intoxication), as opposed to stimulus expectancies (anticipating external consequences such as punishment or praise), and voluntary responses (intentions). The placebo effect suggests that response expectancies are self-confirming[65].

The notion of the placebo effect as a conditioned response has been demonstrated for more than a half a century[52,66–69]. Animal studies have shown that it is possible to have a conditioned response even to injections[70]. The conditioned response is further supported by research demonstrating a greater placebo response when placebo medication is administered after drug treatment rather than when given from the outset[65,70]. One clinical implication of taking advantage of the conditioned aspect of a placebo response was demonstrated in the case report of a child who attained a measurable clinical effect over a 12-month period when chemotherapy agents for lupus were alternated with placebo[58,71]. While expectancy and the conditioned response may play a role in the placebo effect, there has been no evidence to suggest that personality predisposes one to experience a placebo effect[58,72]. Perhaps a more accurate view of the placebo

effect is offered by Moerman[59,73] as a meaning response, rooted in cultural and biological processes. Moerman observes that the placebo effect must be examined in relation to three components of any illness outcome: autonomous response (illness follows a predictable course), specific response (illness responds to a particular treatment) and meaning response (patient associates the particular treatment with cure). Meaning is not limited to the treatment. However, many aspects of the therapy process have symbolic effects[74]. There are three sources of symbolic effect in the therapy process: the explanatory model (the treatment and explanation for the illness make sense to the patient); care and concern (the patient feels concern from the provider); and control and mastery (the patient comes away from the therapeutic process or encounter with a greater sense of control over the illness or its symptoms[74]). This explains how the clinician–patient interaction, messages received from providers, colors of pills and labels on pill bottles all contribute to the placebo effect, because of the meaning assigned to each by the consumer. Nevertheless, 'meaning' is a difficult construct to pin down, because it is difficult to measure experimentally, and it is 'culturally covert'[75].

Understanding the mechanism of a placebo effect is important if we wish to identify this variable accurately in interpreting the results of clinical trials. Ernst and Reich[76] argue that the placebo effect is not always correctly named. The response seen in the placebo arm of clinical trials is not a 'true' placebo effect, but rather, a perceived placebo effect. The true placebo effect is variable, and dependent on factors all of which are not fully understood, whereas the phenomenon involved in a perceived placebo response may be attributed to the natural course of the disease; other time effects; regression towards the mean; and unidentified parallel interventions.

Illness follows a natural course and changes over time, with or without treatment. This natural change may work to exaggerate or obscure a true placebo response. Second, factors that influence a disease outcome are also dynamic. Time effects may include the sense of ease that a patient experiences with repeated visits to his physician's office, thus reflected in a lowering of his/her blood pressure from the first visit to later visits. Another factor inaccurately identified as a placebo response is referred to as regression towards the mean. Most illness is identified at the time when symptoms are greatest and drive the patient to seek medical care. Therefore, measures taken at the initial visit, or baseline measures, are skewed toward the most severe, and will naturally fluctuate with later visits. Because biological measures vary naturally, it is likely that the measure would change. This change can be perceived as a placebo response. Finally, individuals who enter a trial begin to focus on ways to improve their condition, and may contribute either directly or indirectly to their outcome by making lifestyle changes in activity or diet, etc. All of these factors may contribute to exaggerating or masking a true placebo response. The true placebo response can be obtained in a clinical trial by including an untreated control group, i.e. those who receive neither treatment nor placebo. The response exhibited by this group represents the factors listed above. This response can then be subtracted from the placebo group. This leaves the true placebo response. In this way, the natural course of illness, natural fluctuations of outcome measures, peak symptom occurrence and participant behaviors affecting outcome are accounted for in a group that receives no intervention.

Placebo and CAM

The placebo response is especially important in the conduct of CAM clinical trials. Patients generally think of CAM modalities as 'natural' and 'safe'. Many modalities are also characterized by a large amount of time spent with individual practitioners. Most CAM practitioners tend to address the whole person, and therefore numerous recommendations for changes in diet, lifestyle activities, supplements and coping skills may confound the measurable effect of a specific intervention. Further, some CAM practitioners view the placebo effect as a therapeutic tool to use to the patient's advantage by encouraging the patient's expectancy of a positive result, fostering a conditioned response to active treatments, and by creating a positive setting and patient–provider dynamic.

These features of CAM therapy combined with what we know about the placebo response pose challenges to researchers attempting to distinguish between the action or efficacy of a CAM therapy and a placebo response to that therapy that may be induced with other therapies. Moerman and Jonas[74] offer their perspective on the issue of the placebo effect in CAM, in particular homeopathy and acupuncture.

In their thought-provoking article, the authors discuss the irony that homeopathy may provide a means to research the placebo effect since homeopathic dilutions have no discernible substance and the context of the therapeutic interaction imbues the remedy with symbolic power. This would qualify homeopathy as a placebo. Nevertheless, an extensive review of placebo-controlled studies of homeopathy did not support the notion that the effect of homeopathic therapy was the total result of a placebo response[74].

Studies of the effect of acupuncture have faced other challenges. Nearly all research conducted on the use of acupuncture – a complex intervention – involves the use of a placebo-controlled group, despite the fact that other complex interventions such as surgery and physical therapy rarely involve a placebo group. The authors noted that one reason for this was the fact that researchers in the West view acupuncture with more skepticism, therefore a higher level of evidence is required.

Moerman and Jonas argued further that, given the complexity of healing that involves context and symbolic power in addition to active therapy, isolating specific effects of complex interventions may be difficult. If the results of comparing essentially two placebos, i.e. homeopathy and placebo, are occurring in other allopathic (and, for our purposes, other CAM) therapies, we must question the sensitivity of using randomized controlled trials. Our belief in the methodology may in fact blind us to false-positive findings. This is the weakness of a research strategy that focuses on only efficacy, or the identification of specific effects, according to Moerman and Jonas. Rather, we must examine our goals in conducting research and identify the point of diminishing returns in the use of placebo-controlled clinical trials. Outcomes research may be more appropriate in several situations; complex intervention research when the aim is symptomatic and functional improvement, or the quantification of the probability of clinical benefit; and determining the efficacy through randomized controlled trials is difficult or limited due to the nature of the therapy or agent tested[74].

Accounting for the placebo response in CAM therapy poses other challenges. There are legal and ethical considerations, as well as the issue of the nocebo effect, the evil twin of the placebo response. There is no simple answer to the problem of assessing the placebo effect within the regulations of obtaining informed consent. For example, studies of sham surgery among Veterans' Administration (VA) hospital patients involved obtaining informed consent, thus participants knew that they might receive a placebo[74]. Nevertheless, the notion of meaning and symbolic power, context effects and expectation that fuel the placebo effect are probably altered or diminished in a setting of fully informed consent. Each research protocol must be considered individually with regards to the goals and innovative techniques employed to assure that the highest level of science and ethics are maintained[74].

The nocebo effect

Legal and ethical considerations extend to the nocebo effect. The nocebo effect is the occurrence of a negative outcome – sickness or death – caused by the expectation of sickness or death and the emotional state that accompanies such expectation[77]. Nocebo effects may be specific, i.e. a specific outcome is expected and occurs, or generic, i.e. general pessimism or vague negative expectations exist. The nocebo effect can affect a single individual or large numbers of people at once. The most well-known and earliest report of the nocebo effect was voodoo death. Individuals who were the victim of voodoo died as a result of the hex.

A nocebo effect is by definition an expected negative outcome, and therefore should not be confused with placebo side-effects that occur when an individual who expects to be healed develops a negative outcome as well. For example, a participant in a blinded randomized trial of a new antibiotic who develops a rash while on placebo is experiencing a placebo side-effect. Alternatively, if a person is given a drug that actually reduces dyspnea, but is informed that it will cause the condition, and then develops dyspnea, the person has experienced a nocebo effect[58]. In cancer treatment, the nocebo effect may be incited by the communication of poor prognosis (also referred to as medical hexing[58]), or the expectation of a negative effect of some treatment. Expectation of the negative outcome is at the center of the nocebo effect. Distinguishing between nocebo effects and effects directly the result of a CAM therapy may be difficult, but attention to reducing the potential for nocebo effects is important in conducting research in both CAM and conventional therapies.

SAFETY CONSIDERATIONS

The safe use of CAM therapies as a part of integrative oncology is a major priority for future research and public policy. Safety is as important as with prescribed medication, and perhaps even more so, for several reasons. Ernst[78] observes that significant problems exist both in the lack of regulation (of product, providers, etc) and with consumers.

A common example concerns botanical preparations. Product regulation is lacking because the USA (Dietary Health Supplement and Education Act of 1994), UK and Canada classify herbal medicinal preparations as food supplements, thereby eliminating the need for the strict regulation required of pharmaceutical products. Consequently, herbal preparations often do not contain what is stated on the label. This takes the form of contaminants, additives consisting of conventional drugs and underdosing.

Many herbs contain contaminants including microorganisms such as *Staphylococcus aureus*, microbial toxins, pesticides, herbicides, fumigation agents, heavy metals and radioactivity. Furthermore, herbal preparations may contain manufactured drugs or other herbs not noted on the label, such as acetaminophen (paracetamol), phenobarbital and the like. Herbal preparations in Asia are particularly known for containing other drugs. Finally, herbs are frequently underdosed, so that the consumer believes they are receiving a higher dose than the preparation actually contains[78].

Clinical research must give special consideration to contamination of all ingestible preparations. Literature reporting the results of clinical trials using ingestible substances should include a discussion of the procurement process and testing to ensure the dosage and quality of preparations used. Moreover, when considering recommending the use of ingestible CAM therapies to cancer patients, attention should be focused on the potential for CAM therapy side-effects and possible CAM therapy–drug interactions, as well as concerns about treatment efficacy. For many preparations, little is known about the potential interaction with cancer chemotherapy and other cancer therapies; however, there are adverse events reported in the literature as case reports. Two prominent botanical therapies that have significant adverse interactions discussed in the literature are PC-SPES and St John's wort. They illustrate the mechanisms that may account for clinical problems from ingestible agents not subjected to strict regulation, and the danger in proceeding with clinical trials without evaluating for toxicity and drug interactions.

PC-SPES: the case of contaminants

PC-SPES became available in 1996 and is a combination of eight herbs: *Chrysanthemum morifolium*, *Glycyrrhiza glabra* or licorice, *Ganoderma lucidum*, *Isatis indigotica*, *Rabdosia rubescens*, *Serona repens* or saw palmetto, *Scutellaria baicalensis* and *Panax pseudoginseng*[79]. PC-SPES has estrogenic activity and reduces serum testosterone in men with prostate cancer. The herbs that comprise PC-SPES have varying levels of antiproliferative activity as measured in basic science studies, with *Chrysanthemum morifolium* demonstrating the most antineoplastic activity.

Basic science laboratory studies of PC-SPES have demonstrated biologic activity against prostate cancer by inducing cell-cycle arrest of LNCaP, PC-3 and DU145 cell lines and produced a dose-dependent induction of apoptosis[79]. Animal studies have demonstrated that PC-SPES has a dose-dependent effect on suppression of tumor volume and tumor progression[79]. Clinical trials testing PC-SPES in prostate cancer patients have consisted of small numbers of patients. Patients with both androgen-independent, as well as androgen-dependent, cancers showed a drop in PSA levels with PC-SPES. Androgen-dependent patients had a PSA decline of 80% that lasted a median of 57 weeks, whereas 54% of the androgen-independent cancer patients experienced a 50% decline with a median duration of 17 weeks to progression[79,80].

Despite these encouraging findings, PC-SPES was recalled by the manufacturer, and the FDA advised patients to stop taking the supplement in February 2002[81]. Reports of difficulty maintaining normal warfarin ratios in prostate cancer patients taking PC-SPES, and a case of disseminated intravascular coagulation (DIC) occurred in a patient taking the herb. Side-effects of the PC-SPES preparation were posted on the bottle to include increased risk of thromboembolic events such as deep vein thrombosis and pulmonary emboli. Batches of PC-SPES produced by the manufacturer were found to contain warfarin and indomethacin, substances that predispose patients to hemorrhagic events such as DIC. Thus, the side-effects were not due to the botanicals themselves, but due to contaminants in the preparation. Despite the hopeful response in laboratory animal and human studies, the safety concerning preparations of PC-SPES has resulted in its removal from the shelves.

St John's wort: the case of herb–drug interactions

St John's wort has been shown to improve mild to moderate depression. Cancer patients who experience depression following diagnosis may have an interest in St John's wort as a way to improve their mood. However, laboratory studies have shown that despite relieving mild to moderate depression, St John's wort has also been shown to interact with other medications. Specifically, St John's wort induces the expression of the cytochrome P450 enzyme system and drug-transporting proteins. St John's wort induces the expression of the P450 CYP3A4 isoform in intestinal and hepatic cells and induces the expression of MDR1 P-glycoprotein in intestinal cells[82]. Mathijssen and colleagues[82] reported that this

activity had an effect on the absorption of irinotecan, a chemotherapy agent commonly prescribed to colorectal cancer patients. The implications of St John's wort in cancer patients undergoing chemotherapy or other hormonal therapy that metabolizes through these mechanisms are significant. In 2002, an FDA warning was issued about the concomitant use of St John's wort and drugs such as oral contraceptives, warfarin, theophylline, digoxin protease inhibitors and cyclosporine, because of a decrease in concentration or effect of the medications[82]. Other cancer drugs that metabolize through the mechanism include cyclophosphamide, and tamoxifen[83]. In addition, instances of hypertensive crisis have been reported with concomitant use of St John's wort as well as a withdrawal syndrome when the herb was discontinued[83].

The examples of PC-SPES and St John's wort highlight concerns about multiple preparation interactions and herb contamination. The examples also stress the need for phase I trials to determine the safety of herbs alone and in combination with other cancer therapies. These concerns are not unique to botanical therapies, as well tested and standardized pharmaceuticals will often have serious adverse effects or interactions that occur many years after approval. A recent example of this is the anti-inflammatory drug Vioxx, which was pulled off the shelves after being associated with thromboembolic events. However, the lack of regulation of ingestible CAM therapies confounds the situation further.

OTHER ISSUES OF CAM AND SAFETY

Another example of a difficulty in evaluating CAM options concerns providers. Practitioners may not be subject to the same level of licensing regulations demanded of conventional medical providers. CAM practitioners are usually not trained or qualified with regards to conventional medicine. Some practitioners may not adhere to satisfactory standards of clinical practice, because of a lack of such standards in their field. Others may not refer patients to appropriate conventional medical treatment, or may sometimes discourage their patients from seeking this therapy. Prescribed medicines may be ignored, or providers may not account for side-effects of ingestible substances and prescribed drugs taken alone or in combination. Furthermore, CAM providers who lack medical training are at risk of missing signs and symptoms of an undiagnosed condition, and not accounting for it in their treatment regimen[78].

Patients, or consumers of CAM therapies, also contribute to safety concerns. Many users of CAM therapies think of them as less toxic, less dangerous and more natural relative to conventional approaches. Therefore, while a user may report side-effects that arise with a prescribed medication, side effects that develop from CAM use are often ignored[78]. Ernst also cites the lay literature on CAM as a contributor to safety concerns. Many Internet sites and advertisements promote CAM therapies that are unproven and could prove harmful if used[1]. There are laws regulating health claims that can be made for ingestible substances; however, these are often not policed thoroughly[78].

DECISION MAKING IN INTEGRATIVE ONCOLOGY: FACTORS TO CONSIDER IN ANALYSIS OF RISK–BENEFIT AND LEVELS OF EVIDENCE IN CAM CLINICAL TRIALS

We have presented the Kemper classification and how it influences the type of research that can be done concerning certain CAM options. We then discussed the NCI and AHCPR levels of evidence that help to categorize and rank the weight of various types of clinical trial research.

We have presented the integrative oncology (IO) levels of evidence that are used throughout this text. We have also discussed hypothesis-driven research as it pertains to the pyramid of evidence, as well as safety issues that must be addressed in any kind of clinical applications and research.

A final issue to address in the evaluation of CAM therapies is the single-agent versus the systems approach. The discussion in this chapter has focused on research involving single agents, e.g. St John's wort. In contrast, many CAM therapies involve multiple components and are researched as a package or module. Examples of systems approaches might include testing both diet and exercise interventions in which participants receive dietary counseling on a low-fat diet and attend group exercise. This intervention is a 'package' that assumes that the outcome is dependent upon all components rather than any parts taken alone, i.e. adherence to a low-fat diet, diet counseling, exercise instruction, scheduled exercise and group exercise. Similarly, CAM therapies incorporated into conventional cancer treatment may become a package or system type of intervention that may be impossible to test in a randomized controlled trial. In these situations it is important that we do not discourage system-based approaches because of a lack of level I data, especially in the setting of preventive and supportive care options, where the patient risk level is low.

The remainder of the chapter will focus on how we use this knowledge to make clinical decisions about whether to use or recommend a CAM therapy. This is the part of the background that is necessary in deciding whether to invest in services that support CAM therapy in the clinical setting.

THERAPY TYPE AND GOAL

The type of evidence and research needed to make a decision is dependent upon the type of CAM treatment, as defined by the Kemper framework, as well as the therapeutic effect sought. For example, a bioenergetic therapy with little risk, designed to reduce tension or anxiety secondary to a cancer diagnosis, should not require the same level of evidence required to recommend a nutritional or herbal agent with potential side-effects that is purported to cure a type of cancer. Thus, in order to recommend, or not discourage, a CAM therapy, one must consider the risk associated with the agent as well as the primary therapeutic goal, i.e. prevention, supportive care or symptom management, and/or antineoplastic treatment (Figure 2.2).

Individual clinical situation

Clinicians must consider the level of benefit weighed against the risk of a certain treatment in the setting of a specific clinical situation. Again, St John's wort may offer some benefit for depression in moderately depressed individuals, but has been shown to negatively affect the efficacy of certain cancer therapeutic agents, and therefore has safety issues. This botanical should be avoided in patients undergoing chemotherapy. The acuity of a patient's specific clinical situation must be taken into account, i.e. how acute the need for some type of intervention may be. For example, a patient presenting with an acute leukemia cannot afford a treatment delay to begin a yoga class, while a patient presenting with early-stage prostate cancer may have this option. Likewise, a patient presenting with disease that has a high rate of cure or control has different levels of risk and benefit relative to both CAM and conventional care options.

Level of evidence and CAM

Once we understand the intention and practical aspects of treatment delivery, we can define the most appropriate trial, or examine the literature for studies that represent the highest level of evidence possible for a given modality. For example,

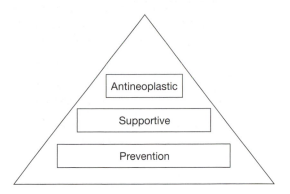

Figure 2.2 Pyramid of therapeutic goals. Higher levels on the pyramid are generally associated with larger risks and benefits and require higher levels of evidence for both safety and efficacy

the safety and efficacy of a herbal, or single agent, used to treat a symptom such as nausea or fatigue, or to treat a solid tumor may be best determined by a randomized double-blinded placebo-controlled clinical trial, after appropriate phase I and II testing with positive results. We would look for NCI level IA–D data or AHCPR and IO level I. On the other hand, a comprehensive lifestyle program, including diet, exercise and mind–body techniques to treat fatigue in breast cancer patients may be tested in a randomized controlled trial. We would then look for NCI level II A–D data or AHCPR and IO level II.

Cohen and Eisenberg[84] presented a helpful framework for clinical decisions involving CAM therapy. The framework, developed in response to a concern for medical liability, consists of five steps that include the following: determine the clinical risk level; document the literature supporting the therapy; ensure that patients receive adequate information about the therapy at the time of consent; maintain standard patient monitoring; and, when considering referral to a CAM practitioner, inquire about the practitioner's competence. For purposes of determining whether to recommend any therapy, one should abide by the following steps:

(1) Determine the goal of the treatment. This helps to define the clinical risk level. If the goal is cancer prevention, symptom control, supportive care during and after treatment, or general health maintenance, then the clinical risk level is lower than if the goal is antineoplastic in nature. The outcome if a patient does not follow advice concerning diet, exercise and coping skills is not as life threatening in the near term as if they do not take proven conventional antineoplastic therapy. This analysis not only gives the oncologist or provider some sense of perspective concerning how immediately important their recommendations may be, but also begins to frame the level of evidence necessary to make a recommendation based on a specific treatment goal. In other words, multiple studies with a high level of evidence concerning safety and efficacy are generally needed to recommend antineoplastic therapies, the risk level to the patient being high – i.e. life or death. Fewer studies with lower levels of evidence may be needed for treatments with preventive or supportive care goals, because the risk level to the patient is considerably lower.

(2) Determine the risk–benefit ratio for a specific therapy in a specific context. In order to determine safety and efficacy, Cohen and Eisenberg[84] classify research findings in one of four ways:

(a) Evidence supports safety and efficacy. The NCI publishes clinical practice guidelines and consensus statements supporting both safety and efficacy of therapies, such as the use of acupuncture for the treatment of nausea in cancer patients. Insurance coverage is appropriate for therapies in this category if found also to be cost effective.

(b) Evidence supports safety, efficacy is inconclusive. Therapies in this category may not be the standard of care but neither are they harmful, therefore the therapy is acceptable with caution and close monitoring for effectiveness.

(c) Evidence supports efficacy, safety is inconclusive. The risk of recommending therapies in this category is higher and therefore less advisable unless there is no biomedical treatment available. Cohen and Eisenberg[84] suggest that, with the lack of scientific knowledge regarding interactions of drugs and herbal therapy, and mechanisms of action of many biomechanical and biochemical therapies, clinicians are counseled to 'consider tolerating, provide caution and closely monitor safety' (p. 598).

(d) Evidence supports neither safety nor efficacy. Therapies falling under this classification are to be avoided and discouraged, particularly with therapies showing evidence of risk, not simply absence of proven safety. Patients who insist on pursuing therapies in this category should be counseled as to the reasons why the approach is not recommended. Physicians should document the session including the fact that there was a discussion of risks, dangers and a proven lack of benefit of the therapy in question.

Weiger and colleagues[85] have proposed criteria for recommending CAM therapy that are based upon the above levels of risk–benefit ratio. The criteria are part of a continuum ranging from 'accept' to 'discourage', based on published research (Table 2.4). While this article provides timely advice on current knowledge of certain CAM therapies which clinicians will find useful, a more important contribution of the article is the framework that clinicians can adapt and use as more is known about these and other therapies.

Table 2.4 Criteria used to determine whether a complementary and alternative medical therapy may reasonably be recommended, accepted or discouraged by physicians

Requirements	Recommend	Accept: may consider recommending	Accept	Discourage
Basic	Evidence supports both efficacy and safety	Evidence supports both efficacy and safety	Evidence on efficacy is inconclusive but evidence supports safety	Evidence indicates either inefficacy or serious risk
Efficacy	≥3 RCTs have evaluated the therapy ≥75% of trials support efficacy or a meta-analysis of trials supports efficacy For ≥3 of the trials that support efficacy: trial has > 50 patients *and* trial is of adequate quality Evidence supporting efficacy must come from > 1 research team	≥1 RCT has evaluated the therapy > 50% of trials support efficacy Evidence supporting efficacy fails to meet the criteria for therapies that may be recommended	Existing evidence is inadequate to conclude whether the therapy is effective or ineffective Data on efficacy fail to meet the criteria for considering recommendation Data on efficacy fail to meet the criteria for discouragement	≥2 RCTs have evaluated the therapy ≥67% of trials suggest that the therapy is ineffective For ≥2 of the trials that suggest lack of efficacy: trial has > 50 patients *and* trial is of adequate quality
Safety	Any documented adverse events associated with the therapy are minor (not life-threatening or permanently disabling) *and* Based on current information, no obvious theoretical potential for major (life-threatening or permanently disabling) adverse events exists	Any documented adverse events associated with the therapy are minor (not life-threatening or permanently disabling) *and* Based on current information, no obvious theoretical potential for major (life-threatening or permanently disabling) adverse events exists	Any documented adverse events associated with the therapy are minor (not life-threatening or permanently disabling) *and* Based on current information, no obvious theoretical potential for major (life-threatening or permanently disabling) adverse events exists	There is reliable documentation of a major (life-threatening or permanently disabling) adverse event occurring in association with the therapy *or* Based on current information, a theoretical potential for major adverse events exists

RCT, randomized controlled trial

CONCLUSION

This aim of this chapter was to offer a framework within which clinicians could make decisions about recommending CAM therapies as a part of integrative oncology. We have reviewed the levels of evidence and the types of research design associated with each level of evidence, as well as the maximum level of evidence that can be expected for certain types of CAM therapy. The clinical trial pyramid of evidence was defined and discussed. Considerations of efficacy and safety that providers should be aware of have been presented. Finally, placing these considerations into the context of patient risk level relative to therapeutic goal, specific clinical situation and levels of evidence concerning treatment safety and efficacy can help to guide oncologists concerning whether to recommend, accept, or discourage CAM use. Clinicians using levels of evidence and knowledge of trial design can review research reports and make informed decisions about the value and risk of CAM therapies for their cancer patients.

ACKNOWLEDGMENT

This work was supported in part by the Comprehensive Cancer Center of Wake Forest University Community Clinical Oncology Program Research Base Grant # 2 U10 CA81851 05.

RESOURCES ON CLINICAL RESEARCH

Ernst E, ed. The Desktop Guide to Complementary and Alternative Medicine: An Evidence Based Approach. London: Mosby, 2001

NCI Office of Complementary and Alternative Medicine (OCCAM):
www.cancer.gov/cam/

Levels of evidence:
www.nci.nih.gov/cancertopics/pdq/levels-evidence-cam/HealthProfessional/page5

Best-case series:
www3.cancer.gov/occam/bestcase. html

USC Norris Library Evidence Based Medicine Web Tutorial:
www.usc.edu/hsc/nml/lis/tutorials/ebm.html

New York Online Access to Health (NOAH):
www.noah-health.org/en/alternative/

Complementary and Alternative Medicine website dedicated to evidence-based medicine:
www.cam.org.nz/

References

1. Ernst E. The current position of complementary/alternative medicine in cancer. Eur J Cancer 2003; 39: 2274–77
2. National Center for Complementary and Alternative Medicine website: http//www.nccam.nih.gov/health/whatiscam
3. Kemper K. Separation or synthesis: a holistic approach to therapeutics. Pediatr Rev 1996; 17: 279–83
4. NCI Levels of evidence for adult cancer treatment studies (PDQ) http://www.nci.cancer.gov; cancerinfo/doc_pdq.aspx?cdrid=62796

5. Mills S. Herbal medicine. In Lewith G, Jonas WB, Walach H, eds. Clinical Research in Complementary Therapies: Principles, Problems and Solutions. London: Churchill Livingstone, 2002: 211–28

6. Browner WS, Newman TB, Cummings SR, et al. Getting ready to estimate sample size: Hypotheses and underlying principles. In Hulley SB, Cummings SR, eds. Designing Clinical Research. Baltimore, MD: Williams and Wilkins, 1988: 128–38

7. Lyn-Cook BD, Rogers T, Yan Y, et al. Chemopreventive effects of tea extracts and various components on human pancreatic and prostate tumor cells in vitro. Nutr Cancer 1999; 35: 80–6

8. Kuroda Y, Hara Y. Antimutagenic and anticarcinogenic activity of tea polyphenols. Mutat Res 1999; 436: 69–97

9. Brown MD. Green tea (Camellia sinensis) extract and its possible role in the prevention of cancer. Altern Med Rev 1999; 4: 360–70

10. Chen D, Daniel KG, Kuhn DJ, et al. Green tea and tea polyphenols in cancer prevention. Front Biosci 2004; 01: 2618–31

11. Blot WJ, Chow WH, McLaughlin JK. Tea and cancer: a review of the epidemiological evidence. Eur J Cancer Prev 1996; 5: 425–38

12. Rogers AE, Hafer LJ, Iskander YS, et al. Black tea and mammary gland carcinogenesis by 7, 12,-dimethyl[benz[a]anthracene in rats fed control or high fat diets. Carcinogenesis 1998; 19: 1269–73

13. Sartippour MR, Heber D, Ma J, et al. Green tea and its catechins inhibit breast cancer xenografts. Nutr Cancer 2001; 40: 149–56

14. Valcic S, Timmermann BN, Alberts DS, et al. Inhibitory effect of six green tea catechins and caffeine on the growth of four selected human tumor cell lines. Anticancer Drugs 1996; 7: 461–8

15. Dvorakova K, Dorr RT, Valcic S, et al. Pharmacokinetics of the green tea derivative, EGCG, by the topical route of administration in mouse and human skin. Cancer Chemother Pharmacol 1999; 43: 331–5

16. Jung YD, Ellis LM. Inhibition of tumor invasion and angiogenesis by epigallocatechin gallate (EGCG), a major component of green tea. Int J Exp Pathol 2001; 82: 309–16

17. Chow HH, Cai Y, Alberts DS, et al. Phase I pharmacokinetic study of tea polyphenols following single-dose administration of epigallocatechin gallate and polyphenon E. Cancer Epidemiol Biomarkers Prev 2001; 10: 53–8

18. Moyers SB, Kumar NB. Green tea polyphenols and cancer chemoprevention: multiple mechanisms and endpoints for phase II trials. Nutr Rev 2004; 62: 204–11

19. Butler K. A Consumer's Guide to Alternative Medicine. A Close Look at Homeopathy, Acupuncture, Faith-Healing, & Other Unconventional Treatments. Buffalo, NY: Prometheus Books, 1992

20. Kaegi E. Unconventional therapies for cancer; 6. 714-X, Task Force on Alternative Therapeutic of the Canadian Breast Cancer Research Initiative. Can Med Assoc J 1998; 12: 1621–4

21. Duda RB, Zhong Y, Navas V, et al. American ginseng and breast cancer therapeutic agents synergistically inhibit MCF-7 breast cancer cell growth. J Surg Oncol 1999; 72: 230–9

22. Amato P, Christophe S, Mellon PL. Estrogenic activity of herbs commonly used as remedies for menopausal symptoms. Menopause 2002; 9: 145–50

23. Punnonen R, Lukola A. Oestrogen like effect of ginseng. Br Med J 1980; 281: 1110

24. Bonham MJ, Galkin A, Montgomery B, et al. Effects of the herbal extract PC-SPES on microtubule dynamics and paclitaxel-mediated prostate tumor growth inhibition. J Natl Cancer Inst 2002; 94: 1641–7

25. Kubota T, Hisatake J, Hisatake Y, et al. PC-SPES: a unique inhibitor of proliferation of prostate cancer cells in vitro and in vivo. Prostate 2000; 42: 163–71

26. Huerta S, Arteaga JR, Irwin RW, et al. PC-SPES inhibits colon cancer growth in vitro and in vivo. Cancer Res 2002; 62: 5204–9

27. Ikezoe T, Chen S, Saito T, et al. PC-SPES decreases proliferation and induces differentiation and apoptosis of human acute myeloid leukemia cells. Int J Oncol 2003; 23: 1203–11

28. de la Taille A, Buttyan R, Hayek O, et al. Herbal therapy PC-SPES: in vitro effects and evaluation of its efficacy in 69 patients with prostate cancer. J Urol 2000; 164: 1229–34

29. Tiwari RK, Geliebter J, Garikapaty VP, et al. Anti-tumor effects of PC-SPES, an herbal

formulation in prostate cancer. Int J Oncol 1999; 14: 713–19

30. Wadsworth T, Poonyagariyagorn H, Sullivan E, et al. In vivo effect of PC-SPES on prostate growth and hepatic CYP3A expression in rats. J Pharmacol Exp Ther 2003; 306: 187–94

31. DiPaola RS, Zhang H, Lambert GH, et al. Clinical and biologic activity of an estrogenic herbal combination (PC-SPES) in prostate cancer. N Engl J Med 1998; 339: 785–91

32. de la Taille A, Hayek OR, Buttyan R, et al. Effects of a phytotherapeutic agent, PC-SPES, on prostate cancer: a preliminary investigation on human cell lines and patients. Br J Urol Int 1999; 84: 845–50

33. Small EJ, Frohlich MW, Bok R, et al. Prospective trial of the herbal supplement PC-SPES in patients with progressive prostate cancer. J Clin Oncol 2000; 18: 3595–603

34. Oh WK, George DJ, Hackmann K, et al. Activity of the herbal combination, PC-SPES, in the treatment of patients with androgen-independent prostate cancer. Urology 2001; 57: 122–6

35. Pfeifer BL, Pirani JF, Hamann SR, et al. PC-SPES, a dietary supplement for the treatment of hormone-refractory prostate cancer. Br J Urol Int 2000; 85: 481–5

36 Sovak M, Seligson AL, Konas M, et al. Herbal composition PC-SPEC for management of prostate cancer: identification of active principles. J Natl Cancer Inst 2002; 94: 1275–8

37. Vickers A. Methodological issues in complementary and alternative medicine research: a personal reflection on 10 years of debate in the United Kingdom. J Altern Complement Med 1996; 2: 515–24

38. Vickers A. How to reduce the number of patients needed for randomized trials: a basic introduction. Complement Ther Med 2001; 9: 234–6

39. Vickers A, Cassileth B, Ernst E, et al. How should we research unconventional therapies? A panel report from the Conference on Complementary and Alternative Medicine Research Methodology, National Institutes of Health. Int J Technol Assess Health Care 1997; 13: 111–21

40. Vickers AJ, de Craen AJ. Why use placebos in clinical trials? A narrative review of the methodological literature. J Clin Epidemiol 2000; 53: 157–61

41. Bloom BS, Retbi A, Dahan S, et al. Evaluation of randomized controlled trials on complementary and alternative medicine. Int J Technol Assess Health Care 2000; 16: 13–21

42. Walker, LG, Anderson J. Testing complementary and alternative therapies within a research protocol. Eur J Cancer 1999; 35: 1614–18

43. Margolin A. Liabilities involved in conducting randomized clinical trials of CAM therapies in the absence of preliminary, foundational studies: a case in point. J Altern Complement Med 1999; 5: 103–4

44. Hyland ME. Methodology for the scientific evaluation of complementary and alternative medicine. Complement Ther Med 2003; 11: 146–53

45. Carter B. Methodological issues and complementary therapies: researching intangibles? Complement Ther Nurs Midwifery 2003; 9: 133–9

46. Verhoef MJ, Casebeer AL, Hilsden RJ. Assessing efficacy of complementary medicine: adding qualitative research methods to the 'gold standard'. J Altern Complement Med 2002; 8: 275–81

47. Block KI, Burns B, Cohen AJ, et al. Point–counterpoint: using clinical trials for the evaluation of integrative cancer therapies. Integr Cancer Ther 2004; 3: 66–81

48. Jonas WB. Safety in complementary medicine. In Ernst E, ed. Complementary Medicine. London: Butterworth-Heinemann, 1996: 132

49. Fisher WB, Cohen SJ, Hammond MK, et al. Clinical trials in cancer therapy: efforts to improve patient enrollment by community oncologists. Med Pediatr Oncol 1991; 19: 165–8

50. Hypericum Depression Study Group. Effect of Hypericum perforatum (St. John's wort) in major depressive disorder: a randomized controlled trial. J Am Med Assoc 2002; 287: 1807–14

51. Bilia AR, Gallori S, Vincieri FF. St John's wort and depression efficacy, safety and tolerability – an update. Life Sci 2002; 70: 3077–96

52. Lasagna L, Mosteller F, von Pellsinger JM, et al. A study of the placebo response. Am J Med 1954; 16: 770–9

53. O'Mathuna DP. The placebo effect and alternative therapies. Alt Med Alert 2003; 6: 1–10

54. Shapiro AK, Shapiro E. The Powerful Placebo: From Ancient Priest to Modern Physician. Baltimore and London: Johns Hopkins University Press, 1997

55. Bensen H, McCallie DP. Angina pectoris and the placebo effect. N Engl J Med 1979; 300: 1424–9

56. Roberts AH, Kewman D, Mercier L, et al. The power of nonspecific effects in medicine and surgery: implication for biological and psychosocial treatments. Clin Psychol Rev 1993; 13: 375–91

57. Chvetzoff G, Tannock IF. Placebo effects in oncology. J Natl Cancer Inst 2003; 95: 19–29

58. Brody H. The Placebo Response. New York, NY: Cliff St. Books, 2000

59. Moerman DE, Jonas WB. Deconstructing the placebo effect and finding the meaning response. Ann Intern Med 2002; 136: 471–6

60. Spiro H. Clinical reflections on the placebo phenomenon. In Harrington A, ed. The Placebo Effect: An Interdisciplinary Exploration. Cambridge, MA: Harvard University Press, 1997: 37

61. Sapirstein G. The effectiveness of placebos in the treatment of depression: a meta analysis. Unpublished doctoral dissertation. University of Connecticut: Storrs, 1995

62. Benson H. Timeless Healing. New York: Fireside, 1997

63. Kuby L. Faith and the Placebo Effect: An Argument for Self Healing. Novato, CA: Origin Press, 2001

64. Kirsch I. Specifying nonspecifics: psychological mechanisms of placebo effects. In Harrington A, ed. The Placebo Effect: An Interdisciplinary Exploration. Cambridge, MA: Harvard University Press, 1997: 166–86

65. Ader R. The role of conditioning in pharmacotherapy. In Harrington A, ed. The Placebo Effect: An Interdisciplinary Exploration. Cambridge, MA: Harvard University Press, 1997: 138–65

66. Wolf S. Effects of suggestion and conditioning on the action of chemical agents in human subjects—the pharmacology of placebos. J Clin Invest 1950; 29: 100–9

67. Knowles JB. Conditioning and the placebo effect. Behav Res 1963; 1: 151–7

68. Evans FJ. The placebo response in pain control. Psychopharmacol Bull 1981; 17: 72–6

69. Gadow KD, White L, Ferguson DG. Placebo controls and double blind conditions. In Breuning SE, ed. Applied Psychopharmacology: Methods for Assessing Effects. New York: Grune and Stratton, 1985

70. Herrnstein R. Placebo effect in the rat. Science 1962; 138: 677–8

71. Olness K, Ader R. Conditioning as an adjunct in the pharmacotherapy of lupus erythematosus. J Dev Behav Pediatr 1992; 13: 124–5

72. Harrington A. Introduction. In Harrington A, ed. The Placebo Effect: an Interdisciplinary Exploration. Cambridge, MA: Harvard University Press, 1997: 1–11

73. Moerman D. Meaning, Medicine and the Placebo Effect. Cambridge, UK: Cambridge University Press, 2002

74. Moerman D, Jonas WB. Toward a research agenda on placebo. Adv Mind Body Med 2000; 16: 33–46

75. Napier AD. Book Review: Meaning Medicine and the Placebo Effect. Med Anth Q 2003; 17: 501–3

76. Ernst E, Resch KL. Concept of the true and perceived placebo effects. BMJ 1995; 311: 551–3

77. Hahn R. The nocebo phenomenon: scope and foundations. In Harrington A, ed. The Placebo Effect: An Interdisciplinary Exploration. Cambridge, MA: Harvard University Press, 1997: 56–76

78. Ernst E. Safety issues in complementary and alternative medicine. In Ernst E, ed. The Desktop Guide to Complementary and Alternative Medicine: An Evidence Based Approach. London: Mosby, 2001: 412–14

79. Wilkinson S, Chodok GW. Critical review of complementary therapies for prostate cancer. J Clin Oncol 2003; 21: 2199–200

80. Small EJ, Frohlich MW, Bok R, et al. Prospective trial of the herbal supplement PC-SPES in patients with progressive prostate cancer. J Clin Oncol 2000; 18: 3595–603

81. Davis NB, Nahlik L, Vogelzang NJ. Does PC SPES interact with warfarin? J Urol 2002; 167: 1793

82. Mathijssen RH, Verweij J, de Bruijn P, et al. Effects of St John's wort on irinotecan metabolism. J Natl Cancer Inst 2002; 94: 1187–8

83. Henney JE. Risk of drug interactions with St. John's wort. J Am Med Assoc 2002; 283: 1697

84. Cohen MH, Eisenberg DM. Potential physician malpractice liability associated with complementary and integrative medical therapies. Ann Intern Med 2002; 136: 596–603

85. Weiger WA, Smith M, Boon H, et al. Advising patients who seek complementary and alternative medical therapies for cancer. Ann Intern Med 2002; 137: 889–90

3

Physician training in integrative medicine

Patrick B. Massey

'The significant problems we face cannot be solved at the same level of thinking we were at when we created them.' – A. Einstein

It would be impossible to discuss the development of an integrative approach to oncology without recognizing the need for medical education. The demand for non-traditional medical therapies is growing rapidly, especially among those who have been diagnosed with cancer[1]. The use of complementary and alternative medicine (CAM) is increasing, in the USA and among cancer patients, with rates varying from 35% up to 85%, depending upon the definition of CAM and the population studied[2-5]. Cancer patients use CAM therapies with or without the knowledge or consent of their conventional provider, often because their physician has little or no experience or education concerning CAM[6,7]. With more than 50% of cancer patients using some form of CAM, it is crucial that physicians have, at least, a working knowledge of these modalities so that they can more effectively communicate with their patients.

The driving force in CAM use has been the consumer: they are demanding greater control of their health and greater access to CAM therapies[8,9]. A result of this consumerism has been an increase in basic science research in herbs and dietary supplements[10], as well as a growing number of well-designed clinical trials for various CAM therapies[11-13]. The relatively small amount of factual information on CAM a decade ago has been replaced with a rapidly expanding mass of clinical information. Many CAM therapies, once considered outside of mainstream medicine, may soon become a part of the standard of care for cancer patients.

There are obvious concerns if patients are using CAM therapies that are contraindicated during chemotherapy and radiation therapy. In contrast are those CAM therapies that may be safe and beneficial even during conventional therapy. Given the scope of CAM, it is impossible for the typical physician independently to keep current with the latest developments in the field. Therefore, physician education through the continuing medical education (CME) process on CAM therapies for cancer is essential.

PHYSICIAN EDUCATION

There are three goals in physician education: to create familiarity; to enhance clinical application; and to establish true expertise. In conventional medicine, this is achieved via three routes: medical school education (to create familiarity), continuing medical education (to enhance clinical application), and advanced education and training (to establish true expertise) (Table 3.1). The goals in CAM education for physicians are the same as those for conventional education. The means to achieving these goals can be found in the methods of traditional medical education.

Medical school

There are a number of steps in physician education, and each step builds upon the last. The first step is medical school. It is in medical school that attitudes toward medicine are formed. It is reasonable to believe that a physician's first introduction to CAM should be as a part of the medical school curriculum. The introduction of CAM therapies in medical school may set a foundation stone of familiarity which will inspire openness toward future learning, communication and patient care.

In response to the need for CAM education in medicine, the majority of medical schools have some form of CAM instruction, either as lectures, symposia, or clinical rotations. In 1997, approximately 64% of the US medical schools offered CAM education. A total of 123 courses were reported, with 68% offered as electives and 31% as a required part of the curriculum[14]. Topics included chiropractic, acupuncture, homeopathy, herbal therapies and mind–body techniques.

One group of medical schools, the Consortium of Academic Health Centers for Integrative Medicine (CAHCIM), has become the vanguard of medical school CAM education[15]. The CAHCIM is composed of 27 medical schools (see Resources section). These members have committed significant resources to CAM in education. The organization promotes the incorporation of CAM education into the core medical school curriculum. They also promote well-designed clinical research into CAM modalities and clinical care. They have developed a syllabus detailing the integration of CAM into physician education that has been distributed to all allopathic and osteopathic medical schools in the USA[15].

The consortium emphasizes the personal/emotional development of the physician as a major part of integrative medicine as well. The CAHCIM recognizes the need to bring balance to medical education, and are active in changing the medical school environment to reflect these values. In their opinion, CAM familiarity can balance medical education so that it becomes a nurturing, holistic experience. This points to the transformational quality of many CAM interventions, especially with regards to self-care.

Through the activity of organizations such as CAHCIM, the hope is that future generations of physicians will have a working knowledge of CAM as they enter their chosen fields of practice. It is also hoped that they will help to create healthy providers and a sustainable health-care system for all involved.

CAM education in residency and fellowship

After medical school, medical education becomes less didactic and assumes more direct clinical

Table 3.1 Conventional physician education: goals and methods

Goal	Method
Create familiarity	Medical school
Enhance clinical application	Continuing medical education
Develop expertise	Advanced education and training

applications. As a result, CAM education is driven by the desire of the physician to learn. Interest in CAM therapies and approaches may be introduced by patient–physician interactions, lectures and symposia. Education takes on the form of independent study and research, akin to continuing medical education. Personal interest by the physician becomes the primary motivating factor in CAM education.

The amount of information associated with CAM is large and rapidly increasing, necessitating physician specialization with the development of CAM fellowships and associate fellowships in order to develop expertise.

Specialized CAM fellowship programs

Fellowship training involves several years of research and clinical training, often with the goal of producing researchers and academicians. Ten years ago, there were no fellowship programs in CAM. In 2004, there are a number of CAM fellowship programs at major medical schools and research centers across the USA (see Resource section). The purpose of these programs is to prepare physicians and scientists for careers as research scholars and clinical investigators in the field of CAM.

The largest supporter of CAM fellowship education is the National Center for Complementary and Alternative Medicine (NCCAM). NCCAM is part of the National Institutes of Health (NIH) and was established in 1992, originally as the Office of Alternative Medicine. NCCAM and the NIH have funded a number of medical schools, universities and medical centers for fellowship training in CAM: Bastyr University, Florida International University, Harvard Medical School, Minneapolis Medical Research Foundation, Morgan State University, University of Arizona, University of Pennsylvania School of Medicine, University of Virginia and Columbia University College of Physicians & Surgeons.

CAM associate fellowship program

Fellowship programs are limited by time and effort, often requiring 2–5 years before completion. In addition, the number of fellows per program is limited. For the majority of physicians interested in serious study of CAM, this type of educational process is simply not realistic. In 2000, the University of Arizona Program in Integrative Medicine initiated its first class for the associate fellowship. This 2-year program was tailored for practicing physicians and nurses. The program makes use of current communications technology and, as a result, most of the program is 'distance' learning. However, there are several 'residential weeks' for didactic education within the 2-year time frame. This program has graduated more than 40 associate fellows per year since 2002, including the editor and several contributors to this text.

CAM and continuing medical education

CME has changed dramatically over the past 20 years. What began initially as books, occasional lectures at the local medical center or a week-long symposium once or twice a year, has developed into an information delivery system that is far more complex and varied[16].

Historically, the majority of physicians get CME from lectures. However, retention of information is low and its effect on changing physician attitudes is limited[17]. Another problem with the conventional CME approach is that, to a large extent, it is detached from the actual practice of medicine. It is limited in that it cannot provide practicing physicians with the information they need, when they need it (usually in the clinical setting)[18,19].

Self-directed learning methods seem to have a greater impact on learning, as measured by changing physician behavior[20,21]. These methods of learning include audiotapes, CD-ROM technology and Internet-based learning. Retention of information and changing physician attitudes requires some degree of repetition. One advantage that self-directed learning programs have over lectures is that the information can be easily retrieved and reviewed. Some CD-ROM and Internet-based programs are designed to enhance clinical decision-making on specific diseases and illnesses, with great potential for changing physician practice and attitudes[22].

The growth of the Internet and computer/telecommunication technologies has dramatically increased the number of options for CME. Continuing medical education programs, as well as expert opinions, can be offered, literally, worldwide with the touch of a button[22]. Timely access to medical research is defining those CAM therapies that may be beneficial in the treatment of cancer and other diseases. Experts can delineate safety and efficacy questions and improve the practicing physician's communication with their patients. Responsible communication is necessary because those advances in technology that have opened the dissemination of medical research findings to the physician have also opened it to the patient. See Table 3.2 for the advantages and disadvantages of various CME approaches.

Ideally, physician education should be from those whose medical practice and/or research focus is on CAM and its clinical integration. Nevertheless, a major shortcoming for CAM education is that there are a limited number of true physician experts. With the increase in CAM fellowships and associated fellowships, there are a growing number of physicians – true experts in CAM – who are beginning to fill these educational needs.

WHAT ARE THE OBSTACLES TO CONTINUING EDUCATION?

The idea of continuing medical education is relatively new. Historically, it has not been a part of the American medical educational process. In a number of studies, it has been found that physicians believe that the practice of medicine, especially now, requires continuous education[23–25]. Medical innovations, medications, therapies and protocols are changing rapidly and it is important that a physician's base of knowledge keeps pace.

Obstacles to CME are:

- Time
  Scarcity of time is possibly the greatest drawback to medical education. Most physicians directly involved with patient care work in excess of 60 hours/week. They may have a number of clinical questions involving patient care every day. Most studies show that at least one medical question is generated for each patient[26]. Thus, over a day, dozens of questions over specific clinical scenarios may be created. Finding answers for clinical questions is central to physician learning and changing behavior.

- CME format
  The method of presentation is important for retention of information and changing practice behavior. At one end of the scale is the lecture, having the least impact on information retention and changing physician practice, and at the other end of the scale is hands-on clinical experience, having the greatest impact on retention and behavior change. Given time restraints, didactic lectures are the most common form of CME, and are a good way to introduce new concepts and present broad overviews on specific topics. CD-ROM and Internet-based learning may play an increasingly important role in physician education at all levels of learning. This may have a greater impact upon retention and behavior changes to the extent that more clinical scenarios are used as teaching and interactive examples[18,27,28]. Barriers to Internet-based CME exist primarily because

computers and the Internet[29] may still be foreign to a number of physicians.

- Cost
  Funding a CME program and individual physician cost to participate may be a significant factor, especially if travel is involved, and expert resources are scarce.

WHAT IMPROVEMENTS HAVE BEEN MADE IN CME OPTIONS?

Technology has significantly increased CME options. Not that many years ago, lectures, journals, textbooks and audiotapes were the only choices. Today, that has expanded with CD-ROM, DVD, on-demand and real-time web-based CME programs[18,27,28]. Many journals are available through the Internet. Journals and textbooks are also available as CD-ROM. These technologies expand learning options and are readily upgradeable to keep current with the changes in medicine. In addition, they can be made interactive with feedback given on whether principles have been learned. See Table 3.2 concerning various CME methods, and the advantages and disadvantages.

The Medical Knowledge Self-Assessment Program (MKSAP®) is a prime example of how technology has changed. The MKSAP has grown from a series of paperback books into a CD-ROM with an Internet website containing questions, immediate feedback, and links to references, radiological studies and more. Another example of advances in information delivery is the Physician's Information and Education Resource (PIER) through the American College of Physicians (ACP). This is an on-line, continuously updated information base for the practicing clinician. It is divided into six categories: diseases, screening and prevention, ethical and legal issues, procedures, drug resources and CAM. However, PIER is only available to members of the ACP.

The Internet will probably become more dominant in the delivery of CME. Retention of information is similar to that for lectures and the convenience advantage is obvious[26]. Because of these advantages, it is possible that paper-based resources may be supplanted as a primary method of CME.

CAM, CANCER AND CONTINUING MEDICAL EDUCATION

Martin Rossman[30] describes three levels of an integrative medicine practice: level one is the accumulation of information and clinical experience concerning integrative medicine; level two is an understanding of CAM therapies and initiation of clinical applications; level three is specialization in one or more specific CAM approaches. I would propose Rossman's 'level one' be divided into two parts, A and B. Level 1A would be defined by a physician who is just beginning to learn about CAM. At this level, the information presented is relatively superficial, leading to an understanding of terms, historical origins and cultural significance. At this level, a physician would be familiar with the terms commonly used in CAM. Level 1B would be analysis of research and data on clinical efficacy, mechanisms of action and safety. At this level, a physician would be able to communicate with patients about CAM use and properly refer patients to CAM providers.

CAM is not commonly used or understood in the traditional medical community. Although the past decade has seen an increase in CAM education, it is safe to say that most physicians have little experience with CAM. As a result, preparatory education must precede meaningful integration of CAM into their medical practices. This would be the level 1A. This preparatory education must concentrate on the history, philosophy and foundation of medicine, both integrative and allopathic, because the practice of

Table 3.2 Common continuing medical education (CME) formats – advantages and disadvantages

Method	Advantages	Disadvantages
Internet		
With the advent of the Internet, a number of corporations are offering CAM CME on line. These can be either as a PowerPoint type of presentation or through specific articles followed by directed questions	Can be free Large selection Conveniently accessed any time Can be downloaded or printed for future reference Potential increased access to experts Current information Low cost	Requires Internet access Requires a minimal level of expertise in computers and the Internet Minimal chance for questions and immediate feedback
CD-ROM		
There are a number of medical schools and corporations offering lectures on CD-ROM that can be conveniently used by the physician. CME credit is available, either by mail or by visiting the specific website and answering directed questions about the lecture	Convenience May be accessed at any time Available for future reference Medical opinions and information from a number of experts on each CD-ROM Information is current Moderate cost	No chance for questions and immediate feedback Requires CD player and some computer expertise and Internet access is beneficial
Seminar and symposium		
Medical schools, medical centers, hospitals, drug companies, publishing houses	Large amounts of information in a specific time frame Networking and discussions with like-minded physicians Travel minimal depending upon location Many opportunities	Time and cost involved in travel and symposium May not meet specific clinical needs and questions
Lectures		
Most commonly presented at local medical schools, medical centers and drug companies	Easily accessible to larger groups of physicians Can be tailored to specific interests Can immediately ask questions of lecturer Variable cost/free	Retention of information limited Not available for future reference
Books and medical journals		
Increasing number of books and journals dealing specifically with CAM and applications Increasing number of CAM articles in common medical journals	Convenience May be accessed at any time Available for future reference Moderate cost	May be more time intensive

Continued…

Table 3.2 *Continued*

Method	Advantages	Disadvantages
Associate fellowship, program in integrative medicine A 2-year training program in CAM for physicians, physician assistants and nurse practitioners Curriculum is presented via web-based learning modules and three week-long symposia	Convenience...may be accessed at any time Available for future reference Continuous access to experts and colleagues	CME limited to week-long symposium Significant time commitment Significant cost
Integrative medicine fellowship 1–2 year, on site, intensive educational experience, resulting in significant expertise	Paid position Significant, in-depth research experience	Often no CME credit Significant time commitment Questionable marketability following graduation

integrative medicine implies more than simply modulating a biomedical system. This type of education would necessitate experiencing those personal aspects of the healing arts not commonly found in medical school and even CME. Mind–body therapies, meditation and discovery of self are probably best done among like-minded peers in relatively small groups. Several such physician support groups and residential retreat organizations exist throughout the country and some are associated with CME offerings. These are available in the Resources section of this text.

Ideally, an oncologist or cancer care provider should have a basic understanding of CAM and know how to refer and discuss patients with CAM providers. At this level, a familiarity of basic CAM concepts by the referring physician is considered necessary. Lectures and seminars may be the best way to acquire a broad, working knowledge of terms, therapies, botanicals and dietary supplements.

For those clinicians interested in a greater understanding and application of CAM therapies in the treatment of cancer, other CME formats, such as symposia, CD-ROM, Internet and even

Table 3.3 CAM education – goals and methods

Create familiarity	Medical school; core curriculum – efforts by the Consortium of Academic Health Centers for Integrative Medicine
	Practicing providers – lectures and seminars
	Personal experience – retreats focused on physician well-being, spas
Enhance clinical application	CME courses – especially symposia, CD-ROM, Internet. Peer-reviewed journals
Develop expertise	Conventional Integrative Medicine Fellowship, Associate Fellowship (e.g. University of Arizona Program)

the Associate Fellowship in the Program in Integrative Medicine at the University of Arizona are available.

Given that cancer patients commonly use CAM, it would be prudent that, at least, an introductory level of CAM education be incorporated as a requirement into all oncology-related fellowships and training programs.

CONTINUOUS CAM EDUCATION FOR COMMUNITY PHYSICIANS

The Alexian Brothers Hospital Network Model

We recognized that, even if a physician does not want to utilize any CAM therapies or approaches, he/she should have an understanding of pertinent terminology, as well as some knowledge about the quantity of research for and against CAM use. There are potential and real contraindications between medications and some dietary supplements. Physicians also need to be able to recognize those medical experts in their geographic area who can serve as a resource.

Even though an increasing number of medical schools, medical centers and physician societies are offering lectures on CAM, either as a stand-alone product or as part of a seminar on a specific disease, the education is generally intermittent. It is difficult for clinicians to learn all that they need to know about CAM when it is not available on a regular basis. Therefore, an ongoing physician education program in CAM was designed to provide needed CME in CAM for clinicians by the Alexian Brothers Hospital Network. They made a commitment to 18–24 2-hour CME CAM lectures over 2–3 years for physicians and nurses. This program began in 2002 and has become one of the most popular CME offerings in the history of the Alexian Brothers Hospital Network.

Clinical physicians who are also experts in various areas of CAM present the lectures. A number of these lectures have been recorded and can be referenced through the medical libraries associated with the hospitals in the Alexian Brothers Hospital Network.

Topics have included:

- Introduction to integrative medicine;
- Dietary supplements;
- Oriental medicine/acupuncture;
- Manual therapies;
- Legal issues in CAM;
- CAM use in the elderly;
- CAM therapies for inflammation;
- Pediatrics and CAM;
- CAM and cancer;
- Dietary supplements and surgery;
- Nutrition: the missing link in medicine;
- Integrative therapies for prostate cancer;
- Integrative approaches to the treatment of Parkinson's disease;
- Acupuncture applications for surgery;
- Alternatives to hormone replacement therapy;
- Qi Gong: Chinese energy medicine – research and clinical applications;
- Boutique medical practice models.

As an outgrowth of this program, CAM therapies are being integrated into a number of lectures and symposia on traditional medicine topics such as prostate cancer, Parkinson's disease and metabolic syndrome. This allows physicians to see how CAM therapies can be safely used in conjunction with traditional medical therapies. It also allows the practicing physician to enter confidently into meaningful discussions with medical experts about CAM therapies for a variety of diseases and health maintenance.

STARTING A CAM CONTINUING MEDICAL EDUCATION PROGRAM

There are a number of different ways to start a CAM CME program at a local hospital and medical center. There may be some resistance from the medical staff. I have included some suggestions based upon my experiences in the CAM CME program through the Alexian Brothers Hospital Network.

(1) Identify medical staff interests in CAM as well as those physicians who are practicing CAM therapies.

(2) Identify specific clinical needs in CAM education for the medical staff.

(3) Approach the CME committee, emphasizing the fact that:

   (a) Education does not equal endorsement.

   (b) The majority of Americans use some form of CAM therapy (in some conditions, such as cancer, CAM use can exceed 75%).

   (c) It is incumbent upon physicians to know what their patients are doing and how this impacts traditional medical care.

(4) Physicians usually prefer CME presentations by physicians. Identify local physicians with expertise/interest in specific CAM therapies for introductory lectures.

(5) Integrate CAM information into traditional medicine lectures, especially in the area of cancer, diabetes and heart disease.

(6) Invite nurses, other health-care personnel and even local CAM practitioners.

(7) Introduce 'non-threatening' CAM therapies such as Tai Chi, yoga and mind–body approaches to both patients and medical

staff for personal experience. Build on that credibility for future CME.

(8) Emphasize that there is a growing body of medical studies on CAM – some positive and some negative.

(9) Detail CAM therapies already part of traditional medicine...mind–body therapies, massage, specific supplements, exercise, hypnosis, nutrition, etc.

SUMMARY

Physician education is a vital aspect of integrative oncology. See Table 3.3 for a summary of education goals and methods concerning CAM. See also the Resources section for information on CME resources, the CAHCIM, postgraduate fellowship training programs in integrative medicine, physician retreats and healing spas, journals and organizations.

RESOURCES FOR COMPLEMENTARY AND ALTERNATIVE MEDICINE (CAM) AND CONTINUING MEDICAL EDUCATION (CME)

CME resources on CAM education

Despite the growing interest in CAM, there are a limited number of CME providers that offer substantial CAM education. Below are a few good starting points.

Biomed Central
www.biomedcentral.com/

Medscape
www.medscape.com/px/urlinfo

Oakstone Medical Publishing
www.oakstonemedical.com

CMEWeb
www.cmeweb.com

American Association of Family Physicians
www.aafp.org

Physicians' Information and Education
Resource (PIER)
http://pier.acponline.org/index.html

CAM and postgraduate medical training (residency and fellowship)

Rosenthal Center, Columbia Medical
Center, NY
www.rosenthal.hs.columbia.edu/Residency.html

CAM Research Fellowship, Harvard Medical
School
www.hms.harvard.edu

B. Macmillen
Phone: +1-617-667-5384
E-mail: bmacmill@caregroup.Harvard.edu

CAM program at Stanford
http://camps.stanford.edu

National Center for Complementary and
Alternative Medicine, NIH
http://nccam.nih.gov/training/t32

Program in Integrative Medicine, University of
Arizona
www.integrativemedicine.arizona.edu

University of Maryland Clinical Fellowship in
Integrative Medicine
www.compmed.umm.edu

Bastyr University, Training in Complementary
and Alternative Medical research
www.bastyr.edu/researchtraininggrant

Florida International University, Training in
Alternative Tropical Botanical Medicine
Sara Chipon

Phone: +1-305-348-3419
E-mail: cenap@fiu.edu

Minneapolis Medical Research Foundation:
training a new generation of CAM clinical
investigators
www.bermancenter.org

Morgan State University: minority research
training
Emmanuel Taylor MSc DrPH
Phone: +1-443-885-4035
E-mail: emtaylor@php.morgan.edu

University of Pennsylvania School of Medicine:
training in complementary and alternative
medicine
www.med.upenn.edu/penncam

University of Virginia: training program in
complementary and alternative medicine
www.healthsystem.virginia.edu/internet/cscat/

Consortium of Academic Health Centers for Integrative Medicine (CAHCIM)

University of Arizona
Program for Integrative Medicine
www.integrativemedicine.arizona.edu

University of Calgary
Canadian Institute of Natural & Integrative
Medicine
www.ucalgary.ca

University of California, Los Angeles
Collaborative Centers for Integrative Medicine
www.uclamindbody.org

University of California, San Francisco
Osher Center for Integrative Medicine
www.ucsf.edu/ocim

Columbia University
Richard and Hilda Rosenthal Center for
Complementary & Alternative Medicine
www.rosenthal.hs.columbia.edu

Duke University
Duke Center for Integrative Medicine
www.dcim.org

Albert Einstein College of Medicine of Yeshiva
University
Continuum Center for Health and Healing
www.healthandhealingny.org

George Washington University
Center for Integrative Medicine
www.integrativemedicinedc.com

Georgetown University
Kaplan Clinic
www.georgetown.edu/schmed/cam

Harvard University
Osher Institute
www.osher.hms.harvard.edu

University of Hawaii at Manoa
Program in Integrative Medicine
www.uhm.hawaii.edu

Thomas Jefferson University
Center for Integrative Medicine
www.jeffersonhospital.org/cim

University of Maryland
Center for Integrative Medicine
www.compmed.umm.edu

University of Massachusetts
Center for Mindfulness
www.umassmed.edu/cfm/

University of Michigan
Complementary & Alternative Research
Center
www.med.umich.edu/camrc

University of Minnesota
Center for Spirituality and Healing
www.csh.umn.edu

University of Medicine and Dentistry of New
Jersey
Institute for Complementary & Alternative

Medicine
www.umdnj.edu/icam

Oregon Health and Science University
Women's Primary Care and Integrative
Medicine, Center for Women's Health
www.ohsu.edu/women

University of Pennsylvania
Office of Complementary Therapies
www.med.upenn.edu/progdev/compmed/
steering.html

University of Pittsburgh
Center for Complementary Medicine
www.complementarymedicine.upmc.com

University of Texas Medical Branch
UTMB Integrative Health Care
cam.utmb.edu

University of Washington
Department of Family Medicine
www.fammed.washington.edu/predoctoral/cam

Physician retreats and healing spas

Many Streams Healing Systems
www.manystreamsheal.org

Innovision
www.alternative-therapies.com

Canyon Ranch Health Resorts
www.canyonranch.com

Buddhist retreats
www.buddhistnetwork.org/welcome.html

Circle of Healers
www.amsa.org/humed/retreat2001.cfm

Omega Institute
www.eomega.org

Miraval
www.miravalresort.com

Sanjevani
www.sanjevani.net

Journals and organizations

Journal of Cancer Integrative Medicine
www.cancerintegrativemedicine.com

Integrative Cancer Therapies
www.sagepub.com/Home.aspx

Society for Integrative Oncology
www.integrativeonc.com

Office of Cancer Complementary and Alternative Medicine, National Cancer Institute
www.cancer.gov

References

1. Weiger WA, Smith M, Boon H, et al. Advising patients who seek complementary and alternative medical therapies for cancer. Ann Intern Med 2002; 137: 889–903

2. Ernst E, Cassileth BR. The prevalence of complementary/alternative medicine in cancer. Cancer 1998; 83: 777–82

3. Wyatt GK, Friedman LL, Given CW, et al. Complementary therapy use among older cancer patients. Cancer Pract 1999; 7: 136–44

4. Kimby CK, Launso L, Henningsen I, Langgaard H. Choice of unconventional treatment by patients with cancer. J Altern Complement Med 2003; 9: 549–61

5. Shumay DM, Maskarinec G, Gotay CC, et al. Determinants of the degree of complementary and alternative medicine use among patients with cancer. J Altern Complement Med 2002; 8: 661–71

6. Frenkel M, Ben-Arye E, Hermoni D. An approach to educating family practice residents and family physicians about complementary and alternative medicine. Complement Ther Med 2004; 12: 118–25

7. Robinson A, McGrail MR. Disclosure of CAM use to medical practitioners: a review of qualitative and quantitative studies. Complement Ther Med 2004; 12: 90–8

8. Haugh R. The new consumer. Hosp Health Netw 1999; 73: 30–4

9. Astin JA. Why patients use alternative medicine: results of a national study. J Am Med Assoc 1998; 279: 1548–53

10. Massey PB. Dietary supplements. Med Clin North Am 2002; 86: 127–47

11. Jonas WB, Anderson RL, Crawford CC, Lyons JS. A systematic review of the quality of homeopathic clinical trials. BMC Complement Altern Med 2001; 1: 12

12. Linde K, ter Riet G, Hondras M, et al. Systematic reviews of complementary therapies - an annotated bibliography. Part 2: herbal medicine. BMC Complement Altern Med 2001; 1: 5

13. Linde K, Vickers A, Hondras M, et al. Systematic reviews of complementary therapies - an annotated bibliography. Part 1: acupuncture. BMC Complement Altern Med 2001; 1: 3

14. Wetzel MS, Eisenberg DM, Kaptchuk DJ. Courses involving complementary and alternative medicine in US medical schools. J Am Med Assoc 1998; 280: 784–7

15. Competencies in integrative medicine for medical students. CAHCIM working group on education. Acad Med 2004; 76: 521–9

16. Manning PR, DeBakey L. Continuing medical education: the paradigm is changing. J Contin Educ Health Prof 2001; 21: 46–54

17. Mamary E, Charles P. Promoting self-directed learning for continuing medical education. Med Teach 2003; 25: 188–90

18. Goodyear-Smith F, Whitehorn M, McCormick R. Experiences and preferences of general practitioners regarding continuing medical education: a qualitative study. NZ Med J 2003; 116: U399

19. Ebell MH, Shaughnessy A. Information mastery: integrating continuing medical education with the information needs of clinicians. J Contin Educ Health Prof 2003; 23 (Suppl 1): S53–62

20. Dooley MJ, Lee DY, Marriott JL. Practitioners' sources of clinical information on complementary and alternative medicine in oncology. Support Care Cancer 2004; 12: 114–19

21. Mamary E, Charles P. Promoting self-directed learning for continuing medical education. Med Teach 2003; 25: 188–90

22. Bennett NL, Casebeer LL, Kristofco RE, Strasser SM. Physicians' Internet information-seeking behaviors. J Contin Educ Health Prof 2004; 24: 31–8

23. Winzenberg T, Higginbotham N. Factors affecting the intention of providers to deliver more effective continuing medical education to general practitioners: a pilot study. BMC Med Educ 2003; 14; 3: 11

24. Booth BJ. Does continuing medical education make a difference? Med J Aust 1997, 167: 237–8

25. Thomson O'Brien MA, Freemantle N, Oxman AD, et al. Continuing education meetings and workshops: effects on professional practice and health care outcomes. Cochrane Database Syst Rev 2001, CD003030

26. Ebell MH, Shaughnessy A. Information mastery: integrating continuing medical education with the information needs of clinicians. J Contin Educ Health Prof 2003; 23 (Suppl 1): S53–62

27. Wutoh R, Boren SA, Balas EA. e-Learning: a review of Internet-based continuing medical education. J Contin Educ Health Prof 2004; 24: 20–30

28. Strasberg HR, Rindfleisch TC, Hardy S. SKOLAR MD: a model for self-directed, in-context continuing medical education. Proc AMIA Symp 2003: 634–8

29. Mamary EM, Charles P. On-site to on-line: barriers to the use of computers for continuing education. J Contin Educ Health Prof 2000; 20: 171–5

30. Rossman ML. Integrating complementary medicine into health systems. In Fass N, ed. Profile: Three Levels of Integrative Practice. San Francisco, CA: Aspen Publication, 2001: 693–5

4

The health of the healer: physician/health-care provider wellness

Danna M. Park

'You have chosen me to watch over the life and health of your creatures. I am about to apply myself to the duties of my profession... Support me in this great work that it may benefit my fellow creatures... Inspire me with love for my occupation and for your creatures... Preserve my physical and spiritual strength that I may cheerfully be of help to rich and poor, good and bad, friend and foe alike. Let me see only the human being in the sufferer'. – Moses Maimonides

INTRODUCTION

I am sitting in a small classroom on the second floor of the medical school with five first- and second-year medical students. The lights are dim; there is a single candle burning at the center of our circle. These students, with 20 of their colleagues, have opted to participate in Rachael Naomi Remen's course 'The Healer's Art', a 5-week elective that is 'an interactive, contemplative and didactic approach [that enables] students to perceive the personal and universal meaning in their daily experience of medicine'[1]. We use discussion and experiential learning, through reflections and drawings, to investigate a variety of topics including 'Discovering and Nurturing Your Wholeness', 'Sharing Grief and Honoring Loss', 'Allowing Awe in Medicine' and 'The Care of the Soul'. The students are inquisitive, worried about what medical training and practice will do to

their sense of self, their compassion and their calling to become a doctor. All five report that, during the long process of applying to medical school, the physicians they encountered urged them not to pursue medicine as a career, citing personal experiences of cynicism, burnout and work environment stressors.

It is rare to see a medical text address health-care provider wellness as a component of patient care. Yet what could be more crucial and critical, especially in today's medical environment? The ongoing health-care crisis has clearly affected practitioners' ability to care for themselves and their patients, families and communities. There is a conflict between self-care and care for others, and a conflict of not enough time – with patients, with family or with self. It is an internal conflict between the life of a healer in medicine and the life of a busy practitioner working with insurance demands and financial pressures that are defining the practice of medicine today.

AN INTEGRATIVE APPROACH TO SELF-CARE

Integrative medicine is defined as healing-oriented medicine that takes account of the whole person (body, mind and spirit), including all aspects of lifestyle. It emphasizes the therapeutic relationship and makes use of all appropriate therapies, both conventional and alternative[2]. An integrative approach to oncology, or to any medical specialty for that matter, recognizes that the provider–patient dyad is a constant back-and-forth, give-and-take, interactive fluctuating relationship, one in which it becomes clear that the provider's own wellness and that of their patient are interlinked. This 'relationship-centered care' is defined by the Fetzer Institute/Relationship-Centered Care Network as being 'an approach to healthcare and healing that places relationship at the core of the therapeutic process. In this approach, all interactions are based upon a fundamental commitment to mutual respect, self-awareness, humility, openness, and caring'[3].

Just as the concept of relationship-centered care is multifaceted, the creation of health and wellness is complex. It necessitates working with interconnected realms that extend beyond the physical body, into emotional, spiritual, interprofessional/institutional and interpersonal spheres. When the practitioner recognizes this and chooses to treat the 'whole patient' and their family, incorporating body, mind, spirit and relationship-centered care into the treatment plan, it brings a powerful component into practicing medicine. The practitioner–patient relationship itself becomes a tool for healing. The health-care provider is invited to be an active participating 'whole provider', one who integrates wellness into their personal and professional life. From an integrative medicine perspective, this is an essential component of being of service to the patient. Data show that personal wellness is good medicine for provider and patient, and it may be more vital in today's challenging environment than ever. To provide this level of integrated care, we as providers need to develop wellness and self-nurturing tools to help sustain and support our physical, emotional, spiritual and social well-being throughout our medical practice. Developing these tools is an investment in self as well as an investment in exceptional care for patients.

Although this chapter uses data and literature from the physician's point of view, it is no less relevant for other health-care practitioners. The stressors and issues inherent in the practice of medicine today affect all health-care providers: doctors, nurses, nurse practitioners and physician assistants alike.

DEFINITIONS OF WELLNESS

Defining wellness is difficult because it is so inherently personal (Tables 4.1 and 4.2). What makes one practitioner feel whole, complete, and healthy on a mind/body/spirit level may be vastly different for another. In addition, it is a fluid state; what we need to balance ourselves changes from day to day. Three definitions capture the complexity of these concepts. The Wellness Definition, from Arizona State University, states

Table 4.1 Components of wellness and challenges

Components	Challenges
Physical wellness	Time pressures
Emotional wellness	Financial pressures
Spiritual wellness	Burnout
Interpersonal relationships	Work environment
Interprofessional relationships	
Institutional wellness	

Table 4.2   Examples of integrating wellness and the challenges

Examples	Challenges
Physical wellness – daily exercise, eating nutritious meals, doctor/dentist appointments	Time, 'provider as patient' issues
Emotional wellness – journaling, counseling, personal development	Time, stigma of 'seeking professional help'
Spiritual wellness – meditation, participating in a church community, connecting with nature	Time, how to connect to something 'bigger than self'
Interpersonal relationships – 'date nights' with spouse/significant other, time with children, counseling	Time, stigma of 'seeking professional help'
Interprofessional relationships – Meaning In Medicine groups, social events, meetings	Time with colleagues is time away from family/other activities
Institutional wellness – vegetarian and low-fat options in cafeteria, gym 'in-house' for employees, stress-reduction programs	Financial considerations/cost

'Wellness is an active, lifelong process of becoming aware of choices and making decisions toward a more balanced and fulfilling life. Wellness involves choices about our lives and our priorities that determine our lifestyles'[4]. The World Health Organization's definition of health emphasizes the multidimensional aspects of wellness: 'Health is a state of complete physical, mental and social well-being and not merely the absence of disease or infirmity'[5]. Ardell and Langdon's definition concentrates on the active role needed to achieve health: 'Wellness is a lifestyle approach to personal excellence. It is a deliberate, conscious decision to pursue optimal well-being. It encompasses the body, mind and spirit. It is a positive choice pursued because it is judged to be a richer way to be alive'[6]. These definitions highlight the fact that we live and work in a complex world, one where health and wellness are not limited to the physical realm; they must also include the spiritual, emotional, interprofessional/institutional and interpersonal dimensions. The idea that health and wellness affect and extend into our relationships (friends, spouse/partner, etc.) is not a new concept, nor is the link between spiritual, emotional and physical health. The impact of the workplace environment on personal wellness has also now been documented (the interprofessional/institutional dimension). Through physician studies, we are starting to understand more about how health-care practitioners' own well-being, satisfaction and health habits have a direct and measurable effect on their patients' health.

PROFESSIONAL SATISFACTION

There is no doubt that the practice of medicine today, no matter what field a practitioner is in, is stressful. Much has been documented in terms of the literal and figurative costs incurred, both personally and professionally, when there is health-care provider 'discontent'. Amazingly, 'provider happiness' may be one of the most important factors we bring into a practitioner–patient relationship.

Studies show that when physicians are 'professionally satisfied' in their work, they provide better quality of care and produce more patient satisfaction[7]. One study's intriguing conclusion was that physicians' global job satisfaction was related to their patients' overall compliance with their treatment plan: 'This study is one of the few to demonstrate that how clinicians feel about their work can influence something as clinically significant as whether their patients carry out instructions, and it is the only study of which we are aware to link physicians' job satisfaction with patient actions that are critical to the management of their chronic diseases'[8]. A national physician survey of 2325 doctors showed associations between high job satisfaction and greater control over the workplace, emphasis on quality of care and support for a balance of work and family life. Low job satisfaction was associated with the perception of time pressure and emphasis on productivity. As might be expected, the more stressed a physician was, the less satisfied they were with their job, and the perceived stress correlated with mental and physical health issues. Age, income and number of complex medical or psychosocial patients in a panel did not correlate with job stress or satisfaction[9].

THE SELF-CARE DEFICIT: LITERAL AND FIGURATIVE COSTS

Literal costs of primary care physician turnover range from $236 000 for family practice to $264 345 for pediatrics[10]. Not only do stressed and unsatisfied physicians have higher job turnover and earlier retirement, but they also have more health complaints and file more disability claims[7]. In addition, practitioners' own personal health care may actually play a role in optimizing their care of their patients. One study showed that primary care physicians who had

good personal health habits provided better preventive medicine counseling and screening for their patients. That study reported[11]:

'This is one of the first demonstrations that physicians' personal health habits are more strongly and consistently correlated with related prevention activities than are many other personal and professional variables…If we value disease prevention, and if physicians' personal health practices are consistent predictors of their likelihood to be more active preventionists, we ought to try to cultivate healthy physicians (in undergraduate, graduate education and in CME).'

Another study showed patients health education videotapes about diet and exercise with and without a physician's personal disclosure of her own healthy diet and exercise patterns. Patients in the personal disclosure video group thought the physician was healthier in general, as well as more motivating and more believable regarding diet and exercise[12].

THE PROVIDER AS PATIENT: CARING FOR OUR PHYSICAL WELL-BEING

Even though we counsel patients daily on healthy habits, lifestyles and preventive health care, it can be difficult to take our own advice. 'Physician, heal thyself' may be a wonderful sentiment, but it is clearly not adequate when it comes to routine health-care maintenance for health-care professionals. One study found that 34% of physicians had no personal health-care provider, 28% did not have regular medical care and 7% self-treated. These data correlated with previous studies that found that anywhere from 35 to 56% of physicians did not have their own personal doctor. In comparison, 14–18% of the general population did not have a routine source of care. Younger age was not a factor, as the mean age in the sample was 61 years. However, physician specialty did matter, with pediatricians and psychiatrists more likely to have a regular provider than pathologists, internists and other specialty physicians. As would be expected, those physicians without a regular provider were less likely to have been screened for colon, breast and prostate cancer. Those who believed chance or fate determined their health outcome were twice as likely not to have a regular provider, as were those who believed 'health-related outcomes are under their own control'[13].

In a study that looked at personal health maintenance care in 1983, 44% of physicians and 74% of non-physicians surveyed reported having their own health-care provider. Those who had their own provider 'were twice as likely to believe they should visit a physician regularly for health maintenance and three times as likely to actually visit a physician for health maintenance as those respondents without a personal physician'[14].

THE RISK OF BURNOUT

Psychological well-being plays an equally important role in overall physician health and good patient care. Burnout in health-care providers has been widely studied as one of the most prevalent psychological issues in medicine today. One definition of burnout is a 'state of mental and/or physical exhaustion caused by excessive and prolonged stress'[15]. Christina Maslach, who created the Maslach Burnout Inventory, takes the definition one step further, emphasizing that burnout has three components: emotional exhaustion, depersonalization and decreased personal accomplishment (Tables 4.3 and 4.4)[16].

Certain personality traits in physicians have been identified that may increase the risk of burnout. A total of 440 physicians took the Minnesota Multiphasic Personality Inventory

Table 4.3	Maslach definition of burnout[16]

Emotional exhaustion
Depersonalization
Decreased personal accomplishment

Table 4.4	Contributing factors to burnout[25]

Autonomy/managed care
Ability to impact work environment
Long hours
Workload
Control over time
Juggling personal and professional life

(MMPI) before medical school and were evaluated for burnout symptoms 25 years later. Those with more indicators of low self-esteem, feelings of inadequacy, dysphoria, obsessive worry, social anxiety, passivity and withdrawal from others had higher burnout scores[17].

BURNOUT IN ONCOLOGY

Oncologists and other cancer care providers seem particularly prone to burnout, with 25–50% of oncologists reporting this problem in various studies. Possible reasons include the emotional stress of caring for patients with terminal illness and perhaps inadequate training on conveying bad news and coping with patients' emotional reactions[18]. One Canadian study evaluated the prevalence of burnout in major providers of medical oncology in Ontario. Using the Maslach Burnout Inventory as one of their assessment tools, researchers found that, of the physicians polled, 53% reported high emotional exhaustion and 48% reported feelings of low personal accomplishment. Oncology-allied health professionals also scored high in these two areas, with high emotional exhaustion (37%) and feelings of low personal accomplishment (54%). Over one-third of the providers in each of these groups reported contemplating changing profession, considering jobs other than cancer care[19].

BURNOUT AND PATIENT CARE ISSUES

Burnout in physicians has been linked to suboptimal patient care. Burnout rates among practicing physicians range from 25–60%[20]. Far from being issues when a practitioner is in the prime of his/her career, depression, stress and other burnout criteria start in residency (and probably in medical school, although studies are lacking in this area). When house officers were polled as to their causes of stress, they included components such as 'pressured work context' with large amounts of paperwork, being on call frequently, high morbidity and mortality to deal with and high patient load. Not surprisingly, lack of sleep was reported as the most important factor contributing to elevated stress levels[21]. One poll of 227 housestaff found that 18% of residents had anxiety and depressive symptoms most of the time[22]. In 115 internal medicine residents, 76% had burnout as defined by the Maslach Burnout Inventory. Not only were those who met the burnout criteria more likely to have a positive screening test for depression, they were also more likely to have reported suboptimal patient care in the previous month or week[20].

MEDICAL TRAINING: A SET-UP FOR BURNOUT?

The data show that mental health issues, which contribute to burnout, start very early in postgraduate medical training. Reported rates of clinical depression in interns vary from 27 to 30%. One review of 20 years' worth of prospective studies on this topic found that mental health symptoms, particularly depression, were highest during the first year of training (PGY-1)[23]. One small study of 61 interns highlighted two concerns. One concern was that, at least during the first year of medical postgraduate training, the decrease in mood and increase in personal distress correlated with a decrease in empathetic concern for others as measured by the Profile of Mood States (POMS) and Interpersonal Reactivity Index (IRI) tools. The second concern was that this combined decline started within the first 4 months of internship and did not reverse itself by the time the second year of training began; a continued downward trend was noted[24].

BURNOUT FACTORS IN MEDICAL PRACTICE

When physicians are finished with their training and continue in their practices, the burnout factors and risks continue to be present. The Physician Burnout Project was a study of 454 physicians by the Sacramento Medical Society that sought to quantify burnout statistics as well as identifying the factors most likely to be responsible. The majority of the clinicians reported that they had thought of leaving their profession at least once in the past 12 months. Many said they would not choose medicine as a career again, nor would they want their children to pursue medicine as a profession; 81% reported burnout as a current issue and 76% stated that it was affecting patient satisfaction on a 'medium to high level'. The top six factors felt to be most contributory to burnout were: autonomy/managed care; ability to impact work environment; long hours; workload; control over time; and juggling personal and professional life (Table 4.5)[25].

Table 4.5 Contributing factors to provider 'discontent'[25,28]

Burnout factors

Sleep deprivation

Delayed gratification

Difficulty setting appropriate limits

Culture of medicine rewards long hours and 'workaholism'

Difficulty asking for help

Stressful practice environment

Time pressures

Financial reimbursement issues

Weakness and vulnerability unacceptable in medical culture

THE COSTS OF BURNOUT, STRESS AND DEPRESSION

Suicide

Given the information on burnout, depression and stress for physicians, it is not surprising that suicide rates for physicians have always been higher than those for the general population. However, the data to identify these rates continue to be difficult to compile, resulting in older research results. One of the more recent estimates is from a 1990 study that showed that physicians have 2.3 times the risk of death by suicide compared to the general population[26]. The overall suicide rate in physicians is estimated to be between 28 and 40 per 100 000 compared to the general population statistic of 12.3 per 100 000. There does not seem to be a difference across specialties, although there is a striking gender difference: female physicians have suicide rates that are four times higher than those of the general female population. In the Women Physicians' Health Study, 19.5% of female physicians reported a history of depression with 1.5% reporting suicide attempts[27]. Social isolation may play a role, as being in a relationship seems to be protective. Physicians who never married or are divorced or widowed have higher suicide rates. Housestaff, probably due to the rates of anxiety, depression and burnout, are also susceptible: 25% of interns have been reported to have suicidal ideation[28]. In a 1980–88 study, suicide was found to be the most common cause of death in young physicians, accounting for 26% of deaths[29].

Drug and alcohol abuse

Abuse of drugs and alcohol is another way in which stress, burnout and depression may manifest. Although physicians do not have an increased prevalence of drug or alcohol abuse compared to the rest of the population, they do have an increased risk of prescription drug abuse[30]. Overall 10–14% of physicians may become addicted to drugs or alcohol during their career; this number decreases to 1–2% when drug addiction alone is considered. Anesthesiology may have the highest incidence of chemical dependence; in one study of anesthesiology training programs, fentanyl was the most common drug abused. Of particular concern, highlighted in the study, was the fact that 18% of individuals died or almost died before substance abuse was even suspected[31]. Nationally, the concern about physician wellness, including substance abuse, alcoholism, physical and mental health, have manifested in state-by-state programs available for confidential health-care provider access. The Federation of State Physician Health Programs (www.fsphp.org) has a list by state of the physician health programs that provide confidential consultation and support to assist health-care providers with a variety of health issues such as the above.

Impact on relationships

Although the issues of substance abuse, depression, suicide and burnout are more acute manifestations of 'dis-ease' in medical practice today, the lack of psychological well-being on interpersonal relationships cannot be overstated. In the medical field, this has often been looked at in the context of marital breakups. There is controversy over whether or not divorce rates among physicians are higher or lower than those among the general population. The National Center for Health Statistics reported from data published in 1996 that, in the general population, 43% of first marriages ended with separation or divorce within 15 years[32]. However, some researchers have estimated divorce rates among physicians to be 10–20% higher than these general statistics[33]. A 1997 study from Johns Hopkins showed a cumulative incidence of divorce of 29% after 30 years of marriage, and found that physician specialty played a role in divorce rates. Cumulative divorce incidence was highest for psychiatrists (50%) followed by surgeons (33%) and 'other' specialties (31%). For internists, pediatricians and pathologists, the incidence ranged from 22 to 24%. Longer work hours, ability to 'displace' issues within the relationship onto outside factors, and personality characteristics that draw physicians to certain specialties were possible explanations. Female physicians had a higher risk of divorce (37%) than their male counterparts (28%). Physicians who had higher levels of anger (as measured by the Habits of Nervous Tension Questionnaire) and those who reported lack of emotional closeness to parents had higher divorce incidence. Interestingly, depression and anxiety were not associated with increased divorce rates, although these and other personality characteristics may not have been adequately assessed[34].

THE ROLE OF 'MEDICAL CULTURE'

Clearly, there is much work to be done in the realm of professional and personal wellness for health-care providers if these studies are any indication. Apart from the stressors in the medical practice environment, there are probably even more subtle factors that contribute to 'provider discontent'. It may be that the health-care profession and training as a whole draws out certain personality facets, such as perfectionism and competitiveness. These traits as well as others may be needed for survival in the 'culture of medicine' in which physicians and other health-care providers-to-be are indoctrinated.

For example, sleep deprivation, which is part of the culture of medical training, can promote cognitive impairment and emotional fragility-staying awake for 24 hours has been found to affect cognitive psychomotor performance as much as having a blood alcohol level of 0.1% (0.08% is the drunk driving limit in most states)[28,35]. One recent study compared medical errors made by interns on a traditional 'every third night' call schedule (up to 34 continuous hours of work) compared to the interns on an 'intervention schedule' where the total amount of consecutive hours worked was approximately 16. When the two groups were compared, the traditional schedule group had 36% more serious medical errors than the intervention schedule group. During the traditional schedule, the total rate of serious errors in the critical care units was 22% higher. There were also 5.6 times more diagnostic errors made and 21% more serious medication errors made in the traditional versus intervention schedule group[36]. Another study showed that, with a similar intervention schedule, attentional failures decreased by more than half[37].

Despite studies like these, medical culture continues to support a practitioner's ability to deny one's own needs (both physical and psychological). In addition, the culture of medicine usually requires delayed gratification (whether subjectively through long training programs or literally through incurred debt), and promotes the inability to set appropriate limits, rewarding long hours and 'workaholic' tendencies.

Revealing weakness and vulnerabilities to others is often felt to be unacceptable, and defense mechanisms are created that make it difficult to ask for help when needed[28].

NAVIGATING THE LABYRINTH: GOING FOR WHOLENESS

When the issues inherent in medical culture are combined with less subtle factors, including medical practice environment, time constraints and financial reimbursement problems, a complex web emerges. Navigating this labyrinth in a way that honors the healer's needs as much as the patients' is a difficult but worthwhile struggle toward wholeness. Rachel Naomi Remen[38] invites us to look beyond the everyday difficulties in medical practice for internal sustenance:

'Part of our responsibility as professionals is to fight for our sense of meaning – against fatigue, numbness, overwork and unreasonable expectations – to find ways to strengthen it in ourselves and in each other…It has become vital to remember the essential nature of this work and renew our sense of calling to preserve the meaning of the work for ourselves and for those who will follow.'

It may well be, as the Association for Healing Healthcare Projects' motto states, that, as we heal ourselves, we in turn heal our relationships and our communities[39]. As each provider commits to their own healing and wellness in mind, body, spirit and relationship, the choices and changes created extend beyond the individual into the larger domain of their medical practice and community circles. Renewing our sense of calling and meaning in medicine may require, at the very core level, focusing attention on ourselves by exploring our own self-care in these areas. As the studies show, both our patients and we benefit on a personal and professional level from this work (Table 4.6).

THE CHALLENGE OF WELLNESS

Given the data, few would argue with the need for physician self-care as an integral part of professional practice. However, there are countless

Table 4.6   Benefits of provider wellness

When physicians are 'professionally satisfied' in their work, they provide better quality of care and produce more patient satisfaction[7]

Physicians who had good personal health habits provided better preventative medicine counseling and screenings for their patients[11]

The happier a physician is in their job, the more satisfied their patients[7,8]

When a physician gives positive verbal support, patients adhere better to their treatment plans and medication schedules[8]

Patients receive better care when physicians are not feeling depressed or burned out[20,25]

Satisfied and less stressed physicians have less job turnover, less health complaints and less disability claims[7]

Physicians who share or model their own health practices are more motivating and more believable to their patients regarding diet and exercise[12]

barriers. Health-care providers by definition are busy – it is the nature of the job. There are financial pressures and time management issues, further complicating caring for ourselves and working on our own wellness, yet our own personal well-being is essential. Zeev Neuwirth, an Assistant Professor of Medicine at Tufts University who writes about physician well-being and the doctor–patient relationship, sums up this need clearly: 'If we are physically, emotionally and spiritually exhausted, it is unlikely that we will be able to provide the type of medical care and healing that our patients want and need'[40].

The Institute of Medicine, in the report *Improving Medical Education: Enhancing the Behavioral and Social Science Content of Medical School Curricula*[41], emphasizes the integral nature of emotion, behavior, social and psychological factors in health:

'Although the scientific evidence linking biological, behavioral, psychological, and social variables to health, illness and disease is impressive, the translation and incorporation of this knowledge into standard medical practice appear to have been less than successful. To make measurable improvements in the health of Americans, physicians must be equipped with the knowledge and skills from the behavioral and social sciences needed to recognize, understand, and effectively respond to patients as individuals, not just to their symptoms…'

Obviously, the medical environment's 15-minute office visit is not set up to be able to incorporate behavioral and social medicine into patient care effectively. How do we teach and incorporate these biopsychosocial factors into our practices and medical school curricula when we are stuck between a rock and a hard place? In addition, how do we teach that which we struggle with in our own lives to our patients and students?

WORKING WITH THE IMPOSSIBLE

Once we acknowledge the impossible, whether that is the medical system we work in, the financial strain, the tight schedule, the overwork, or the myriad of other issues that abound in the medical culture, we may choose to act. The system may be on the verge of collapse, but that does not mean that we need to be. It does mean that we need the best parts of ourselves – the creative, compassionate, flexible, caring, determined parts – to create ways to circumvent the impossible. Perhaps one place to start is the cultivation of compassion for ourselves. It takes a different sort of discipline and focus to create a healthy lifestyle as a health-care provider immersed in the culture of medicine today. It requires caring for ourselves as much as we care for our patients. Cultivating the ability to see beyond the challenges and impossibilities may create exciting possibilities.

THE TRANSFORMATION OF 'SICKCARE' INTO HEALTH CARE: A CALL TO ACTION

There are many groups that are actively working on wellness issues from the perspective of transforming the health-care environment. One working group, in addressing these issues, created a list of guidelines entitled 'Principles to Transform Healthcare'. These principles, which follow, are described as being '…a distillation of the wisdom of the many members of the Association of Healing Health Care Projects and the Relationship-Centered Care Network [Fetzer Institute]'[42]:

(1) Create caring relationships. Acknowledge the importance of self-awareness, self-care, and self-growth. Beginning with self, establish an ethic of love, forgiveness, unconditional positive regard, and service; then extend this ethic as the core of all

relationships in health care. Develop these relationships to sustain health of self, patients, heath care team, organization, community, and environment.

(2) Respect each person's experience as valid. Respect the practice of relationship-centered care and healing health care in all its unique representations, without bias toward or against any religion, race, sex, position or rank, community, or culture. All change toward creating health and healing is valued, great or small.

(3) Respect the person's own power and self-healing processes. Place control with the person receiving the care. Appreciate the patient's meaning of the health–illness condition, and base care on his or her needs and values.

(4) Value and practice personal responsibility for health, intentions, and actions. Individual lifestyle choices, actions, and practices largely determine the outcome of health. Provide information to support the person/patient in being an informed decision-maker.

(5) Honor the sacred. Pay attention to and respect the most precious aspects of each person and place. Respect the person's dignity, uniqueness, and integrity (mind–body–spirit unity). Create sanctuary – space and time to reconnect with wholeness and something greater than oneself. Honor the ancient as well as the visionary.

(6) Hold economic models responsible and accountable to the outcome of health. Acknowledge and attend to the relationship between wise use of economic resources and health.

(7) Adopt an attitude and practice of continuous learning and improvement. Challenge ideas; remain open-minded and receptive to innovation and experimentation; respond to the changing environment with unchanging commitment to these principles.

(8) Connect with others. Build and sustain conscious connections/partnerships with other individuals and groups who share this intention for transforming health care.

(9) Create a compelling vision that is inclusive of all providers and citizens. Respect the integrity of the community, and participate actively in community development and dialogue. A sustained intention with action for the well-being of others endures all obstacles.

(10) Start now, act locally, keep going, and support each other. Many local actions are global action – the transformation of health care.

These principles reflect similar visions of health and well-being that have been proposed in the past by many authors. In 1978, Dale Garell proposed a similar construct for physicians' optimal well-being[43], asking: 'Can we learn a way of life that not only minimizes the "risk" of being a physician, but also maximizes the opportunity to provide the highest quality of medical care while at the same time encouraging our own satisfaction and professional and personal development?'

CONNECTING WITH SELF: THE FIRST STEP

These principles are a call to action. Instead of their being 'one more thing on our plates' to accomplish externally, they compel us to start with introspection and honest self-evaluation, honoring the fact that the individual is at the heart of change (Table 4.7). There may be many areas that lack attention; choosing where to start may be as simple as asking one's self: 'What would nurture me the most? What would allow me to grow personally and professionally? What would help me to sustain the day-to-day challenges and to connect with my work's meaning?'

Zeev Neuwirth uses the following questions as a way to further this introspection, emphasizing the need to re-evaluate 'our personal philosophies toward medicine and healing': 'How do I define health and healing? How do my behaviors and relationships reflect and represent those values? What values would I want my patients and colleagues to recognize in my behaviors? What might I do to increase the likelihood of those values being expressed?'[40]

Starting with one's own personal philosophy and beliefs may be ideal, but since wellness spans multiple realms (physical, spiritual, emotional, interprofessional/institutional and interpersonal), the starting place will be highly individual. In a medical culture that repeatedly taught us to put others' needs before our own, it takes a special kind of discipline and compassion to reconnect with ourselves. The most important action may be just to start in whatever area seems most appropriate at the time, realizing that once 'human being' starts occurring in one realm of wellness, it will catalyze changes in other areas too.

PROVIDERS' WELLNESS PRACTICES: WHAT WE KNOW

Just as Remen emphasizes remembering our connection and our calling to practice medicine as a way to sustain ourselves[38], other researchers and authors have identified certain individual practices that physicians carry out in order to create optimal well-being.

One study, looking at predictors of psychological well-being among physicians, found that a high level of support from the practitioner's closest relationship, lower levels of practice stress and the ability to maintain one's individual identity around family members were the most

relevant factors[44]. This group of authors questioned why there is so much information about physician impairment but so little information on positive practices that physicians incorporate to improve their well-being. Their later study, which qualitatively assessed physicians' wellness-promotion practices, found that responses clustered into five primary areas. The first was relationships, including involvement with community, family, friends and colleagues. The second was religion or spirituality, participating in church activities, attending services, praying or reading the Bible. The third was self-care, including various self-care actions such as taking vacation, exercising, meditating, having a hobby, being nutritionally mindful, avoiding drugs and alcohol, obtaining counseling and treatment for depression, and leaving unhealthy relationships. The fourth was work practices, including creating meaning and satisfaction from work, limiting practice or choosing a certain type of medical practice. The fifth was philosophical approaches, ranging from concentrating on success and being positive to creating and maintaining balance in one's life (Table 4.8)[45].

THE POWER OF PERSONAL NARRATIVE

Another study used a narrative approach to see what experiences in physician's practices increased their sense of meaning and the purpose of their work. Researchers identified common themes in narrative analyses of physicians' stories written during 'Meaningful Experiences in Medicine' workshops. Three major themes emerged when stories were analyzed for commonalities in providers' professional experiences: a difference the provider made in someone's life, a connection made with a patient and a change in the provider's perspective[46]. A daily practice that health-care providers might use as a way to

Table 4.7 Questions for professional growth[40,47]
How do I define health and healing?
What values would I want my patients and colleagues to recognize in [me]?
What would allow me to grow personally and professionally?
What would help me to sustain the day-to-day challenges and connect with my work's meaning?
What surprised me today?
What moved/touched me today?
What inspired me today?

Table 4.8 Wellness promotion practices[45]
Relationship   involvement with friends, family, community and colleagues
Spiritual or religious activities   participation in church activities, attending services, praying
Self-care   vacation, exercise, counseling, hobbies, eating nutritious food, avoiding drugs/alcohol
Work practices   creating meaning/satisfaction in work, limiting practice, choosing certain type of practice
Philosphical approaches   concentrating on success, being positive, maintaining balance in one's life

connect with their own meaningful work experiences is highlighted by Remen in one story from her book, *My Grandfather's Blessings*[47]. Three questions may be used as a journaling tool, as in the story, or simply as a personal ritual for daily meditation or reflection: 'What surprised me today? What moved or touched me today? What inspired me today?'

THE 'BIG PICTURE': USE OF SPIRITUALITY FOR HEALING AND RENEWAL

There is much literature on the impact of spirituality, religion and prayer on medical conditions and outcomes. Spirituality and religion are two distinct concepts; one definition of spirituality that highlights the difference between the two is:

'Religion organizes the collective spiritual experiences of a group of people into a system of beliefs and practices…Spirituality is a broader concept than religion and is primarily a dynamic, personal, and experiential process. Features of spirituality include quest for meaning and purpose, transcendence

(the sense that being human is more than simple material existence), connectedness (e.g. with others, nature, or the divine), and values (e.g. love, compassion, and justice).[48]

Religious practices and health benefits

Studies have shown that patients who are involved in religious activities live longer, have less cardiovascular disease and hypertension, have less risk of depression, anxiety, substance abuse and suicide and have better coping skills with illness[48]. One study found that prayer was identified as a coping strategy in 84% of cancer patients[49]. Although physicians struggle with how and when (and even whether it is appropriate) to include a discussion of spirituality in medical care, a Newsweek poll showed that 72% of Americans said they would welcome a conversation with their physician about faith[50]. Especially in end-of-life care in oncology, there is need for further research to address the impact of spirituality.[51]

SPIRITUAL WELLNESS: A LIGHT IN THE DARKNESS

Spirituality may be good medicine for patients and providers. The practitioner's spiritual wellness can play a particularly supportive role in self-care, especially because of the stressors inherent in communicating bad news and working with terminally ill and dying patients. One group of researchers describes the darkness of oncology practice this way:

> 'Oncologists are confronted daily with transcendence, suffering, uncertainty and mortality. These forces occasionally create moments of epiphany that help us redefine our values and purpose. More often, they make life seem meaningless and bewildering. Mistakenly, physicians often feel alone with these challenges and struggle in silence and isolation. This solitude limits opportunities to connect with colleagues and gain insight from the experience of others.'[18]

Practitioners face their own emotions of grief, loss and pain daily, in addition to being the 'bearer of bad news', being witness to suffering, and dealing with patients' and families' emotions and reactions. Having a 'spiritual outlet', in addition to other wellness practices, may be a way to cope constructively and thrive in the midst of these intense life experiences. In addition, spirituality can strengthen connection to a 'higher power', to self and to others. Identifying transcendent experiences (ones that extend beyond the usual limits of ordinary experience) with patients and families can provide a different and vastly larger context and viewpoint for daily work and life. For some providers, this may be a personally fulfilling way to move beyond the silence and isolation described by the researchers above. It can also serve as a way for practitioners to cope with their own grieving, pain and loss.

Without a larger context for their work, clinicians can become hardened and callous, clinical and brusque. Not only is this painful to the practitioner, it can be devastating to the patient and family when empathic care is required. For example, one patient's oncologist came into his room, stood in front of friends and family, and told the patient that he had unresectable pancreatic cancer with metasteses, that he should get his affairs in order, and that chemotherapy was not effective for treating his cancer. The oncologist left the room quickly, leaving a stunned patient and very angry onlookers. Another patient was told of her unresectable adenocarcinoma by phone.

Clearly, these are not examples of patient-centered, relationship-centered care, but they do highlight some of the more dramatic ways providers' stress, burnout, grief and loss may impact patient care. Spirituality can increase our sense of connectedness, meaning, purpose and transcendence, and be another way of promoting our own healing. In addition, more training in compassionate care may be useful. The National Cancer Institute is funding an OncoTalk retreat program for oncology fellows to learn effective and empathic communication skills for patients and families especially during the transition from curative to palliative care – see www.depts. washington.edu/oncotalk/program.html for more information.

Spiritual self-inquiry

Cultivating spiritual wellness is intensely personal. One medical model for inquiring about patients' spirituality, the HOPE Questions, can be used as a starting point for providers' self-inquiry as well. The first step (H) is to assess basic spiritual resources, and identify sources of hope, meaning, comfort, strength, peace, love and connection. The second and third steps (O and P) identify any use of organized religion and/or personal spirituality and practices. The fourth step (E), in patients is used to assess the effects of personal spirituality and practices on their medical care and end-of-life issues.[52] For practitioners, the fourth step could be used in a variety of ways, from inquiry into how spirituality might be an asset in their clinical care to how it could be used personally as a source of connection and renewal.

Spirituality and healing versus curing

Remen describes the essence of the spiritual realm in the following way:

> '...the spiritual is inclusive. It is the deepest sense of belonging and participation. We all participate in the spiritual at all times, whether we know it or not...The most important thing in defining spirit is the recognition that the spirit is an essential need of human nature. There is something in all of us that seeks the spiritual. This yearning varies in strength from person to person but it is always there in everyone. And so, healing becomes possible...[53]

When a clinician is able to hold the larger viewpoint and context that spirituality provides, the concept of healing versus curing emerges. There may be many rich opportunities to be present and to be of service to a 'non-curable' patient in ways that facilitate healing, whether that is coming to terms with illness, family dynamics, financial concerns, the dying process, or other issues. This can be healing to practitioner and patient alike.

Psychosocial support for the provider

As the stories above illustrate, the impact of unexplored physician/provider emotions as well as the balance of emotional give-and-take between provider and patient can have ramifications on both patient care and practitioner well-being[54]. Certainly with the high rates of burnout, oncology providers need to pay particular attention to their own psychological and emotional well-being. There are many ways in which providers can care for themselves in this important area; for some practitioners, this may be the most important area of wellness in which to start.

Balint groups

One study showed that incorporating psychosocial support, in the form of a Balint group (an interactive provider-led group usually focusing on doctor–patient interactions) in one hematology–oncology training program, improved fellows' comfort level in dealing with emotional clinical situations with patients and improved the fellow's view of him/herself as a physician[55].

Personal emotion work: a medical model

Another method advocates using a medical model, with a clinically oriented multi-step process created for 'detecting and working with physicians' personal emotions'. The first step is to assess clinical situation risk factors that may be unbalancing the emotional give-and-take in the physician–patient relationship and may be affecting patient care. This ranges from the physician's having a long-standing relationship or identifying with the patient to time pressures and uncertainty about medical care goals. The second and third steps are to identify behaviors and feelings of emotion, and to keep in mind that emotional responses and reactions are normal parts of the professional practice of medicine. The fourth step involves reflecting on the emotion as a way of 'stepping back' and looking at one's potential behavioral responses. A useful part of this fourth step is to 'consult a trusted professional colleague' for further reflection and feedback.[54]

BREAKING THE SILENCE: CONNECTING WITH OTHER PROVIDERS

Sharing difficult professional experiences with another colleague may seem at first to be extremely difficult because of the medical culture in which we are immersed. Sharing a difficult situation and asking for help may be seen as revealing personal and professional weakness. It is important to transcend this barrier, to realize that this is one of the biggest façades in medicine, and to realize that the culture will only change as much as individual providers are willing to risk connecting with each other. Thankfully, there are now many formal and informal programs supporting this connection.

Residential retreat programs

Residential retreats for physicians to reconnect with the meaning of their work are available through several sources. The Institute for the Study of Health and Healing (ISHI) and Many Streams Healing Systems (MSHS) offer two excellent examples. In these workshops, physicians can connect on a deeper level with colleagues, reconnect with their original desire to become doctors, experience health-promoting modalities and learn new self-care skills. Continuing medical education (CME) credits are available. Other organizations offer workshops and retreats for a wider range of healthcare providers, such as Harmony Hill – see www.harmonyhill.org/retreats/healthprof.html.

Example of a formal program: Schwartz Center Rounds

One formal program often used in oncology is the Schwartz Center Rounds, which is independent of medical or ethics rounds. Now implemented in a variety of medical environments from academic centers to outpatient settings, the

Rounds were developed as a way to promote compassionate care and sharing between providers. 'The Rounds…offer caregivers a safe, open and relaxed place where they can share their concerns and fears, both for their patients and themselves. The premise is that caregivers are better able to make a personal connection with patients when they have greater awareness of and insight into their own responses and feelings'[56] Two excellent Rounds on 'Breaking Bad News' and 'Burnout' are published in transcript form in the journal *The Oncologist*, and emphasize the power of provider–provider interaction and sharing about these difficult topics[57,58].

Informal program examples: Finding Meaning in Medicine®, and Doctoring to Heal

Informal programs are usually held outside the hospital environment, and convened by a group of interested physicians. Two examples of this type of program are Finding Meaning in Medicine and Doctoring to Heal. Finding Meaning in Medicine is a physician outreach program started by Rachael Naomi Remen and the Institute for the Study of Health and Illness (ISHI). Able to be easily started by any interested clinician with support materials available from ISHI (www.commonweal.org/ishi), this program revolves around story-telling, sharing and reflection on a set topic. Doctoring to Heal, started by Michael Rabow and Stephen McPhee in 1996, is another easily established personal reflection program where providers' written narratives about clinical experiences around a set topic are shared and discussed. Practitioners who have participated in the Doctoring to Heal program report a strengthening of their personal and professional identity, improved connectedness with their colleagues, gleaning of useful techniques for their practice from others' experiences, and improved balance and well-being (Table 4.9)[59].

Table 4.9	Programs/activities to enhance personal wellness

Relationship-Centered Care Network   www.fetzer.org/rcc

Kenneth B. Schwartz Center (Schwartz Center Rounds)   http://www.theschwartzcenter.org/rounds.asp

Doctoring to Heal Program – see *West J Med* 2001; 174: 68–9.

OncoTalk Retreat Program for Oncology Fellows   www.depts.washington.edu/oncotalk/program.html

Balint Groups   http://www.balint.co.uk/groups.html

Institute for the Study of Health and Healing (ISHI)   www.commonweal.org/ishi

Finding Meaning in Medicine Physician Groups   www.meaninginmedicine.org

Many Streams Healing Systems   http://www.manystreamsheal.org/html/media.html

The Association of Healing Healthcare Projects   http://www.healinghealthcareassoc.org/

Harmony Hill retreats for healthcare providers   www.harmonyhill.org/retreats/healthprof.html

Western Journal of Medicine 2001; 174 January issue – dedicated to physician well-being

American Academy on Physician and Patient   http://www.physicianpatient.org/

The Federation of State Physician Health Programs (www.fsphp.org) – confidential consultation and support for a variety of health issues

Women in medicine: stresses and solutions – excellent article for women physicians – see *Western Journal of Medicine* 2001; 174: January issue

AN INVITATION

Personal wellness is essential for providing excellent patient care, especially in oncology. How a practitioner's self-care evolves is very personal, and may include emotional and spiritual aspects in addition to attention to physical well-being, and interpersonal relationships. When providers work together to create interprofessional and institutional support for well-being, the possibility emerges for the entire medical system to change.

As our 5 weeks of 'The Healer's Art' course comes to a close, the medical students participate in the last session, entitled 'The Care of the Soul'. We talk about medicine as a calling, the power of service and possibility for a sense of mission in the work. The students write their own version of the Hippocratic Oath, as a reflection of the following questions: 'If your work were simply an opportunity for you to express your highest values in the world, what would your work look like? Ask for help in bringing this dream of service closer to your everyday work life. Ask for help for what you would like to be able to do or be, for whatever needs to change in yourself, for what you want to do differently…'[60]

One fourth-year student's work eloquently describes his desire for self-care and professional well-being:

May I always remember that my patients are people with full and rich lives no matter where they come from, and that they are people deserving of my care.

May I never become burnt-out as a physician because of my desire to earn more money, see more patients, practice as if on an assembly line, or because I've lost my empathy.

May I at least try and care for people as I would my own loved ones, particularly my wife and family.

73

May I never sacrifice too much time with my children for the sake of my career.

May I always be able to laugh a little and lighten up especially when life is difficult.

Allow me to take better care of myself and to remember that it will make me a better doctor, not a selfish person.

Allow me to create a practice where I'm fulfilled and which serves my need to ask questions, ponder difficult cases, get to know my patients and which is family-friendly.

May I seek out more mindfulness and compassion in all that I do.[61]

As we continue the work outwardly, treating patients and families, keeping abreast of the latest medical developments and treatments, and finding ways to continue providing excellent care within the financial constraints of an ailing health-care system, we must also remember to turn inward. Now more than ever, learning how to sustain and nurture ourselves in the escalating demands of medical practice is a requirement, not a privilege or selfish act. Practitioners, patients and the health-care system will all benefit from providers' investment in self-care.

References

1. The Healer's Art – Resource Guide. ©Rachael Naomi Remen, MD, 2002
2. Definition of Integrative Medicine. ©Program in Integrative Medicine, University of Arizona, 2003
3. Definition of relationship-centered care from www.fetzer.org/rcc, accessed 1 July, 2004
4. Arizona State University Wellness Definition. ©Arizona Board of Regents, 2000
5. Preamble to the Constitution of the World Health Organization as adopted by the International Health Conference, New York, 19–22 June, 1946; signed on 22 July 1946 by the representatives of 61 States (Official Records of the World Health Organization, no. 2, p.100) and entered into force on 7 April 1948
6. Ardell DB, Langdon JG. Wellness: The Body, Mind and Spirit. Dubuque, Iowa: Kendall/Hunt Publishing Company, 1989
7. Haas JS. Physician discontent: a barometer of change and need for intervention. J Gen Intern Med 2001; 16: 496–7
8. DiMatteo MR, Shelbourne RD, Hays L, et al. Physicians' characteristics influence patients' adherence to medical treatment: results from the Medical Outcomes Study. Health Psychology 1993; 12: 100
9. Williams ES, Konrad TR, Linzer M, et al. SGIM Career Satisfaction Study Group. Health Serv Res 2002; 37: 121–43
10. Buchbinder SB, Wilson M, Melick CF, et al. Estimates of costs of primary care physician turnover. Am J Manage Care 1999; 5: 1431–8
11. Frank E, Rothenberg R, Lewis C, Belodoff B. Correlates of physicians' prevention-related practices. Arch Fam Med 2000; 9: 359–67
12. Frank E, Breyan J, Elon L. Physician disclosure of healthy personal behaviors improves credibility and ability to motivate. Arch Fam Med 2000; 9: 287–90
13. Gross CP, Mead LA, Ford DE, et al. Physician, heal thyself? Regular source of care and use of preventive health services among physicians. Arch Int Med 2000; 160: 3212
14. Kahn KL, Goldberg RJ, DeCosimo D, et al. Health maintenance activities of physicians and nonphysicians. Arch Intern Med 1988; 148: 2433–6

15. Definition from Girdino DA, Everly GS, Dusek DE. Controlling Stress and Tension. Needham Heights, MA: Allyn & Bacon, 1996, accessed from www.texmed.org/cme/phn/psb/burnout.asp on 1 July, 2004

16. Maslach C, Jackson SE. Maslach Burnout Inventory – Manual, 2nd edn. Palo Alto, CA: CPP/Consulting Psychologists Press, 1986

17. McCranie EW, Brandsma JM. Personality antecedents of burnout among middle-aged physicians. Behav Med 1988; 14: 30–6

18. Shanafelt T, Adjei A, Meyskens FL. When your favorite patient relapses: physician grief and well-being in the practice of oncology. J Clin Oncol 2003; 21: 2617

19. Grunfeld E, Whelan TJ, Zitzelsberger L, et al. Cancer care workers in Ontario: prevalence of burnout, job stress and job satisfaction. J Can Med Assoc 2000; 163: 166–9

20. Shanafeldt TD, Bradley KA, Wipf JE, et al. Burnout and self-reported patient care in an internal medicine residency program. Ann Intern Med 2002; 136: 358–67

21. Schwartz AJ, Black ER, Goldstein MG, et al. Levels and causes of stress among residents. J Med Educ 1987; 62: 744–53

22. Hendrie HP, Claire DK, Brittain HM, et al. A study of anxiety/depressive symptoms of medical students, housestaff and their spouses/partners. J Nerv Ment Dis 1990; 178: 204–7

23. Tyssen R, Vaglum, P. Mental health problems in young doctors: an updated review of prospective studies. Harvard Rev Psychiatry 2002; 10: 154–65

24. Bellini LM, Baime M, Shea JA. Variation of mood and empathy in internship. JAMA 2002; 287: 3143–6

25. Snider M, Svenko D. The Physician Burnout Project. Sacramento, CA. El Dorado-Sacramento Medical Society, January 1997

26. Stack S. Occupation and Suicide. Soc Sci Quarterly June 2001; 82: 392

27. Frank E. The Women Physicians' Health Study: Background, Objectives and Methods. JAMWA 1995; 50: 64–6

28. Miller MN, McGowen KR, Quillen JH. The painful truth: physicians are not invincible. Southern Med J 2000;93:966–73

29. Samkoff JS, Hockenberry S, Simon LJ, et al. Mortality of young physicians in the United States, 1980-1988. Acad Med 1995; 70: 242–4

30. O'Conner PG, Spickard A. Physician impairment by substance abuse. Med Clin North Am 1997; 81: 1037–52

31. Booth JV, Grossman D, Moore J, et al. Substance abuse among physicians: a survey of academic anesthesiology programs. Anesth Analg 2002; 95: 1024–30

32. Kreider RM, Fields JM. Number, timing and duration of marriages and divorce: 1996. US Census Bureau Current Population Reports, February 2002: 18

33. Sotile WM, Sotile MO. The Medical Marriage: A Couple's Survival Guide. New York, Carol Publishing, 1996

34. Rollman BL, Mead LA, Wang N, et al. Medical specialty and the incidence of divorce. N Engl J Med 1997; 336: 800–3

35. Dawson D, Reid, K. Fatigue, alcohol and performance impairment. Nature 1997; 388: 235

36. Landrigan CP, Rothschild JM, Cronin JW, et al. Effect of reducing interns' work hours on serious medical errors in intensive care units. N Engl J Med 2004; 351: 1838–48

37. Lockley SW, Cronin JW, Evans EE, et al. Effect of reducing interns' weekly work hours on sleep and attentional failures. N Engl J Med 2004; 351: 1829–37

38. Remen RN. Recapturing the soul of medicine. West J Med 2001; 174: 4–5

39. The Association of Healing Healthcare Projects. Accessed from www.healinghealthcareassoc.org 27 July, 2004

40. Neuwirth ZE. Reclaiming the lost meanings of medicine. Med J Aust January 2002; 176: 78

41. Improving Medical Education: Enhancing the Behavioral and Social Science Content of Medical School Curricula ©2004, 2001. The National Academy of Sciences. Accessed from http:www.nap.edu/openbook/030909142X/html/16.html on August 13, 2004

42. From Impasse to Breakthrough: A National Summit: 'Principles to Transform Health Care: Healing Health Care and Relationship-Centered Care'. Accessed from http://www.breakthroughsummit.org/principles.cfm August 13, 2004

43. Garell DC. Some reflections on physicians' well-being. New Physician 1978; 27: 32–3

44. Weiner EL, Swain GR, Gottlieb M. Predictors of psychological well-being among physicians. Fam Syst Health 1998; 16: 419–30

45. Weiner EL, Swain GR, Gottlieb M. A qualitative study of physicians' own wellness-promotion practices. West J Med 2001; 174: 19–23

46. Horowitz CR, Suchman AL, Branch Jr., WT et al. What do doctors find meaningful about their work? Ann Int Med 2003; 138: 772–5

47. Remen, RN. My Grandfather's Blessings: Stories of Strength, Refuge and Belonging. New York: Riverhead Books, 2000: 116–19

48. Mueller PS, Plevak DJ, Rummans TA. Religious involvement, spirituality, and medicine: implications for clinical practice. Mayo Clin Proc 2001; 76: 1225–35

49. Sodestrom KE, Martinson IM. Patients' spiritual coping strategies: a study of nurse and patient perspectives. Oncol Nurs Forum 1987; 14: 41–6

50. Kalb C. 'Faith and Healing' Newsweek 2003 10 November. Accessed from http://msnbc.msn.com/id/3339654/site/newsweek/ on 27 September, 2004

51. 'ASCO Releases Position Statement on End-Of-Life Care.' News Bulletin in The Oncologist, 1998; 3: 204–5

52. Anandarajah G, Hight E. Spirituality and medical practice: using the HOPE questions as a practical tool for spiritual assessment. AFP 2001; 63: 86

53. Remen RN. On defining spirit. Noetic Sciences Review Winter 1998; 47: 64. Accessed from http://www.noetic.org/publications/review/issue47/r47_Remen%20.html on 28 September, 2004

54. Meier DE, Back AL, Morrison RS. The inner life of physicians and care of the seriously ill. JAMA 2001; 286: 3007–14

55. Sekeres MA, Chernoff M, Lynch TJ Jr, et al. The impact of a physician awareness group and the first year of training on hematology-oncology fellows. J Clin Onc 2003; 21: 3676–82

56. The Kenneth B. Schwartz Center. Accessed from http://www.theschwartzcenter.org/rounds.asp on 24 September, 2004

57. Penson RT, Dignan FL, Canellos GP, et al. Burnout: caring for the caregiver. Oncologist 2000; 5: 425–34

58. Dias L, Chabner BA, Lynch TJ, et al. Breaking bad news: a patient's perspective. Oncologist 2003; 8: 587–96

59. Rabow MW, McPhee SJ. Doctoring to heal: fostering well-being among physicians through personal reflection. West J Med 2001; 174: 68–9

60. The Healer's Art – Resource Guide. ©Rachel Naomi Remen, MD, 2004, page 69

61. Used with permission from Stephen Turner, MS 4, University of Virginia School of Medicine

5

Models of care

Judith Boyce

HIPPOCRATES MEETS THE MEDICINE WHEEL

'Above All, Do No Harm

I swear by Mother Earth, Father Sky, Powers of the Four Directions, and All My Ancestors to uphold this Oath.

I will take the time to listen without judgment and to ask the right questions.

I make peace with the fact that there will be challenging patients, and I will see them through fresh eyes at each visit.

I pledge to remain firm in my commitment to honor my patients' right to choice, and will partner in decision-making in their efforts to find optimum health, regardless of diagnosis or prognosis.

I will learn from past experience and teachers, and pass on what I have learned to future practitioners.

I will incorporate healing silence into my practice.

I say yes! to listening to Spirit and to practicing with Heart.

I will seek and store wisdom by participating in research and evaluating my practice.

I vow to do my part to protect The Earth, the children, and the children's children until the sun no longer sets and the moon no longer rises'. – Aho

Judith Boyce MD

(Adapted from the Native American Medicine Wheel as taught by Reverend Rosalyn Bruyere, Arizona, April 2003)

INTRODUCTION

This revision of the Hippocratic Oath evolved during an exercise at a transformational retreat where a number of physicians gathered to explore and reconnect with the meaning in their work. Many physicians who feel strained by the demands of managed care organizations, insurers and administrators feel a loss of connection to the people they serve and to their call to serve, and seek ways to enrich their practice. Patients, meanwhile, are turning to complementary and alternative medicine (CAM) therapists because they find the time, talk and touch approaches they may be missing in conventional medical settings. Health-care administrators, both hospital-based and in managed care organizations, have noticed this trend and are beginning to take steps to partner with CAM as consumer demand increases[1]. Particularly in oncology, conventional providers may feel pressure to address CAM use, as cancer patients are some of the heaviest users – anywhere from 30 to 83% according to a recent review[2]. The blending of CAM and conventional medical care is becoming a hot area of interest among physicians, administrators and insurers alike[1].

But what does this blend look like? The concept of integrating CAM with conventional care has been described using a number of terms – for example, integrative medicine, integrated medicine, integrative health care, multidisciplinary care. A standardized and accepted definition of this integration will make such tasks as developing standards of care, teaching and conducting research, and developing health policy more achievable[3]. The National Center for Complementary and Alternative Medicine (NCCAM) currently defines integrative medicine as health care that 'combines mainstream medical therapies and CAM therapies for which there is some high-quality scientific evidence of safety and effectiveness'.[4] This author prefers a definition of integrative medicine that emphasizes the importance of the patient–practitioner relationship, such as the one developed by the Working Group of the Consortium of Academic Health Centers for Integrative Medicine (Kligler *et al.*[5] p. 522): '...an approach to the practice of medicine that makes use of the best-available evidence, taking account of the whole person (body, mind, and spirit), including all aspects of lifestyle. It

emphasizes the therapeutic relationship and makes use of the rich diversity of therapeutic systems, incorporating both conventional and complementary/alternative approaches'.

It is important to differentiate between alternative therapies and complementary therapies – especially in cancer care where patients may be seeking a cure for their disease. Alternative therapies are defined as those used *in place of* conventional medicine, whereas complementary or integrative approaches are considered those that can be safely *combined with* mainstream medical care[2]. For the sake of this discussion, complementary and alternative therapies, taken together, refer to the latter. In the USA, integrative oncology centers that have been developed in association with hospitals and medical centers tend to focus on supportive, complementary care.

Integrative oncology is a natural outcropping of the integrative medicine movement due to the high rates of CAM usage among people with cancer. There has been a movement by some oncologists and primary care physicians to offer these services to patients in a safe, healing environment in answer to the patients' question, 'What *else* can *I* do?'. Likewise, comprehensive cancer centers and community hospitals around the country are developing programs of integrative care to meet the desires, needs and expectations of people with cancer[6]. Hospice and palliative care settings can make particularly good use of an integrative approach to help relieve pain and suffering by addressing the physical, emotional and spiritual needs of patients in the advancing stages of cancer[7]. Pediatric oncology is another natural and appropriate combination with integrative medicine (S. Sencer, oral communication, April 2004).

For administrators and/or physicians engaged in the start-up phase of an integrative oncology or integrative medicine program, one place to turn for guidance is those who have gone before. There is a growing number of integrative medicine centers in North America, according to a 2002 American Hospital Association survey. These centers are being developed both in association with hospital systems and as free-standing ventures, and tend to add CAM services to existing conventional care; that is, medical care remains a priority. Most are directed by a physician, and those that are directed by naturopaths, osteopaths, or PhDs most often have a physician on the staff[1]. Several of these centers are listed in the Examples of Models of Care section with websites for easy reference and contact.

Developing an integrative medicine center is not without significant obstacles: concerns about financial viability due to uncertain reimbursement; questionable effects on hospital and physician image; medicolegal issues; and the difficulty of rallying medical staff and community physician support. A conventional medical practice business plan should be adapted and followed to guide decision making (Table 5.1). To circumvent some of the obstacles, it may be helpful to address the following questions[8,9]:

(1) What do you wish to accomplish?

(2) Which patient population do you want to reach (gender, disease)?

(3) How will you reach the patient population (marketing, access to services)?

(4) Where will it be located (on-site hospital, off campus but still associated with the hospital, freestanding)?

(5) Who will organize and run it (nurses, social workers, physicians)?

(6) How will you gain trust from the medical community?

(7) How will you establish a referral stream to CAM services?

(8) Who will pay for it (hospital or cancer center, self-supporting, grants and

Table 5.1   Selecting an appropriate model of care for your community: what fits?

An integrative medicine business plan template

Market analysis
- Community needs and preferences
- Community physician attitudes
- Needs of the target patient population

Mission
- Concept of the final product/goals

Program description
- Sketch of innovative programs and services
- Addition of education and research

Market and promotion plan
- To reach target patient population

Physician relations
- Champions and supporters
- Building trusting relationships and a positive public image

Management, organization and staffing
- Appropriate administrative staff
- Availability of trained CAM providers

Facility, equipment and licenses
- Healing environment
- Location, location, location
- Availability of space

Phasing and schedule
- Realistic time-line

Financial analysis
- Financial resources
- Generating a referral stream
- Proforma

Risk assessment
- Identify and quantify risks

Legal review
- Medicolegal issues
- Credentialing guidelines

Evaluation
- Method for reviewing program performance

Adapted from Kaiser Institute Integrative Medicine Tools: Business Plan Outline [www.kaiser.net]

endowments, insurance) and will financing be sustainable?

These and other issues specific to individual centers and communities can now be tackled with the help of a growing number of integrative medicine business consultants and successful clinic founders around North America. The Resources section provides a list of a number of consultants and useful websites.

MODELS OF INTEGRATIVE MEDICINE CARE

There are at least two currently existing methods for describing the various ways integrative care is delivered in North America today. One, developed over the past number of years by Novey[8], is loosely based on the location and type of integrative medical care offered. The second, recently published by Mann et al.[10] and backed by an NCCAM grant, is based on the CAM education and interest of the physician involved and the complexity of CAM services rendered. There is a great deal of cross-over, but each descriptive method has unique categories that readers may be able to adapt to their own particular situations. Both are presented here with a brief discussion of the benefits and limitations of each model (Tables 5.2 and 5.3).

NOVEY'S SIX MODELS OF INTEGRATIVE MEDICAL CARE

Consultation-based integrative medicine

Specific patient population

In this model, integrative medicine expertise is focused on a single type of illness or service line; for example, oncology or supportive cancer care, chronic pain, or cardiac risk reduction and

Table 5.2 Novey's six models of integrative medicine care[8]

1. (a) Consultation-based – specific patient population
   (b) Consultation-based – general patient population
2. Integrative primary care
3. Integrative medicine – 'clinic without walls'
4. Integrative medicine in a fitness center
5. Virtual model of integrative medical care
6. Integrative medicine in a spa or health resort

Table 5.3 Seven models of integrative care by Mann et al.[10]

1. The informed clinician
2. The informed, networking clinician
3. The informed, CAM-trained clinician
4. Multidisciplinary integrative group practice
5. Interdisciplinary integrative group practice
6. Hospital-based integration
7. Integrative medicine in an academic medical center

rehabilitation. The advantage is that the practice is usually part of a larger hospital or community system, so there is a built-in referral base. A disadvantage is that success is dependent upon an active referral system, although patients can usually self-refer for such specialized integrative services.

General patient population

In this type of practice, a physician with special training or interest in integrative medicine sees patients for integrative medicine consultations as an adjunct to primary or specialist care, then returns the patient to the primary physician for ongoing care. An advantage to this approach is that the service is seen as a non-competitive, valued resource. The disadvantages are mainly financial. CAM providers working within the practice must maintain high volumes, as traditionally the bulk of revenue is brought in by integrative medicine consultations.

Integrative primary care

This type of practice provides integrative medicine within the context of continuing primary care. For example, a primary care practitioner – a family physician, internal medicine specialist or pediatrician – incorporates an integrative approach at each patient visit with added CAM services on site. The advantage of this approach is that revenues come from both CAM and billable primary medical care. A disadvantage is that this comprehensive model may compete with existing practices.

Integrative medicine – 'clinic without walls'

This model may be carried out as a primary care or a consultative practice, but the integrative medicine physicians do not have CAM providers on site. Instead, referrals are made to researched, certified and experienced CAM providers in the community. The advantage is that there is typically lower overhead with fewer medicolegal and administrative issues. A significant disadvantage is the loss of a team approach, and care may be fragmented if concerted efforts to communicate are not made by all involved practitioners.

Integrative medicine in a fitness center

This model has integrative medicine services located within or in association with a fitness center. The advantages are high visibility, the interest of a population focused on wellness, and an environment that is more likely to promote merchandising. A disadvantage is that medical patients may not be inclined to seek care in a fitness center model and services may be limited to those who are generally well.

Virtual integrative medicine services

A 'virtual' integrative care model has CAM services that are scattered throughout a facility or health-care system. The advantage is that it can be a truly integrated system, with conventional and CAM practitioners working side by side, generating minimal excess overhead, and using existing personnel. This approach can 'ease in' CAM services without committing to a centralized facility. If planning is not thorough, the disadvantages are numerous: no image of a central resource, lack of the team meeting approach, limited communication between practitioners, lack of a 'healing space' and difficulty monitoring individual CAM providers' practices.

Integrative medicine in a spa or health resort

The emerging health resort model is a vacation destination focusing on relaxation, recreation, and total health and well-being. Traditional spa services, such as massage and skin and nail treatments, are incorporated into an expanded menu of offerings including medical and behavior science consultations, fitness and outdoor sports, nutrition consultations and education – including healthy gourmet meals – and spiritual development with modalities such as yoga and Tai Chi. There is often a retail outlet on site. Like a fitness center model, the health resort tends to attract a population motivated to be fit and well, and who have the resources to pay for it. In addition, patrons are a captive audience while at the resort, open to learning experiences and stress reduction. A disadvantage is the relatively high cost of such health vacations, which precludes access for most North Americans.

SEVEN MODELS OF INTEGRATIVE CARE AS DESCRIBED BY MANN *ET AL.*

The informed clinician

This model represents the simple case of a conventional physician becoming knowledgeable about CAM, making a practice of asking patients about CAM use, and informing and educating patients about CAM therapies. Because this approach requires more time for discussion and history-taking, information and communication become key areas of focus. This informed clinician may recommend certain CAM therapies depending on his or her personal experience and belief system and, ideally, after experiencing any recommended therapies at first hand. Benefits of this approach are improved patient communication and an added service to patients, potentially resulting in increased patient and physician satisfaction. Limitations are difficulty with CAM decision-making due to lack of depth of knowledge in the particular area, little or no communication with CAM providers and difficulty tracking outcomes of patients using CAM.

The informed, networking clinician

This model is similar to the first, except that the clinician has become familiar with local CAM resources and develops an informal referral network. As in the 'clinic without walls' model, this clinician has visited a number of CAM practitioners, looked at credentials and licenses, and has accessed patient feedback before deciding on who will make up the network. There is ongoing communication set up between the physician and CAM providers in the network. An advantage to this system is an increase in the range of CAM options available. Limitations may include gaps in communication and documentation of the CAM therapy and inconvenience for patients traveling to off-site locations.

The informed, CAM-trained clinician

In this case, the physician has obtained extra training in a CAM therapy, such as acupuncture, that has led to expertise and, often, a license to provide the therapy. Advantages include control over documentation of patient progress and outcomes, and an added source of income. There is little added risk except for the addition of an uninsured service, which can increase practice management costs.

Multidisciplinary integrative group practice

All practitioners, conventional and CAM, work in the same center or clinic, share space, cross-refer, and may focus on a particular service line, such as oncology. They may see the same patients, but do so separately and without conferring in a formal, team meeting approach to plan care together. Main advantages are the ability to offer comprehensive services to a particular patient population, and potentially lower overhead and increased income due to space-sharing and expanded support personnel. There is potential for a great deal of information-sharing among the disciplines, which benefits staff and patients. This model will lend itself more readily to research. Limitations are financial and legal: there may be increased start-up costs, inconsistency in productivity of CAM providers and/or ability to collect fees, and possible medicolegal issues around credentialing of CAM providers.

Interdisciplinary integrative group practice

This model represents a high level of integration. Not only do conventional and CAM practitioners share the same office space, they may share a common patient record and hold meetings to discuss individual cases and develop integrative care plans. There may be emphasis on a specific service line, such as oncology, or some centers may choose to offer general integrative health care. Advantages for patients include a broad perspective on their illness and a comprehensive care plan; for practitioners, this model offers frequent learning opportunities – especially in the context of the integrative patient conference. Disadvantages may be centered around difficulties reaching consensus on patient care and inconsistencies in financial reimbursement. The operation may cost more owing to larger staff and office space, and the abovementioned medico-legal credentialing issues may arise.

Hospital-based integrative care

In this model, conventional medicine and CAM care are delivered within the same hospital system or medical center. Generally, the hospital administration demonstrates a commitment to provide integrative medical care, with the added goal of improving the patient and family in-patient experience. Benefits include improved patient care and satisfaction, and increased retention of nursing and support staff with resulting improvements in public image. Most limitations, such as increased costs for extra staff, are offset by a competitive edge; however, medicolegal issues must be considered.

Integrative medicine in an academic medical center

Three areas of focus – teaching, research and clinical care – exist in the context of evolving understanding of and access to CAM. This setting is optimal for cancer care to the extent that much cutting-edge conventional oncology is in academic centers. The emphasis is on evidence-based care rendered by professionals who combine clinical, teaching and research responsibilities. Advantages include the availability of government research grant monies to enhance program funding, comprehensive patient care,

ability to expose students to CAM, and opportunities for practitioners to participate in research. Limitations include difficulties in credentialing CAM providers and the high cost of providing services within a center that provides care in an educational setting.

EXAMPLES OF INTEGRATIVE MEDICINE CENTERS

The following examples of successful clinics and centers represent a blending of the descriptive models of care, and each is labeled accordingly (Table 5.4). They are provided for use as a resource to the interested reader who may be planning an integrative oncology project. Features such as mission statement, targeted service line, referral base, reimbursement structure, practitioners involved, and research and education initiatives are detailed. The data for this section were gathered by questionnaire after initial permission was granted to feature the program as an exemplary model of care.

There is a collegial attitude of sharing among those working in integrative medicine, and the contact persons for each of these centers – medical directors or clinic coordinators – were more than willing to provide this information. Some inconsistencies may appear from example to example, as there was considerable variance in the responses, reflecting the uniqueness of these innovative models of health-care delivery.

Consult-based integrative oncology – academic centers

Leonard P. Zakim Center for Integrated Therapies, Dana-Farber Cancer Institute, Boston, MA (Zakim Center)

Affiliated with Dana-Farber Cancer Institute and Harvard University, the Leonard P. Zakim

Table 5.4   Examples of models of care

Consult-based integrative oncology – academic centers

Leonard P. Zakim Center for Integrated Therapies
Dana-Farber Cancer Institute, Boston, MA
www.dana-farber.org/pat/support/zakim_default.asp

Place...of wellness

MD Anderson Cancer Center, Houston, TX
www.mdanderson.org/departments/wellness

Consult-based integrative oncology – freestanding centers

Multidisiplinary group practice

California Hematology Oncology Medical Group
Los Angeles and Torrance, CA
www.CHOMG.com

Informed, networking, CAM-trained clinicians

Regional Radiation Oncology Center (Harbin Clinic
 Radiation Oncology)
Rome, GA
www.harbinclinic.com

Interdisciplinary group practice

Center for Integrated Healing
Vancouver, BC, Canada
www.healing.bc.ca

Hospital-based integrative oncology

Cancer Treatment Centers of America
Zion, IL and Tulsa, OK
www.cancercenter.com

Hospital-based pediatric integrative oncology

Children's Hospital and Clinics
Minneapolis, MN
www.childrenshc.org/communities/integrativemed.asp

Consult-based general integrative medicine

Interdisciplinary group practice

Carolinas Integrative Health
Charlotte, NC
www.carolinas.org/services/cih

Integrative primary care

Multidisciplinary group practices

Family Practice Center of Integrative Health and
Healing
Burlington, ON, Canada
www.fpcihh.com

Center for Integrative Medicine and Healing
Therapies
Largo, FL
Office: 727-584-8777

'Clinic without walls' – the informed, networking, CAM-trained clinician

Integrative Internal Medicine Clinic
San Diego, CA
www.SDIntMed.com

Integrative primary care medicine in a fitness center

Multidisciplinary group practice

Alitus Integrative Health and Wellness
Vernon Hills, IL
www.northshorehealth.com

Virtual model of integrative medical services

Gwinnett Health System
Lawrenceville, GA
www.gwinnetthealth.org/programs/programs.asp

Integrative medicine in a spa or resort

Canyon Ranch
Tucson, AZ and Lenox, MA
www.canyonranch.com

Center for Integrated Therapies is dedicated to enhancing the quality of life for cancer patients and families by incorporating CAM into traditional cancer care. The Center provides afford-able clinical services for pediatric and adult patients and their families, educates and empowers patients about use of CAM, and conducts peer-reviewed research.

In-house therapists include an acupuncturist, massage therapist, Therapeutic Touch and Reiki therapist, a nutritionist and a music therapist. The medical director does integrative medicine consultations for patients who request them. CAM experiences are separated into group and individual sessions (for example, meditation, Chi Gong, music and dance), and expressive arts are experienced in a group setting, while appointments for massage and acupuncture are individually booked. At team meetings held once a month, clinical issues are discussed and physicians are invited to present patient cases.

At the Zakim Center, CAM providers may be employed on a 'casual' basis or salaried, with the various therapies being offered to patients fee-for-service, but at lower than community rates. There is some philanthropy, which may be used to offset costs of CAM therapies for patients. There is no retail operation at this center.

Patient referrals come in different ways and are currently in a state of flux. In the past, patients self-referred for center services. Now, a letter of consent from the oncologist is required before patients may access CAM therapies. The response to this approach has been favorable; in addition to building relationships with colleagues, referrals are now coming to the Zakim Center from the oncologists at Dana-Farber.

There is an active CAM research program at the Zakim Center, with a number of projects ongoing at one time, including patient usage surveys. Examples include exercise and immunity, acupuncture and neutropenia, and effects of Chi Gong, music and Reiki therapy.

In terms of education, there is a resident rotation, and special lectures are provided for fellows in Harvard University's MD/MPH program, who rotate through the Zakim Center as part of their curriculum. There are also education programs for patients, families and staff.

Innovative programs include the Lenny Lecture series, which is a once yearly lecture featuring well-known speakers in the field of integrative medicine. Currently, Zakim Center staff members are making plans to expand programming to offer CAM services to inpatients at Dana-Farber.

For more information about the Leonard P. Zakim Center for Integrated Therapies, please see www.dana-farber.org/pat/support/zakim_default.asp.

Place…of wellness, MD Anderson Cancer Center, Houston, TX

This supportive cancer care program aims to create an environment where all persons touched by cancer may enhance their quality of life through programs that complement medical care and focus on mind, body and spirit. Although the target service line is oncology, *all persons touched by cancer* means that the programs are offered to family and friends as well as patients.

Place…*of wellness* offers over 100 programs; many are on site while others are held at outreach locations. CAM services include acupuncture, mind–body therapy, yoga and Tai Chi, as well as a vast array of support and discussion groups and lectures on complementary and integrative therapies.

All practitioners are credentialed and programs are rigorously screened for appropriateness and safety for people with cancer. As part of the credentialing procedure, each CAM provider is assigned to a health-care professional on staff at MD Anderson in a field most closely resembling the particular CAM therapy. For example, massage therapists are assigned to physical therapists and acupuncturists are assigned to anesthesiologists. This staff member acts as a mentor and a resource to the CAM provider for questions or concerns. Three MD Anderson staff physicians – a psychiatrist, an anesthesiologist with expertise in pain management, and a rehabilitation medicine physician – oversee practitioners and activities at Place...*of wellness*, and plans are underway to recruit a physician to provide integrative oncology consultations at the center.

The Place...*of wellness* administration team meets weekly to discuss operational issues, and the staff meets weekly for announcements and to discuss projects and patient/provider issues. Team meetings to discuss or plan individual patient care are not held at this time.

There is an extensive research program at MD Anderson for investigating CAM therapies and cancer in conjunction with the NCCAM. Place...*of wellness* educates physicians and patients via a CAM education website called CIMER (Complementary/Integrative Medicine Education Resources) (www.mdanderson.org/departments/CIMER). Relationships with other health-care professionals are built by providing a continuing medical education (CME) lecture series for physicians, physician assistants, nurses and dietitians. This population is also enthusiastically targeted with marketing material.

A unique offering to Place...*of wellness* is a set of two CD ROMs which contain lectures on CAM therapies and programs – one aimed at patients, the other at health-care providers. These materials may be distributed to individuals and organizations anywhere in the USA.

For more information on Place...*of wellness* at MD Anderson Cancer Center, please see www.mdanderson.org/departments/wellness.

Consult-based integrative oncology – freestanding centers: multidisciplinary group practice

California Hematology Oncology Medical Group, Los Angeles and Torrance, CA

The California Hematology Oncology Medical Group (CHOMG) has been a provider of medical oncology services in the Los Angeles and South Bay area for 15 years. Dedicated to healing the whole person in a physical and emotional crisis, CHOMG has partnered with B'Shert Integrative Oncology Services (BIOS) to create an Integrative Cancer Center. CHOMG and BIOS work in harmony to provide highly individualized cancer care. CHOMG provides and coordinates allopathic (conventional) oncology care, while BIOS provides supportive and complementary functions such as Healing Touch, massage therapy, and group support.

CHOMG has as its mission to enhance the physical, emotional and spiritual well-being of patients and families through individualized treatment plans, education, and the blending of conventional and complementary practices. It is an adult medical oncology practice, with the main component being conventional cancer treatment. BIOS, a subdivision of the group, plans and oversees the integrative program, holds the retail license for the sale of herbs and supplements, and also accepts charitable donations. There is one shared chart for each patient, although the CAM portion is kept separately in order to thin the chart. All practitioners have access to all parts of the chart, however. The staff works together in a team approach, with some staff members providing both conventional and complementary care. For example, the director of nursing also practices Healing Touch.

CHOMG also houses a massage therapist, an acupuncturist, a nutritionist, a Bowen Therapist (a gentle system of body work for pain control – www.bowentherapy.com), and a cancer guide. The person who acts as a cancer guide provides guidance and resources for patients looking for innovative treatments and trials, as well as CAM services for themselves and their families. Most of the complementary providers were already part of the traditional team. That is, these individuals were employed in conventional roles and were retrained, so there is not an additional cost to the practice. For example, the office manager was offered the opportunity to become a massage therapist, so she is now part of the health-care team as well as continuing her position as an administrator.

Care is co-ordinated by case conferences that include physicians and practitioners who discuss conventional and complementary therapies for individual patients. The staff has also used in-service presentations and written communications to maintain their team approach.

Patients are referred to the integrative program by the conventional oncology service. The integrative services at CHOMG are reimbursed by a blended system. Patients pay for services if no coverage is available. Insurance pays for some services, particularly acupuncture and nutrition and occasionally massage. Some treatments are funded by donations and some are subsidized. There are plans to make BIOS a non-profit organization in the future.

There is a retail component through BIOS that provides supplements and herbs to patients who find this service convenient. The staff is careful to avoid a 'hard sell' approach; patients benefit by purchasing through the clinic as it is a tax-free event. Further savings are passed on through wholesale pricing of products. There is no attempt to subsidize the integrative oncology program through retail items.

CHOMG participates in conventional oncology clinical trials; there is no CAM research program at this time. The staff provides CME presentations occasionally, but does not educate students of health professions at this time. The group members make themselves available to speak to the public, to hospital groups, and at private functions. Relationships within the group are built and supported by a strong team approach, while every effort is made to work in collaboration with private physicians and specialists outside the group, to ensure that optimum communication and care are achieved.

As part of its innovative program, CHOMG offers patient seminars on CAM topics, provides copies of CAM articles in the waiting room and publishes a monthly newsletter. An open house to introduce patients to CAM therapies was held, and center staff members have taken support group participants on outings to meditation workshops, healers and movies.

CHOMG was founded by Dr Lorne Feldman, a graduate of the Associate Fellowship Program in Integrative Medicine at the University of Arizona. Dr Feldman was a long-term cancer survivor and an inspiration to his patients and colleagues. He died in November 2003 secondary to complications of advancing disease.

For more information about CHOMG, please see www.CHOMG.com.

Consult-based integrative oncology – informed, networking, and CAM-trained clinicians

Regional Radiation Oncology Center, Rome, GA

The Regional Radiation Oncology Center (RROC) is a freestanding radiation oncology center offering state-of-the-art radiation therapy treatment and integrative oncology consultations. Care is customized to meet patients' physical, emotional and general health needs and includes advanced cancer treatment blended with proven supportive complementary therapies and psychosocial counseling. The mission at RROC is to be a caring, loving and quality center, meeting the needs of patients, families and staff.

RROC staffs two radiation oncologists (one is trained in integrative medicine), an integrative medicine-trained family practitioner, a psychologist, two nurses trained in Reiki, and the full complement of radiation technologists, dosimetrists and physicists. Physicians refer out to well-known CAM practitioners in the community for such services as massage, chiropractic, acupuncture and Reiki therapy.

As part of the Comprehensive Cancer Care Program, RROC provides, at no extra charge, an integrative medicine consultation to patients who are interested in CAM or who are flagged at intake as candidates for this service. The center is currently developing a menu of weekly educational and experiential CAM offerings that patients may access as desired. Topics will include nutrition and cancer, movement therapy and physical activity, stress reduction, spirituality and health.

The integrative medicine team, which comprises the physicians, the psychologist, two nurses and the office manager, meets once weekly, during which case presentations are made, care is co-ordinated and literature concerning integrative oncology is reviewed. There is a single medical record for all patients that includes the integrative assessment and recommendations.

Patients are referred by local physicians for conventional radiation oncology treatment, and come to the integrative team by way of referral by in-house physicians or nurses. Some patients are self-referred, usually for a second opinion or because they are seeking an integrative approach. This is a conventional practice that bills insurance and Medicare/Medicaid, except for the integrative medicine consults which, as above, are provided to patients as a complimentary service. Mind–body assessments and counseling are billed to the appropriate payor. RROC does not have an on-site retail operation, but has made arrangements with manufacturers of several high-quality supplements to sell products to their patients at wholesale prices.

Research and education are important at RROC. The center actively participates in conventional and CAM clinical trials, and CME conferences are held in the community concerning an integrative approach. In addition, there is an opportunity for integrative approaches to be discussed at conventional tumor board meetings. RROC also hosts visiting medical students and radiation oncology residents and fellows. Patient and family relationships are built and strengthened by clear communication and the availability of practitioners to answer questions. Relationships with community physicians are maintained by CME presentations, participation in hospital committees and consult letters. The integrative family physician regularly attends tumor conferences and has built alliances with community medical oncologists through that venue.

In addition to the program at RROC, and unique to Rome, GA, is Many Streams Healing Systems (MSHS), a non-profit 501c3* organization whose mission is to provide safe and supportive group education for cancer patients and their families. MSHS provides workshops concerning a variety of healing options which address the whole person. The organization also presents transformational residential retreats for people with cancer, for physicians and for corporate health care workers.

Floyd College in Rome, GA offers a program for nurses to obtain certification as an Oncology Nurse Navigator. The Nurse Navigator is trained to assist patients to navigate the complex system of cancer care from diagnosis through treatment and supportive care. Another local support is the Floyd Center for Health and Healing (www. floyd.org/services/health/healing.htm). This interdisciplinary group practice offers integrative medicine consults, medical acupuncture, massage, mind–body programs, therapeutic yoga and energy medicine, and is located close-by and is mandated to serve cancer patients. All of these programs were initiated by support from the Georgia Cancer Coalition (www.georgiacancer coalition.org).

As of March 2005, RROC became Harbin Clinic Radiation Oncology. For more information, please see www.harbinclinic.com.

---

* Internal Revenue Code meaning that donations made by individuals or groups/companies are tax-deductible.

Consult-based integrative oncology – interdisciplinary group practice

Center for Integrated Healing, Vancouver, British Columbia, Canada

The Center for Integrated Healing (CIH) is a non-profit society that provides an integrated cancer care program for people with cancer and their families. It was founded by a family physician with a life-long interest in nutrition, natural healing and complementary therapies in cancer care. The Center's medical staff members are the first physicians in Canada to be funded by a provincial government to provide complementary care.

CIH aims to empower people with cancer and their families to explore options in CAM therapies in a safe environment, to document research on the effectiveness of these therapies, to inspire change in the health-care system and to contribute to the reduction of cancer incidence and mortality. Care at CIH is based on an integrative concept; one primary chart is used and each CAM practitioner may keep additional notes. CIH is not affiliated with a hospital or with an oncology group, it provides an adjunctive cancer care program working closely with the British Columbia Cancer Agency (BCCA).

The physicians at the center are funded through the provincial government by way of BCCA to see cancer patients only. The CAM practitioners, however, will treat people with or without cancer for health promotion and prevention, as well as various other health concerns.

CIH has on staff five primary care physicians, full-time and part-time, with experience incorporating CAM into conventional practice. Other providers see patients on a part-time basis. These include a naturopath, a Doctor of Traditional Chinese Medicine, a massage therapist, a nutritionist and a Therapeutic Touch practitioner. Off-site services that are recommended include counseling, yoga, meditation, support groups and a variety of classes and programs. The care team meets regularly to discuss business and to connect with each other, and select patient cases may be reviewed.

Patients come to CIH by way of referral by physicians, by CAM providers, and by self-referral. Physician services at CIH are billed to the British Columbia Medical Services Plan. CAM practitioners are not insured by the government, so 60% of funding for those services comes from private donations. The patient is required to pay the balance out of pocket. There is no retail operation at CIH.

CIH is active in CAM research and has two researchers on staff. In addition, abstracts describing new research are regularly distributed to practitioners. The Center will be initiating a pilot study in 2005 to evaluate the benefit of an integrative oncology approach for patients with incurable cancer.

The Center hosts medical students, Family Practice residents and PhD students who may choose electives at CIH. Two of the integrative physicians teach an undergraduate course on integrated healing for the University of British Columbia's Faculty of Medicine.

CIH builds relationships with patients, families and other caregivers through a focus on communication; for example, consult letters are sent to primary care physicians. At this time, there is no CME program underway at CIH. The focus is primarily patient-centered with some emphasis on the healing community – family, caregivers and community at large.

Because CIH is able to see only 400 patients a year, owing to funding constraints, the staff has developed an Outreach Program within British Columbia and The Yukon to bring information on their healing programs (prevention-based) to the public and to school children. This program also includes research information and education on CAM and conventional therapies.

Another unique program at CIH is their 2-day introductory program, which patients and family members attend prior to the integrative physician visit. This program is run every 2 weeks and consists of 12 hours of seminars and workshops on topics such as complementary cancer care and healing, meditation, visualization, healthful nutrition, vitamins, supplements, group sharing and decision-making, and is an opportunity to meet and chat with the center's various practitioners. The goal of the program is to provide a framework for people to explore ways that the mind, body and soul can contribute to healing, and to provide support as they create their comprehensive healing program. The cost of the 2-day introductory program, which includes an individualized 2-month supply of vitamins and supplements valued at $200, is $240 CDN. This fee includes the attendance of a family member or other support person. There is a limited number of bursaries available for those in need of financial assistance.

The initial visit with the center's physicians is 3 hours in total. The first 90 minutes is spent discussing the patient's life, social support, fears, concerns, illness and treatments. A complete medical history and physical examination is undertaken at this time, including an exploration of all conventional and complementary therapies that have been or are being used.

The second visit – the treatment planning visit – takes place at least 1 week later, after the patient has kept a 7-day history of food intake, sleep habits, exercise and relaxation, and bowel habits. To fully prepare for the treatment planning visit, patients and families are encouraged to attend the 2-day introductory program. During the second visit, remaining questions and concerns are addressed, and an individualized complementary cancer care program is created. This program is initiated once the patient feels comfortable with treatments suggested and all questions have been answered.

For more information on the Center for Integrated Healing, please see www.healing.bc.ca.

Integrative oncology in a hospital-based system

Cancer Treatment Centers of America, Zion, IL and Tulsa, OK

Founded in 1975, this institution has an exclusive focus on integrated and individualized cancer care. Their approach combines the latest medical, surgical and radiological therapies with supportive modalities such as nutrition, mind–body medicine, physical therapy, naturopathy and spiritual wellness.

The mission at the Cancer Treatment Centers of America (CTCA) is to seek out and provide powerful and innovative therapies to heal the whole person; its vision is to be recognized as the premier center for healing and hope by people with cancer. Integrative medicine at CTCA is a team approach to patient care, blending conventional and CAM therapies under one roof, individualized to meet the needs of the whole person. Medical, radiation and surgical oncologists work alongside CAM providers – all work as a team, sharing one patient record in a patient-centered medical model. It is a hospital-based system with two locations, one in Zion, IL and one in Tulsa, OK, and an outpatient clinic in Seattle, WA.

Alongside standard therapies such as surgery, chemotherapy and radiation, are CAM therapies such as clinical nutrition, vitamin and mineral supplementation, naturopathic medicine, herbal medicine, homeopathy, acupuncture, hydrotherapy, detoxification, exercise and rehabilitation programs, mind–body medicine and spiritual support. The physicians work as part of the integrative team, with the medical oncologist typically serving as the attending physician. Team meetings are held two to three times a week to discuss all inpatients. Complicated outpatient cases are discussed in the same manner.

The full range of support services, such as laboratory, radiology, respiratory therapy, rehabilitation therapy, pain management and pharmacy, is available in the main hospitals. In the outpatient site in Seattle, medical oncologists are supported by naturopaths, nutritionists, acupuncturists, Traditional Chinese Medicine practitioners, mind–body experts and massage therapists.

Approximately 50% of patients come to CTCA via referral by MDs, CAM practitioners or patients, and the rest are self-referred as a result of direct marketing through the Internet website. New oncology patients are required to have a thorough intake and assessment on their first visit. They are seen initially by a nurse who carries out a complete nursing assessment (vital signs, medications, allergies, etc.) and a history including chart review. A chronological summary of the patient's story is created from diagnosis to intake, including tests, scans, pathology, laboratory findings, surgeries, etc. The patient is then seen by an appropriate oncologist, depending upon disease type and stage, who reviews this history and takes his or her own history and physical examination. All necessary tests and scans are ordered and are completed within 48 hours. During those first two days, woven around the test schedule, the patient will meet with a naturopathic physician, nutritionist, mind–body therapist, exercise/rehabilitation physiologist, pastoral carer and a case manager. All of these providers also perform an initial assessment. Typically on day 3, the patient will meet again with the oncologist who presents the patient with results of the testing and recommendations for treatment. Once the treatment plan has been determined and begun, patients have regular follow-up with both CAM practitioners and oncologists.

CTCA hospitals and clinics are reimbursed by private insurance and Medicare and, occasionally, cash. All of the CTCA facilities have a supplement center on site, although they differ in structure. At one site, the retail component is part of the hospital pharmacy, while at the other it is a stand-alone walk-in store where supplements are sold. A new subsidiary company called Cancer Nutrition Centers of America is being developed to sell high-quality vitamins and supplements especially formulated for cancer patients. Sales are expected to add significantly to the bottom line over the next few years.

Both CTCA hospitals are actively engaged in CAM research and have trials open for patients on an ongoing basis. CTCA helps support the Cancer Treatment Research Foundation, which provides funding for clinical research in several major university hospitals around the country. CTCA is also actively involved in education. There is a naturopathic medicine residency program at both hospitals. This is the only naturopathic hospital residency program focusing on oncology in the USA. CTCA also offers many classes and seminars for patients and the public in communities where the hospitals are located. The forums are designed to focus on prevention and early detection. There is also a Cancer Resource Center that provides information for the public on all types of cancer and treatments.

Building and maintaining relationships is a priority at CTCA. Patients and families benefit from clear explanations and respect for individual decisions. CTCA has found that the best way to build relationships between CAM providers and medical doctors is continually to educate the physicians on the scientific evidence behind the CAM therapies that are recommended. All physicians and CAM providers attend the same educational forums at CTCA, so they learn together and also from each other.

CTCA is unique in that it is the only cancer hospital system known that has naturopathic physicians working side by side with medical doctors. The naturopath treatment program focuses on building the patient's immune system and managing symptoms and side-effects of treatments and of the disease itself. The mind–body program helps patients deal with the emotional impact of cancer, and the goal of the nutrition program is to reverse the weight loss and immune system decline so often associated with malignancy and anti-neoplastic treatment.

For more information about Cancer Treatment Centers of America, please see www.cancercenter.com.

Pediatric integrative oncology in a hospital-based system

Children's Hospitals and Clinics, Minneapolis, MN

The integrative medicine program at Children's Hospitals and Clinics (Children's) offers families a broad range of health-care choices, blending traditional, cultural and complementary medical practice and treatment. Along with being a national leader in offering integrative treatment options to families, Children's is sensitive to cultural differences. Trans-cultural services are offered to Hispanic, Somali and Hmong groups.

The Integrative Medicine and Cultural Care Departments offer services to all patients, regardless of the type of illness. Oncology patients may be seen as inpatients or outpatients by the Integrative Team, which has been operational in the hospital since 2001. This team is composed of an integrative oncologist, a behavioral pediatrician, a psychologist, a clinical nurse specialist and acupuncturists.

Referrals to the integrative team are not automatic. Once a child is diagnosed with cancer, there is a waiting period of 1–2 weeks while the patient and family adjust. Then, if it suits the child, the diagnosis, the family and their coping style, a referral is made to the Integrative Medicine Department. At intake, available integrative medicine services are explained to the family; for example, acupressure wrist-bands or aromatherapy may be used for nausea. Acupuncture is used only occasionally, as many children are afraid of needles, and it was not found to be economically viable on a large scale.

According to the center's pediatric oncologist, self-hypnosis, guided imagery and biofeedback are very useful therapies for children. Child Life Specialists at Children's who work with all patients use guided imagery extensively. The integrative team will also refer to a community energy healer if requested by the family.

The Integrative Medicine Department relies heavily on philanthropy (memorial funds, some grants) for payment of services, as it is part of a larger non-profit hospital organization; however, Children's does bill insurance where appropriate. Creative reimbursement strategies such as offering a set number of complimentary introductory massages, then working with families to begin paying, have worked well. There is also a sliding fee scale. As for outpatient integrative medicine physician services, they are billable, as the integrative consult occurs during regular oncology follow-up visits. All CAM programs are fee-for-service.

Children's is actively involved in both conventional and CAM research trials. According to one pediatric oncologist, the field of pediatrics has not been extensively studied during CAM development, and the pediatricians at Children's feel a sense of responsibility to contribute to the science of pediatric integrative medicine. The integrative medicine team is also involved in educating students of the health professions and they provide regular educational offerings through hospital Grand Rounds and CME activities locally and nationally. The integrative physicians communicate with conventional colleagues via comprehensive consult letters.

Children's provides a comprehensive education program for parents, including a folder of plainly written materials on CAM therapies. This includes information on biofeedback, clinical aromatherapy, stress management, mental imagery, massage, yoga, exercise, nutrition, Traditional Chinese Medicine, herbal medicine, Healing Touch and spirituality. One particularly innovative program is the Academic Therapy program, which is overseen by the Integrative Medicine department. A specially trained coach works with children with learning difficulties to build on strengths and develop strategies to overcome weaknesses.

For more information about Children's, please see www.childrenshc.org/communities/integrativemed.asp.

Consultation-based general integrative medicine – interdisciplinary group practice

Carolinas Integrative Health, Charlotte, NC

In association with Carolinas HealthCare System, Carolinas Integrative Health (CIH) offers complementary and alternative therapies at an off-site but central location under the supervision of a physician with fellowship training in integrative medicine. CIH aims to offer the highest quality health care possible and in doing so, change the practice of medicine in North Carolina for the better – by embracing all people, being clinically and economically effective, including a range of therapies critically appraised through research and/or experience, and based on a foundation of knowledge, possibility, and hope. The clinic is integrative in concept, with practitioners sharing one chart.

CIH is a consultative service, working closely with patients' primary care and specialty practitioners, seeing patients with a range of ages and complaints. The most common conditions seen are chronic pain, autoimmune disorders, behavior issues in children, menopause, depression/anxiety, heart disease, obesity and cancer.

For cancer patients, CIH has a program of yoga for cancer survivors and provides cancer prevention consults. Wellness and prevention consultations are also provided for well persons.

In addition to the integrative medical physician onsite, CIH houses two massage therapists,

a Doctor of Traditional Chinese Medicine (who also teaches Tai Chi), a mind–body therapist (also a Reiki practitioner), a nutritionist and a yoga instructor. Patients can book individual assessments with any of the providers (that is, they are not required to have an integrative medicine assessment first). However, CAM practitioners will consult a physician if they are uncomfortable with any medical situation. All practitioners meet once a week and occasionally they discuss selected patients. There is ample opportunity for practitioners to discuss patients at any time if there are questions or concerns.

Most patients are self-referred, with 20–25% being practitioner-referred. CIH accepts Medicare, but is mainly fee for service. Patients are provided with a billing sheet with all the necessary codes on it (ICD-9, CPT and ABC codes), which they may submit to their insurer for consideration. These sheets also include a brief description of the center for the information of the insurance companies. The center feels that this is one way to educate the insurance companies about integrative medicine.

CIH operates a small retail outlet offering supplements that have been researched fully, with regards to both manufacturer and data on safety and efficacy. The clinic also carries some specialty products, such as skin creams, candles and dark chocolate. Although these items are sold at a marginal mark up, retail sales do not contribute greatly to the financial success of the center.

CIH is actively involved in research projects and has put together several grant proposals. The clinic works closely with the research and epidemiology department at the parent hospital, Carolinas HealthCare System. CIH also hosts medical students, interns and residents for 1–5 days at a time. The staff members at CIH participate in Grand Rounds and CME/staff education events throughout the hospital, and give public lectures on a frequent basis. Communication lines with community physicians are kept open and by consult notes sent by the integrative physician.

Innovative programming is under development. A recent pilot weight loss program was both popular and effective, and plans are currently in place to develop specific programs to target the indigent populations served by Carolinas HealthCare System.

For information about Carolinas Integrative Health, please see www.carolinas.org/services/cih.

Integrative primary care – multidisciplinary group practices

The Family Practice Center of Integrative Health and Healing, Burlington, Ontario

The Family Practice Center of Integrative Health and Healing (FPCIHH) works to integrate the highest standard of conventional, complementary and alternative medicine in the context of a family practice setting. The focus is empowerment and partnership with patients and community. Its vision is to serve as a model for a new paradigm of patient-centered health care, engaging in evidence-based research and education in integrative medicine.

FPCIHH is owned by a sole family physician proprietor with fellowship training in integrative medicine. She has admitting privileges at the community hospital and is part-time faculty at McMaster University. There are two other physicians in the practice: one family physician with experience in CAM therapies, and another integrative medicine-trained physician who provides consultations. The integrative medicine consultant provides energy medicine treatments, guided imagery and hypnosis in addition to integrative medicine consultations. The center also houses a chiropractor, a naturopath, a Doctor of Traditional Chinese Medicine (DTCM), massage therapist and a psychotherapist who does Heart-Math™ assessments (www.heartmath.org).

Each provider has a separate chart, but patients may sign a consent form to have their information shared with the other practitioners in the center. Patients may book for individual services – it is not necessary to see one of the physicians first. CAM providers pay the center a rental fee based on space, administrative services and supplies provided. The team meets monthly and chooses selected cases for discussion.

Patients come to FPCIHH by way of self-referrals and physician- and CAM practitioner-referrals. This practice is located in Canada, therefore payment for services is a blend of government funding and patients paying out-of-pocket for services not covered by the provincial health plan. This innovative system is generally working well, with some challenges. The DTCM and naturopath both sell products that do not contribute to the bottom line of the center.

FPCIHH is actively involved in medical education and plans to participate in CAM research. At present, the integrative family practitioner is in discussion with the Family Practice Research Department at McMaster University regarding possible research projects, and regularly gives lectures to family practice residents on integration of CAM into conventional family practice. Medical students and family practice residents may do elective rotations at the center, where they spend time with the integrative family practitioner and the other providers.

Relationships are built and maintained by one-on-one communication, monthly newsletters, letters to community physicians, consult letters and speaking to the media.

For more information about FPCIHH, please see www.fpcihh.com.

Center for Integrative Medicine and Healing Therapies, Largo, FL

This is a practice consisting of an integrative internal medicine physician providing primary care services in association with several CAM providers sharing space. Although they refer to one another and confer occasionally on patient cases, there is no affiliation otherwise.

The Center for Integrative Medicine and Healing Therapies (CIMHT) mission is to create an integrated physician-managed center where patients have access to the best practices in conventional and complementary medicine to promote healing and total wellness. Patients are invited to be actively involved in their healing process, which focuses on the whole person - body, mind and spirit.

In addition to primary care medical services, the physician provides individual preventive assessments and nutrition and exercise counseling. A licensed acupuncturist and two massage therapists share the clinic space. The providers may also refer patients to known and trusted CAM practitioners in the community on an as-needed basis.

The center receives physician and CAM provider referrals, and patients may self-refer. Reimbursement is by third-party billing, including Medicare. There is no retail operation at CIMHT.

The clinic has a major interest in participating in CAM trials and clinical phase II, III and IV trials – there are four research nurses on staff. At this time, there is no student education program, but plans are being made to provide a 2-week rotation for family practice residents.

The medical director is actively involved in hospital medicine in the community, and through this route the clinic has developed relationships with a number of physicians in the area. Friendly relations with CAM practitioners have come as a result of staff visits to them and subsequently referring patients. The medical director gives community talks, but has not provided CME to date.

Unlike many fee for service integrative medicine centers, this practice sees all medical patients including indigents, the uninsured and illegal aliens. Medications and laboratory work are offered to this population free of charge through a liaison with a nearby free clinic and hospital. CAM services are separate and remain fee-for-service for this population.

For more information about the Center for Integrative Medicine and Healing Therapies, please call 727-584-8777.

Integrative medicine 'clinic without walls' – the informed, networking and CAM-trained clinician

Integrative Internal Medicine Clinic, San Diego, CA

The Integrative Internal Medicine Clinic (IIMC) is a solo primary care practice. The mission is to become the center of excellence for integrative medicine in San Diego by providing state-of-the-art integrative health care.

At the present time, a physician with fellowship training in integrative medicine is the solo practitioner. She will soon be joined by a Nurse Practitioner with an integrative background. The main focus is internal medicine, but the practice has a particular emphasis on women's health care, which fits well with integrating CAM modalities. In addition to regular primary care, whole health assessments are provided on request. A primary care relationship is often established at that preventive visit.

The physician refers out to acupuncturists, a Traditional Chinese Medicine practitioner, biofeedback and guided imagery therapists, a homeopath, massage therapists, nutritionists, chiropractors, osteopaths, hypnotherapists and some others. She has met with most and reviewed their credentials, as she prefers to use licensed practitioners. Most practitioners provided a demonstration therapeutic session.

At the present time, this physician is reimbursed by insurance and Medicare, with some fee-for-service billing of patients who choose to see her outside their HMO or those who are uninsured. Her business plan is to build a strong reputation in the community, and then move to an integrative consultation-based model that is purely fee for service. There is no retail operation at IIMC.

Patient referrals come from a number of sources. Some self-refer for integrative services, and a number of patients come from local acupuncturists and other colleagues in the community. The physician is listed on the hospital physician finder under 'Integrative Medicine', and people find her on the Internet. Patients also come via public speaking presentations and the hospital's marketing efforts, which comprise television, radio appearances and newspaper articles. Most new referrals are family and friends of existing patients.

Development of a research program is in the business plan for the future, particularly after an associate physician joins the practice. IIMC also has plans to participate actively in community education and teaching of health-care professionals.

Patient relationships are built by inviting family members to be included in intake and often in the examination room, according to patient wishes. With other physicians, lines of communication are kept open and care is taken not to be aggressive with CAM until a consultation is sought.

The IIMC office uses a 'soft touch' – there is no voice mail. A pleasant medical assistant answers the telephone or returns calls promptly. Care has been taken to create a healing environment. Every effort is made to be on time and to demonstrate in other ways that patient interests are most important. For example, intake assessments are done in a quiet consultation room, and every patient is offered bottled water on arrival. Patients comment on how relaxed they feel in the office, which is the intent.

For more information about Integrative Internal Medicine Clinic, please see www.SDInt Med.com.

Integrative primary care within a fitness center – multidisciplinary group practice

Alitus Integrative Health & Wellness, Vernon Hills, IL

This comprehensive medical and fitness center integrates traditional family medicine with complementary medical services. Led by family physicians, the emphasis is on a holistic, personalized approach to family health care. Both physicians are fellowship-trained in integrative medicine. They are committed to being high-quality health-care providers when patients are ill, and wellness advisors to keep them feeling their best as a baseline.

In addition to primary medical care, Alitus Integrative Health & Wellness (Alitus) offers acupuncture, massage, naturopathy, yoga, Tai Chi, nutritional counseling, personal fitness training, podiatry and mental health services – all on site. The group does not hold team meetings, but do speak informally about patient and clinic issues. Referrals to Alitus come from patients, physicians and the CAM community.

Alitus has developed an innovative model of reimbursement under the heading of a 'retainer-style' program, with plans to blend fee-for-service and Medicare payments in the near future. Currently, each patient is assigned an annual fee (membership) and is offered a package, as described below. This ensures availability of the time and resources needed to provide for a personal relationship with a physician, grounded in a comprehensive, integrative approach to health and wellness. Alitus has a small retail operation selling a limited number of supplements – the most commonly recommended, such as multivitamins, omega-3 fatty acids and probiotics.

Alitus members may utilize their annual investment/package according to their individual needs and goals. The package consists of a specified number of visits for the fee – including an annual health maintenance visit – and they may redeem those visits with a practitioner of their own choosing. The physicians strongly encourage patients to take advantage of the personal training program. All patients are invited to consult a primary health-care team that not only treats current symptoms in the context of conventional medical care, but also serves as a resource to maintain total body wellness.

Alitus educates medical students and the physicians provide public education lectures. There is no research program at this time.

This innovative clinic model builds relationships with patients by providing time, easy access and attention to communication. Community speaking helps build community relationships. Alitus is not providing a CME program at this time.

To learn more about Alitus, please see www.northshorehealth.com.

A virtual model of integrative health care

Gwinnett Health System, Lawrenceville, GA

Gwinnett Health System (GHS) is a not-for-profit healthcare network serving Gwinnett County and the surrounding areas northeast of Atlanta, GA. The system includes three hospitals and other supporting medical facilities, more than 3800 employees, and 700 affiliated physicians. Their goal is to be the leading health system in the community by offering services to treat disease and injury, and to provide early intervention and preventive care.

Integrative medical services are offered throughout the system, but there is no particular center or clinic. A freestanding outpatient Community Health and Wellness Clinic provides an extensive array of programs such as nutrition and lifestyle counseling, corporate wellness, diabetes education, health and wellness programs, fitness classes and workshops, expressive arts and massage therapy. These programs are operated out of the Health and Wellness Clinic, but are offered at various locations around the hospital system. Practitioners such as nutritionists, health educators, nurses and massage therapists are both in-house and outreach. The health and wellness services are offered only to outpatients at present.

The integrative medicine committee at GHS is led by the director of health education and includes a representative from the fields of nutrition, clinical nursing, oncology nursing and marketing. Physicians, although encouraged to be involved, are not represented on the committee at this time, and integrative consultations with a physician are not a part of the program. Administrative support comes from the chief executive and operating officers, who are strongly in favor of health education services.

Reimbursement for the many health education and wellness services is largely fee for service. For inpatients, music therapy provided by a Celtic harpist in the hospital, and guided imagery sessions provided by some nurses, are free of charge. Patients and community members may self-refer for services and classes. The hospital gift shop sells essential oils and guided imagery CDs as a service to patients and program participants.

There is an active community health education program, and corporate health and wellness programs are taken to off-site workplaces. However, there is no CME program at this time. Nurses, health educators and administrators build relationships with each other by sitting on committees together; efforts are being made to engage physicians in the program.

GHS has a number of unique projects under way. A pilot program of guided imagery relaxation tapes for ventilated patients in the intensive care unit was carried out with positive outcomes at night time. A phase two study is under way in the daytime hours. The expressive arts program for women with breast cancer is enjoying much success, and a labyrinth was recently completed on the hospital grounds.

For more information about the health and wellness services at Gwinnett HealthCare System, please see www.gwinnetthealth.org/programs/programs.asp.

Integrative medicine in a health resort

Canyon Ranch, Tucson, AZ

Canyon Ranch is a system of health resorts and spa clubs committed to providing guests with an experience that combines relaxation and pampering with personalized health education. There are two main health resorts, in Tucson, AZ and Lenox, MA, and spa clubs in resorts in Las Vegas and Florida. There is also a Canyon Ranch spa aboard the Queen Mary 2 cruise ship. The goal at Canyon Ranch is to inspire and motivate guests to translate healthy intentions into sustainable action.

Health-conscious vacationers at Canyon Ranch design their own experience – choosing such areas as nutrition, preventive medicine, stress reduction, weight management, spiritual awareness, exercise and/or rest and relaxation. On-site practitioners at the main resorts include physicians, chiropractors, podiatrists, acupuncturists, a Traditional Chinese Medicine practitioner, nurses, behavioral health practitioners, exercise physiologists, spiritual guides, movement and aquatic therapists, nutritionists, massage therapists, estheticians and health educators.

Some guests choose to have a health and fitness assessment or their annual physical examination performed at Canyon Ranch. These people spend significant one-on-one time with a physician, have laboratory testing and investigations performed, and receive an in-depth evaluation and integrative health plan prior to check out. Canyon Ranch does not bill insurance for services offered; payment is fee for service with detailed receipts issued to patients.

Canyon Ranch participates in CAM research by donating funds for such research to two major universities. It is an accredited site for CME for physicians and nurses, offering the Life Enhancement Program, which is specifically designed to help health professionals make lasting lifestyle changes. Other courses, such as weight management, stress reduction and specific disease management are available in group-oriented 7-day programs that include time with a physician, laboratory work, nutrition and exercise counseling, and cardiometabolic testing (EKG stress testing that includes basal metabolic rate). Lectures on a number of topics from new medical research to special interest areas are provided. Physicians can earn CME credit for learning preventive practices in a clinical setting, learning how to teach patients about self-care and prevention, and learning how an interdisciplinary team can work together toward wellness goals.

There are a number of special programs available at Canyon Ranch, some focusing on chronic disease problems such as arthritis and diabetes, others on wellness such as heart health, woman's health and optimal aging.

For more information about Canyon Ranch, please see www.canyonranch.com.

CONCLUSION

Several models of integrative medical care have been presented. Each practice is unique, and reflects the philosophies and experiences of the leaders and visionaries involved, and – hopefully – the needs and desires of the patients being served. Development of an integrative medicine/oncology practice or center must be approached in the same fashion as any medical business, considering all aspects of a conventional business plan. For guidance in start-up, the physician or administrator can look to colleagues in existing integrative care centers, use integrative medicine consultants, search the Internet and attend conferences addressing the business of integrative medicine.

Integrative cancer care can be provided in any of the settings presented here. Persons with cancer seeking an integrative approach might quite conceivably appear at a family practitioner's office, a fitness center, a health resort, a multidisciplinary cancer center or an academic center. As long as the oncology practitioner is committed to honoring the whole person, as well as incorporating appropriate CAM therapies, that person is practicing integrative oncology.

ACKNOWLEDGMENTS

I wish to thank Donald Novey, MD, Nancy Schulman, MBA and Michael Cohen, JD for their help and direction in preparing this chapter: Dr Novey graciously shared his expertise on identifying and categorizing models of care, Ms Schulman reviewed the chapter and Mr Cohen was a valuable resource for specific historical information. My gratitude also goes to the directors of the clinics and centers featured as examples; they were more than willing to share their experiences. Many thanks to you all.

RESOURCES FOR MODELS OF CARE

Integrative medicine – business consultant

Nancy Schulman MBA
Integrative Health Solutions Boulder, CO
nancy@ihsolutions.info
www.ihsolutions.info

Integrative medicine – clinical consultants

Donald Novey MD
Medical Director, The Center for Complementary Medicine, Park Ridge, IL
President, Integrative Medicine Associates, Evanston, IL
dnovey@medicalmediasystems.com
www.medicalmediasystems.com/IMA

Bradly Jacobs MD MPH
Assistant Clinical Professor of Medicine, Osher Center for Integrative Medicine, Mail Box 1726,
University of California–San Francisco, San Francisco, CA 94143-1726
jacobsb@ocim.ucsf.edu
www.ucsf.edu/ocim

Integrative medicine – medicolegal consultant

Michael H. Cohen JD
Assistant Professor of Medicine and Director of Legal Programs, Harvard Medical School Osher Institute, 401 Park Drive, 22-W, Boston, MA 02215
www.camlawblog.com

Integrative medicine in the United Kingdom

The Prince of Wales's Foundation for Integrated Health
www.fihealth.org.uk

References

1. Ruggie M. Marginal to Mainstream: Alternative Medicine in America. UK: Cambridge University Press, 2004

2. Basch E, Ulbricht C. Natural Standard special report: CAM therapies in cancer and cancer prevention. J Cancer Integrative Med 2004; 2: 111–24

3. Boon H, Verhoef M, O'Hara D, et al. Integrative healthcare: Arriving at a working definition. Altern Ther Health Med 2004;10: 48–56

4. Definition of integrative medicine [online]. 2002 [accessed 28 November 2004]. Available from URL: http://nccam.nih.gov/health/whatis cam/index.htm#3

5. Kligler B, Maizes V, Schacter S, et al. Core competencies in integrative medicine for medical school curricula: A proposal. Acad Med 2004; 79: 521–31

6. Gordon J. Introductory remarks. The new medicine and the healing journey. CancerGuides®

Professional Training Program. 24–30 January 2004; Berkeley, California

7. Lewis C, de Vedia A, Reuer B, et al. Integrating complementary and alternative medicine (CAM) into standard hospice and palliative care. Am J Hosp Palliat Care 2003; 20: 221–8

8. Novey D. Integrative medicine delivery systems: Trends, lessons, and strategies. Proceedings of the 2nd Annual Integrative Medicine for Healthcare Organizations: Business Strategies, Practical Tools, and Best Practices. 22–24 January 2004; San Diego, California

9. Tepper J. Integrative modalities and their utility in cancer care. Proceedings of the 1st International Conference of the Society for Integrative Oncology. 17–19 November 2004; New York

10. Mann D, Gaylord S, Norton S. Moving toward integrative care: Rationales, models, and steps for conventional-care providers. Complementary Health Pract Rev 2004; 9: 155–72

6

Legal issues

Michael H. Cohen and David Rosenthal

'Those who think they know, do not know. Those who know they do not know, know.' – Upanishads

INTRODUCTION

The practice of integrative oncology raises important legal issues for clinicians and institutions. Integrative oncology can be defined as a comprehensive, evidence-based approach to cancer care which addresses the whole person. An integrative approach will often use a combination of conventional with complementary and alternative (CAM) therapies. In general, institutions must consider potential liability issues involved in hiring CAM providers as part of an integrative care team[1], as well as credentialing mechanisms for these providers[2]. Most clinicians are less involved in credentialing decisions but remain keenly concerned about the possibility that they might share liability with other members of the integrative care team (e.g. the neurologist and chiropractor, or the oncologist and acupuncturist, or the osteopath and massage therapist, each sharing liability for the other's negligence)[3].

This chapter focuses on the clinician – specifically, the oncologist whose patient seeks therapeutic advice concerning CAM therapies, is enrolled in a clinical trial that uses such therapies, or, perhaps, has determined to use such therapies with or without medical advice. Each of these scenarios presents differing yet parallel complexities; overall, the advent of integrative care presents situations in which clinicians sometimes can find themselves caught between the different demands of patient expectations, clinical judgement and liability considerations. Such complex scenarios often leave the clinicians with legitimate concern yet little professional guidance, either from their home institutions or from relevant professional groups. This is because clinical algorithms or pathways for integrative care do not yet exist; nor have many US hospitals, by and large, created a system of rational policies and procedures to help guide their clinicians through various liability dilemmas[4].

This environment might seem discouraging at first. The good news is that the field of CAM therapies has sufficiently shifted past the black-and-white rhetoric of 'proven' and 'unproven', 'conventional' and 'unconventional', 'orthodox' and 'unorthodox,' to serious, clinical considera- tion of integrative strategies, with appropriate disclosure and discussion of risks and benefits[5]. This means that the decision as to how to guide the patient deserves serious, extended discussion; it is no longer a matter of simply approving or disapproving of inclusion of CAM therapies generically. In short, a century of rhetoric has shifted into a fluid conversation of how to engage multiple clinical disciplines in a way that is 'clin- ically responsible, ethically appropriate, and legally defensible'[6].

The National Center for Complementary and Alternative Medicine (NCCAM) at the National Institutes of Health (NIH) currently defines integrative medicine as health care that 'combines mainstream medical therapies and CAM therapies for which there is some high- quality scientific evidence of safety and effective- ness'[7]. Such a definition implicitly recognizes the potential value of combining conventional and CAM therapies, provided that such therapies have 'some high-quality' evidentiary base. The NCCAM definition does not set an evidentiary threshold, thus leaving the clinician to make del- icate judgements at the borderland of good clin- ical and legal sense.

THE LAW RELEVANT TO INTEGRATIVE CARE

As a starting point, the law governing CAM providers and therapies (and, by extension, inte- grative care) grows out of, and overlaps with, sev- eral different areas of law governing conventional care (Table 6.1). The major areas are these seven: (1) licensure; (2) scope of practice; (3) malprac- tice liability; (4) professional discipline; (5) access to treatments; (6) third-party reimbursement; and (7) fraud[1].

'Licensure' refers to the requirement in most states that health-care providers maintain a cur- rent state license to practice their professional

Table 6.1 Overlapping areas of law concerning conventional and CAM therapies
Licensure
Scope of practice
Malpractice liability
Professional discipline
Access to treatments
Third party reimbursement
Fraud

healing art. While a few states recently have enacted statutes authorizing non-licensed CAM providers to practice[8], in most states licensure serves as the first hurdle to professional practice. Licensure of CAM providers varies by state; chi- ropractors, for example, are licensed in every state, whereas massage therapists and acupunc- turists are licensed in well over half the states, and naturopaths in about a dozen states[2].

'Scope of practice' refers to the legally author- ized boundaries of care within the given profession. State licensing statutes usually define a CAM provider's scope of practice; regulations by the relevant state licensing board (for example, the board of chiropractic) often supplement or interpret the relevant licensing statute; and both statutes and administrative regulations are interpreted by courts (see reference 1, pp. 39–46). For example, chiropractors can give nutritional advice in some states but not others; typically, massage therapists are prohibited from mental health counseling. (For a list of state licensing statutes, see reference 9*). Licensing and scope of practice definitions can serve as general guidelines for reasonable CAM practices.

'Malpractice' refers to negligence, which is defined as failure to use due care (or follow the standard of care) in treating a patient, and thereby injuring the patient. Generally, each CAM profession is judged by its own standard of care – for example, acupuncture, chiropractic,

*These statutes can change over time and the authors are not aware of any current Web listing, although individual professional organizations may maintain current lists. For addresses of CAM professional organizations, see reference 2.

physical therapy, massage therapy[1]. In cases where the provider's clinical care overlaps with medical care – for example, the chiropractor who takes and reads a patient's X-ray – then the medical standard might be applied[1]. 'Professional discipline' refers to the power of the relevant professional board – in the oncologist's case, the state medical board – to sanction a clinician, most gravely by revoking the clinician's license. The concern over inappropriate discipline, based on medical board antipathy to inclusion of CAM therapies, has led consumer groups in many states to lobby for 'health freedom' statutes – laws providing that physicians may not be disciplined solely on the basis of incorporating CAM modalities. (See reference 1, pp. 92–95. For a listing of current states, see http://www.healthlobby.com/statelaw.html.) More recently, the Federation of State Medical Boards has issued Model Guidelines for Physician Use of Complementary and Alternative Therapies, reaffirming this same principle[10]. The opening paragraph of this document states 'a full and frank discussion of the risks and benefits of all medical practices is in the patient's best interest.' The text continues with an analysis of practice criteria for both conventional and CAM treatments based on safety and efficacy data. The document then states 'the Board recognizes that a licensed physician shall not be found guilty of unprofessional conduct for failure to practice medicine in an acceptable manner solely on the basis of utilizing CAM' (see reference 1, pp. 66–67).

'Access to treatments' refers to the interest by patients in obtaining therapeutic substances outside typical clinical delivery. These generally fall into two categories: dietary supplements, and drugs not approved by the federal Food and Drug Administration (FDA) (see reference 1, pp. 73–86). The Dietary Supplement Health and Education Act of 1994 (DSHEA) provided that 'dietary supplements' – containing vitamins, minerals, amino acids, and herbs – generally were to be regulated as foods, not drugs, and therefore could be sold in interstate commerce without prior proof of safety or efficacy.

Since the enactment of the DSHEA, case reports have emerged in the medical literature concerning safety issues associated with various herbal products; studies have shown the possibility for serious adverse herb–drug interactions; and the efficacy of popular supplements such as St John's wort has been called into question. Regarding non-FDA-approved drugs, federal legislation has been introduced several times in Congress authorizing patient access (the Access to Medical Treatment Act), but the legislation has not been approved. Meanwhile, if no viable, approved conventional treatment exists, the FDA has provided several mechanisms for expedited access to non-approved drugs, under certain circumstances, to patients enrolled in clinical trials (see reference 1, pp. 73–77).

'Third-party reimbursement' involves a number of insurance policy provisions, and corresponding legal rules, designed to ensure that reimbursement is limited to 'medically necessary' treatment; does not, in general, cover 'experimental' treatments; and is not subject to fraud and abuse (see reference 1, pp. 96–108). In general, insurers have been slow to offer CAM therapies as core benefits – largely because of insufficient evidence of safety, efficacy and cost-effectiveness – though a number of insurers have offered policyholders discounted access to a network of CAM providers, such as chiropractors and acupuncturists.

'Health-care fraud' refers to the legal concern for preventing intentional deception of patients. Overbroad claims sometimes can lead to charges of fraud, and its related legal theory, misrepresentation (see reference 1, pp. 68–70). Legal recovery under these theories also can potentially cover advertising that makes unsubstantiated claims of efficacy for specific uses of CAM therapies. Further, if the clinician or institution submits a reimbursement claim for care that the clinician knew, or should have known, was medically unnecessary, this also might be grounds for a finding of fraud and abuse under federal law (see reference 1, pp. 104–108).

CLINICAL CASES

With these general legal rules as background, consider the following hypothetical clinical cases.

Case one: the clinical trial with a contaminated herbal product

The Department for Integrative Oncology at Dewey Medical Center (DIODMC) received a three-million-dollar grant from the NIH to run a phase III clinical trial comparing the best conventional treatment with Formula X, an herbal formula that had considerable anecdotal evidence of success in Asia, and no evidence of causing patient harm. Together with his outstanding team of co-investigators and research assistants, Paul Plympton, MD, an oncologist, Professor of Medicine at Dewey Medical, and principal investigator of the clinical trial, recruited 300 patients to participate in the trial. Appropriate informed consents were given to each patient in accordance with recruitment procedures approved by Dewey Medical's institutional review board.

The protocol provided that patients who would otherwise receive a therapeutic recommendation of chemotherapy or radiation were to take Formula X for a period of 2 weeks, while their tumors were conventionally monitored. If any patient's tumor progressed past a certain pre-defined point, the patient was to be taken off Formula X and given chemotherapy or radiation as medically necessary and appropriate.

As part of his grant application, Professor Plympton had included a colleague who would use various assays and screens to break Formula X into its component parts, in an attempt to find the active ingredient.

Two months into the clinical trial, the data showed that, of the 39 patients enrolled to date who had received Formula X, a statistically significant number had benefited from the formula's use (the rate of tumor growth expected was diminished by a statistically significant constant). However, the trial's 'power' was not yet significant; Formula X would not be proven effective until results were achieved for at least 80% of the targeted recruitment population.

Professor Plympton was treating his 40th patient when he received a call from his co-investigator, alerting him that the brand of Formula X that he had purchased from an Asian manufacturer had a contaminant. This contaminant carried a small risk of harming the patient enrollees. Professor Plympton, fearing the consequences, hesitated to call the hospital's legal counsel before consulting internally with his team. In subsequent internal discussions, he learned that: (1) contamination of the Formula X sample made the herbal product legally 'adulterated' under relevant FDA law and regulations; (2) even if the investigators managed to obtain non-contaminated Formula X from another supplier, the variability of the formula's constituents from batch to batch made it difficult to offer patients any quality assurance; and (3) even if the contaminant posed a small risk to enrollees, that risk had not been disclosed and discussed, and therefore the informed consent was tainted.

Professor Plympton felt torn. On one hand, Formula X seemed to be helping his patients improve, and appeared to be outperforming the other arm of the study or conventional therapy. Nobody else in the country was testing the formula, and he was nearing a statistically significant sample size. On the other hand, he had to be guided by the ethical obligation to 'do no harm'. He told his team: 'I'm reluctant to abandon the trial and reluctant to abandon our patient enrollees, yet hesitant to continue treatment with a contaminated herbal product'. He wondered about his legal and ethical obligations to his patients in the clinical trial, and about the consequences of either continuing or stopping the trial.

Case two: the patient who abandons chemotherapy

Dr Plympton put three patients on a course of traditional chemotherapy. All three, however, had read a report featured on the Internet site MSN.com that week, opining that energy healing, combined with a unique nutritional protocol, can reduce tumors faster than chemotherapy. The report quoted an oncologist who did not provide any medical evidence to back up his assertion. All three patients were refusing chemotherapy and insisting on trying the alternative protocol featured on the website.

Dr Plympton was troubled by his patients' request. He tried to argue – unsuccessfully with each – that the patients were biased by what they had seen on the Internet, and that there was no medical evidence to support the Texas oncologist's claim. Each patient insisted on rejecting Dr Plympton's advice. Dr Plympton, feeling the tug of this conflict between his patients' wishes, and his obligation to 'do no harm', was uncertain of his legal and ethical responsibility.

He contacted the hospital's attorney and reported his dilemma, then added a series of questions:

- What do I do when patients demand and expect to use CAM therapies that lack a sufficient base in the medical evidence to justify my recommending these therapies?

- What do I do when patients insist on making their own decisions, against medical advice?

- Am I responsible if patients use CAM therapies without informing me, and are thereby injured?

- The first patient, John Runyon, has early-stage Hodgkin's disease, a condition curable by traditional radiation therapy or chemotherapy. The second patient, Jane Hernandez, has newly diagnosed acute leukemia. The third, Doug Smith, has advanced refractory non-small-cell lung cancer stage IV. John Runyon has done a lot of his own research and understands the risks and benefits of trying the CAM approach, whereas Jane Hernandez and Doug Smith state that they are willing to try anything.

- Does it make a difference if we are facing potentially curable disease versus an incurable disease? Does it matter if we are using the intervention as supportive care versus as an antineoplastic agent?

- What are my obligations to discuss the risks and benefits in each scenario?

- What if the patient does not abandon conventional therapy but has a complication from the interaction of conventional therapy with the CAM therapy, and there is little, if any, medical literature to inform the clinician (for example, concerning the combination of chemotherapy and high-dose antioxidants)?

- What if the patient asks me for a referral to a CAM therapist and I feel this is not in the patient's best medical interest?

- What is the liability of the Texas oncologist making the claim for an unproven treatment? What is the liability of the Internet site?

Theories of malpractice liability

Essentially, there are two basic theories on which clinicians typically are found liable for professional malpractice. The first involves negligence, or lack of due care. Under this theory, 'medical malpractice' is defined as providing clinical care below generally accepted professional standards, and thereby causing the patient injury.

The second theory involves a failure of informed consent. The legal obligation of informed consent is to provide the patient with all the information material to a treatment decision – in other words, that would make a difference in the patient's choice to undergo or forgo a given therapeutic protocol. These two theories of malpractice apply across the board, whether CAM or conventional therapies are involved (see Table 6.2) (see reference 1, pp. 56–62).

In Case One, if Professor Plympton were to continue the clinical trial, knowing that the herbal product was unsafe, he would probably be violating the professional standard of care owed to enrolled patients, and this violation of care would most likely injure the patient. Hence, malpractice concerns would suggest stopping the trial.

The case states that the contaminant in Formula X poses a 'small' risk to enrollees. The greater the risk of injury to enrollees, the greater the likelihood of a lawsuit, and the greater the likelihood that Dr Plympton will be liable for malpractice. If no patient is injured, then by definition a lawsuit will be unsuccessful.

There are several additional concerns. The first is that the presence of the contaminant, and its hazards, were not disclosed to the patients enrolled in the trial. Since such a risk would probably be material to a patient's decision to take or not to take Formula X, such failed disclosure would be likely to constitute inadequate informed consent, the second theory of malpractice liability. However, as urgently, the informed consent required for human research subjects is even more stringent than that required for clinical care generally. The hospital's institutional review board would be most likely to require that the trial be halted.

Adulteration of dietary supplements also violates federal food and drug law. Dr Plympton would be well advised to stop the clinical trial, and to inform any enrollees who had received Formula X about the contaminant and its attendant risks and benefits. (He would also have been wise to perform a thorough analysis of the Formula X compound prior to initiating the trial for

Table 6.2 Malpractice liability
Standard of care violation
Failure to obtain adequate informed consent

two reasons: to identify any contaminants; and to ensure that if the study were positive, the results could be replicated by using a similar compound. This, however, is not always possible.)

Having analyzed the legal issues, we are left with some ethical complications in the case. The clinician has a duty of beneficence (benefiting the patient) as well as of non-maleficence (doing no harm). In the case, Dr Plympton is torn between the desire to keep patients on Formula X, since it seems to be helping, and the concern for the small risk of harm from the contaminant. The concern for patient safety, however, usually trumps the possibility that there might be a benefit, unless the evidence of efficacy is unusually strong, in which case physician and patient together may be willing to accept more risk.

Abandoning patients is ethically proscribed and legally yet another ground for suit[11]. Dr Plympton need not abandon his patients, but rather should offer them the option of continuing conventional care for their condition; however, he will be unable to offer them Formula X, unless he has resolved both the informed consent and the FDA adulteration issues.

Suppose one of the patients insists on obtaining and continuing to use Formula X outside the clinical trial – say from a naturopathic physician unaffiliated with the medical center. If Dr Plympton plans to continue monitoring and treating that patient, he needs to consider the liability implications in more detail (discussed in the following section). If Dr Plympton feels uncomfortable continuing to monitor and treat that patient conventionally, then again, abandonment is not an option; Dr Plympton should refer the patient to another oncologist who would be able to see the patient under these conditions[11]. He should be sure to report use of the drug and details of its adulteration so that appropriate warnings could be posted.

A framework for assessing potential liability

A useful and more detailed framework for assessing the potential exposure for malpractice liability involves reviewing the medical evidence regarding safety and efficacy for any CAM therapies included in the patient's therapeutic regimen. This framework is applicable across clinician specialties and applicable whether the oncologist is practicing within an integrative clinical care center styled as such, a hospital oncology department, or a freestanding clinic.

Specifically, clinicians seeking to assess their potential malpractice liability risk in counseling patients concerning CAM therapies should evaluate whether the medical evidence: (1) supports both safety and efficacy; (2) supports safety, but evidence regarding efficacy is inconclusive; (3) supports efficacy, but evidence regarding safety is inconclusive; or (4) indicates either serious risk or inefficacy[12]. Figure 6.1 expresses possible permutations.

Thus, if (1) the medical evidence supports both safety and efficacy, liability is unlikely, and clinicians should recommend the CAM therapy; if (4) the medical evidence indicates either serious risk or inefficacy, liability is probable, and clinicians should avoid and actively discourage the patient from using the CAM therapy; if the medical evidence (2) supports safety, but evidence regarding efficacy is inconclusive, or (3) supports efficacy, but evidence regarding safety is inconclusive, then clinicians should caution the patient and, while accepting the patient's choice to try the CAM therapy, continue to monitor efficacy and safety respectively[12]. In either case (2) or (3), liability is conceivable but probably unlikely, particularly in case (2) where the product is presumably safe[12].

A specific example that comes up frequently is the use of acupuncture and herbs, which can fall in the gray region of (2) and (3). Again, these categories are flexible. Thus, for example, if the CAM therapy is supportive or preventive, the physician might feel comfortable recommending it in region (2), while discouraging it in region (3); whereas if using an antineoplastic goal, the physician might be willing to tolerate either case with caution, depending upon the patient's situation and options.

To address the questions in Case Two in this analysis, if patients demand and expect to use CAM therapies that lack a sufficient base in the

Therapies that may be recommended:	Therapies that may be accepted:	Therapies that should be discouraged:
Evidence supports efficacy	Evidence regarding efficacy is inconclusive	Evidence indicates inefficacy
and	but	or
Evidence supports safety	Evidence supports safety	Evidence indicates serious risk

Figure 3.1 Guidelines for advising patients based on evidence of efficacy and safety. (Adapted from reference 13)

medical evidence to justify the clinician's recommending these therapies, then the clinician should decide whether the therapy fits within categories (2), (3), or (4) in the above framework, and accordingly either (2) caution and monitor efficacy; (3) caution and monitor safety; or (4) avoid and discourage.

In general, if patients insist on making their own decisions, against medical advice, the clinician should document this in the medical record[12]. There is a legal doctrine known as 'assumption of risk'. The doctrine can, under some circumstances, provide a defense to medical malpractice where the patient has chosen a therapeutic course despite the physician's efforts to dissuade and discourage (see reference 3, pp. 26–31).

In some states, if patients continue to use a CAM therapy against the physician's advice, and this is documented in the medical record, there may be a defense to a malpractice action (see reference 3, pp. 26–31). Some attorneys might advise physicians to have the patient sign a waiver, expressly stating that the patient knowingly, voluntarily, and intelligently chose the CAM therapy or regimen – for example, energy healing and a nutritional protocol – instead of the recommended conventional treatment. Courts, however, tend to disfavor waivers of liability in medical malpractice cases, taking the perspective that medical negligence cannot be waived away, and that the physician remains responsible for the patient's treatment. Thus, signed waivers are not always enforceable.

Case Two also asks whether Dr Plympton is responsible if his patients use CAM therapies without informing him, and are thereby injured. At first blush, Dr Plympton should not be responsible. He should, however, take due care in getting an accurate and adequate medical history, inquiring into use of CAM therapies, including all dietary supplements. Such a full history is especially important because of the possibility of adverse herb–drug interactions. One might even reasonably argue that it would be negligent *not* to

inquire into use of CAM therapies or any OTC medication. Assuming Dr Plympton has performed this due diligence, in a thorough way, it is up to the patient to report honestly; Dr Plympton should not be liable for adverse interactions with CAM therapies the patient is using that the patient fails, after reasonable inquiry by Dr Plympton, to disclose.

Further considerations

The next part of the case offers three variations: a patient (John Runyon) with early-stage Hodgkin's disease, a condition curable by traditional chemotherapy; a second patient (Jane Hernandez) with newly diagnosed acute leukemia; and a third (Doug Smith) with non-small-cell lung cancer, Stage IV. The case asks whether these patients are distinguishable in terms of the way liability concerns might shape Dr Plympton's clinical choices.

From a liability perspective, the more acute and severe the condition, the more important it would be to monitor and treat conventionally. Again, the definition of medical malpractice emphasizes failure to follow the standard of care, and patient injury. The greater the disease's severity, the more likely the patient injury will result from over-relying on a CAM therapy – and thus the greater possibility for a lawsuit with concomitant malpractice liability; as well, the more likely the oncologist will be held liable for failure to insist on standard, conventional care. Further, the more curable the condition conventionally, the more likely a court would be to see failure to provide (or even, perhaps, insist on) such care as negligent. The first discussion of treatment by a physician could make the difference between acceptance or rejection by the patient. Careful thought needs to be placed here by the oncology team.

Therefore, Dr Plympton should strongly advise John Runyon (whose condition is curable with chemotherapy) and Jane Hernandez (who has an acute condition that can rapidly progress, and also has curative intent with conventional treatment options), to consider conventional care. If either of these patients insists on trying CAM therapies instead of chemotherapy, Dr Plympton may choose to try to persuade them to accept a time-limited approach, monitored conventionally, with conventional care as an option if specific results do not occur within a specified time. This period of time may vary based on the patients' specific disease stage and natural history. Most importantly, Dr Plympton should provide education and counseling concerning the natural history of their disease, and risks that may be associated with a delay in proven conventional therapy. An integrative approach would also educate the patient concerning CAM methods that are supportive in nature, and can assist in improving quality of life and tolerance of conventional therapies. Other members of the integrative team, including a nutritionist, psychologist, nurse and social workers, may be especially helpful as a part of this discussion. Again, integrative care should include integration of the conventional caregivers who can offer supportive services as part of the team.

One could argue that Doug Smith is in a different category. His condition is incurable, so the benefit of chemotherapy is purely palliative in nature. In fact, in his situation, the side-effects could outweigh the benefit – he may live longer, but be more sick while he is alive – the proverbial 'cure that is worse than the disease'. Or, even if the side-effects are endurable, the benefit would be palliative and not curative. Because levels of evidence are ever-changing and patients may make individual choices, strong emphasis should be placed on a respectful dialogue that attends to and incorporates the patient's wishes.

As a caveat, oncologists should consider the case of *U.S. v. Rutherford*, in which terminally ill cancer patients sought to obtain laetrile, a non-FDA-approved drug[14]. These patients argued that they had a right to obtain the treatment of their choice, since they were dying of cancer. The US Supreme Court affirmed a lower court ruling denying these patients access to the treatment they sought. The Court reasoned that Congress, in enacting the relevant federal statute, had intended to shield even terminally ill patients from potential fraud. *Rutherford* suggests that some courts may make no distinction between patients with curable versus incurable conditions, particularly when the case involves a therapy (such as laetrile) where the evidence shows no efficacy.

A deeper ethical analysis

Another cut at Dr Plympton's question with regard to these different patients is a detailed ethical analysis of his obligation. Adams *et al.* offer seven factors to consider in assessing whether or not to offer the patient CAM therapies[11]:

(1) Severity and acuteness of illness;

(2) Curability with conventional treatment;

(3) Invasiveness, toxicities, and side-effects of conventional treatment;

(4) Quality of evidence of safety and efficacy of the CAM treatment;

(5) Degree of understanding of the risks and benefits of conventional and CAM treatments;

(6) Knowing and voluntary acceptance of those risks by the patient;

(7) Persistence of patient's intention to utilize CAM treatment.

Applying these factors, all three patients have a severe and/or acute illness; John Runyon's and Jane Hernandez's are potentially curable with chemotherapy. This treatment, however, has severe toxicities and side-effects. On the other hand, the quality of evidence for efficacy of the CAM treatment they seek is low, although there is no evidence of harm. John Runyon's early-stage Hodgkin's disease can progress but is certainly less immediately life threatening than the acute leukemia of Jane Hernandez. The case supposes that, while all three strongly intend to use CAM therapies, only one of the patients understands the risks and benefits of trying the CAM approach, and knowingly and voluntarily accepts the risks of that approach.

It is sometimes difficult to apply a multifactorial approach, but this is the reality of most clinical situations (Table 6.3). It seems clear, however, that at least for Jane Hernandez, it is ethically compelling to try the CAM approach for a limited period of time, if at all. The oncologist must ensure that she understands the natural history of her disease and implications of treatment delay. The entire integrative oncology team should ensure that the patient understands the risks and benefits, is willing to assume the risk of trying such an approach, and insists on this route; with full disclosure that the corresponding conventional approach carries toxicities and side-effects (e.g. nausea, hair loss, etc.), but has proven life-saving benefits. John Runyon's early-stage Hodgkin's disease may be treated more reasonably with a monitored, wait-and-see approach. His disease is not nearly as acute or life threatening, but all of the above communications must also take place. Finally, Doug Smith's metastatic lung cancer presentation has no current curative intent conventional treatment option, and yet a phase I/II new experimental therapy may have significant side-effects. Certainly, a monitored approach in this situation would be the most reasonable of the three cases.

It is clear that the patients' individual circumstances – including the stage of their disease, performance status and goal of therapy – enter significantly into any treatment recommendation. It is of the utmost importance that patients have a clear understanding of the risks and benefits of the approach they advocate. The ethical scales would be further evened if Dr Plympton engaged them in a conversation about these risks and benefits.

Table 6.3 Clinical issues related to the legalities of integrative oncology
Delay of effective treatment (conventional or CAM)
Patient abandonment
Level of evidence of treatment concerning safety and efficacy
Benefiting patient versus doing no harm
Liability of Integrative Team for individual member's actions
Referral to CAM practitioners
Interactions of CAM and CAM, CAM and conventional
Cost
Shared decision making including the patient

Intent of therapy
  curative versus palliative
  supportive care or symptom control
  prevention

On the whole, integrative oncology suggests the need for such conversations. Even though the legal obligation of informed consent *mandates* disclosure of risks and benefits, the premise of integrative care suggests the importance of engaging patients in shared decision making, rather than the physician only choosing between the three possibilities suggested in the liability analysis above: recommend, tolerate, or reject. Most importantly, Dr Plympton, with the oncology team, should review all the clinical options with each patient. In the scenario of 'tolerating' (or accepting) the patient's persistent interest in using CAM therapies, he should be ready to step in with conventional medical care if and when appropriate, in shared decision making with the patient. Involving the entire integrative oncology team will also prove helpful, in the least as a supportive care measure, and to ensure patient understanding of medical concepts.

Complications

Case Two also asks what happens if the patient does not abandon conventional therapy, but rather, has a complication from the interaction of conventional therapy with the CAM therapy, and there is little, if any, medical literature to inform the clinician (for example, concerning the combination of chemotherapy and high-dose antioxidants). This presents a paradox of integrative medicine: the effort to engage in shared decision making can be frustrated not only by different perspectives, but also by lack of sufficient evidence to inform a decision. Once again, looking at the intent of a therapy, and its risks and benefits, may help to guide levels of evidence needed to recommend a therapy or avoid an interaction. Individual oncologists may have particular biases toward or against certain practices (for example, choosing to avoid all antioxidants during definitive radiation, and instead recommending non-ingestible supportive care measures that have general efficacy with regards to supportive care endpoints, such as group support and individual counseling, guided imagery, etc. during conventional radiation). Currently, much of the evidence is so conflicting that the best practice may be to inform the patient of that fact until studies document efficacy or not, safety or not.

The liability framework presented earlier presents a reasonable initial screening guide for the clinician. If there is little evidence of safety or efficacy, and on the other hand none of harm or inefficacy, then the CAM therapy can be accepted for a period of time, while the oncologist continues to monitor conventionally, given that clinical information specific to that individual case allows for a reasonable fit, considering all the criteria noted above. If the therapy turns out to be either unsafe or ineffective, then the oncologist accordingly should advise the patient to discontinue its use (with the caveat that early intervention may be warranted, since otherwise the oncologist may not learn of an adverse effect until it is too late). Since research regarding CAM therapies is ongoing and the medical evidence can change rapidly, the oncologist should communicate regularly with the patient regarding any new developments. If, for example, it turns out that high-dose antioxidants negatively interact with chemotherapy, then this information may change the decision to continue using high-dose antioxidants during chemotherapy, or to rely on them as part of a CAM regimen for a period instead of chemotherapy. It is important to bear in mind that integrative oncology has three general goals – preventive, supportive and antineoplastic – and that these must be discussed with patients, educating them that most CAM therapies are supportive and preventive in nature.

Updating the patient about changes in medical evidence also is an important part of the informed consent obligation. If the discussion involves an herbal product (such as Formula X in Case One), the oncologist should try to deconstruct the notion that 'natural' necessarily means 'safe'. It should be noted that some patients are more deferential/compliant to clinical authority, whereas others are resistant. In any event, from the perspective of the ethical framework presented above, informing the patient about the changing medical evidence may shift (in one direction or another) the patient's willingness to accept the known risks and benefits of the CAM therapy, or even to use this therapy.

Parenthetically, the discussion so far largely involves advising clinicians in situations in which patients are making choices contrary to medical advice. An interesting question is how the law might treat clinicians who fail to make recommendations for patients regarding nutrition, mind–body treatments or other readily accepted CAM therapies as adjuncts to conventional care. As medical evidence begins to show safety and efficacy for such therapies, and these therapies become more generally accepted within the medical community, there may be liability for clinicians who fail to make helpful, adjunctive recommendations involving CAM therapies (reference 1, p. 59).

Consider the following scenario.

111

Case three: failure to inform about viable CAM options

A 45-year-old woman is being treated with adjuvant chemotherapy for breast cancer and develops significant nausea. She has an extrapyramidal reaction to Compazine and has to pay out of pocket for Zofran, which costs her over $1000 for her entire course. She learns, through a support group, about complementary modalities that may have been used to help her nausea, and begins using acupuncture with a 'Relief Band'; this results in total resolution of her symptoms. She feels that this therapy, which an NIH Consensus Statement has determined to be effective, should have been offered to her (this would still be an out of pocket cost, but much less). She seeks legal counsel concerning expenses for the other drugs, including pain and suffering.

In this case, one could argue that there was failure of informed consent, as well as failure to treat with a safe and effective CAM option. Again, the patient's successful claim would probably depend on the court's view of whether the medical profession generally accepted the CAM therapy as safe and effective for her condition, and indeed, as a safer and more effective therapeutic option than the conventional drug for which she had incurred expense (reference 1, pp. 60–62). This case points out the need for dissemination of information concerning the efficacy and safety of proven CAM treatment options, as well as a need to teach physicians how to discuss and refer patients with CAM providers.

REFERRALS

While there are few judicial opinions setting precedent regarding referrals to CAM therapists, the general rule in conventional care is that there is no liability merely for referring to a specialist. There is no particular reason why this rule

should not be applied to any referral, whether for conventional or CAM care (see reference 3, pp. 47–58).

One of the exceptions to this general rule, however, involves 'joint treatment', in which various clinicians collaborate to develop a treatment plan and to monitor and treat the patient. Such co-ordinated care is a premise of integrative care. It suggests that liabilities may be shared within the integrative care team – for example, between the oncologist and the acupuncturist, whether or not they are employed by or operating within the same health-care institution.

If, in Case Two, Dr Plympton feels that the requested referral to a CAM therapist is not in the patient's medical interest, Dr Plympton can decide not to provide such a referral. So long as he continues conventional monitoring and care, Dr Plympton would not thereby be abandoning the patient. On the other hand, if the patient insists on a referral to a CAM provider, such a referral should not in itself necessarily make Dr Plympton liable for negligence by such a provider. This statement must be modified by the following caveats: first, when patients sue, they tend to sue up and down the chain of providers, and immunity from being named as a defendant is not guaranteed; second, Dr Plympton should not refer to a CAM provider whom he knows or should have reason to know could be dangerous; third, he should document in the medical record that he and the patient have discussed the referral, and his opinion about whether the referral for CAM therapies would be likely to be safe and/or effective.

CAM THERAPIES AVAILABLE WITHIN THE INSTITUTION

Some institutions offer CAM therapies outside the setting of the oncology center. For example, many hospitals may have acupuncturists, credentialed and hired to work within the pain unit. The question arises as to how the oncologist should handle requests for referral to an acupuncturist within such a unit.

One approach is to contact the patient's primary care physician (PCP), and inform the PCP that the patient has requested the CAM therapy (in this case, acupuncture). Appendix 1 provides a sample guideline and form used at Dana-Farber Cancer Institute (DFCI). The guideline lists conditions that are known potentially to benefit from acupuncture, as well as those that may not benefit from acupuncture.

By involving the PCP, the oncologist can reduce the risk of liability. Such a form helps involve the oncologist and reduces the possibility that the patient will over-rely on acupuncture to the detriment of necessary medical care, or suffer from contraindications or adverse reactions. While shared liability for negligence may still be the rule, the overall risk of liability is reduced.

LIABILITY FOR DELAY

As suggested, if a condition readily can be cured by conventional care, there is a strong ethical imperative to provide such care, in balance with the other ethical factors noted above. Consider the following case).

Case four: delay of curative conventional care

A 45-year-old woman with locally advanced breast cancer comes to our radiation oncology office with a 3-year history of breast cancer. She was advised by a friend to seek out help from alternative medicine in order to avoid the toxicities of conventional medicine. She went to a clinic in the USA specializing in CAM therapies and has been treated with intravenous chelation, a variety of herbs and homeopathic remedies, nutritional supplements and some rudimentary mind–body interventions (guided imagery tapes). Her cancer has progressed and the head of the clinic has told her that it is her fault because she 'cannot visualize her disease' and has not followed their recommendations concerning buying their proprietary supplements.

She now learns of an integrative approach and is using conventional medicine and supportive CAM therapies with good results. She is quite angry about the delay in receiving this therapy and wants to know whether she has any legal recourse against the CAM clinic and its practitioners.

This case can be analyzed by returning to the definition of medical malpractice: violation of the professional standard of care, with injury to the patient. Because the clinic this patient visited purported to treat her disease (cancer), it would probably be held to the medical standard of care. Failing to monitor conventionally and to provide necessary conventional care could be considered violation of the standard of care.

Delay in itself is not negligent, but delay that aggravates the patient's condition or leads to irreversible progression of the disease might be considered negligent. If the patient 'knowingly, voluntarily, and intelligently' assumed the risk of trying CAM therapies for a time, and as a result, deteriorated, a court might find in such 'assumption of risk' a defense to malpractice. Again, states vary, as do the results of individual cases.

Certainly, blaming the patient for her disease progression (with reference to visualization) is not a good strategy, nor is it ethically responsible. From a liability perspective, poor communication between doctor and patient often leads to litigation. The clinic specializing in CAM therapies would have been well advised to provide full disclosure (and discussion) of risks and benefits for various therapeutic options, and to engage the patient in shared decision making. Finally, many states would view the clinic's selling dietary supplements to their patients as presenting an unethical conflict of interest, and would have legislation banning such sales of supplements. Again, blaming the patient for refusing to purchase these supplements could give a jury a strong negative impression about the clinic's commitment to its patients' health. Other issues in integrative oncology include physician selling or branding of substances; and assumption of risk as potential defense to malpractice.

FEDERATION OF STATE MEDICAL BOARD GUIDELINES

As noted, the Federation has passed model guidelines for: '(1) physicians who use CAM in their practices, and/or (2) those who co-manage patients with licensed or otherwise state-regulated CAM providers'[15]. These guidelines are not binding, but rather offer a framework for individual state medical boards to regulate physicians integrating CAM therapies. They should be read in conjunction with existing medical board guidelines in the state in which the oncologist practices, as the guidelines may provide ways for medical boards to think about integrative practices.

In general, the guidelines 'allow a wide degree of latitude in physicians' exercise of their professional judgment and do not preclude the use of any methods that are reasonably likely to benefit patients without undue risk'. The guidelines also recognize that 'patients have a right to seek any kind of care for their health problems', and that 'a full and frank discussion of the risks and benefits of all medical practices is in the patient's best interest'. To this extent, the guidelines implicitly recognize both shared decision making and patients' interest in integrative care.

At the same time, in trying to assess whether an integrative care practice is violative and should trigger physician discipline, the guidelines ask whether the therapy selected is:

- Effective and safe? (having adequate scientific evidence of efficacy and/or safety or greater safety than other established treatment models for the same condition);

- Effective, but unsafe? (having evidence of efficacy, but also significant adverse side-effects);

- Inadequately studied, but safe? (having insuficient evidence of clinical efficacy, but reasonable evidence to suggest relative safety);

- Ineffective and unsafe? (proven to be ineffective or unsafe through controlled trials or documented evidence or as measured by a risk/benefit assessment).

These guidelines deal only with the level of data concerning a specific therapy: the details of the patient's clinical situation, the goals of the intended therapy, the costs, and their understanding of the situation are equally important items for consideration, even if a therapy is proven effective and safe. Note that the Federation standards are similar to the malpractice guidelines offered earlier, although the guidelines leave greater ambiguity. For example, the first category is stated in terms of the CAM therapy having proven 'efficacy and/or safety or greater evidence of safety' than the applicable conventional treatment. There may or may not be adequate levels of available evidence to suggest whether this condition is met. Moreover, the guidelines list these four categories but do not offer suggestions for how to utilize the categories in clinical decision making.

In addition to the above standards, the guidelines provide an extensive checklist of items to which the physician must attend when providing CAM therapies. The oncologist practicing integrative care should review these items with legal counsel and determine which are advisable and practical. For example, these items include documentation regarding[15]:

- What medical options have been discussed, offered or tried, and if so, to what effect, or a statement as to whether or not certain options have been refused by the patient or guardian;

- That proper referral has been offered for appropriate treatment; that the risks and benefits of the use of the recommended treatment to the extent known have been appropriately discussed with the patient or guardian;

- That the physician has determined the extent to which the treatment could interfere with any other recommended or ongoing treatment.

The guidelines also provide that the CAM treatment should[15]:

- Have a favorable risk/benefit ratio compared to other treatments for the same condition;

- Be based upon a reasonable expectation that it will result in a favorable patient outcome, including preventive practices;

- Be based upon the expectation that a greater benefit will be achieved than that which can be expected with no treatment.

Again, the guidelines are suggestive but not binding in any given state, unless adopted by that state's medical board. (You may find out whether your state medical board has adopted this, or another policy, by contacting them directly.)

If these guidelines were applied to the integrative care clinic in Case Four, the head of the CAM center would probably receive discipline. Among other things, the case suggests that the chosen treatment was not based on a reasonable expectation of a favorable outcome, did not necessarily have a more favorable risk/benefit ratio than the applicable conventional care alone, and may in fact have interfered with recommended treatment. The case also suggests that the patient was not engaged in a full and fair conversation regarding the potential benefits and risks of the integrative treatment plan provided in the clinic.

CONCLUSION

Integrative oncology can present clinicians with legal and ethical dilemmas when their preferences and perspectives clash with those of their patients. This chapter has attempted to illustrate ways to handle these situations, using cases drawn from the authors' experience. We have drawn on liability and ethical frameworks to analyze situations that are likely to come up in practice.

The caveat is given that, although such situations can be generalized, it may be useful to ask legal counsel to give legal advice or opinion in any given situation. Oncologists practicing in a hospital will have the benefit of guidance from the hospital's legal counsel, and those in freestanding integrative care clinics, from their attorneys. Medical and other professional organizations have begun to craft guidelines for clinicians in integrative care practices, but these guidelines must be refined as medical evidence changes and integrative care develops. Medical organizations may wish to consider the suggestions in this chapter as input for continued reflection.

ACKNOWLEDGMENTS

This chapter was funded by grants from the Greenwall Foundation (New York) and the Rudolph Steiner Foundation (San Francisco).

NOTE

Cases three and four were taken from the actual practice of Matt Mumber MD.

APPENDIX 1: DFCI CLINICIAN CONTACT/PERMISSION

Hello Dr Jones,

One of your patients, John Smith, MRN: 193158, has requested an acupuncture visit. I tentatively scheduled him for Wednesday, January 7th, 2004 pending your approval. The following is a guideline used to determine patient eligibility for acupuncture.

At this time, acupuncture treatment is NOT recommended to cancer patients with the following conditions:

(a) Absolute neutrophil count (ANC) less than 500/ml;

(b) Platelet count less than 25 000/ml;

(c) Altered mental state;

(d) Clinically significant cardiac arrhythmias;

(e) Other unstable medical conditions.

The following conditions may benefit from acupuncture treatment:

(a) Chronic pain (e.g. cancer-related, postoperative, musculoskeletal);

(b) Headaches (e.g. tension headaches or migraine headaches);

(c) Depression and anxiety;

(d) Chemotherapy-induced nausea and vomiting;

(e) Low WBC count;

(f) Immune deficiency;

(g) Constipation;

(h) Insomnia;

(i) Various musculoskeletal pain.

I'd appreciate you letting me know if your patient, MRN: 193158, is eligible for acupuncture by replying to this email. In case you'd like more information on acupuncture, I'm attaching a link to the NIH Consensus Statement on Acupuncture. *http://odp.od.nih.gov/consensus/cons / 107/107_statement.htm.*

APPENDIX 2: A MODEL STANDARD CONSENT FORM* FOR USE OF CAM THERAPIES (REPRINTED WITH PERMISSION FROM REFERENCE 16)

Documentation of informed consent

By signing this form, I, [name of patient], agree that [name of clinician] has disclosed to me sufficient information, including the risks and benefits, to enable me to decide to undergo or forgo [name of therapy or course of treatment] for [name of patient's condition].

Our discussion has included: (1) the nature of my condition and procedures to be performed; (2) the nature and probability of material risks involved; (3) benefits to be reasonably expected of the procedure; (4) inability of the provider to predict results; (5) irreversibility of the procedure, if that is the case; (6) the likely result of no treatment or procedure; and (7) available alternatives, including their risks and benefits. [Name of clinician] has informed me that he or she has recorded an accurate, written description of the above in my medical record.

I have [refused the following recommended diagnostic and therapeutic interventions, and] elected to use the following [CAM] therapies [list therapies]. [I understand that treatment X is not approved by the federal Food and Drug Administration.]

My consent to this course of treatment is given voluntarily, without coercion, and may be withdrawn, and I am competent and able to understand the nature and consequences of the proposed treatment or procedure.

Assumption of risk and release of liability

The specific risks in making this choice of treatment are: [list of risks provided by clinician]. I knowingly, voluntarily, and intelligently assume these risks and agree to release, indemnify, and defend [name of clinician] and his or her agents from and against any and all claims which I (or my representatives) may have for any loss, damage, or injury arising out of or in connection with my treatment.[*]

I have carefully read this form and acknowledge that I understand it. No representations, statements, or inducements, oral or written, apart from the foregoing written statement, have been made. This form shall be governed by the laws of the state of [name of state] which shall be the forum for any lawsuits filed under or incident to this form. If any portion of this form is held invalid, the rest of the document shall continue in full force and effect.

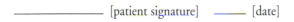

———————— [patient signature] ——— [date]

———————— [clinician signature] ——— [date]

MAJOR RESOURCES FOR LEGAL AND ETHICAL ISSUES IN INTEGRATIVE CARE

Articles

Adams KE, Cohen MH, Jonsen AR, Eisenberg DM. Ethical considerations of complementary and alternative medical therapies in conventional medical settings. Ann Intern Med 2002; 137: 660–4

Astin JA. Why patients use alternative medicine: results of a national study. J Am Med Assoc 1998; 279: 1548–53

Cohen MH, Eisenberg DM. Potential physician malpractice liability associated with complementary/integrative medical therapies. Ann Intern Med 2002; 136: 596–603

Cohen MH. Malpractice considerations affecting the clinical integration of complementary and alternative medicine. Curr Pract Med 1999; 2: 87–9

Cohen MH. Of rogues and regulation: a review of accommodating pluralism: the role of complementary and alternative medicine. Vt L Rev 2003; 27: 801–15

Cohen MH. Healing at the borderland of medicine and religion: regulating potential abuse of authority by spiritual healers. J Law Relig 2004; 18: 373–426

Cohen MH, Ruggie M. Integrating complementary and alternative medical therapies in conventional medical settings: legal quandaries and potential policy models. Cinn L Rev 2004; 72: 671–729

Dietary Supplements Health Education Act, 103 P.L. 417; 108 Stat. 4325; 1994

Dumoff A. Protecting ACM physicians from undeserved discipline: legislative efforts in Maryland. Altern Complement Ther 2002; 8: 120–6

Dumoff A. Coding system for alternative and complementary therapies: it's not as easy as ABC. Altern Complement Ther 2002; 8: 246–52

Dumoff A. The Federation of State Medical Boards' New Guidelines for ACM Practice: improvements and concerns. Altern Complement Ther 2002; 8: 303–9

Dumoff A. A collision between principles and law: a case study in why integration is so [damn] difficult. Altern Complement Ther 2002; 8: 8–9

Dumoff A. State Medical Board prohibitions on physician sale of supplements. Physician Consult 2000

[*]This form is a model, which must be adapted by an attorney licensed to practice law within the client's state. It includes elements of both informed consent and assumption of risk. As noted, in some states physicians are not allowed to include an assumption of risk clause, and inclusion of such a clause could, potentially, invalidate the entire agreement.

Dumoff A. Regulating professional relationships: kickback and self-referral restrictions on collaborative practice. Altern Complement Ther 2000; 6: 41–6

Dumoff A. Understanding the Kassebaum–Kennedy Health Care Act: addressing legitimate concerns and irrational fears. Altern Complement Ther 1997; 3: 309–13

Dumoff A. Protecting your practice: myth v. fact. Altern Complement Ther 1996; 2: 186–91

Eisenberg DM, Cohen MH, Hrbek A, et al. Credentialing complementary and alternative medical providers. Ann Intern Med 2002; 136: 660–4

Eisenberg DM. Advising patients who seek alternative medical therapies. Ann Intern Med 1997; 127: 61–9

Ernst EE, Cohen MH. Informed consent in complementary and alternative medicine. Arch Intern Med 2001; 161: 19: 2288–92

Executive Summary, Final Report, White House Commission on Complementary and Alternative Medicine Policy (2002)

Federation of State Medical Boards, Guidelines for Complementary and Alternative Therapies in Medical Practice (2002) (available at www.fsmb.org)

Federal Trade Commission. Dietary Supplements: An Advertising Guide for Industry (available on-line at www.ftc.gov)

Food and Drug Administration. Regulations on Statements Made for Dietary Supplements Concerning the Effect of the Product on the Structure or Function of the Body, 21 CFR Part 101, 65:4 Fed Reg 1000 (6 January 2000)

Hathcock J. Dietary supplements: how they are used and regulated. J Nutr 2001; 3 (Suppl) 131: 1114S–7S

Kaptchuk TJ. Varieties of healing 1: medical pluralism in the United States. Ann Int Med 2001; 135: 189

Kaptchuk TJ. Varieties of healing 2: a taxonomy of unconventional healing practices. Ann Int Med 2001; 135: 196

Kemper K, Cohen MH. Ethics in complementary medicine: new light on old principles. Contemp Pediatr 2004; 21: 321

Marcus DM, Grollman AP, Botanical medicines: the need for new regulations. N Engl J Med 2002; 347: 25

McNamara SH. Regulation of dietary supplements. N Engl J Med 2000; 343: 1270

Pelletier KR, Astin JA, Haskell WL. Current trends in the integration and reimbursement of complementary and alternative medicine by managed care organizations (MCOs) and insurance providers: 1998 update and cohort analysis. Am J Health Promot 1999; 14: 125–33

Pelletier KR, Marie A, Krasner M, Haskell WL. Current trends in the integration and reimbursement of complementary and alternative medicine by managed care, insurance carriers, and hospital providers. Am J Health Promot 1997; 12: 112–23

Studdert DM, Eisenberg DM, Miller FH, et al. Medical malpractice implications of alternative medicine [see comments]. J Am Med Assoc 1998; 280: 1610

Young AL. Bass IS. The Dietary Supplement Health and Education Act. Food Drug Law J 1995; 50: 285–92

Books

Callahan D, ed. The Role of Complementary & Alternative Medicine: Accommodating Pluralism. Washington, DC: Georgetown University Press, 2002

Cohen MH. Complementary and Alternative Medicine: Legal Boundaries and Regulatory Perspectives. Baltimore: Johns Hopkins University Press, 1998; 1–180

Cohen MH. Beyond Complementary Medicine: Legal and Ethical Perspectives on Health Care and Human Evolution. Ann Arbor: University of Michigan Press, 2000; 1–214

Cohen MH. Future Medicine: Ethical Dilemmas, Regulatory Challenges, and Therapeutic Pathways to Health and Human Healing in Human Transformation. Ann Arbor: University of Michigan Press, 2003; 1–359

Ernst EE, Pittler MH, Stevinson C, White A. The Desktop Guide to Complementary and Alternative Medicine: An Evidence-based Approach. London: Harcourt Publishers, 2001; 1–444

Faas N, ed. Integrating Complementary Medicine into Health Systems. Gaithersburg, MD: Aspen Publishers, 2001; 1–763

Humber JM, Almeder RF, eds. Alternative Medicine and Ethics. Atlanta: Humana Press, 1998; 1–220

Slater V, Rankin-Box D. The Nurses' Handbook of Complementary Therapies. New York: Churchill-Livingstone, 1996

Websites

Michael H. Cohen publishes current informational resources at
www.camlawblog.com

Websites specifically pertaining to regulation of dietary supplements

American Dietetic Association
www.eatright.org/gov/supplements.html

Berkeley Wellness Letter
www.berkeleywellness.com/html/ds/dsSupplements.html

Food and Drug Administration
http://vm.cfsan.fda.gov/~dms/supplmnt.html

Labels
www.fda.gov/bbs/topics/NEWS/NEW00678.html

FTC
www.ftc.gov/bcp/conline/pubs/buspubs/dietsupp.htm

NIH
http://dietary-supplements.info.nih.gov/

Database
http://ods.od.nih.gov/databases/ibids.html

Facts
www.cc.nih.gov/ccc/supplements/intro.html

NIH Press Release
www.nih.gov/news/pr/oct99/ods-06.htm

NLM
www.nlm.nih.gov/services/dietsup.html

Dietary Supplement Information Bureau
www.supplementinfo.org

USDA
www.nalusda.gov/fnic/etext/000015.html

Books
www.nalusda.gov/fnic/pubs/bibs/gen/dietsupp.html

USP
www.usp.org/frameset.htm? www.usp.org/dietary/

Federation of State Medical Boards. Model guidelines for physician use of complementary and alternative therapies in medical practice
www.fsmb.org

Other websites

White House Commission on Complementary and Alternative Medicine Policy:
www.whccamp.hhs.gov/

Legal Resources – Michael H. Cohen
www.michaelhcohen.com

References

1. Cohen MH. Complementary and Alternative Medicine: Legal Boundaries and Regulatory Perspectives. Baltimore: Johns Hopkins University Press, 1998; 56–72

2. Eisenberg DM, Cohen MH, Hrbek A, et al. Credentialing complementary and alternative medical providers. Ann Intern Med 2002; 137: 965–73

3. Cohen MH. Beyond Complementary Medicine: Legal and Ethical Perspectives on Health Care and Human Evolution. Ann Arbor: University of Michigan Press, 2000

4. Cohen MH, Ruggie M. Integrating complementary and alternative medical therapies in conventional medical settings: legal quandaries and potential policy models. Cinn L Rev 2004; 72: 671–729

5. Ernst EE, Cohen MH. Informed consent in complementary and alternative medicine. Arch Intern Med 2001; 161: 2288–92

6. Cohen MH. Legal Issues in Alternative Medicine. Berne, NC: Trafford Publishing, 2003

7. NCCAM website (available at www.nccam.nih.gov, accessed 02/04/04)

8. Cohen MH. Healing at the borderland of medicine and religion: regulating potential abuse of authority by spiritual healers. J Law Relig 2004; 18: 373–426

9. Cohen MH. A fixed star in health care reform: the emerging paradigm of holistic healing. Ariz State L J 1995; 27: 79–173

10. Federation of State Medical Boards, Model Guidelines for Physician Use of Complementary and Alternative Therapies in Medical Practice (available at www.fsmb.org, accessed 02/05/04)

11. Adams KE, Cohen MH, Jonsen AR, Eisenberg DM. Ethical considerations of complementary and alternative medical therapies in conventional medical settings. Ann Intern Med 2002; 137: 660–4

12. Cohen MH, Eisenberg DM. Potential physician malpractice liability associated with complementary/integrative medical therapies. Ann Intern Med 2002; 136: 596–603

13. Weiger WA, Smith M, Boon H, et al. Advising patients who seek complementary and alternative medicine therapy for cancer. Ann Intern Med 2002; 137: 889–903

14. 438 F. Supp. 1287 (W.D. Okla. 1977), remanded, 582 F.2d 1234 (10th Cir. 1978), rev'd, 442 U.S. 544 (1979), on remand, 616 F.2d 455 (10th Cir. 1980), cert. denied, 449 U.S. 937 (1980), later proceeding, 806 F.2d 1455 (10th Cir. Okla. 1986)

15. Federation of State Medical Boards. Model Guidelines for Physician Use of Complementary and Alternative Therapies in Medical Practice (available at www.fsmb.org, accessed 02/05/04)

16. Cohen MH. Legal Issues in Alternative Medicine. Berne, NC: Trafford Publishing, 2004

7

Business assessment

Joan Kines

' Ideals are like stars: you will not succeed in touching them with your hands, but like the seafaring man on the ocean desert of waters, you choose them as your guides, and following them, you reach your destiny.' – Carl Schurz

WHY PROVIDE?

Integrative medicine, as defined by the National Center for Complementary and Alternative Medicine (NCCAM), combines mainstream medical therapies and complementary and alternative medicine (CAM) for which there is some high-quality scientific evidence of safety and effectiveness. Integrative oncology can be defined in this context as the combination of conventional (mainstream) medical treatments and therapies and evidence-based complementary and alternative therapies. An integrative oncology business assessment begins by asking 'Why provide integrative oncology services?'

The answer will establish the goals and objectives for the program. There are a multitude of reasons that may be given for developing an integrative oncology program. Some of these reasons include: giving patients a sense of control, providing access through medical doctors

for patients who wish to use CAM, providing patients strong spiritual and psychological benefits, addressing the whole person, and remaining competitive with other practices offering similar services. Other reasons to consider are improved patient satisfaction, improved staff performance and lower rates of burnout. Additionally, improved prevention and support can result in cost savings for the provider as well as patients.

Dr Barrie Cassileth, chief of the Integrative Medicine Services at Memorial Sloan Kettering Hospital, acknowledged that by 2010 the supply of alternative practitioners, e.g. chiropractors, naturopaths and practitioners of oriental medicine, would grow by 88%. This is compared to the supply of traditional medical physicians increasing by only 16%[1]. Dr Cassileth suggests that the following issues also be considered before establishing integrative services for patients:

- What services to provide?

- Where and who is the patient population to be served?

- What licensures and certifications will be required of CAM practitioners?

- What will be reimbursed?

- What will it cost you to offer these services?

- How will access be handled?

- What referrals will be required (if outsourcing is required)?

- Who manages the program?[1]

WHO WILL USE INTEGRATIVE ONCOLOGY SERVICES

As a part of its educational outreach to local communities, the NCCAM of the National Institutes of Health (NIH) held several town meetings. At the first gathering in 2000, David M. Eisenberg, MD, stated: ' More than 80 million adults routinely use CAM therapies. In 1997, Americans made more than 600 million office visits to CAM providers and spent an estimated $30 billion on CAM related treatments and products.' To evaluate the effectiveness of American's increased use of CAM, the NIH has committed research funding to NCCAM[2]. In fiscal year 2000, NCCAM had a budget of $8.7 million and in fiscal year 2005 the estimated budget is $121.1 million[3]. On 30 November 2004, there were 29 CAM cancer clinical trials listed on the NCCAM website[4].

Who is using CAM? Approximately one in four persons in the USA use some type of CAM. Out-of-pocket costs of CAM rival medical treatment at $21.2 to $32.7 billion versus $29.3 billion, respectively[5]. Users of CAM tend to have high incomes and high levels of education. Most users of CAM have medical conditions not easily treated by modern medicine such as

chronic pain, poor mental health, human immunodeficiency virus infection and cancer[6]. Over 40% of patients with depression and anxiety reported that they used CAM for their medical conditions[6].

Several surveys of CAM use by cancer patients have been conducted with small numbers of patients. One study published in the February 2000 issue of the journal *Cancer* reported that 37% of 46 patients with prostate cancer used one or more CAM therapies as part of their cancer treatment[7]. These therapies included herbal remedies, vitamins and special diets. A study of CAM use in patients with different types of cancer was published in the July 2000 issue of the *Journal of Clinical Oncology*[8]. This study found that 69% of 453 cancer patients had used at least one CAM therapy as part of their cancer treatment.

COSTS

Luther W. Brady, MD, stated in the Foreword of the American College of Radiology *Practice Management Guide* 2004, 'the imminent future in radiation oncology will be driven by financial considerations'[9]. The field of oncology has been impacted significantly by improved technology, pharmaceuticals and clinical research. Cancer care providers must balance the high costs of technology and staffing with reduction in reimbursement. This creates significant challenges regarding the incorporation of CAM services not reimbursed by third-party payors.

To recruit and retain well-trained and experienced oncology physicians, nurses, pharmacists, physicists, radiation therapists and other allied health professionals, salaries have to remain competitive, driving up the practice cost. Cost increases from vendors, suppliers, office and facility utilities and repairs, along with more cost associated with staff salaries and benefits, are not offset by Medicare's 1.5% increased reimbursement for physicians effective in 2005. There has been a focus in recent years on reducing Medicare payment for drugs by eliminating the use of average wholesale price (AWP). In 2005, the new Average Sales Price (ASP) system will be implemented with much uncertainty surrounding the accuracy of ASP prices. Lower drug reimbursement, along with the under-reimbursed practice expense, are critical issues faced by medical oncology in 2005.

In order to establish a successful model for integrative oncology services, it is important to know both the potential patient population to be served, and their ability to pay for traditional medicine as well as CAM. If the practice is already established, historical data can be reviewed. If no practice data are available (or if the practice plans to increase market share), estimates of new cancer cases and payment patterns can be determined based on the total population served.

In the USA, the American Cancer Society estimates that over 19 000 000 new cancer cases have been diagnosed since 1990. Excluding approximately 1 000 000 skin cancers, an estimated 1 334 100 new cancer cases were diagnosed in 2003[10].

The American Cancer Society's *Cancer Facts and Figures 2003* has detailed information on how to estimate new cancer cases locally. The incidence for new cancer cases for all sites can be determined by taking the total population served multiplied by 0.0047[10]. Example: 100 000 patient population × 0.0047 = 470 estimated new cancers for all sites. The number of new cases of breast, colorectal, lung, and prostate cancer can also be determined (Table 7.1).

Using the estimated potential number of cancer patients, it is helpful to analyze the population demographics of health care coverage by the state where CAM services will be offered. Federal and state demographic categories are available at http://ferret.bls.census.gov/macro/032003/healt h/h05_000.htm. These data are helpful in determining how CAM services/providers are paid. Medicare and Medicaid do not reimburse physicians/providers for most CAM services. For a state (or community) with a higher population covered by Medicare and Medicaid, and no insurance, cancer patients may not be able to pay out-of-pocket for non-covered CAM services.

The nations uninsured, along with declines in the percentage of people covered by employment-based health insurance, create added cost to providers who accept responsibility to provide care to those who cannot pay for services. In 2002, those without health insurance increased to 43.6 million people with an increase of 2.4 million people over the prior year[11]. While Medicaid insured 14.0 million people in poverty,

Table 7.1	Determination of new cases of cancer				
	All sites	Female breast	Colon and rectum	Lung	Prostate
New cancer cases	0.0047	0.0015	0.0005	0.0006	0.0016
People who will eventually develop cancer	0.4085	0.1333	0.058	0.0671	0.1661
Based on 100 000 population					
New cancer cases	470	150	50	60	160
People who will eventually develop cancer	40 850	13 330	5800	6710	16 610

10.5 million other people in poverty had no health insurance[12].

REIMBURSEMENT ANALYSIS

According to data from the *CPS Annual Social and Economic Supplement* for 2002 Income, formerly called the March Supplement, the percentage of covered lives with health insurance in the USA was 84.8% (285 933 000) with 15.2% (43 574 000) without any health insurance. These data include the population covered by government insurance (Medicare, Medicaid and military health care). Of those 65 and older and more at risk for cancer, 38 448 000 were covered by Medicare[13].

Medicare is the national health insurance program for over 40 million Americans, including those aged 65 or older, some under the age of 65 with disabilities, and those with end-stage renal disease. Centers for Medicare and Medicaid Services (CMS) administer the Medicare Program[14]. Medicare's health-care insurance coverage is divided into four parts:

- Part A covers hospital, hospice, nursing home and home health services;

- Part B covers physician services, laboratory and diagnostic tests, durable medical equipment and hospital outpatient services;

- Part C covers beneficiaries receiving Medicare benefits through a managed care plan;

- Part D, recently added by Congress, refers to the new prescription drug benefit under Medicare[15].

Medicare Part A reimburses hospital-based costs for Diagnosis Related Groups (DRGs). DRGs includes the types of patients a hospital treats by taking the 10 000 plus listed International Classification of Diseases, 9th Revision, Clinical Modification (ICD-9-CM) diagnosis codes and

breaking them down to a more manageable number (close to 500)[16]. Patients within each DRG are similar both clinically and with regards to the resources needed to provide their inpatient care. Hospitals are reimbursed based on the inpatient's DRG. Hospitals must carefully monitor their resource utilization for Medicare inpatients to keep their cost at or below the DRG amount.

Medicare Part B reimburses physicians for more than 7000 services and procedures using a national physician's fee schedule. Rather than pay what a physician charges, payment is based on a fee allowance for a procedure determined by the relative value units (RVU) (consisting of physician work, practice expense and malpractice expense) that is adjusted by locality cost differences and multiplied by a conversion factor that determines the dollar value of the RVU[17]. Physicians must enroll in the Medicare Program and be issued a Unique Provider Identification Number (UPIN) before submitting claims to be reimbursed for services provided to patients with Medicare.

Medicare Part B reimburses hospitals for outpatient services using the hospital outpatient prospective payment system (HOPPS) and ambulatory payment classifications (APCs). The payment rate is determined for each APC and does not carry a professional component for physician services. New codes may be added by CMS using temporary G codes that have a temporary payment rate for hospital outpatients only. An example is: G0173 Stereotactic radiosurgery: complete course of therapy in one session. Physicians who bill globally for radiation therapy services and perform this same service cannot bill Medicare Part B using this G code, as it is meant only for hospitals.

State Medicaid programs receive state and federal funding to provide health-care coverage to children and adults under age 65 based on income and other eligibility requirement. Medicaid providers participate with the Medicaid program and receive a Medicaid provider number to bill for services. Medicaid coverage of health-care services and reimbursement varies from state to state.

From employer-based plans to private individual insurance plans, the types of plans, costs and coverage can vary significantly. The plans that provide the most coverage and are most affordable are usually employer based. To keep costs down, employers are increasingly moving to managed care plans. Managed care plans include:

- Health Maintenance Organizations (HMOs) are prepaid health plans with the insured paying a monthly premium in exchange for comprehensive health services that require co-payments at the time of service.

- Preferred Provider Organizations (PPOs) directly insure clients to receive care from physicians and providers that participate with the PPO.

- Point of Service (POS) Plans require the insured to select a participating primary care physician who will manage their care and obtain pre-certification before referring for certain diagnostic tests or referring the insured to a specialist.

Other types of employer health benefit plans include:

- Cafeteria Plans, defined under Section 125 of the Internal Revenue Code as plans maintained by an employer to allow each participant to select among cash and one or more qualified non-taxable benefits – this is sometimes called a flexible spending account.

- Flexible Spending Accounts, allowing the employee to set aside pre-taxed monies to be used for covered health-care services paid out of pocket.

- Medical Savings Accounts (also available to individuals), benefiting individuals with low health-care costs who can take advantage of low premiums and pay high deductibles with the advantage of accumulating large savings accounts that can be used for covered services.

With the risk for being diagnosed with cancer increasing with age, the Medicare population (usually 65 and older) will usually be significant for most cancer care providers. With few CAM services reimbursed by Medicare, the next step is to identify major employers and small businesses that can be contacted to determine the insurance plans/managed care organizations within the practice's primary service area. The local Chamber of Commerce can provide a list of area employers and their telephone numbers. Identifying plans that may offer employees access to CAM providers and services is an important part of the business assessment.

CPT® CODES

The Health Insurance Portability and Accountability Act (HIPPA) now requires all payers, including Medicare, to use a standard nomenclature system established by the American Medical Association (AMA), called Current Procedure Terminology (CPT®) codes. Although coverage, documentation, payment and billing protocols can vary across plans, claims are required to be filed for services using CPT® codes.

The AMA's CPT® codes have been published since 1966, and is now in its 4th edition[18] (all CPT codes, descriptions and material only ©2004 American Medical Association). CPT IV codes are used to bill professional and technical services, as well as outpatient hospital services. The Relative Value System (RVS) attaches value modifiers, called Relative Value Units (RVU), to the CPT® codes. The RVU Update Committee (RUC) determines the Relative Value Unit (RVU) then makes their recommendations to CMS. RUC recommendations for the RVU associated with the CPT® code are based on the following components: 55% physician work (time intensity), 42% practice expense (staff, supplies, equipment), and 3% liability[19]. Along with conversion factors (determined annually by Congress based on using an established formula) and locality modifiers, the dollar reimbursement for each code is then determined[18].

Not all ©2004 American Medical Association (AMA) CPT® IV codes are reimbursed by Medicare and third-party carriers. For integrative services that do not currently have a CPT® IV code with assigned RVUs, services are considered non-covered. This means that there is no reimbursement from Medicare, most state Medicaid plans, and fee for service insurance plans. Some types of medical insurance may cover services that are not covered by Medicare and other third-party carriers. These include Managed Care Plans (usually requiring preauthorization before service is provided), Medical Savings Accounts (a state-approved savings account that the employer and/or insured pays into), Flexible Spending Accounts (an employer-sponsored account that the employee contributes to before tax monies to uses for covered health care service) and other types of employer Cafeteria Plans (an employer offering of various options for employees to select from and use before tax monies for covered services).

Why is it important to understand how conventional health-care services are billed to and reimbursed by Medicare and other third-party payors? Because CAM services that do not have CPT® IV codes make it challenging for conventional health-care providers to integrate some types of CAM modalities and practitioners into their practices. Physicians who participate with Medicare cannot bill patients for non-covered services without informing the patient before the service is delivered that the service is not covered by Medicare, the amount the patient will be charged, and that the patient is responsible for paying for the service. Documentation must be on file that the patient has been informed that Medicare will not pay for the service, agrees to have the service, understands the cost and agrees to pay out-of-pocket for the non-covered service. Managed care contracts are typically based on the RVU system used by Medicare and reimbursement is a percentage of the Medicare allowable for each code. Hospitals receive payment from Medicare Part A based on DRGs and may not have additional resources to provide CAM services.

HOW TO GET A CPT® CODE ADDED

For traditional and CAM services that are not defined by a CPT®-IV code, there is a mechanism to get a new code added. The AMA website (http://www.ama-assn.org/ama/pub/article/3866-3862.html) provides assistance with the process to revise or create a new CPT® code. The CPT®-5 Executive Project Advisory Group provides recommendations to the AMA CPT® Editorial Panel[20]. 'The CPT-5 Project is structured to address challenges presented to emerging user needs including changes to enhance the use of CPT® by practicing physicians, managed care and other payor organizations, and researchers'[20].

The AMA has a review process through which new CPT® codes can be added. There are three types of CPT® codes:

(1) Category 1 CPT® codes are a five-digit CPT® code and descriptor nomenclature of a procedure consistent with contemporary medical practice. The procedure must have well-established and documented clinical efficacy with the specific devices or drugs approved by the Food and Drug Administration (FDA) and be performed by many physicians in multiple locations across the country[20]. Intensity-modulated radiation therapy (IMRT) is a recent example of a relatively new category I CPT® code.

(2) Category II CPT® codes are used to facilitate data collection of services and/or test results that have been agreed upon to contribute to better health outcomes and quality care. These are used to track codes for performance measurements (typically included in Evaluation and Management service codes)[20]. An example of a category II code is 0003F: tobacco use, cessation intervention, counseling[21].

(3) Category III CPT® codes collect data for assessment of new services and procedures with the purpose of substantiating widespread use, or in the FDA approval process (with the service/procedure having relevance for research)[20]. Category III CPT® codes are removed and cannot be reused if not accepted for placement into the category I CPT codes within 5 years[20]. An example of a category III code is 0060T: an electrical impedance scan of the breast (bilateral risk assessment device for breast cancer)[22].

Anyone can submit a new code, although most physician subspecialties have legislative committees to initiate the development of a new code. Once a service obtains a category I CPT code, it goes to the RVU Update Committee (RUC) for determination of the Relative Value Unit (RVU) that is then recommended to CMS. The therapy must then be approved by Medicare through a process called national coverage determination. An example: acupuncture is a potential integrative service that received national non-coverage determination first in 1980, and again upon review in April 2004[23].

Medicare provides information regarding covered and non-covered services at the following website: http://www.medicare.gov/Coverage/Home.asp. In order to determine whether Medicare reimburses a therapy, you may select state and service to determine the reimbursement and coverage for Medicare beneficiaries. For example: the state of Georgia Medicare Part B has issued coverage determinations for the following services: nutrition therapy (medical), alternative therapies, chiropractic services, non-physician health care provider services, and massage therapy. Please see the Appendix[24–28] (pages 135–138). The full text is available online.

CAM AND REIMBURSEMENT

A medical oncologist, Dr Jeremy R. Geffin, MD FACP, testified to the United States Congress Committee on Government Reform Hearing on Integrative Oncology: Cancer Care for the New Millennium on 7 June, 2000. He stated:

'We need vastly more significant funding, and reimbursement, for modalities of healing that honor and address the needs of the whole person … In my opinion, there is something deeply flawed about a healthcare system in which I, as an oncologist, can readily spend tens of thousands of dollars of Medicare funds to extend the life of an elderly man with advanced lung cancer for perhaps three or four months, utilizing expensive chemotherapy treatments, growth factors, blood transfusions, CT Scans, MRI Scans, and other costly diagnostic procedures … but I cannot find $100 dollars, or even $50 dollars, for an acupuncture treatment, a therapeutic massage, or a private counseling session for a frightened, terrified single mother of three children who is battling metastatic breast cancer – and who is sitting in the very next room[29].

Geoffrey Cowley in his cover story for *Newsweek Magazine* (2 December 2002), points out:

'From Medicare down to the smallest private health plan, the reimbursement system is still strongly biased against holistic care. The

nation's insurers spend $30 billion a year on bypass and angioplasty for cardiovascular disease, for example, but only 40 of them cover the lifestyle-based program developed by Dr. Dean Ornish – despite repeated demonstrations that it is safe, effective and vastly less expensive than surgery... [30]

Forty-two states require private insurers to cover chiropractic treatment, six states mandate acupuncture coverage, and California requires insurers to offer an acupuncture rider[31]. In the September/October 2000 issue of *Managed Care & Cancer*, John L. Surprenant, Corporate Executive Director of Oncology of St. John Health System, Detroit, Michigan, cited the Landmark Healthcare report on public perceptions of alternative care: four out of ten adults surveyed said their view of the importance of using CAM services has improved in the past five years. Suprenant stated,

'Insurers and managed-care companies are now evaluating the potential benefits of incorporating integrative health-care services into their plans...major insurers Aetna/US Healthcare, BlueCross/Blue Shield, Kaiser Permanente, United and Oxford Health now have integrative healthcare Products, or are exploring how to develop them. [32]

In 1997, Oxford Health Plans of Connecticut was the first major Health Maintenance Organization (HMO) that responded to consumer interest for CAM. One key feature of the Oxford's benefit and management plan was the research and outcomes partnership with David Eisenberg, MD at Harvard University. Another feature of Oxford's plan for CAM services is the credentialing requirements of alternative providers (Table 7.2). The cost for the alternative benefits was an additional premium of 2–3%.

An additional avenue for funding would be in large corporate environments. Many large corporations look to Employee Wellness programs to improve current employees' overall health and to attract new talent to the organization. A well thought out plan or program to improve employee wellness using integrative services can create an entirely new population of potential clients. Corporate sponsorship would also provide the needed funding that integrative medicine requires. Persuading corporate organizations to proceed down this path is a long-term commitment to the process. There are many levels of approval to pass before one of these programs can move forward. Working from the top of the organization – at the level of the Chairman, CEO, VP-HR – is a good potential strategy for jump starting the process.

As insurance companies and HMOs respond to legislation and consumer interest to provide reimbursement, there is increased importance placed on the credibility of the CAM disciplines. With increased use of CAM, it is anticipated that insurance companies and HMOs will give more value to the outcomes of increased patient satisfaction, functionality, quality of life and productivity.

Prudential Insurance developed an assessment of CAM that traced the history of acupuncture, chiropractic, massage, midwifery, and naturopathy. The development assessment traced these alternative professions for accrediting, educational recognition, number of schools, creation of standardized examination, and malpractice insurance coverage. Table 7.3 demonstrates several significant data points concerning accreditation and standardization of acupuncture, chiropractic, massage, midwifery and naturopathy[33]. Formalized education and licensure requirements similar to conventional approaches make it more feasible to offer reimbursement.

A 1995 Washington State law mandated all health care plans must include 'every category of provider.' The mandate required insurance coverage of licensed chiropractors, massage therapists, acupuncturists, naturopathic physicians and

Table 7.2 Oxford Health Plan's alternative medical benefits

Market research
- Poll of 750 members revealed that 35% had visited an alternative provider in the previous 2 years
- Poll of large employers showed that 75% were interested in the product

Start
- Roll-out 1 January 1997, in NY, NJ, CT (ND only in CT, where the profession is licensed)

Provider groups
- Initially DC, ND, acupuncturists
- Second phase adds clinical nutritionists, RDs, licensed massage practitioners, yoga instructors

Number of providers
- 2000 by 31 December 1997

Patient access
- Direct to credentialed member of the provider categories
- No PCP referral required

Limitations
- Ceiling on benefit not announced

Provider fees
- Schedule not released; expected to be at a discounted rate

Research and outcomes
- Partner with David Eisenberg, MD, Harvard University

Core credentialing criteria
- Licensed in state of practice
- Graduate of a fully accredited professional training program

- At least 2 years of clinical experience
- Ongoing CE credits required (unspecified number)
- Proper malpractice insurance (unspecified levels)
- Onsite visits 'may' be required

Internal operations and management
- 12-member department
- Advisory boards for DC, ND, and acupuncture
- Leading practitioner in each discipline chair board

Cost
- Price as a supplement 2–3% added to premium

Target market
- Large group clients

Excluded market
- Individuals, to protect against expected adverse selection

Natural medicinals
- Vitamins, botanicals and other natural agents are not covered
- Available at a discounted rate through a health plan mail order service

Member self-care
- Natural health educational materials (books, tapes, videos, etc.) available via discounted mail order service
- Facilitated access to online information on alternative medicine and self-care

Special programs
- Educational seminars on menopause and senior citizen health concerns to start, others to follow

---

ND, naturopathic physician; DC, chiropractor; RD, registered dietician; PCP, primary care physician; CE, continuing education. St. Anthony's Business Report on Alternative and Complementary Medicine, November 1996, Copyright © 1996, St. Anthony's Publishing Inc.

midwives[33]. Prudential Insurance limited coverage of all CAM services to the provider's licensed scope of practice, based upon the performance of a formal technology assessment. Washington State's Group Health Task Force responded to the 'every category of provider' mandate by setting up initial benefit limits. HMOs established guidelines for patient access, coverage and utilization review of acupuncture, massage therapy and naturopathy[33].

A 1998 survey of 37 insurance companies showed an increase in national coverage for some

				Standardized		
		US		national		
	Accrediting	Department		examination		
	agency	of Education	Recognized	examination	State	Malpractice
Profession	established	recognition	schools	created	regulation*	insurance
Acupuncture	1982	1990	15	1982	33 states	Early 1980s
Chiropractic	1971	1974	16	1963	50 states	1960s
Massage	1982	Application under consideration	Uncertain	1994	24 states	1993
Midwifery	1990s	Application fall 1996	First school accredited 1995	First certification examination 1994	18 states	Off-and-on since 1980s
Naturopathy	1978	1987	4	1986	11 states	1988

Table 7.3 Development of standards for complementary professions

* For chiropractors and naturopathic physicians, this category uniformly represents licensing statutes; for acupuncture, massage, and direct-entry midwifery, a mixture of licensing, certification, and registration.

Copyright © 1997, John Weeks/Integration Strategies for Natural Healthcare, Seattle, WA

CAM therapies. Ten of the 16 insurance companies with coverage available nationally reimbursed for acupuncture and chiropractic. Insurance companies that reimburse for CAM therapies are located in Connecticut, Massachusetts, California and Arizona.

Most evidence-based CAM methods provided in hospital clinics and integrative medicine practices are provided as fee for service[34]. The integrative care clinics provide patients with a billing sheet with the correct Classification of Diseases Ninth Edition (ICD9), CPT and/or APC codes. Memorial Sloan-Kettering Cancer Center has posted on their website concerning Integrative Medicine: 'all Memorial Sloan-Kettering Integrative Medicine Services, therapies and classes are fee for service and payable by cash, check, or credit card'[35].

Dick Roberts, Administrator of Columbus Regional Medical Center in Columbus, Indiana, was a speaker at the 1999 *Society for Radiation Oncology Administrators' Annual Meeting*. He addressed over 400 radiation oncology

administrators saying: 'It (integrative medicine) isn't voodoo medicine…Academia is now doing randomized clinical trials. It's going to become conventional medicine and then reimbursable'[36]. Many other cancer centers have instituted complementary medicine units. The M.D. Anderson Cancer Center in Houston, Texas, Dana-Farber Cancer Institute in Boston, Massachusetts, and Memorial Sloan-Kettering Cancer Center New York, New York have integrated CAM into their traditional oncology services. Funding sources to pay for CAM are different at each of these cancer centers. Clem Bezold, PhD, Consultant and President of the Institute for Alternative Futures, states that 'providing CAM lowers costs, which should drive what gets on the list of reimbursable care'[37].

Memorial Sloan-Kettering's Integrative Medicine Service found that most outpatients preferred not to receive CAM services at the location they received their outpatient chemotherapy and radiation therapy services. Simone B. Zappa, RN, MBA said that patients preferred CAM being at a separate site. It helped them feel good about their CAM experience and 'not like cancer patients'[37].

Three nationally recognized cancer centers, long considered medical Meccas, have instituted different types of integrative practices into their oncology services.

Dana-Farber's Zakim Center was formed as a coalition of Brigham & Women's Hospital, Massachusetts General Hospital, Children's Hospital, Beth Israel Hospital and the Massachusetts College of Pharmacy. The Zakim center offers 'relaxation techniques, mindful meditation, guided imagery, yoga, Therapeutic Touch and Reiki.' Memorial Sloan-Kettering uses some of these therapies 'as well as reflexology, mind/body work, acupuncture (performed only by MDs) and inpatient music therapy.' M.D. Anderson offers yoga, Tai Chi, meditation, art, music, humor therapy, support groups, nutrition, stress management, relaxation, guided imagery and educational forum[37].

Ms Zappa, program director of the Memorial-Sloan Kettering CAM program, believes their success is a result of sticking to 'evidence-based therapies, structuring the unit on a medical model, and collaborating closely with the health care team'[37].

Another consideration important to the successful integration of CAM services is how referring physicians view an integrative approach. The oncology practice should evaluate the potential revenue losses or gains associated with the decision to integrate CAM. When services were being planned at our local institution, a community survey was performed. This found that a majority of people surveyed had used some form of CAM in the preceding year, and most did not discuss this with their physician[38]. A similar survey of physicians within the community found that 80% thought that an integrative approach to medicine was reasonable and a large majority of the physicians surveyed were interested in learning more about integrative medicine[39].

Radiation and medical oncology are specialties that depend on referrals from other physicians. A strategic initiative should be developed to educate referring physicians about evidence-based CAM. Communication to build the referring physician's trust and confidence in evidence-based integrative oncology services helps to remove the risk of alienating referring physicians.

Below is a list of selected evidence-based CAM services that may be included in an integrative oncology practice. Additionally, reimbursement sources are listed if known, and are subject to different health plan specifics and different states laws.

MASSAGE THERAPY

- Chiropractors are currently billing insurance, Medicare and Medicaid.

- Medicare and Medicaid usually do not cover services billed by physicians or CAM providers (verify coverage by state).

- Medical Savings Accounts & Flexible Spending Accounts may cover this service.

- Many insurance plans reimburse if billed by chiropractor.

- Physical therapy departments are reimbursed if ordered by a physician (with documention of medical necessity using ICD-9 codes).

Example: lymphedema management for postoperative breast cancer.

NUTRITIONAL COUNSELING REIMBURSEMENT

- Limitations to Medicare reimbursement based on diagnosis of diabetes, kidney disease (but not on dialysis), or after a transplant when referred by a doctor. These services can be given by a registered dietician or Medicare-approved nutrition professional and include nutritional assessment and counseling.

- Medical Savings Accounts & Flexible Saving Accounts may cover this service.

- Check major insurance and managed care plans in market area (determine if registered dietician is required to perform service and if coverage is based on diagnoses).

HERBS AND DIETARY SUPPLEMENTS REIMBURSEMENT

Dietary supplements were defined by Congress in a law passed in 1994. A dietary supplement is a product (other than tobacco) taken by mouth that contains a 'dietary ingredient' intended to supplement the diet. Dietary ingredients may include vitamins, minerals, herbs or other botanicals, amino acids and substances such as enzymes, organ tissues and metabolites. Under current law, dietary supplements are considered foods, not drugs[40].

- Not covered by Medicare and Medicaid.

- Medical Savings Accounts & Flexible Savings Accounts may cover.

- Check major insurance and managed care plans in market area (determine if supplier is designated by plan).

MIND–BODY (STRESS REDUCTION) REIMBURSEMENT

Examples are meditation, guided imagery, relaxation techniques, support groups not delivered or billed by a clinical psychologist (see Psychosocial).

- Not covered by Medicare and Medicaid.

- Medical Savings Accounts & Flexible Savings Accounts may cover this service.

- Check major insurance and managed care plans in market area (determine if physician's order is required and if direct physician supervision is required).

PSYCHOSOCIAL SERVICES REIMBURSEMENT

Services provided and billed for by a licensed clinical psychologist which can include a wide array of mind–body relaxation and stress management therapies, as deemed clinically appropriate as a part of therapy.

- Examples of CPT IV codes that may be used are:

    - 90801 Initial Individual Assessment (first session).

    - 90804 Individual Psychotherapy (20–30 minutes).

    - 90806 Individual Psychotherapy (45–50 minutes).

    - 90808 Individual Psychotherapy (approximately 75–80 minutes).

    - 90847 Family Psychotherapy (40–50 minutes).

- Medicare covers the services of specially qualified non-physician practitioners such as clinical psychologists.

- Most major insurance and managed care plans in market area.

- Medical Savings Accounts & Flexible Savings Accounts may cover these services.

PREVENTIVE MEDICINE REIMBURSEMENT

Weight and lifestyle management, smoking cessation, energy medicine and health education are a few examples of preventive medicine (excluded here are the 2005 preventive medicine evaluation and management codes).

- Not covered by Medicare and Medicaid.

- Medical Savings Accounts & Flexible Savings Accounts may cover some of these services.

- Check major insurance and managed care plans in market area.

NON-CONVENTIONAL PROVIDERS

Conventional medicine is defined as medicine as practiced by holders of an MD (medical doctor) or DO (doctor of osteopathy) degree and by their allied health professionals, such as physical therapists, psychologists, physician's assistants, nurse practitioners, social workers and registered nurses. Other terms for conventional medicine include allopathy, Western, mainstream, orthodox, regular medicine and biomedicine. Some conventional medical practitioners are also practitioners of CAM[40].

- Medicare covers the services of specially qualified non-physician practitioners such as clinical psychologists (see above), clinical social workers, nurse practitioners, clinical nurse specialists, physician assistants, certified registered nurse anesthetists, certified nurse midwives, and speech–language pathologists, as allowed by state and local law for medically necessary services[27].

- Medicare and Medicaid do not pay for services provided by non-conventional providers.

- A few national insurance plans provide a list of non-conventional providers who offer discounted rates to their insured (no reimbursement from the insurance company and the patient pays out of pocket).

CONCLUSION

Based upon the current mechanisms for billing traditional oncology services, reimbursement for most CAM therapies and services by third-party payors is limited. Health-care providers and insurance companies use a standard set of codes (physicians use CPT® IV codes and hospital outpatient departments use CPT IV and APCs) in billing for medical services.

For CAM services such as art therapy, biofeedback, dance, hypnotherapy, interactive guided therapy, meditation therapy, music therapy, color therapy, magnetic field therapy, and energy medicine that do not have specific CPT® codes, costs will have to be absorbed within the oncology practice or outsourced to CAM providers. When no CPT® code is assigned to a service, it is inappropriate to fit the service with a CPT® code that is similar (for billing purposes only). While petitioning the AMA to establish new codes for CAM therapies is an option, the criteria for category I coding may be difficult to establish. Petitioning the AMA for category II status would be a good method to gather data on usage and efficacy patterns. For services such as massage therapy and acupuncture that have established AMA CPT® codes, careful documentation and billing within the established guidelines is required.

Medicare (usually the largest payor for oncology services) does not generally reimburse for CAM services, unless clinically indicated and performed by conventional professionals using established and appropriate CPT codes. Some insurance companies in various states may provide varying levels and mechanisms for reimbursement to CAM service providers. Oncology practices with a large Medicare population may find it difficult to provide CAM services and absorb the associated costs. Oncologists can outsource recommended services to CAM providers, taking into careful consideration the legal ramifications and the impact upon relationships with referring physicians. CAM providers usually receive payment at the time of service (for services covered by insurance a statement is provided to the patient to file directly with their insurance plan). Community and hospital cancer centers that have incorporated CAM services generally expect payment at the time of service and provide billing information to patients who wish to file a claim with their insurance. Cancer programs (with foundations that support CAM) use donations to provide CAM services at no cost to patients.

A valuable tool for CAM consumers is available online at http://nccam.nih.gov/health/financial/index.htm#2. The National Center for Complementary and Alternative Medicine (NCCAM) 'Get the Facts' *Consumer Financial Issues in Complementary and Alternative* gives consumers NCCAM's definition of CAM services and how patients pay for these services (out of pocket or limited coverage by a few insurance plans). Also provided is a list of recommended questions for patients to ask their insurance plan before seeking CAM therapies[41].

An estimated one in four Americans are already using some type of CAM and a majority do not discuss using CAM with their physician. Integrating CAM services that provide value to oncology patients, selecting the right CAM providers, and keeping CAM services affordable to patients (including those who may have already incurred huge health-care costs), is challenging but possible. The financial assessment is just one part of a successful integrative oncology program.

DISCLAIMER

Caution: reimbursement policies are subject to change and may vary significantly from insurer to insurer and in different geographical locations within the USA. All CPT codes and descriptions, guidelines and instructions are copyright 2004 of the American Medical Association. DRG guidelines determine reimbursement for inpatient Medicare patients.

Physicians and hospitals should bill for the specific services performed by the health-care provider (with appropriate documentation maintained in the patient's medical record). It is recommended that providers contact the insurer (Medicare, Medicaid or private insurance companies) to verify appropriate codes and reimbursement levels. The final decision for coding and billing for medical services, including CAM services, must be made by the oncologist (or provider) with consideration of regulations of insurance carriers and any local, state or federal laws that apply to the physician's and/or provider's practice.

Mention or discussion of any programs or materials does not constitute endorsement, promotion or criticism. Information in this chapter is intended to be purely informational; the author does not assume responsibility for the consequences related to the use of the information contained in this chapter.

APPENDIX

Nutrition Therapy Services (Medical)	
Coverage under Medicare	Medical nutrition therapy services are covered for people with diabetes, kidney disease (but not on dialysis), and after a transplant when referred by a doctor. These services can be given by a registered dietician or Medicare-approved nutrition professional and include nutritional assessment and counseling
The amount you need to pay	You pay 20% of Medicare-approved amounts
The part of Medicare that pays for this service or supply	Part B Benefit
Medicare contact for additional information	State of Georgia Carrier: 1-800-727-0827
Important notes	(1) You must pay an annual $100 deductible for Part B services and supplies before Medicare begins to pay its share
	(2) Actual amounts you must pay may be higher if a doctor, health care provider, or supplier does not accept assignment
Additional information	There are 2 Local Medical Review Policies (LMRPs) and 1 National Coverage Determinations (NCDs) written that explain when services or supplies are covered, including when they are considered medically necessary. For more information about LMRPs and NCDs for these services or supplies, please visit the Medicare Coverage Database on www.cms.hhs.gov.

Reference 24

Alternative Therapies	
Coverage under Medicare	Alternative therapies (including acupuncture, chelation therapy, biofeedback and holistic medicine) are not covered by Medicare
The amount you need to pay	You pay 100%
The part of Medicare that pays for this service or supply	Not currently a Medicare benefit
Medicare contact for additional information	Not applicable
Important notes	No important notes to display
Additional information	There are 1 Local Medical Review Policies (LMRPs) and 1 National Coverage Determinations (NCDs) written that explain when services or supplies are covered, including when they are considered medically necessary. For more information about LMRPs and NCDs for these services or supplies, please visit the Medicare Coverage Database on www.cms.hhs.gov

Reference 25

Chiropractic Services

Coverage under Medicare	Medicare covers manipulation of the spine to correct a subluxation, when provided by chiropractors or other qualified providers
The amount you need to pay	You pay 20% of Medicare-approved amounts
The part of Medicare that pays for this service or supply	Part B Benefit
Medicare contact for additional information	State of Georgia Carrier: 1-800-727-0827
Important notes	(1) You must pay an annual $100 deductible for Part B services and supplies before Medicare begins to pay its share
	(2) Actual amounts you must pay may be higher if a doctor, health care provider, or supplier does not accept assignment
Additional information	There are 1 Local Medical Review Policies (LMRPs) and 0 National Coverage Determinations (NCDs) written that explain when services or supplies are covered, including when they are considered medically necessary. For more information about LMRPs and NCDs for these services or supplies, please visit the Medicare Coverage Database on www.cms.hhs.gov

Reference 26

Non-Physician Health Care Provider Services

Coverage under Medicare	Medicare covers the services of specially qualified non-physician practitioners such as clinical psychologists, clinical social workers, nurse practitioners, clinical nurse specialists, physician assistants, certified registered nurse anesthetists, certified nurse midwives, and speech-language pathologists, as allowed by state and local law for medically necessary services
The amount you need to pay	You pay 20% of Medicare-approved amounts
The part of Medicare that pays for this service or supply	Part B Benefit
Medicare contact for additional information	State of Georgia Carrier: 1-800-727-0827
Important notes	(1) You must pay an annual $100 deductible for Part B services and supplies before Medicare begins to pay its share
	(2) Actual amounts you must pay may be higher if a doctor, health care provider, or supplier does not accept assignment
Additional information	There are 1 Local Medical Review Policies (LMRPs) and 0 National Coverage Determinations (NCDs) written that explain when services or supplies are covered, including when they are considered medically necessary. For more information about LMRPs and NCDs for these services or supplies, please visit the Medicare Coverage Database on www.cms.hhs.gov

Reference 27

CMS policy on massage therapy is found under physical therapy.

PHYSICAL THERAPY CMS POLICY

Massage therapy (CPT code 97124)

(1) Massage is the application of systemic manipulation to the soft tissues of the body for therapeutic purposes. Although various assistive devices and electrical equipment are available for the purpose of delivering massage, use of the hands is considered the most effective method of application, because palpation can be used as an assessment as well as a treatment tool.

(2) Massage therapy, including effleurage, petrissage, and/or stocking compression, percussion, may be considered reasonable and necessary if at least one of the following conditions is present and documented:

    (a) The patient having paralyzed musculature contributing to impaired circulation;

    (b) The patient having sensitivity of tissues to pressure;

    (c) The patient having tight muscles resulting in shortening and/or spasticity of affected muscles;

    (d) The patient having abnormal adherence of tissue to surrounding tissue;

    (e) The patient requiring relaxation in preparation for neuromuscular re-education or therapeutic exercise; and

    (f) The patient having contractures and decreased range of motion.

Joint mobilization (peripheral or spinal) (CPT code 97140): manual therapy techniques (e.g. mobilization manipulation, manual lymphatic drainage, manual traction)

(1) The goal of this type of therapy is to reduce lymphedema of an extremity by routing the fluid to functional pathways, preventing backflow as the new routes become established, and to use the most appropriate methods to maintain the reduction of the extremity after therapy is complete. This therapy involves intensive treatment to reduce the size of the extremity by a combination of manual decongestive therapy and serial compression bandaging, followed by an exercise program.

    (a) It is expected that during these sessions, education is being provided to the patient and/or caregiver on the correct application of the compression bandage.

    (b) It is also expected that after the completion of the therapy the patient and/or caregiver can perform these activities without supervision.

(2) This procedure may be considered reasonable and necessary if restricted joint motion is present and documented. It may be reasonable and necessary as an adjunct to therapeutic exercises when loss of articular motion and flexibility impedes the therapeutic procedure.

Therapeutic procedure(s), group (2 or more individuals) (CPT 97150)

Group therapeutic procedures involve constant attendance of the physician or therapist, but by definition does not require one-on-one patient contact by the physician or therapist. Since most group procedure(s) do not require the professional skills of a therapist, coverage of this procedure will be determined on an individual case basis. Documentation must identify the specific treatment technique(s) used in the group, how the treatment technique will restore function, the frequency and duration of the particular group setting and the treatment goal in the individualized plan. The number of persons in the group should be documented. Case management techniques such as 'dove tailing' could constitute group therapy[28].

References

1. Bien A. 'What is Complementary Medicine's Place in Oncology?' Medical Group Management Assembly/Society News and Views. 15 July, 2000: 2

2. National Center for Complementary and Alternative Medicine. General Information.' 15 October 2000. http://nccam.nih.gov/nccam/an

3. NCCAM Funding. National Center for Complementary and Alternative Medicine. 30 November 2004. http://nccam.nih.gov/about/appropriations/index.htm

4. Cancer Clinical Trials. National Center for Complementary and Alternative Medicine. 30 November 2004. http://nccam.nih.gov/clinical-trials/cancer.htm

5. General Information. National Center for Complementary and Alternative Medicine. 15 October 2000. http://nccam.nih.gov/nccam/an

6. Cauffield JS. The psychosocial aspects of complementary and alternative medicine. Pharmacotherapy 2000; 20.11: 1289–94

7. Kao GD, Devine P. Use of complementary health practices by prostate carcinoma patients undergoing radiation therapy. Cancer 2000; 88: 615–19

8. Richardson MA, Sanders T, Palmer JL, et al. Complementary/alternative medicine use in a comprehensive cancer centre and the implications for oncology. J Clin Oncol 2000; 18: 2505–14

9. American College of Radiation Oncology. Practice Management Guide. Bethesda, MD: ACRO, 2004: 3

10. American Cancer Society. Cancer Facts and Figures. Atlanta, GA: ACS, 2003: 1–2, 13

11. http://www.census.gov/hhes/hlthins/hlthin02/hlth02asc.html12 Last revised: 21 April 2004

12. http://www.census.gov/hhes/hlthins/hlthin02/hlth02asc.html13 Last revised: 21 April 2004

13. Source: US Census Bureau, Current Population, 2003 Annual Social and Economic Supplement

14. http://www.cms.hhs.gov/about/history/ Last modified 24 September 2003

15. The ASTRO/ACR Guide to Radiaton Oncology Coding 2005: 8

16. http://www.umanitoba.ca/centres/mchp/concept/dict/drg.define.htm, December 2004

17. The ASTRO/ACR Guide to Radiation Oncology Coding 2005: 8

18. Brogardus CA. A User's Guide for Radiation Oncology Management & Billing Procedures, 6th edn. Oklahoma City, OK: Cancer Care Network, 2004: 19

19. Coding and Reimbursement Seminar, ASTRO, Atlanta, GA, 2 October 2004

20. http://www.ama-assn.org/ama/pub/article/3866-3862.html 17 March 2004

21. The 2004 CPT Expert. Baltimore, MD: Ingenix Inc., 2003: 327.

22. The 2004 CPT Expert. Baltimore, MD: Ingenix Inc., 2003: 328.

23. http://www.cms.hhs.gov/mcd/viewncd.asp?ncd_id=30.3.2&ncd_version=1

24. http://www.medicare.gov/Coverage/Search/Results.asp?State=GA%7CGeorgia&Coverage=43%7CNutrition+Therapy+Services+%28Medical%29&submitState=View+Results+%3E

25. http://www.medicare.gov/Coverage/Search/Results.asp?State=GA%7CGeorgia&Coverage=

1%7Calternative+Therapies&submitState=View+results+%3E

26. http://www.medicare.gov/Coverage/Search/Results.asp?State=GA%7CGeorgia&Coverage=10%7CChiropractic+Services&submitState=View+Results+%3E

27. http://www.medicare.gov/Coverage/Search/Results.asp?State=GA%7CGeorgia&Coverage=41%7CNon-Physician+Health+Care+Provider+Services&submitState=View+Results+%3E

28. http://www.cms.hhs.gov/mcd/viewlmrp.asp?lmrp_id=2695&lmrp_version=5&basket=lmrp%3A2695%3A5%3AOutpatient+Physical+Therapy%3AF1%3AMutual+of+Omaha+Insurance+Company+%2852280%29%3A

29. http://www.geffencenter.com/congress1.html

30. Crowley G. 'Now, Integrative Care', Newsweek, Dec 02, 2002. http://vienna-doctor.com/ENG/Articles_ENG/integrative_care.html

31. Novellino T. 'Modern Shamans.' Good Morning America. ABC. New York. 4 February 2001. http://more.abcnews.go.com/sections/gma/goodmorningamerica/gma001205alternative_medicine_two.html

32. Surprenant J. The emergence of integrative oncology: a new approach to providing cancer care. Managed Care Cancer September–October 2000; 9.4: 12–15

33. Weeks J. The emerging role of alternative medicine in managed care.' Drug Benefit Trends 1997; 9.4: 14–28

34. Survey of cancer programs performed by Judith Boyce MD, 2004

35. http://www.mskcc.org/mskcc/html/1985.cfm

36. General Session at Society for Radiation Oncology Administrators Annual Meeting, San Antonio, TX, 31 October 1999

37. Hatfield S. Cancer and healing – exploring top centers and integrative options. Advance for Administrators in Radiology & Radiation Oncology 10.10

38. Survey performed and data provided by PRN, Inc.

39. Survey performed and data provided by PRN, Inc.

40. http://nccam.nih.gov/health/decisions/index.htm

41. http://nccam.nih.gov/health/financial/index.htm#2, December 2004

Section II

Practice

Practice

The practice of integrative oncology has yet to be clearly defined. This portion of the text will attempt to build a decision making guideline for physicians, who are considered to be the 'conductors' of the integrative approach. We will then discuss methods available to motivate change in individuals, especially as it pertains to changing lifestyle related behaviors. The section on modalities will initially describe each field and then present a general review of preventive, supportive and antineoplastic options related to cancer care. The intention in presenting information under the heading of a specific clinical goal was to develop a framework whereby all of the interventions could be considered together as a part of an integrated approach, rather than merely running in parallel. Specific clinical situations – tobacco and alcohol cessation and palliative/end-of-life care are presented separately. The five most common malignancies are presented with tables listing modalities and interventions along with levels of available evidence.

An integrative oncology must address all involved with the process at all levels of their being and experience. This type of comprehensive approach recognizes the needs of cancer patients, their families and health-care providers. The blending of preventive, supportive and antineoplastic options in a setting which respects the life changing nature of the cancer care process, while at the same time accomplishing quality targeted interventions, represents the art of an integrative approach.

8

Clinical decision analysis

Matthew P. Mumber

Several attempts have been made to develop an approach to clinical decisions in an integrative setting[1–3]. There are limited clinical data available concerning most complementary and alternative medicine (CAM) treatment options. Despite this, consistent judgments have to be made as to the value and evidence level for CAM therapies in order to make recommendations for or against use. This has been deemed necessary because, unlike conventional treatment options in which conventional providers are gatekeepers of therapy, patients have access to CAM services on their own. This unlimited access can result in both significant benefit (improved care) and harm (dangerous interactions). Of course, this is a view that looks at these issues from a paternalistic perspective. There is also a perspective that honors patient choice given full information and disclosure. Please see Chapter 6 for further discussion.

A comprehensive approach to decision making in integrative oncology will address multiple issues (Table 8.1). It will address these issues in all participants at all levels of their being and experience. It will take into account prevention, supportive care and antineoplastic treatment. It will make rational recommendations based on the specific situation of the patient, the general and specific goals of therapy, the levels of evidence concerning safety and efficacy for specific interventions, and a resulting risk–benefit analysis.

Previous attempts to develop clinical guidelines have been limited in scope. Weiger *et al.* proposed a method to evaluate and recommend CAM interventions based on levels of evidence, concentrating on safety and efficacy data[1]. This guideline did not differentiate the patient's clinical status (acute versus sub-acute presentation and need for intervention, disease stage and type, or prognosis). It also did not take into account the therapeutic goal (prevention, supportive care, or antineoplastic intent), or the subsets of treatment goals within prevention, supportive and antineoplastic care. Adams *et al.*[2] came closer to a comprehensive approach, outlining seven important factors to consider when recommending CAM approaches. They are presented with a detailed discussion in Chapter 6 and are listed below:

(1) Severity and acuteness of illness;

(2) Curability with conventional treatment;

(3) Invasiveness, toxicities and side-effects of conventional treatment;

Table 8.1 Factors to consider in clinical decision tree formation for integrative oncology

Factor	Definition
Patient's clinical situation	Acute versus subacute presentation and need for intervention
	Disease stage and type
	Prognosis
Specific treatment goals	Prevention
	Supportive care
	Antineoplastic care
General preventive approach	Primary
	Secondary
	Tertiary
General supportive care approach	Translational versus transformational utility
	Improved tolerance of antineoplastic therapy
	Symptom control
	General quality of life
	End-of-life care
General antineoplastic approach	Curative versus palliative
Level of evidence for therapy	Data levels I–IV, for both safety and efficacy
	Risk/benefit ratio – including cost, toxicity, chances of beneficial and harmful outcome

(4) Quality of evidence of safety and efficacy of the CAM treatment;

(5) Degree of understanding of the risks and benefits of conventional and CAM treatments;

(6) Knowing and voluntary acceptance of those risks by the patient;

(7) Persistence of the patient's intention to utilize CAM treatment.

Preventive and supportive interventions, and the categories within these areas, are not mentioned in this work. There also appears to be a bias in both of these analyses toward thinking of CAM in the light of antineoplastic alternative medicine only – something that patients do instead of rational, evidence-based conventional approaches.

The Federation of State Medical Board guidelines 'allow a wide degree of latitude in physicians' exercise of their professional judgment and do not preclude the use of any methods that are reasonably likely to benefit patients without undue risk'. The guidelines emphasize shared decision-making.[4] (For further discussion of these guidelines, please see Chapter 6.)

With all of the above in mind, an attempt to construct a comprehensive integrative oncology decision tree has been made (Decision Trees 1–4). This analysis is done from a case-based, patient-focused standpoint at a specific point in time. An integrative approach also includes all participants at all levels of their being and experience. While this may seem to be a daunting task for one individual, the physician can accomplish this through several avenues: by being the 'conductor' of a team of providers with specific, well-defined skills; by having the knowledge and ability to discuss and refer among providers; and by adherence to the guiding principles of integrative medicine. The decision tree also revolves around points that are listed as black and white options – for example, high versus low chance of cure, control or response; and acute versus subacute need for intervention. The majority of clinical situations are not as easily defined and may require difficult clinical judgments. However, these caveats do not preclude the utility of decision tree analyses, which are seen to be useful in conventional oncology approaches where similar ambiguities may exist.

Another concept has arisen for assessing interventions that have limited data: it has been coined the 'Precautionary Principle'. This principle was developed in order to address situations in which the collection of data that would absolutely prove efficacy and safety was prohibitive[5,6]. Using the Precautionary Principle should not be seen as an excuse to advance one's hypotheses without evidence, but can allow us to act in situations where limited data are available, if that action is almost certainly safe and deemed necessary.

This decision-making guide is an attempt to explore the new territory of integrative oncology. These are, by definition, exploratory tools – and are not meant to be firm clinical guidelines.

There are four decision trees presented here. The four major groups represent variations on patient and disease characteristics – localized versus metastatic disease; and high versus low rates of disease control or response. Each group then has a separate decision pathway for the specific intervention goals of prevention, supportive and antineoplastic care. A standardized method is used to decide upon a recommendation for or against use of a specific modality based upon level of evidence for safety and efficacy. If a therapy can be recommended based upon the data, a further risk benefit discussion with the patient must take place, including the signing of an informed consent document, where appropriate.

DECISION TREE 1

Information needed: disease type and stage, health situation, prognosis

Specific situation: localized disease, high rates of cure, disease control or response

Specific goal: prevention:

1. Primary
2. Secondary
3. Tertiary

Research evidence concerning modality: data level (I–IV) for safety and efficacy

Data level I   Data level II   Data level III   Data level IV

Note: Level IV data only are considered unknown, pending further evidence, unless the Precautionary Principle is used, in which case one could consider the data preliminarily positive or negative and make appropriate recommendation. Strength of positive or negative data escalates with level I (strongest), followed by level II and level III

Use preponderance of data for safety and efficacy to arrive at a recommendation:

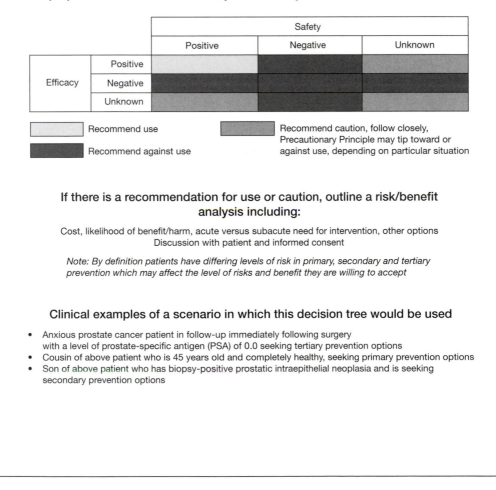

If there is a recommendation for use or caution, outline a risk/benefit analysis including:

Cost, likelihood of benefit/harm, acute versus subacute need for intervention, other options
Discussion with patient and informed consent

Note: By definition patients have differing levels of risk in primary, secondary and tertiary prevention which may affect the level of risks and benefit they are willing to accept

Clinical examples of a scenario in which this decision tree would be used

- Anxious prostate cancer patient in follow-up immediately following surgery with a level of prostate-specific antigen (PSA) of 0.0 seeking tertiary prevention options
- Cousin of above patient who is 45 years old and completely healthy, seeking primary prevention options
- Son of above patient who has biopsy-positive prostatic intraepithelial neoplasia and is seeking secondary prevention options

DECISION TREE 1

Information needed: disease type and stage, health situation, prognosis

Specific situation: localized disease, high rates of cure disease, control or response

Specific goal: supportive care:

1. Translational
2. Transformational

Translational: therapy and outcome discrete and easily measurable

Two separate groups: Symptom control and quality of life *during* conventional antineoplastic therapy
Symptom control and quality of life *after* antineoplastic care

Research evidence concerning modality: data level (I–IV) for safety and efficacy

Data level I   Data level II   Data level III   Data level IV

Note: Level IV data only are considered unknown, pending further evidence, unless the Precautionary Principle is used, in which case one could consider the data preliminarily positive or negative, and make appropriate recommendation. Level IV data are unusual in supportive care options. Strength of positive or negative data escalates with level I (strongest), followed by level II and level III

Use preponderance of data for safety and efficacy to arrive at a recommendation:

		Safety		
		Positive	Negative	Unknown
Efficacy	Positive			
	Negative			
	Unknown			

☐ Recommend use   ☐ Recommend caution, follow closely, Precautionary Principle may tip toward or against use, depending on particular situation

☐ Recommend against use

If there is a recommendation for use or caution, outline a risk/benefit analysis including:

Cost, likelihood of benefit/harm, acute versus subacute need for intervention, other options
Discussion with patient and informed consent

Note: Significant differences exist in these two groups of patients. This is especially true in a situation such as this, in which the patient presents with localized disease in which the probability for cure, response or control is high. During antineoplastic therapy, the Precautionary Principle should apply to withholding any substance that could alter the effectiveness of known active therapeutics. Following active antineoplastic therapy, this distinction vanishes, and therefore the Precautionary Principle could be used to recommend with caution supportive therapies in which unknown or inadequate data exist

Clinical examples of a scenario in which this decision tree would be used

- 60-year-old woman with early stage-breast cancer undergoing adjuvant postoperative radiation, asking about antioxidant vitamin supplements during treatment to help with fatigue
- Same patient asking about relaxing massage to help with anxiety during and after treatment
- Same patient asking about vitamins after radiation

DECISION TREE 1

Information needed: disease type and stage, health situation, prognosis

Specific situation: localized disease, high rates of cure disease, control or response

Specific goal: supportive care:

1. Translational
2. Transformational

Transformational: difficult to measure, difficult to define cause and effect

Efficacy is difficult, if not impossible, to measure for transformational interventions, other than by qualitative, testimonial-type feedback. In this situation, it is also possible that there is no single outcome that defines the presence or absence of a transformational experience. Therefore, safety is the primary concern. If an intervention is safe, then it can be recommended with caution and monitoring

If there is a recommendation for use or caution, outline a risk/benefit analysis including:

Cost, likelihood of benefit/harm, acute versus subacute need for intervention, other options
Discussion with patient and informed consent

Note: In this scenario, the patient has localized disease with a high likelihood of cure, control or response. A transformational-type intervention would therefore seem to be of lower priority relative to other possible interventions, and the Precautionary Principle would dictate that definitive antineoplastic interventions take priority. On the other hand, beginning a specific practice with transformational intent could be pursued simultaneously if no delays would be expected

Clinical examples of a scenario in which this decision tree would be used

- A 49-year-old white male with T1N0M0 non-small-cell lung cancer eligible for resection wants to delay surgery so that he can go on a residential retreat for several weeks in order to experience yoga, massage, vegetarian nutrition and group support with the ultimate goal of greater self-understanding
- The same patient who wants to begin a yoga and prayer practice in order to increase self-understanding but does not wish to delay antineoplastic therapy

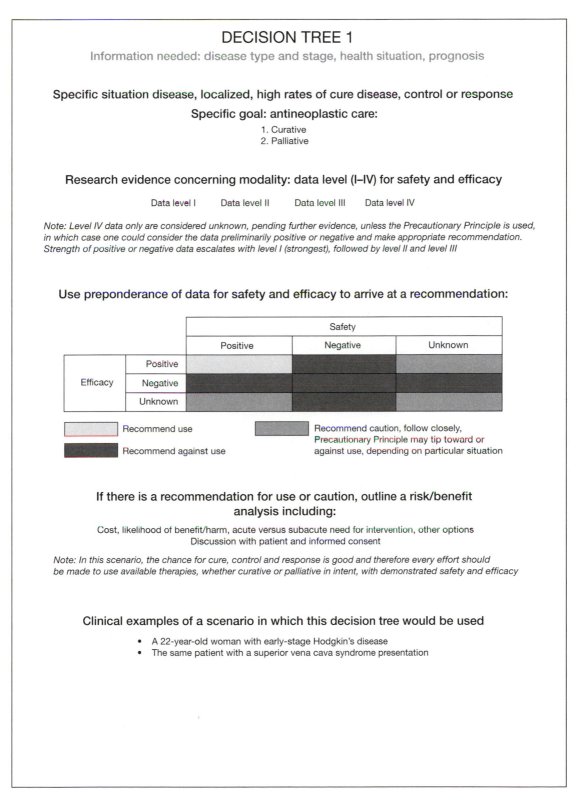

DECISION TREE 1

Information needed: disease type and stage, health situation, prognosis

Specific situation disease, localized, high rates of cure disease, control or response

Specific goal: antineoplastic care:

1. Curative
2. Palliative

Research evidence concerning modality: data level (I–IV) for safety and efficacy

Data level I   Data level II   Data level III   Data level IV

Note: Level IV data only are considered unknown, pending further evidence, unless the Precautionary Principle is used, in which case one could consider the data preliminarily positive or negative and make appropriate recommendation. Strength of positive or negative data escalates with level I (strongest), followed by level II and level III

Use preponderance of data for safety and efficacy to arrive at a recommendation:

		Safety		
		Positive	Negative	Unknown
Efficacy	Positive			
	Negative			
	Unknown			

Recommend use

Recommend against use

Recommend caution, follow closely, Precautionary Principle may tip toward or against use, depending on particular situation

If there is a recommendation for use or caution, outline a risk/benefit analysis including:

Cost, likelihood of benefit/harm, acute versus subacute need for intervention, other options
Discussion with patient and informed consent

Note: In this scenario, the chance for cure, control and response is good and therefore every effort should be made to use available therapies, whether curative or palliative in intent, with demonstrated safety and efficacy

Clinical examples of a scenario in which this decision tree would be used

- A 22-year-old woman with early-stage Hodgkin's disease
- The same patient with a superior vena cava syndrome presentation

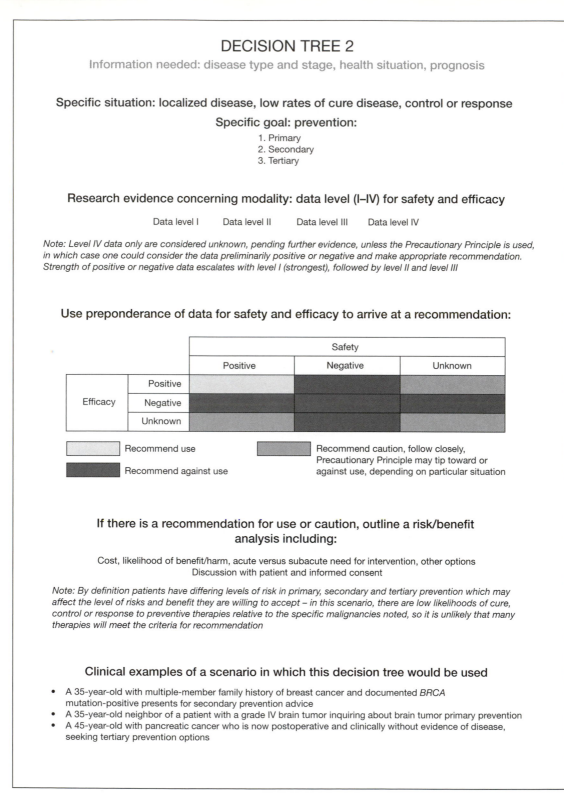

DECISION TREE 2

Information needed: disease type and stage, health situation, prognosis

Specific situation: localized disease, low rates of cure disease, control or response
Specific goal: prevention:
1. Primary
2. Secondary
3. Tertiary

Research evidence concerning modality: data level (I–IV) for safety and efficacy

Data level I   Data level II   Data level III   Data level IV

Note: Level IV data only are considered unknown, pending further evidence, unless the Precautionary Principle is used, in which case one could consider the data preliminarily positive or negative and make appropriate recommendation. Strength of positive or negative data escalates with level I (strongest), followed by level II and level III

Use preponderance of data for safety and efficacy to arrive at a recommendation:

		Safety		
		Positive	Negative	Unknown
Efficacy	Positive			
	Negative			
	Unknown			

Recommend use

Recommend against use

Recommend caution, follow closely, Precautionary Principle may tip toward or against use, depending on particular situation

If there is a recommendation for use or caution, outline a risk/benefit analysis including:

Cost, likelihood of benefit/harm, acute versus subacute need for intervention, other options
Discussion with patient and informed consent

Note: By definition patients have differing levels of risk in primary, secondary and tertiary prevention which may affect the level of risks and benefit they are willing to accept – in this scenario, there are low likelihoods of cure, control or response to preventive therapies relative to the specific malignancies noted, so it is unlikely that many therapies will meet the criteria for recommendation

Clinical examples of a scenario in which this decision tree would be used

- A 35-year-old with multiple-member family history of breast cancer and documented *BRCA* mutation-positive presents for secondary prevention advice
- A 35-year-old neighbor of a patient with a grade IV brain tumor inquiring about brain tumor primary prevention
- A 45-year-old with pancreatic cancer who is now postoperative and clinically without evidence of disease, seeking tertiary prevention options

DECISION TREE 2

Information needed: disease type and stage, health situation, prognosis

Specific situation: localized disease, low rates of cure disease, control or response

Specific goal: supportive care:

1. Translational
2. Transformational

Translational: therapy and outcome discrete and easily measurable

Symptom control and quality of life *during* conventional antineoplastic therapy
Symptom control and quality of life *after* antineoplastic care
End-of-life care

Research evidence concerning modality: data level (I–IV) for safety and efficacy

Data level I   Data level II   Data level III   Data level IV

Note: Level IV data only are considered unknown, pending further evidence, unless the Precautionary Principle is used, in which case one could consider the data preliminarily positive or negative, and make appropriate recommendation. Strength of positive or negative data escalates with level I (strongest), followed by level II and level III

Use preponderance of data for safety and efficacy to arrive at a recommendation:

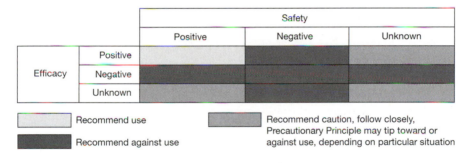

		Safety		
		Positive	Negative	Unknown
Efficacy	Positive			
	Negative			
	Unknown			

☐ Recommend use   ▨ Recommend caution, follow closely, Precautionary Principle may tip toward or
■ Recommend against use   against use, depending on particular situation

If there is a recommendation for use or caution, outline a risk/benefit analysis including:

Cost, likelihood of benefit/harm, acute versus subacute need for intervention, other options
Discussion with patient and informed consent

Note: Significant differences exist among these patients. End-of-life care may be an option in patients with locally advanced disease in whom therapy has poor results and offers significant toxicity, and the patient has a very poor performance status. In the first two subsets of patient, despite the fact that cure, control or response rates are low, the disease is still localized. During antineoplastic therapy, the Precautionary Principle should apply to withhold any substance that could alter the effectiveness of known active therapeutics in this patient with localized disease. Following active antineoplastic therapy, this distinction vanishes, and therefore the Precautionary Principle could be used to recommend with caution therapies in which unknown or inadequate data exist

Clinical examples of a scenario in which this decision tree would be used

- A 60-year-old with locally advanced pancreatic cancer undergoing postoperative radiation asking about antioxidant vitamin supplements during treatment to help with fatigue
- The same patient asking about relaxing massage to help with anxiety during and after treatment
- The same patient who is bed bound, unable to eat and drink, and had significant locally advanced disease who desires end-of-life care through a hospice and is inquiring about supportive diet, physical activity and mind–body stress reduction techniques

DECISION TREE 2

Information needed: disease type and stage, health situation, prognosis

Specific situation: localized disease, low rates of cure disease, control or response

Specific goal: supportive care:

1. Translational
2. Transformational

Transformational: difficult to measure, difficult to define cause and effect

Efficacy is difficult, if not impossible, to measure for transformational interventions, other than by qualitative, testimonial-type feedback. In this situation, it is also possible that there is no single outcome that defines the presence or absence of a transformational experience. Therefore, safety is the primary concern. If an intervention is safe, then it can be recommended with caution and monitoring

If there is a recommendation for use or caution, outline a risk/benefit analysis including:

Cost, likelihood of benefit/harm, acute versus subacute need for intervention, other options
Discussion with patient and informed consent

Note: In this scenario, the patient has localized disease with a low likelihood of cure, control or response. Despite this fact, a transformational-type intervention would seem to be of lower priority relative to other possible interventions, and the Precautionary Principle would dictate that definitive antineoplastic interventions take priority. On the other hand, beginning a specific practice with transformational intent could be pursued simultaneously if no delays would be expected, especially if the need for therapy is subacute

Clinical examples of a scenario in which this decision tree would be used

- A 49-year-old white male with locally advanced non-small-cell lung cancer who wants to delay initiation on a protocol using chemotherapy, radiation and surgery so that he can go on a residential retreat for several weeks in order to experience yoga, massage, vegetarian nutrition and group support with the ultimate goal of greater self-understanding
- The same patient who wants to begin a yoga and prayer practice in order to increase self-understanding but does not wish to delay antineplastic therapy

DECISION TREE 2

Information needed: disease type and stage, health situation, prognosis

Specific situation: localized disease, low rates of cure disease, control or response

Specific goal: antineoplastic care:

1. Curative
2. Palliative

Research evidence concerning modality: data level (I–IV) for safety and efficacy

Data level I   Data level II   Data level III   Data level IV

Note: Level IV data only are considered unknown, pending further evidence, unless the Precautionary Principle is used, in which case one could consider the data preliminarily positive or negative and make appropriate recommendation. Strength of positive or negative data escalates with level I (strongest), followed by level II and level III

Use preponderance of data for safety and efficacy to arrive at a recommendation:

		Safety		
		Positive	Negative	Unknown
Efficacy	Positive			
	Negative			
	Unknown			

- Recommend use
- Recommend against use
- Recommend caution, follow closely, Precautionary Principle may tip toward or against use, depending on particular situation

If there is a recommendation for use or caution, outline a risk/benefit analysis including:

Cost, likelihood of benefit/harm, acute versus subacute need for intervention, other options
Discussion with patient and informed consent

Note: In this scenario, the chance for cure, control and response is poor but the disease is localized, therefore every effort should be made to use available therapies, whether curative or palliative in intent, with demonstrated safety and efficacy

Clinical examples of a scenario in which this decision tree would be used

- A 55-year-old man with postobstructive pneumonia and locally advanced non-small-cell lung cancer
- The same patient with a diagnosis of superior vena cava syndrome and chest pain related to his tumor

DECISION TREE 3

Information needed: disease type and stage, health situation, prognosis

Specific situation: metastatic disease – poor prognosis for disease control or symptom response

Specific goal: prevention:
1. Primary
2. Secondary
3. Tertiary

Research evidence concerning modality: data level (I–IV) for safety and efficacy

Data level I   Data level II   Data level III   Data level IV

Note: Level IV data only are considered unknown, pending further evidence, unless the Precautionary Principle is used, in which case one could consider the data preliminarily positive or negative and make appropriate recommendation. Strength of positive or negative data escalates with level I (strongest), followed by level II and level III

Use preponderance of data for safety and efficacy to arrive at a recommendation:

		Safety		
		Positive	Negative	Unknown
Efficacy	Positive			
	Negative			
	Unknown			

☐ Recommend use

■ Recommend against use

☐ Recommend caution, follow closely, Precautionary Principle may tip toward or against use, depending on particular situation

If there is a recommendation for use or caution, outline a risk/benefit analysis including:

Cost, likelihood of benefit/harm, acute versus subacute need for intervention, other options
Discussion with patient and informed consent

Note: By definition patients have differing levels of risk in primary, secondary and tertiary prevention which may affect the level of risks and benefit they are willing to accept. In this case, the patient has a poor prognosis, and few effective options, therefore prevention will consist of counseling and symptom prevention

Clinical examples of a scenario in which this decision tree would be used

- An anxious prostate cancer patient with metastatic hormonally refractory disease and multiple visceral metastases, seeking counseling, wishing to prevent complications and manage stress related to his disease in the future

DECISION TREE 3

Information needed: disease type and stage, health situation, prognosis

Specific situation: metastatic disease – poor prognosis for disease control or symptom response

Specific goal: supportive care:
1. Translational
2. Transformational

Translational: therapy and outcome discrete and easily measurable

Symptom control and quality of life during conventional antineoplastic therapy
Symptom control and quality of life after antineoplastic care

Research evidence concerning modality: data level (I–IV) for safety and efficacy

Data level I   Data level II   Data level III   Data level IV

Note: Level IV data only are considered unknown, pending further evidence, unless the Precautionary Principle is used, in which case one could consider the data preliminarily positive or negative, and make appropriate recommendation. Level IV data are unusual in supportive care options. Strength of positive or negative data escalates with level I (strongest), followed by level II and level III

Use preponderance of data for safety and efficacy to arrive at a recommendation:

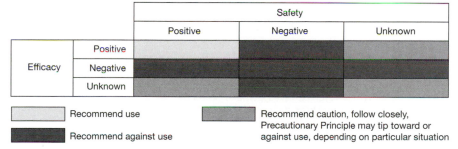

If there is a recommendation for use or caution, outline a risk/benefit analysis including:

Cost, likelihood of benefit/harm, acute versus subacute need for intervention, other options
Discussion with patient and informed consent

Note: Significant differences exist in these two groups of patients. This is less significant, however, in a situation such as this in which the patient presents with metastatic disease in which the probability for cure, response or control is low. Still, during antineoplastic therapy, the Precautionary Principle should apply to withholding any substance that could alter the effectiveness of known active therapeutics. Following active antineoplastic therapy, this distinction vanishes, and therefore the Precautionary Principle could be used to recommend with caution supportive therapies in which unknown or inadequate data exist

Clinical examples of a scenario in which this decision tree would be used

- A 60-year-old with advanced metastatic non-small-cell lung cancer undergoing palliative radiation asking about antioxidant vitamin supplements during treatment to help with fatigue
- The same patient asking about relaxing massage to help with anxiety during and after treatment
- The same patient asking about vitamins after radiation

DECISION TREE 3

Information needed: disease type and stage, health situation, prognosis

Specific situation: metastatic disease –
poor prognosis for disease control or symptom response

Specific goal: supportive care:

1. Translational
2. Transformational

Transformational: difficult to measure, difficult to define cause and effect

Efficacy is difficult, if not impossible, to measure for transformational interventions, other than by qualitative, testimonial-type feedback. In this situation, it is also possible that there is no single outcome that defines the presence or absence of a transformational experience. Therefore, safety is the primary concern. If an intervention is safe, then it can be recommended with caution and monitoring

If there is a recommendation for use or caution, outline a risk/benefit analysis including:

Cost, likelihood of benefit/harm, acute versus subacute need for intervention, other options
Discussion with patient and informed consent

Note: In this scenario, the patient has metastatic disease with a low likelihood of control or response. A transformational-type intervention would therefore seem to be of higher priority relative to other possible interventions, and the Precautionary Principle would dictate that definitive antineoplastic interventions are less relatively indicated

Clinical examples of a scenario in which this decision tree would be used

- A 49-year-old patient with metastatic pancreatic cancer who is asymptomatic and wants to delay palliative intent chemotherapy so that he can go on a residential retreat for several weeks in order to experience yoga, massage, vegetarian nutrition and group support with the ultimate goal of greater self-understanding
- The same patient who wants to begin a yoga and prayer practice in order to increase self-understanding at the same time as palliative chemotherapy

DECISION TREE 3

Information needed: disease type and stage, health situation, prognosis

Specific situation: metastatic disease – poor prognosis for disease control or symptom response

Specific goal: antineoplastic care
1. Curative
2. Palliative

Research evidence concerning modality: data level (I–IV) for safety and efficacy

Data level I   Data level II   Data level III   Data level IV

Note: Level IV data only are considered unknown, pending further evidence, unless the Precautionary Principle is used, in which case one could consider the data preliminarily positive or negative and make appropriate recommendation. Strength of positive or negative data escalates with level I (strongest), followed by level II and level III

Use preponderance of data for safety and efficacy to arrive at a recommendation:

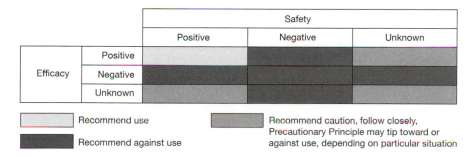

		Safety		
		Positive	Negative	Unknown
Efficacy	Positive			
	Negative			
	Unknown			

☐ Recommend use

■ Recommend against use

▨ Recommend caution, follow closely, Precautionary Principle may tip toward or against use, depending on particular situation

If there is a recommendation for use or caution, outline a risk/benefit analysis including:

Cost, likelihood of benefit/harm, acute versus subacute need for intervention, other options
Discussion with patient and informed consent

Note: In this scenario, the chance for control and response is poor and therefore every effort should be made to focus on symptom control and quality of life. Antineoplastic therapy should be initiated only with proven efficacy and safety regarding these measures

Clinical examples of a scenario in which this decision tree would be used

- A 62-year-old woman with metastatic cervical cancer who has failed three types of chemotherapy and is asymptomatic
- The same patient who is symptomatic

DECISION TREE 4

Information needed: disease type and stage, health situation, prognosis

Specific situation: metastatic disese – good prognosis for disease control or symptom response

Specific goal: prevention:

1. Primary
2. Secondary
3. Tertiary

Research evidence concerning modality: data level (I–IV) for safety and efficacy

Data level I   Data level II   Data level III   Data level IV

Note: Level IV data only are considered unknown, pending further evidence, unless the Precautionary Principle is used, in which case one could consider the data preliminarily positive or negative and make appropriate recommendation. Strength of positive or negative data escalates with level I (strongest), followed by level II and level III

Use preponderance of data for safety and efficacy to arrive at a recommendation:

		Safety		
		Positive	Negative	Unknown
Efficacy	Positive			
	Negative			
	Unknown			

Recommend use

Recommend against use

Recommend caution, follow closely, Precautionary Principle may tip toward or against use, depending on particular situation

If there is a recommendation for use or caution, outline a risk/benefit analysis including:

Cost, likelihood of benefit/harm, acute versus subacute need for intervention, other options
Discussion with patient and informed consent

Note: By definition patients have differing levels of risk in primary, secondary and tertiary prevention which may affect the level of risks and benefit they are willing to accept. In this case, the patient has a metastatic disease, but there are effective options, therefore prevention will consist of counseling and symptom prevention

Clinical examples of a scenario in which this decision tree would be used

- An anxious prostate cancer patient with metastatic disease which is newly diagnosed wishing to manage stress from his treatment and disease in the future

DECISION TREE 4

Information needed: disease type and stage, health situation, prognosis

Specific situation: metastatic disese –
good prognosis for disease control or symptom response

Specific goal: supportive care:
1. Translational
2. Transformational

Translational: therapy and outcome discrete and easily measurable

Symptom control and quality of life during conventional antineoplastic therapy
Symptom control and quality of life after antineoplastic care

Research evidence concerning modality: data level (I–IV) for safety and efficacy

Data level I   Data level II   Data level III   Data level IV

Note: Level IV data only are considered unknown, pending further evidence, unless the Precautionary Principle is used, in which case one could consider the data preliminarily positive or negative, and make appropriate recommendation. Level IV data are unusual in supportive care options. Strength of positive or negative data escalates with level I (strongest), followed by level II and level III

Use preponderance of data for safety and efficacy to arrive at a recommendation:

		Safety		
		Positive	Negative	Unknown
Efficacy	Positive	Recommend use	Recommend against use	Recommend caution
	Negative	Recommend against use	Recommend against use	Recommend against use
	Unknown	Recommend caution	Recommend against use	Recommend caution

■ Recommend use   ■ Recommend caution, follow closely, Precautionary Principle may tip toward or
■ Recommend against use   against use, depending on particular situation

If there is a recommendation for use or caution, outline a risk/benefit analysis including:

Cost, likelihood of benefit/harm, acute versus subacute need for intervention, other options
Discussion with patient and informed consent

Note: Significant differences exist in these two groups of patients. This is less significant, however, in a situation such as this, in which the patient presents with metastatic disease in which the probability for cure, response or control is still high. Still, during antineoplastic therapy, the Precautionary Principle should apply to withholding any substance that could alter the effectiveness of known active therapeutics. Following active antineoplastic therapy, this distinction vanishes, and therefore the Precautionary Principle could be used to recommend with caution supportive therapies in which unknown or inadequate data exis

Clinical examples of a scenario in which this decision tree would be used

- A 60-year-old woman with advanced metastatic breast cancer newly diagnosed undergoing palliative radiation asking about antioxidant vitamin supplements during treatment to help with fatigue
- The same patient asking about relaxing massage to help with anxiety during and after treatment
- The same patient asking about vitamins after radiation

DECISION TREE 4

Information needed: disease type and stage, health situation, prognosis

Specific situation: metastatic disese –
good prognosis for disease control or symptom response

Specific goal: supportive care:

1. Translational
2. Transformational

Transformational: difficult to measure, difficult to define cause and effect

Efficacy is difficult, if not impossible, to measure for transformational interventions, other than by qualitative, testimonial-type feedback. In this situation, it is also possible that there is no single outcome that defines the presence or absence of a transformational experience. Therefore, safety is the primary concern. If an intervention is safe, then it can be recommended with caution and monitoring

If there is a recommendation for use or caution, outline a risk/benefit analysis including:

Cost, likelihood of benefit/harm, acute versus subacute need for intervention, other options
Discussion with patient and informed consent

Note: In this scenario, the patient has metastatic disease with a high likelihood of control or response. A transformational-type intervention would therefore seem to be of modest priority relative to other possible interventions, and the Precautionary Principle would dictate that definitive antineoplastic interventions are probably still indicated as a priority, especially if the need is acute (i.e. the patient is symptomatic)

Clinical examples of a scenario in which this decision tree would be used

- A 49-year-old patient with metastatic prostate cancer, newly diagnosed, who is asymptomatic and wants to delay palliative intent hormonal therapy so that he can go on a residential retreat for several weeks in order to experience yoga, massage, vegetarian nutrition and group support with the ultimate goal of greater self-understanding
- The same patient who wants to begin a yoga and prayer practice in order to increase self-understanding at the same time as hormonal therapy

DECISION TREE 4

Information needed: disease type and stage, health situation, prognosis

Specific situation: metastatic disese – good prognosis for disease control or symptom response

Specific goal: antineoplastic care:
1. Curative
2. Palliative

Research evidence concerning modality: data level (I–IV) for safety and efficacy

Data level I   Data level II   Data level III   Data level IV

Note: Level IV data only are considered unknown, pending further evidence, unless the Precautionary Principle is used, in which case one could consider the data preliminarily positive or negative and make appropriate recommendation. Strength of positive or negative data escalates with level I (strongest), followed by level II and level III

Use preponderance of data for safety and efficacy to arrive at a recommendation:

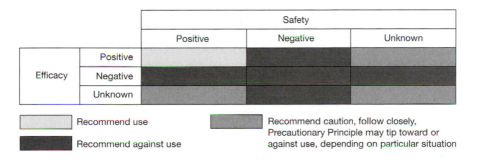

		Safety		
		Positive	Negative	Unknown
Efficacy	Positive			
	Negative			
	Unknown			

☐ Recommend use

■ Recommend against use

▨ Recommend caution, follow closely, Precautionary Principle may tip toward or against use, depending on particular situation

If there is a recommendation for use or caution, outline a risk/benefit analysis including:

Cost, likelihood of benefit/harm, acute versus subacute need for intervention, other options
Discussion with patient and informed consent

Note: In this scenario, the chance for control and response is still good, despite the presence of metastatic disease, and therefore every effort should be made to focus on symptom control and quality of life through the use of safe and effective antineoplastic therapy

Clinical examples of a scenario in which this decision tree would be used

- A 62-year-old woman with painful metastatic, breast cancer who is asymptomatic and the disease is newly diagnosed
- The same patient who has bone metastases and is in pain

References

1. Weiger WA, Smith M, Boon H, et al. Advising patients who seek complementary and alternative medical therapies for cancer. Ann Intern Med 2002; 137: 889–903

2. Adams KE, Cohen MH, Eisenberg D, Jonsen AR. Ethical considerations of complementary and alternative medical therapies in conventional medical settings. Ann Intern Med 2002; 137(8): 660–4

3. Cohen MH, Eisenberg DM. Potential physician malpractice liability associated with complementary and integrative medical therapies. Ann Intern Med 2002; 136: 596–603

4. Federation of State Medical Boards. Model guidelines for physician use of complementary and alternative methods in medical practice. Federation of State Medical Boards. Accessed 5 February 2004. Available from URL: www.fsmb.org

5. Davis DL, Axelrod D, Bailey L, et al. Rethinking breast cancer risk and the environment: the case for the precautionary principle. Environ Health Perspect 1998; 106: 523–9

6. Richter ED, Laster R. The Precautionary Principle, epidemiology and the ethics of delay. Int J Occup Med Environ Health 2004; 17: 9–16

9

Stages of change

Robert B. Lutz

The world of a cancer patient is filled with change – from the diagnosis of a potentially life-threatening disease to the initiation of often toxic antineoplastic therapies. While cancer patients may be highly motivated to make lifestyle-related changes in order to support them through the treatment process and potentially help with recovery and prevention of recurrence, it can prove more difficult to counsel high-risk individuals successfully concerning cancer-prevention activities. Cancer patients may also have different levels of readiness for supportive care options, depending upon their ability to cope with multiple changes all at the same time. For example, recommendations for psychotherapy may have negative connotations for patients who feel they have their situation 'under control' and would rather focus on conventional antineoplastic therapy only. It is important to evaluate patient needs through appropriate screening. Once a need is identified, counseling should begin with an assessment of the individual's level of readiness for change.

The 'stages of change' model is one that many health-care providers are familiar with. It identifies five stages that relate to an individual's readiness to initiate a new behavior:

(1) Pre-contemplation;

(2) Contemplation;

(3) Preparation;

(4) Action;

(5) Maintenance.

This model was proposed by Prochaska *et al.*[1,2] to understand smoking and substance usage behavior. It has been adapted to address a number of behaviors and is commonly applied to physical activity/exercise promotion. It emphasizes the process of change as a function of an individual's readiness (motivation) to change. Individuals spiral through five distinct stages of readiness. They progress through these stages at different rates in a non-linear fashion, often going back and forth before achieving maintenance. Progress may be slow, but individuals spiraling through these stages rarely return completely to their previous stage.

The following defines the stages of change and suggests an appropriate clinical application for individulas in each stage with regards to a variety of wellness choices.

PRE-CONTEMPLATION

There is no intention to change behavior in the foreseeable future. 'It isn't that they can't see the solution. It is that they can't see the problem.' (G.K. Chesterton)

Application

Increase awareness of the benefits of beginning to implement changes, for example, an exercise program or modifying their diets. Encourage the individual to give consideration to this behavior; acknowledge the challenges that exist and express willingness to assist in overcoming these barriers.

CONTEMPLATION

There is an awareness of a problem and a willingness to address it, but individuals have not made a commitment to take action. A weighing of pros and cons of the problem and the solution commonly occurs during this stage.

Application

Encourage the formulation of a specific plan of action – e.g. identification of an up-coming charity running event to raise money for a worthwhile cause; decide closely to monitor calorie intake and learn how to read food labels.

PREPARATION

Individuals intend to take action within the next month and may have unsuccessfully taken action in the past year. They may have partially addressed their desired behavior, but insufficiently so as to achieve effective action.

Application

An action plan is created with goals and objectives that are realistic and attainable; short- and long-term goals are discussed with timelines created. Example: an up-coming 5-k and fun walk is identified that is 4 months in the future. A program is created that identifies an immediate action plan and short-term goals leading up to the event.

ACTION

Initiation/modification of a behavior. The environmental context or experience occurs during this stage. It is of significant quality to be perceived as 'successful' and demonstrates sufficient effort to change.

Application

Return visits where feedback, reinforcement and solution identification occur; identification of social support; checking occurs regularly, either in person or by phone.

MAINTENANCE

Individuals work to prevent relapse, creating stabilizing behaviors that serve to perpetuate the behavior change.

Application

Identification of coping strategies for inevitable slips and relapses; providing appropriate reminders; consider alternate solutions if barriers prove formidable.

COUNSELING PATIENTS

A model of counseling that incorporates the above elements has been proposed. This was originally developed to address physical activity, but may be generalized to other modalities as well[3].

ASSESSMENT

There are four key subheadings under this stage.

Quality-of-life concerns, goals and expectations

This is potentially the most important consideration in the assessment stage. It seeks to identify and/or assist the individual in identifying reasons for making a change (e.g. relaxation, vitality, disease prevention, well-being).

Current health status/fitness status

What is an individual capable of achieving, given his/her current physical, emotional, social and mental condition?

Health practices and attitudes

What has the individual done in the past, and what do they currently do, and why? What new activities may be of interest? What are the skills and what is needed to go forward and/or try something new? How might other behaviors (e.g. nutrition, stress level, social activities, employment, family support, hobbies) affect current health status as well as affecting the initiation of new behaviors?

Life situation and environment

What is their current employment status? What type of work do they do (e.g. amount of work-related physical activity, nutrition, stress in the workplace)? Is their current job primarily sedentary and, if so, are there opportunities for adding activity to the work day? Are there hobbies that entail activity or promote relaxation and group support? Are there significant time constraints that will need to be addressed, and, if so, how can potential solutions be identified? What does the individual's physical environment look like – urban vs. suburban vs. rural; access to trails, parks and green spaces; proximity and access to recreation facilities; weather considerations; access to fresh fruits and vegetables, faith-based organizations, complementary providers? What are current dietary patterns? What is their relationship to food – i.e. as stress reliever? How do they deal with stress? How do they relax?

TARGET IDENTIFICATION

Using the information gained during the initial assessment, providers partner and assist in identification of a realistic 'target' for behavior initiation. This must be attainable and amenable to available resources. For example, it may be the actual behavior, or it may be a preliminary step, such as finding a fitness center, or locating a market that has fresh fruits and vegetables. Recognition of the individual's readiness to change assists the provider in tailoring the appropriate message.

PLANNING

What is a reasonable starting point, to include amount of time being spent and the frequency of performance? What venue will be chosen for this activity? Will it be done in an individual setting or with a group, and, if the latter, where is this group and how can the individual become connected? Are there seasonal considerations that need to be factored into the program? What kind of support exists, if any?

IMPLEMENTATION

Getting started can sometimes be challenging, but approaching behavior initiation according to the above lays the necessary groundwork to address potential obstacles.

EVALUATION AND REFORMULATION

The program should be periodically re-evaluated, with acknowledgment of barriers and challenges that need to be overcome. Feedback and encouragement should be provided for overcoming obstacles and goal achievement. Every visit should serve as an opportunity to check in. Recognizing that individuals cycle through the stages of change, reassessment of an individual's current stage should be performed. This will allow for program and message modification if necessary. Monitoring of physical and health-related parameters, such as weight and mood, may provide important reinforcement. Determination of how the program has affected an individual's perceived quality of life should be at the core of this step.

This general approach to evaluating and counseling individuals can be helpful both to the patient and to the provider. Through a step-wise approach to counseling, the individual's unique situation can be addressed, realistic expectations met and frustrations minimized.

Physicians who 'walk the talk' and have healthy lifestyle habits themselves will probably be better able to provide meaningful counseling (see Chapter 4). By speaking from personal experience and demonstrating an appreciation for the unique situation for which they are providing recommendations, providers may find their patients more able and willing to incorporate these recommendations into their lives.

References

1. Prochaska JO, DiClemente CC. The Transtheoretical Approach: Crossing Traditional Boundaries of Change. Homewood, IL: Dorsey Press, 1984
2. Prochaska JO, DiClemente CC, Norcross JC. In search of how people change. Am Psychol 1992; 47: 1102–14
3. Laitakari J, Asikainen TM. How to promote physical activity through individual counseling – a proposal for a practical model of counseling on health-related physical activity. Patient Educ Counsel 1998; 33: S13–24

10

Modalities – overview

In this section, we will review the modalities to be presented as a part of an integrative oncology. Each modality will include a general introduction, followed by cancer research background and the major current questions facing that field. This will be followed by a general summary, including tools for practice, and a glossary of modality-specific terminology.

The authors for the modalities remain the same for the prevention, supportive and antineoplastic care sections. It should be noted that the authors did not collaborate with regards to content on modalities other than their own.

10a

Physical activity

Robert B. Lutz

> 'All parts of the body that have a function, if used in moderation, and exercised in labors to which each is accustomed, become healthy and well developed and age slowly; but if unused and left idle, they become liable to disease, defective in growth and age quickly.' – Hippocrates

> Every US adult should accumulate 30 minutes or more of moderate-intensity physical activity on most, preferably all, days of the week[1].

INTRODUCTION

Although separated by millennia, the authors of the above statements share a common understanding – physical activity is essential for good health. No distinction is made for individuals who may be diagnosed with an illness, such as cancer. Rather, health is defined as a multidimensional concept that engages all elements of an individual. The World Health Organization defines health as '…a resource for everyday life, not the object of living. It is a positive concept emphasizing social and personal resources as well as physical capabilities'[2]. Using this definition, health can be achieved, even when experiencing illness, and its presence may allow individuals to achieve their potential.

Physical activity is a natural element of living and is fundamental to the construct of 'lifestyle'.

A healthy lifestyle dynamically reflects behaviors that change over time for individuals, dependent upon their life's context. Physical activity is an important foundation of an integrative approach to medicine that is healing-oriented, engages the whole person (body, mind and spirit), and includes all aspects of lifestyle.

Recommending or prescribing physical activity and/or exercise to patients remains a somewhat empiric endeavor. Even the terminology can be confusing. Physical activity represents all forms of bodily movement while exercise is defined as a form of physical activity dedicated to improving fitness and inclusive of the training components of intensity, duration, mode of activity and frequency. Please refer to the glossary at the end of this section for some definitions and examples of physical activity-related terms.

PHYSICAL ACTIVITY AND CANCER RESEARCH – BACKGROUND

It has been suggested that sedentary lifestyles may be one explanation for the differences in cancer rates between specific groups identified in population and migration studies[3]. Research concerning the role of physical activity and cancer prevention is relatively new. Conclusions are based primarily upon animal studies and supported by observational occupational epidemiologic studies[4]. For example, a study reported in 1975 found that 'professionals' were at increased risk for colorectal cancer as compared to those with careers requiring more physical activity[5]. Subsequent occupational studies identified a common finding: individuals employed in 'low-activity' occupations were at increased risk for colon cancer[6]. In 1994, an often-cited study was published linking physical activity with reduced risk of breast cancer[7]. Likewise, studies linking prostate cancer and physical activity were reported[8]. There are few epidemiologic studies that have looked at this association in other cancer types, however – often as a function of lower cancer incidence rates.

The research to date is encouraging in its findings for an association between physical activity and cancer. This relationship is certainly more robust for some cancers (e.g. colon cancer) than for others (e.g. ovarian cancer), and more research is necessary to determine the role of physical activity in cancer prevention. Although cancer is currently the second leading cause of mortality in the USA, increasingly it is acknowledged that the 'actual' causes of death in this country are not diseases, but rather the lifestyle behaviors that often influence their incidence[9].

Currently, there are few cancer prevention studies that address physical activity prospectively as an intervention. The data that are available have often been obtained as secondary outcomes from studies of other diseases[10]. Logistical considerations preclude using cancer incidence as an endpoint, owing to the length of follow-up as well as loss to follow-up that would occur.

As survival rates for cancer have steadily increased (5-year survival for all cancers and stages, 62%; for the most common cancers with early detection, 90%[11]), there is increasing interest in the role of physical activity in affecting the quality of life (QOL) for people with cancer, both during and after treatment[12]. Whether or not such supportive interventions affect traditional outcome measures of response, relapse rates and survival remains an unknown, but it certainly provides a rich area for future research.

As the body of research exploring the relationship between physical activity and cancer expands, clinicians will be better able to provide evidence-based recommendations to their patients.

CURRENT QUESTIONS FOR RESEARCH

Whereas the exact biological mechanisms defining the relationship between physical activity and cancer remain unknown, many plausible explanations have been identified. It is equally as important to realize that questions still exist, such as, 'What is the best type of exercise – aerobic, endurance, flexibility associated, or resistance?' 'When is the best time in an individual's life to be physically active for prevention?' 'What is the best 'dose' of exercise for prevention or supportive care?' 'Can physical activity affect prevention of recurrent disease in cancer survivors?'

CONCLUSION

The available research supports a role for physical activity in cancer prevention and treatment, as will be explored in later chapters. Although the exact mechanisms for this association may not be clearly known, there are multiple plausible biological mechanisms that have been identified through animal and epidemiological studies. As treatment options improve survival in patients with cancer, more research is necessary to clarify these mechanisms as well as to address how physical activity may be implemented as a treatment that affects both recurrence and supportive care issues.

Integrative medicine fundamentally approaches health care through an emphasis on the primacy of the patient–provider relationship. Individuals are strongly encouraged to become active participants in their own health care, in both the absence and the presence of a disease. Health, viewed as a 'resource for everyday life, not the object of living'[2], can be experienced by all individuals, irrespective of their disease status. It is through a mutual commitment to exploration that physical activity promotion can identify the wealth of potential that may exist for people with cancer, providers and society in general.

TOOLS FOR PRACTICE

Please see Chapter 9 and the Glossary below.

GLOSSARY OF TERMS

Physical activity   Broadly defined as any bodily movement that is produced by the contraction of skeletal muscle and that substantially increases energy expenditure.

Leisure-time physical activity   Physical activity undertaken during discretionary time.

Occupational or vocational activity   Work-related physical activity. It can include activities that are done at home, such as housework and gardening, as well as those activities that are directly work-related, such as lifting boxes while stocking shelves.

Exercise   Leisure-time physical activity that is conducted with the intention of developing and/or improving physical fitness. It requires consideration of several training components, including intensity, duration, mode of activity and frequency.

Exercise testing   Maximal oxygen consumption or VO_{2max}, refers to the body's maximal ability to utilize oxygen. It is considered the gold standard for determining aerobic fitness. VO_{2max} is determined by a graded exercise test on a treadmill or stationary bicycle (ergometer). The test is conducted as a person exercises while the workload is gradually increased until the person can no longer continue (approximately 12–15 minutes). During the test, the person breathes through a mouthpiece and their expired air is analyzed for oxygen content by a computer to evaluate VO_{2max}. These tests may be performed by trained health-care professionals or exercise physiologists. Submaximal testing is a more readily available option as it can be performed without measuring expired air. Predictive submaximal tests are used to predict maximal aerobic capacity, while performance submaximal tests involve measuring the responses to standardized physical activities that are typically encountered in everyday life. These are performed by a variety of exercise specialists, such as personal fitness trainers. As they are not performed at a maximal level, they carry less risk for the patient with known medical problems.

Physical fitness   A set of attributes that people have or achieve relating to their ability to perform physical activity. The American College of Sports Medicine defines physical fitness as 'The ability to perform moderate-to-vigorous levels of physical activity without undue fatigue and the capability of maintaining this capacity throughout life'[13].

Health-related physical fitness   There are five components of health-related physical fitness.

They have been associated with lowering the risk for disease and improving quality of life. These components are exclusive but interrelated:

(1) **Body composition** The relative amounts of body fat and lean body tissue/fat-free mass (i.e. muscle, bone and water). A common measure of this is body mass index (BMI), calculated by: Weight (kg)/Height (m)^2, or alternatively as the Weight (lbs)/Height (in)$^2 \times 703$. The current recommendations are that a healthy weight be defined by a BMI of 19–24.9 kg/m^2; overweight BMI $\geq$ 25–29.9 kg/m;^{2} and obesity BMI > 30 kg/m^2.

(2) **Cardiovascular fitness** It is also known as cardiovascular endurance, aerobic fitness or cardiorespiratory fitness. It is the ability of the circulatory and respiratory systems to extract oxygen and deliver it to working muscles during sustained physical activity and to adjust to, and recover from, the effects of physical activity. It is generally regarded as the key component of health-related fitness.

(3) **Musculoskeletal fitness** It has three components: flexibility, muscular strength, and muscular endurance.

   (a) **Flexibility** A functional capacity of the joints to move through a full range of movement. It is affected by the muscles and connective tissues surrounding the joints, and is specific to each joint.

   (b) **Muscular endurance** The ability to apply a submaximal force repeatedly, or to sustain a submaximal contraction for a specified period of time. More simply, it is a measure of the muscle's ability to perform without fatigue. As seen with flexibility, this measure is specific for each muscle. It can be measured both isometrically (static muscular contraction) or isotonically (dynamic muscular contraction).

   (c) **Muscular strength** Relates to the ability of a muscle to exert a maximal force. It is muscle-specific. Muscular strength can be measured both isometrically and isotonically.

MET (metabolic equivalent) Activities are often provided a unit of measure as a gauge of intensity, where 1 MET is defined as the resting metabolic rate (RMR) during quiet sitting (approximately 3.5 ml O_2/kg per min). The MET for a given activity therefore represents a ratio of the associated activity divided by the RMR. See Table 10.1 for examples of activities and their metabolic equivalent categorized as level of intensity.

Table 10.1 Examples of types of exercise and intensity

Light (< 3 MET or < 4 kcal/min)	Moderate (3–6 MET or 4–7 kcal/min)	Vigorous (> 6 MET or >7 kcal/min)
Slow walking (1–2 mph)	Brisk walking (2–4 mph)	Brisk walking uphill/with load
Stationary cycling (< 50 W)	Cycling (< 10 mph)	Cycling (10 mph or greater)
Swimming, slow treading	Swimming, moderate effort	Swimming, paced effort
Mowing lawn – riding mower	Mowing lawn – power mower	Mowing lawn – hand mower
Home care – carpet cleaning	Home care – general cleaning	Home care – moving furniture
Gardening – watering	Gardening – raking, weeding	Gardening – shoveling

Light exercise Intensity less than 3 MET or < 4 kcal/min

Moderate exercise Intensity of 3–6 MET or 4–7 kcal/min

Vigorous exercise Intensity of greater than 6 MET or > 7 kcal/min

RESOURCES FOR PHYSICAL ACTIVITY

Linking to the American College of Sports Medicine (www.acsm.org/index.asp) is a good starting point to access further information. Likewise, contacting local hospitals will provide additional resources. Some other web resources follow.

www.aicr.org/index.lasso

http://cancer.stanfordhospital.com/healthInfo/overview.html

www.cancer.umn.edu/page/patients/riskred3.html

www.cancer.org/docroot/MIT/MIT_2_1x_ExerciseToStayActive.asp

www.ncpad.org/disability/fact_sheet.php?sheet=38&section=270

www.hsph.harvard.edu/cancer/index.html

References

1. Pate RR, Pratt M, Blair SN, et al. Physical activity and public health. A recommendation from the Centers for Disease Control and Prevention and the American College of Sports Medicine. JAMA 1995; 273: 402–7

2. World Health Organization. Ottawa Charter for Health Promotion. Copenhagen, Denmark: World Health Organization, European Regional Office, 1986

3. Thune I, Furberg AS. Physical activity and cancer risk: dose-response and cancer, all sites and site-specific. Med Sci Sports Exerc 2001; 33 (Suppl): S530–S550

4. Shepard RJ, Futcher R. Physical activity and cancer: how may protection be maximized? Crit Rev Oncol 1997; 8: 219–72

5. Berg JW, Howell MA. Occupation and bowel cancer. J Toxicol Environ Health 1975; 1: 75–9.

6. Garabrant DH, Peters JM, Mack TM, et al. Job activity and colon cancer risk. Am J Epidemiol 1984; 119: 1005–14

7. Bernstein L, Henderson BE, Hanisch R, et al. Physical exercise and reduced risk of breast cancer in young women. J Natl Cancer Inst 1994; 86: 1403–8

8. Lee I-M, Paffenbarger RS Jr, Hsieh CC. Physical activity and risk of prostatic cancer among college alumni. Am J Epidemiol 1992; 135: 169–79

9. Mokdad AH, Marks JS, Stroup DF, et al. Actual causes of death in the United States, 2000. JAMA 2004; 291: 1238–45

10. Mctiernan A. Intervention studies in exercise and cancer prevention. Med Sci Sports Exerc 2003; 35: 1841–5

11. American Cancer Society. Cancer Facts and Figures 2003. Atlanta, GA: American Cancer Society, 2003: 48

12. Courneya KS. Exercise in cancer survivors: an overview of research. Med Sci Sports Exerc 2003; 35: 1846–52

13. American College of Sports Medicine. www.acsm.org/index.asp

10b

Nutrition

Cynthia Thomson and Mara Vitolins

'Let food be thy medicine and medicine be thy food.' – Hippocrates

INTRODUCTION

Dietary patterns and food selections have been estimated to account for the development of 30–50% of all cancers[1]. Generally diets high in fat and processed carbohydrate or simple sugars, low in vegetables, fruit and fiber, and excessive in energy are associated with a high incidence of cancer. What we eat is a choice each of us makes each and every day (if not multiple times each day), and yet the complexity of food intake and its relationship with the development of chronic disease, including cancer, continues to evade us. Diet, however, is a *modifiable* risk factor for disease, and thus holds significance in efforts both on the individual and public health levels in terms of reducing the cancer burden.

Discussions throughout this text will explore the role of nutrition in integrative oncology care. Historically, tissue/body wasting was well recognized as one of the sequelae of cancer progression. In addition, during the 1970s and 1980s there was increasing concern that providing nutrition/feeding to patients with cancer might

'feed the tumor' thus contributing to the patient's demise. However, more recently there has been recognition of the importance of supporting cancer patients nutritionally throughout the care process. In addition, there are well-documented changes in nutrient metabolism which warrant the ongoing involvement of well-trained nutrition professionals in the provision of nutritional care for oncology patients[2,3].

NUTRITION AND RESEARCH – BACKGROUND

There is strong evidence in support of cancer incidence being influenced by environmental factors. Observational studies illustrate the wide variation in international cancer mortality rates, which are particularly high in Northern Europe and North America, and much lower in Japan and other Asian countries[4]. An example of the influence of environmental factors comes from the observation of people who migrate from a country with low risk for cancer to a country with higher risk. The level of risk for the migrant becomes similar to that in the country to which they migrate. For example, immigrants from Poland and Japan, where the incidence of prostate cancer is low, exhibit a significant increase in the risk of developing prostate cancer when they reside in the USA[5–7]. The rate of breast cancer also increases among Japanese women who immigrate to the USA[8].

It has been suggested that many cancer deaths may be preventable through dietary means. Researchers estimate that between 30 and 40% of all cancers could be prevented if people maintained a healthy body weight, ate nutritious foods and increased their physical activity[9].

Nutrition may also have a distinct role in supportive care, as well as prevention of recurrence of disease for cancer survivors. However, conducting research regarding cancer (prevention, survival, death) and nutrition is very difficult, for a variety of reasons (e.g. amount of funding required, large sample size, length of follow-up to reach outcomes such as recurrence or death).

CURRENT RESEARCH QUESTIONS

Can specific phytonutrients provide benefit in primary, secondary and tertiary prevention? What is the optimal route of delivery – whole foods or supplements?

What is the role of antioxidant supplements during active antineoplastic therapy? What is the role of nutraceuticals as supportive care? What is the role of a diet with a low glycemic index in cancer prevention and supportive care?

CURRENT RESEARCH TRIALS

The following is a list of current research trials:

- SELECT trial – supplemental selenium and vitamin E as primary prevention for prostate cancer.

- Cancer-preventing qualities of broccoli sprouts tea – study sponsored by the National Center for Complementary and Alternative Medicine (NCCAM).

- Macrobiotic diet and flax seed – effects on estrogens, phytoestrogens and fibrinolytic factors – NCCAM sponsored.

- Weight loss counseling for African American breast cancer survivors – NCCAM sponsored.

- The American Cancer Society Prevention Study II Nutrition cohort – a large cohort of 84 000 men and 97 000 women being followed prospectively since 1992.

SUMMARY

There are foods, micronutrients and phytochemicals that may have cancer-preventive actions, and these will be discussed in detail in later sections. In addition, nutrition should be an integral part of supportive and palliative care. There may even be some role for certain foods as antineoplastic agents; however, research here is currently lacking.

GLOSSARY OF TERMS

Adjuvant therapy Treatment given in addition to the primary treatment to enhance the effectiveness of the primary treatment.

Antioxidant Any substance that delays or inhibits oxidative damage (the attack upon biological molecules of oxygen containing 'free radicals'). All molecules in living organisms are potential targets of oxidative damage: lipids, proteins, nucleic acids, connective tissue and carbohydrates. Antioxidants work primarily by donating or 'sacrificing' an electron to the free radical thereby stabilizing the free radical. Found in: many plants – especially those rich in bioflavonoids. Vitamins A, C and E, superoxide dismutase (SOD), glutathione peroxidase, selenium, zinc, copper, manganese have antioxidant activity.

Apoptosis   A normal cellular process involving a genetically programmed series of events leading to the death of a cell.

Body mass index (BMI)   A mathematical formula to assess body weight relative to height. The measure correlates highly with body fat. Calculated as weight in kilograms divided by the square of the height in meters (kg/m^2).

Calorie   A unit of measure, like an inch or a pound. Calories measure the amount of energy the body gets from food. You need energy to be physically active and for your body to grow and function. Carbohydrates, fat and protein provide the energy from food.

Cancer   A term for diseases in which abnormal cells divide without control. Cancer cells can invade nearby tissues and can spread through the bloodstream and lymphatic system to other parts of the body.

Carbohydrate   The body's most readily available source of energy. Each gram of carbohydrate provides 4 calories of energy. The main forms of carbohydrate are sugars and starches. Sugars are simple carbohydrates. Starches, as in breads, cereals and pasta, are complex carbohydrates.

Carcinogen   Any substance that is known to cause cancer.

Carcinogenesis   The process by which normal cells are transformed into cancer cells.

Diet history   The respondent is questioned about 'typical' or 'usual' food intake in an interview format. The aim is to construct a typical 7-day eating pattern. The interviewer may discuss each meal and inter-meal eating in turn or each

day of the week consecutively. Questions are usually open-ended, although a fully structured interview may be used. The diet history may be preceded by a 24-hour recall and/or supplemented by a checklist of foods usually consumed.

Dietary records   'Gold standard' record of intake of foods. It self-reports beverages and food consumed for 1 or more days. A blanket term for all record methods. It is often used without qualification and with quantification using 'household measures'. A record is of actual food and drink consumed on specified days after the first contact by the investigator. The number of days recorded classically is 7, but may be fewer or more.

Dietary 24-hour recall   Face-to-face or telephone interview which attempts to remember and report all intake from the preceding day. The respondent is asked to recall the actual food and drink consumed on specified days, usually the immediate past 24 hours (24-hour recall) but sometimes longer periods.

Fat   A concentrated energy source. Fat provides 9 calories per gram, more than twice as much energy as protein and carbohydrate. Fat also provides essential fatty acids, is an important component of cell structure, and transports vitamins A, D, E and K.

Fiber   A form of carbohydrate which your body cannot digest. Fiber helps your digestive tract work.

> **Insoluble fiber** – cellulose, hemicellulose and lignin – is not soluble in water. Foods which contain insoluble fibers are wheat bran, whole grain products, and vegetables. Insoluble fibers are responsible for increased stool bulk and help to regulate bowel movements.

> **Soluble fiber** – gums, pectins and mucilages – becomes gummy in water. When eaten, these fiber sources actually slow the passage of food through the digestive system. Some researchers believe this action helps to regu-

late cholesterol and glucose (sugar) levels in the blood by affecting absorption rates. Food sources of soluble fibers are dried beans, oats, barley and some fruits and vegetables.

Food frequency questionnaires The respondent is presented with a list of foods and is asked how often each is eaten in broad terms, such as *x* times per day, per week, per month, etc. The foods listed are usually chosen for the specific purposes of a study and generally assess the total diet. The questionnaire may be interviewer-administered or self-completed. Assessment of the quantities of food consumed on each eating occasion or day may also be included.

Functional foods Foods designed to promote health beyond the normal nutrient benefits. Also referred to as nutraceuticals. Examples include orange juice with calcium, soy chips, beverages with ginseng.

Glycemic index The glycemic index (GI) is a numerical system of measuring how much of a rise in circulating blood sugar a carbohydrate triggers – the higher the number, the greater the blood sugar response. Thus a low GI food will cause a small rise, while a high GI food will trigger a dramatic spike.

Macronutrient A chemical element required by plants in relatively large amounts. Macronutrients contain carbon, hydrogen and oxygen, and include carbohydrates, fats and proteins.

Micronutrient A chemical element required in relatively small quantities. Micronutrients are typically found in cofactors and coenzymes. They include copper, zinc, molybdenum, manganese, cobalt and boron and vitamins.

Phytochemicals Compounds other than nutrients which are naturally present in foods (predominantly foods of plant origin) and which have the potential to improve health.

Protein A major component of all body tissue. Your body needs protein to grow and repair itself. Protein is also a necessary component of hormones, enzymes and hemoglobin.

Resting energy expenditure (REE) Expenditure represents the amount of calories required for a 24-hour period by the body during a non-active period. Energy cost of physiological functions to maintain homeostasis.

Saturated fat Type of fat found in foods of animal origin and a few of vegetable origin; they are usually solid at room temperature. Abundant in meat and dairy products, saturated fat tends to increase low-density lipoprotein (LDL) cholesterol levels, and it may raise the risk of certain types of cancer.

Trans fat Created when hydrogen is forced through an ordinary vegetable oil (hydrogenation), converting some polyunsaturates to monounsaturates, and some monounsaturates to saturates. Trans fat, like saturated fat, tends to raise LDL cholesterol levels, and, unlike saturated fat, trans fat also lowers high-density lipoprotein (HDL) cholesterol levels at the same time, and may increase the risk of certain cancers.

Waist circumference The distance around the natural waist (just above the navel) measured in the standing position with tape measure parallel to the floor.

RESOURCE FOR NUTRITIONAL INFORMATION

American Cancer Society publishes information on nutrition before, during and after cancer therapy (www.cancer.org).

Nutrition.gov – general source for nutritional information.

References

1. Doll R, Peto R. The causes of cancer: quantitative estimates of avoidable risks of cancer in the United States today. J Natl Cancer Inst 1981; 66: 1191–308

2. Laviano A, Meguid MM. Nutritional issues in cancer management. Nutrition 1996; 12: 358–71

3. The need for dietary counseling of cancer patients as indicated by nutrient and supplement intake. J Am Dietetic Assoc 1995; 95: 1319–22

4. Wynder EL, Mabuchi K, Whitmore WF Jr. Epidemiology of cancer of the prostate. Cancer 1971; 28: 344–60

5. Dunn JE. Cancer epidemiology in populations of the United States – with emphasis on Hawaii and California – and Japan. Cancer Res 1975; 35: 3240–5

6. Haenszel W, Kurihara M. Studies of Japanese migrants. I. Mortality from cancer and other diseases among Japanese in the United States. J Natl Cancer Inst 1968; 40: 43–68

7. Staszewski J, Hainszel W. Cancer mortality among the Polish-born in the United States. J Natl Cancer Inst 1965: 35; 291–7

8. Shimizu J, Ross RK, Berstein L, et al. Cancers of the prostate and breast among Japanese and white immigrants in Los Angeles Country. B J Cancer 1991: 63; 963–6

9. WCRF/AICR. Food, Nutrition and the Prevention of Cancer: a Global Perspective. Washington, DC: World Cancer Research Fund/American Institute for Cancer Research, 1997

10c

Mind–body interventions

Linda E. Carlson and Shauna L. Shapiro

> 'We shall not cease from exploration
> And the end of all our exploring
> Will be to arrive where we started
> And know the place for the first time.
> Through the unknown, remembered gate
> When the last of earth is left to discover
> Is that which was the beginning…'
> – T.S. Eliot

INTRODUCTION

Any overview of integrative therapies for cancer care would be remiss not to address the widespread use of mind–body interventions. A recent survey of American households found 19% of respondents had used a mind–body therapy in the last year[1]. When looking specifically at cancer patients, that number ranges widely, depending on the type of therapy assessed, the group of patients, the year and the geographical region. Values range anywhere between 12% usage of mind–body therapies in a nationwide Canadian sample (Leis, personal communication), 14% for psychological therapies in the USA[2], 16.9% use of relaxation in an Israeli sample[3], 28% use of relaxation/meditation and 13% use of imagery and support groups in an American breast cancer

sample[4], to a high of 81.6% use of 'mind–body' therapies in Hawaii[5]. This range in values could also conceivably be due to what is included in the definition of 'mind–body' therapies.

Indeed, any effort to summarize research documenting effects of mind–body interventions faces the difficult question of definition. Mind–body interventions are usually defined by default in the literature, using examples of therapies that are commonly used or thought to be effective as exemplars. However, it is essential to have a precise and agreed-upon definition in order for the research to move forward. The National Institutes of Health (NIH) Center for Complementary and Alternative Medicine (NCCAM) define mind–body medicine as using 'a variety of techniques designed to enhance the mind's capacity to affect bodily function and symptoms'[6]. For purposes of this chapter, we define a 'mind–body intervention' as any treatment that addresses the interaction between the mind (thoughts, feelings) and body (physical processes). Some techniques that were categorized as complementary and alternative medicine (CAM) in the past have become mainstream (for example, patient support groups and cognitive–behavioral therapy). Other mind–body techniques are still considered CAM, including meditation, prayer, mental healing and therapies that use creative outlets such as art, music, or dance[6].

In practice, a number of therapies have been identified in this area that are commonly used within oncology, including relaxation, meditation, guided imagery, hypnosis, biofeedback, cognitive behavioral therapy and psychoeducational approaches[7]. The inclusion of more traditional psychotherapies as mind–body interventions may seem questionable to some, since they have become mainstream, as in the NCCAM definition. In oncology, however, their use is still often considered adjunctive, and we believe they are not fully accepted and/or utilized by mainstream practitioners. Hence, we have chosen to include them in this review.

Therefore, the areas that will be covered throughout this text are those that have a body of empirical support in an oncology context. These include hypnosis, imagery, relaxation, meditation, yoga, psychotherapy and creative therapies (dance, music therapy, writing/journaling, painting/drawing, sculpting). Other interventions, such as biofeedback, healing prayer and autogenic training could also be included. However, owing to both space constraints and limited empirical research in these areas, we have chosen to focus on the aforementioned as the major important mind–body treatments in oncology. The literature will be briefly reviewed in each section, but the intention is simply to summarize the general findings in each area so the appropriate use of these mind-body interventions can be identified.

MIND–BODY THERAPY – CANCER RESEARCH BACKGROUND

Mind–body interventions have been used in cancer care for centuries, particularly those related to prayer. Early reports of the use of meditation in the scientific literature began to emerge in the late 1960s and early 1970s, with the growing popularization of transcendental meditation in the West. Herbert Benson is an early scientific researcher who published extensively on the physiological benefits of induction of the relaxation response via meditation[8]. In cancer, Ainsley Meares in Australia reported a series of case studies in the late 1970s and early 1980s detailing the beneficial effects of meditation for regression of cancer tumors (for example, see reference 9). After that point there was somewhat of a lull in research related to meditation, although the hypnosis literature continued to thrive, owing to its association with psychodynamic psychotherapy. Meditation and relaxation research in oncology became more mainstream in the 1990s with the popularization of the mindfulness-based stress-reduction paradigm of Jon Kabat-Zinn at the University of Massachusetts[10].

Research supports the utilization of mind–body interventions in cancer care, especially in the area of supportive care. Interventions such as hypnosis, music and imagery have been found particularly useful for controlling symptoms such as pain and nausea. Meditation and yoga programs have applicability in areas of decreasing anxiety, mood disturbance and potentially enhancing sleep, as well as enhancing vitality for both patients as well as family members, caregivers and health-care providers. The most significant amount of literature support overall is in the application of psychotherapy, meditation, hypnosis and imagery/relaxation for supportive care of cancer patients.

There is clearly a great deal of interest in the possible antineoplastic potential of mind–body interventions, as evidenced by the growing body of literature investigating the impact of a variety of interventions on outcomes such as immune function, stress hormone levels and survival. Further work in this emerging area of interest will hopefully link specific mind–body therapies with particular antineoplastic effects.

In general, the area of mind–body intervention research suffers from methodological weaknesses such as small sample sizes (leading to low power and increased chance of type II error (defined as the likelihood of finding negative trial results when in fact the intervention is helpful), lack of randomized controlled trials, low control over intervention structure and integrity, and unstandardized outcome measures. These factors combine to result in an inconsistent literature that is most likely to underestimate the efficacy of mind–body interventions because of flaws in trial design. In addition to applying methodological rigor in future studies, the area would be strengthened by expanding the paradigm of research from the Western reductionistic model it is steeped in. Some examples of this are to incorporate patients' own stories and lived experience through the use of qualitative research methods such as narrative, phenomenology and case studies.

Mind–body interventions clearly have the potential to reduce pathology and negative symptomatology, but they can also be used for health enhancement and positive growth. It is important that future researchers explore the positive aspects of mind–body interventions, examining whether they can perhaps help persons facing cancer find greater meaning and value in their current circumstances.

CURRENT QUESTIONS

Can stress management provide preventive benefits, both for new onset of disease as well as to prevent recurrence? If so, what are the biological mechanisms of such action? What is the optimal method of mind–body intervention for patients with specific types of malignancy, and what are the mechanisms specific to carcinogenesis of different types of cancer that may be altered? How can mind–body therapy best be a part of end-of-life care?

ONGOING CLINICAL TRIALS

A search of NIH-funded studies indicates a fair number of trials currently under way investigating mind–body interventions in cancer care. One of the largest, a multi-site trial of 'mindfulness relaxation' – really mindfulness meditation – versus relaxing music and standard symptom management for patients with solid tumors undergoing chemotherapy, is currently under way at MD Anderson University and the University of Toronto. A total of 400 patients will be followed for up to 5 years for effects not only on treatment tolerance and quality of life, but also on immune outcomes and survival. Another large multi-site study of stress management for patients undergoing radiation therapy is under way at centers in eight states, led by researchers at the H. Lee Moffitt Cancer Center in Florida.

Interestingly, another study currently recruiting patients in Temple, Texas, is investigating the efficacy of hypnosis for the treatment of hot flashes in breast cancer survivors, a common side-effect of hormonal treatments. Patients will either receive hypnosis or usual care, and record daily diaries of the frequency and severity of their hot flashes. In a similar vein, self-hypnosis is being investigated in a trial at Beth Israel Medical Center as a relief for pain and anxiety associated with invasive procedures in 390 uterine cancer patients.

Other studies of more psychotherapeutic interventions are also under way, including one at Memorial Sloan Kettering in New York City, investigating meaning-centered psychotherapy in advanced cancer. Researchers will compare this new type of therapy to a standard support group and investigate its effects on psychological and spiritual well-being.

Some studies are close to completion and may be reported within the next few years. A randomized study of transcendental meditation in older women with stage II–IV breast cancer has recently been completed at St Joseph's hospital in Chicago, with outcomes of quality of life and survival time being measured. However, no results have yet been released.

Mindfulness-based art therapy, a combination of mindfulness meditation and creative therapy, has also been investigated in a randomized controlled trail at Thomas Jefferson University Hospital in Philadelphia, with outcomes of quality of life, stress symptoms and coping responses.

GENERAL SUMMARY

Mind–body therapies have an important role in integrative oncology. Recommendations for prevention of cancer include investigating mind–body interventions that help to decrease symptoms of depression and encourage emotional expression. Clinicians treating cancer patients may want to consider the use of hypnosis, imagery/relaxation or music therapy during active treatment and/or palliation to help with symptoms of pain, discomfort and anxiety, as well as interventions such as meditation, imagery, relaxation and yoga for reduction in stress symptoms and improved coping skills. Psychotherapy is also useful in dealing with symptoms of anxiety and depression and to enhance coping skills, and interventions such as creative therapies, yoga and meditation may also help after treatment with recovering vitality and personal growth. Many of the mind–body therapies have potential impact on the immune and endocrine systems, but the evidence is strongest currently for the beneficial effects of psychotherapy and meditation.

As growing numbers of cancer patients explore these widely available and cost-effective mind–body interventions[11], it behooves both researchers and clinicians to become educated as to the evidence of their efficacy, and indications for treatment.

With such a large breadth of different mind–body interventions available to the cancer patient, it can seem difficult if not overwhelming for individuals and their caregivers to choose appropriate options at different points in the cancer trajectory. Given that patients have differing psychosocial needs as they move through the stages of diagnosis, active treatment and recovery or palliation and death, the practitioner would be well advised to consider matching the intervention to patient needs common at these different time points. For example, around the time of initial diagnosis, patients have high information needs and high anxiety levels. Psychoeducation and relaxation are appropriate interventions at this time point. During active treatment patients are engrossed with trying to tolerate toxic treatments and are primarily using direct problem-focused coping, so interventions such as cognitive behavioral therapy with a focus on active coping strategies, imagery and relaxation are again beneficial. After active treatment and during the recovery phase, patients are trying to regain physical strength and figure out how to move on with life after cancer. This phase is often accompanied by existential angst and questions about spirituality, life priorities, and meaning and purpose in life. Interventions such as meditation and yoga are ideal at this point. For patients dealing with issues around death and dying, meditation, guided imagery, and hypnosis as well as spiritual counseling are often helpful (Table 10.2).

Other patient-related variables that are helpful to take into account when assessing which interventions may be appropriate include the patients' personality characteristics, their spiritual/religious beliefs, their physical limitations, as well as simple preference and comfort with dif-

Table 10.2 Varying needs of cancer patients over time and appropriate mind–body approaches

Situation	Needs	Therapeutic possibilities
Diagnosis	Information, address anxiety levels	Psychoeducation, relaxation
Active treatment	Treatment tolerance	Cognitive behavioral therapy with focus on active coping strategies, imagery, hypnosis, relaxation, creative arts
Recovery	Regain strength, existential issues (meaning, purpose)	Meditation, yoga, creative arts therapies
Survivorship	Promote health, address fear of recurrence	Support groups, retreats
Palliation	Symptom control, quality of life	Coping strategies, imagery, hypnosis
End-of-life care	Transition, transcendence	Address spirituality and symptom control, meditation, creative therapies

ferent modalities. Psychosocial oncology practitioners should conduct a thorough evaluation of each patient, including screening for clinical pathology such as mood and anxiety disorders, before referral to mind–body interventions. Many patients, particularly those with a history of psychopathology and little social support, are vulnerable to major depression and/or anxiety disorders and may require psychiatric consultation and perhaps psychotropic medication prior to participation in mind–body interventions.

GLOSSARY OF TERMS

Cognitive–behavioral therapy (CBT) Therapeutic intervention that focuses on how thoughts and interpretations mediate the relationship between life events and feelings and behavior. The target of interventions is to change maladaptive thoughts that maintain negative feelings such as anxiety and depression, and negative behavioral patterns such as addictions.

Creative therapy Intended to integrate physical, emotional and spiritual care by facilitating creative ways to respond to illness. Creative therapies include the following techniques: drawing, painting, writing, sculpting, music, photography and dance.

Hypnosis A natural state of aroused, attentive focal concentration coupled with a relative suspension of peripheral awareness, involving three main factors: absorption, dissociation and suggestibility.

Imagery Use of the imagination to create sensory experiences through any of the sense modalities (vision, olfaction, taste, touch, sound), for a particular purpose.

Meditation A family of techniques that involve intentionally training the mind in awareness and attention.

Mind–body interventions A variety of techniques designed to enhance the mind's capacity to affect bodily function and symptoms.

Relaxation A state wherein the 'relaxation response' is evoked, resulting in a decrease in autonomic sympathetic arousal and corresponding increase in parasympathetic control.

Physiologically, heart rate and respiration decrease, blood pressure decreases and muscles relax. This is often accompanied by a psychological state of quietness and decreased anxiety.

Yoga Derived from the Sanskrit word *yug*, meaning 'to yoke' or 'union'. The intent of yoga practice is to yoke or unite the individual with the totality of the universe. The techniques of yoga include ethical practice (do's and don'ts of daily living), physical exercise (*asanas*), breathing techniques (*pranayama*) and meditation training.

RESOURCES FOR MIND–BODY CLINICAL INTERVENTIONS

Borysenko J. Minding the Body, Mending the Mind. Reading, MA: Addison-Wesley. 1987

Cousins N. Head First: The Biology of Hope and the Healing Power of the Human Spirit. New York: Penguin Books, 1990

Kabat-Zinn J. Full Catastrophe Living: Using the Wisdom of Your Body and Mind to Face Stress, Pain, and Illness. New York: Bantam Doubleday, 1990

Khalsa DS, Stauth C. Meditation as Medicine: Activate the Power of Your Natural Healing Force. New York: Simon and Schuster, 2001

Martin P. The Healing Mind: The Vital Links Between Brain and Behavior, Immunity and Disease. New York: St. Martin's Press, 1997

Rossi EL. The Psychobiology of Mind–Body Healing: New Concepts of Therapeutic Hypnosis. New York: WW Norton, 1986

Graham H. A Picture of Health: How to Use Guided Imagery for Self Healing and Personal Growth. London: Judy Piatkus, 1995

Carrico M. Yoga Journal's Yoga Basics. New York: Henry Holt, 1997

Weil A. Spontaneous Healing. New York. Fawcett Columbine, 1995

Simonton OC, Mathews-Simonton S, Creighton, J. Getting Well Again. Los Angeles: JP Tracher, 1978

Center for Mindfulness in Medicine Health Care, and Society: University of Massachusetts Medical School (www.umassmed.edu/cfm/). Main page for the Center has links to other sites, training opportunities, and information on the annual mindfulness conference in Worcester.

Mindfulness Tapes (www.mindfulnesstapes.com/). Site to order tapes with yoga and meditation exercises by Jon Kabat-Zinn.

North Wales Centre for Mindfulness Research and Practice (www.bangor.ac.uk/mindfulness/index.html). Site developed in the UK by Mark Williams and colleagues involved in Mindfulness-based Cognitive Therapy. Includes many links and references.

References

1. Wolsko PM, Eisenberg DM, Davis RB, Phillips RS. Use of mind–body medical therapies. J Gen Intern Med 2004; 19: 43–50

2. Jordan ML, Delunas LR. Quality of life and patterns of nontraditional therapy use by patients with cancer. Oncol Nurs Forum 2001; 28: 1107–13

3. Paltiel O, Avitzour M, Peretz T, et al. Determinants of the use of complementary therapies by patients with cancer. J Clin Oncol 2001; 19: 2439–48

4. Henderson JW, Donatelle RJ. Complementary and alternative medicine use by women after completion of allopathic treatment for breast cancer. Altern Ther Health Med 2004; 10: 52–7

5. Shumay DM, Maskarinec G, Gotay CC, et al. Determinants of the degree of complementary and alternative medicine use among patients with cancer. J Altern Complement Med 2002; 8: 661–71

6. National Centre for Complementary and Alternative Medicine. What Is Complementary and Alternative Medicine (CAM)? http://nccam.nih.gov/health/whatiscam/#4. 2004

7. Astin JA. Mind–body therapies for the management of pain. Clin J Pain 2004; 20: 27–32

8. Benson H. The Relaxation Response. New York: Morrow, 1975

9. Meares A. Regression of recurrent carcinoma of the breast at mastectomy site associated with intensive meditation. Aust Fam Physician 1981; 10: 218–19

10. Kabat-Zinn J. Full Catastrophe Living: Using the Wisdom of Your Body and Mind to Face Stress, Pain and Illness. New York: Delacourt, 1990

11. Simpson JSA, Carlson LE, Trew M. Impact of a group psychosocial intervention on health care utilization by breast cancer patients. Cancer Practice 2001; 9: 19–26

10d

Botanicals

Lise Alschuler

> 'Only to him who stands where the barley stands and listens well, will it speak and tell, for his sake what man is.' – Masanobu Fukoka, co-creator of Findhorn Garden

INTRODUCTION

The estimated use of herbal preparations is 13–63% among patients with cancer[1]. Botanical therapies include the use of a plant-derived compound or compounds for a specific health indication. Botanical therapies are consumed as herbal teas, herbal condiments, herbal tinctures (alcohol-extracted liquid concentrates), herbal capsules, tablets and pills, topical applications and pharmaceutical grade injectables.

While these preparations are widely available to the general public, there are relatively few health-care professionals trained to competently recommend botanical therapies. The following health-care providers have training, albeit at varying levels, in botanical medicine: naturopathic doctors, certain certified herbalists and acupuncturists with additional certification in Chinese Herbal Medicine. Additionally, Native American healers, and some other health-care providers, such as allopathic physicians, chiropractic doctors and pharmacists obtain additional certification training in botanicals, lending them credibility in making recommendations.

BOTANICALS AND CANCER RESEARCH: BACKGROUND

The data on the use of botanical medicines and cancer care are largely experimental. There are certainly encouraging results and developing trends in the research. It is also true, however, that the likelihood of large randomized trials with herbs is remote, given the lack of funding, financial incentive and expertise for designing these trials. This leaves the clinician in the uncomfortable place of making decisions about the inclusion of botanical remedies into an integrative cancer care plan based upon largely insufficient data. It is, nonetheless, important to maintain an open mind to the existing information available. The data hold promising trends, compelling physiological discoveries and reliable clinical information. It is equally important to regard unfounded claims regarding the antineoplastic or chemoprevention properties of herbal therapies warily until some evidence, albeit preliminary, is available.

The US Food and Drug Administration's Dietary Supplement Health and Education Act (DSHEA) of 1994 has laid the framework for the regulation of herbal products. This law received the greatest amount of grassroots advocacy of any law passed by Congress. The DSHEA regulates labeling, manufacture and marketing of dietary supplements, including herbal products. Using the authority of the Food and Drug Administration (FDA) and Federal Trade Commission (FTC), this act:

- Limits claims to structure and function.

- Requires full disclosure on labels.

- Requires adequate safety data in advance for any new ingredients (not sold prior to 1994).

- Requires good manufacturing practices (GMP).

- Outlaws unfair, deceptive or inadequately substantiated advertising.

- Investigates complaints or questionable trade practices.

- Maintains sentinel systems for complaints on product quality, safety, effectiveness and labeling.

However, the question remains, is DSHEA enough? There are no official standards of quality for herbal products. There is minimal government monitoring of labeled identity or potency. After much work by industry groups in cooperation with the FDA, more stringent GMPs were published by the FDA in 2003. These requirements are scheduled to go into effect by 2005. Additionally, legislation for a mandatory reporting system for serious Adverse Event Reports (AERs) is very likely within the next year. Many herbal manufacturers and industry groups have been drafting appropriate language

and guidelines for this AER system, as the current FDA system is widely viewed as inadequate for botanical products.

The proposed GMP requirements, while necessary, will be challenged by significant complexity in the regulation and analysis of herbal products. Dried herbs and herbal tinctures are difficult to standardize and may contain contaminants that are difficult to detect (e.g. pesticides, micro-organisms and heavy metals). The marker standards utilized to make standardized extracts do not guarantee or standardize the method of extraction and concentration. Products with the same amount of a standardized constituent may be very different products. The standardization process is often proprietary. The standardized ingredient may not be an active constituent (e.g. hypericin versus hyperforin in *Hypericum perforatum*). In addition, herb research lacks a uniform set of criteria for evaluating its research substances. Many published studies on herbs do not specify the type of herbal product, degree or method of herbal concentration, or verification of identity of the product. This has led to erroneous conclusions regarding efficacy and contraindications in marketing and literature, and therefore in public use.

Finally, there is an emerging, but currently scant, pool of information regarding herb–drug interactions. Much of this information is currently gleaned from isolated case reports which are difficult to analyze given the variance of herbal products, and the inherent limitations of using one or a few incidences to establish universal precautions. The remaining guidance in the area of drug–herb interactions is derived from a theoretical perspective. Based upon the known pharmacology and pharmacokinetics of certain plants and their constituents, this information is compared to that of pharmaceutical compounds. This process has resulted in a tentative data bank of cautionary herb–drug interactions. Clearly, this is an area that needs additional research attention, and one which has direct implications in oncology patients using botanicals who are also receiving any form of conventional care.

CURRENT AIMS FOR RESEARCH

- Establishment of practical, ethical and useful study designs to determine the role of botanicals in the co-management and treatment of malignancies.

- Characterization of botanical agents – based upon available scientific literature – in terms of therapeutic potential for each cancer type, in order to prioritize subsequent human intervention trials.

CURRENT RESEARCH

The following trials, related to the use of herbs in the context of cancer or cancer care, are of particular interest:

- A prospective study of healthy volunteers to determine whether the use of herbal products interferes with normal anticoagulation. Stephen Bent, MD is the principal investigator and is sponsored by the National Center for Complementary and Alternative Medicine (NCCAM). This trial is expected to be completed in January 2006.

- A randomized, single-blind controlled trial to assess the potential for adverse interactions between St John's wort extract and oxycodone and fentanyl is expected to be complete in May 2005. The principal investigator is Danny Shen, PhD and sponsored by NCCAM.

- A randomized phase III trial to determine the effect of valerian for improving the quality of sleep in patients with cancer receiving adjuvant therapy is expected to be completed in 2006. The study is sponsored by the North Central Cancer Treatment Group and the National Cancer Institute (NCI).

- A phase III randomized, double-blind study to determine the efficacy of St John's wort in treating mild to moderate depression compared to sertraline in patients with cancer. The study began enrolling patients in 2004 and is sponsored by the Comprehensive Cancer Center of Wake Forest University and the NCI.

- A phase II randomized study of ginger in patients with cancer and chemotherapy-induced nausea and vomiting began enrolling patients in 2004 and is sponsored by the University of Michigan Comprehensive Cancer Center and the NCI.

- A phase II randomized trial to study the effectiveness of silymarin in treating patients who have acute lymphoblastic leukemia with chemotherapy-related side-effects to the liver began recruiting patients in 2004 and is sponsored by the Herber Irving Comprehensive Cancer Center and the NCI.

- A phase I/II trial to study the effectiveness of *Scutellaria barbatae* in treating women who have metastatic breast cancer began recruiting patients in 2004 and is sponsored by the University of California, San Fransisco and the NCI.

- A phase I study of Huang Lian (Chinese herb) in patients with advanced solid tumors began recruiting patients in 2004 and is sponsored by the Memorial Sloan-Kettering Cancer Center and the NCI.

- A randomized phase I/II trial to study the effectiveness of herbs used in traditional Chinese medicine in decreasing the side-effects of chemotherapy after surgery in women who have stage I, stage II, or early stage III breast cancer completed patient enrollment in 2004 and is sponsored by the University of California, San Francisco and the NCI.

SUMMARY

The role of botanicals in chemoprevention is most promising and deserves particular attention. Botanicals may also provide excellent co-management options for patients receiving conventional treatments. The antineoplastic actions of botanicals remains their most understudied and tenuous application. Future research into the use of botanicals in the context of cancer care remains an exciting and critical need.

A novice to botanical medicine is entering an exciting, but overwhelming world. The interface of botanical medicine with conventional medicine, particularly in the context of oncology, is at once promising and perilous. It is critical to gather expertise in the form of practitioners and references to help navigate these explorations. Expertise in herbal medicine resides in the professions of naturopathic medicine, acupuncture with Chinese Herbal Medicine, ethnobotany, pharmacology and herbalism. There are also excellent resources now available in the form of books, journals, published literature and medical conferences (see Resources section).

GLOSSARY OF TERMS

Botanical   Of plant origin.

Botanical medicine   Plant-derived substances used in the prevention or management of a human condition.

Chemoprevention   In the context of botanicals, this is defined as the use of a naturally derived substance to prevent or delay the onset or progression of malignancy.

Constituent   Molecular compound found in a plant.

Herbal medicine   Synonymous with botanical medicine.

Phytochemicals   Molecular compounds found in plants, many of which are studied to determine their physiological effects on living tissue.

Phytotherapy   The study of the medicinal use of plants.

Standardized extract   Botanical preparation in which one or several marker constituents are present in the final product at pre-determined concentration(s).

RESOURCES FOR BOTANICALS

Books

The Complete German Commission E Monographs – Therapeutic Guide to Herbal Medicine. Austin TX: Blumenthal, 1998

The ABC Clinical Guide to Herbs. Austin TX: Blumenthal, 2003

Mosby's Handbook of Herbs and Natural Supplements, 2nd edn. St Louis, MO: Skidmore-Roth, 2004

Mosby's Handbook of Drug–Herb and Drug–Supplement Interactions. St Louis, MO: Harkness and Bratman, 2003

Clinical Botanical Medicine. Larchmont, NY: Yarnell, Abascal and Hooper, 2003

Journals

HerbalGram. American Botanical Council

Planta Medica. Thieme Publications

PhytoMedicine. Gustav Verlag Stuttgart

Journal of Cancer Integrative Medicine. Prime National Publishing Corp.

Conferences

Society for Integrative Oncology

International Botanical Congress

American Association of Naturopathic Physicians

Reference

1. Sparreboom A, Cox MC, Acharya MR, Figg WD. Herbal Remedies in the United States: potential adverse interactions with anticancer agents. J Clin Oncol 2004: 22: 2489–503

10e

Manual therapy

J. Michael Menke

> 'I am not a mechanism, an assembly of various sections. And it is not because the mechanism is working wrongly that I am ill.' – D.H. Lawrence

INTRODUCTION

An integrative oncology approach should have a healthy regard for the role of the ancient and venerable skills of hands-on therapies for improving function and reducing anxiety and pain[1]. Massage, osteopathic manipulation (not the profession, but the manipulative skill set practiced by some osteopaths) and the chiropractic profession (simply called chiropractic) are sometimes organized as manual 'medicines', although the three professions and therapies do not serve as complete and distinct healing systems that can replace conventional medicine's diagnostics and care[2]. A 'medicine' in this context implies a complete and exhaustive system of diagnosis and treatment. Traditional Chinese Medicine is one such system. Today's rational osteopaths, chiropractors and massage therapists would never consider their training in manual techniques a substitute for conventional medical care[3]. Therefore, many prefer to call hands-on therapies 'manual therapies' rather than medicines, or complete systems of healing.

Simply put, massage practitioners practice massage, so their skill set is nearly equivalent to and defines the activities of a massage professional. Chiropractic and osteopathy are not so easily described. Chiropractors are trained in imaging, clinical history taking, review of systems and physical, neurological and orthopedic examination to arrive at differential diagnoses. Listening to hearts and looking at retinas and tympanic membranes with oto-ophthalmoscopes, for example, are aspects of chiropractic clinical competency. Chiropractic manipulation, called the adjustment, is a therapy employed by chiropractors depending on patient need and chiropractor philosophy. Practitioners of these therapies see a great deal of skin, so there are many opportunities to detect skin cancers[4].

Osteopaths practice medicine, but today only a small proportion provide manipulative services that were the foundation of osteopathy at its inception in 1874[5]. Osteopathic manipulation is then a skill set, not the entire osteopathic profession.

Massage, chiropractic and osteopathy refer to the hands-on and manipulative aspects and skill sets of each[2]. The manual therapies of massage, chiropractic and osteopathic manipulation treat from the 'outside-in' – via the musculoskeletal system. Manual therapies are sought to treat primarily pain and dysfunction; they each also offer various degrees of supportive care for a few non-musculoskeletal syndromes depending on practitioner predilection, training and legal scope[6–9]. Manual medicines, in restoring structural and mechanical function, appear to reduce pain, disability and concomitant inflammation.

The treatment of cancer with the use of manual therapies as an antineoplastic goal has no evidence of efficacy and lacks any plausible mechanisms. There is also no role for prophylactic musculoskeletal treatment to prevent cancer or to reduce cancer risk, although a link between inflammation and cancer is compelling[10]. There is no support for the idea that neuromusculoskeletal lesions contribute to mutagenicity or neoplasms, nor that the removal of such lesions could effect progression of malignant disease. It is often assumed that 'hands-on' therapies are contraindicated for cancer patients, because of acceleration of the course of the disease[11]. On the contrary, modern manual therapists and therapies can offer risk assessment[3,12–16], preventive[13,17,18], early detection[4], supportive[19–22], and rehabilitative services[23] as part of an integrative oncology. This includes focused and well-considered manipulation and massage. Certain clinical situations do necessitate careful consideration, including patients with bony metastases in whom one would need to avoid direct pressure over involved bone that could result in pathologic fracture.

With additional training, manual medicine practitioners could serve some other roles for the general population: as evidence-based cancer prevention advisors for high-risk individuals and populations[3,4,17,18]; and as screeners and early detectors of cancer in the musculoskeletal system, integument and related palpable and visible structures. When cancer develops, manual therapists may work with medical specialists to provide palliative care for anxiety, pain, lymphedema, restlessness, nutrition and other co-management advice. Symptom prevention in cancer patients may also be possible. In addition, each non-medical encounter with cancer patients can be the eyes and ears for oncologists and primary care physicians in monitoring adverse events, unexpected side-effects of cancer therapies, sudden changes in symptoms and the general course of the disease.

CURRENT RESEARCH QUESTIONS

Can massage, chiropractic adjustment or strain–counterstrain techniques help with non-malignant musculoskeletal aches, pains and anxiety in cancer patients? Can manual therapies help in palliative care and symptom prevention?

CURRENT RESEARCH

- *Massage therapy for the treatment of cancer-related pain* – National Center for Complementary an Alternative Medicine (NCCAM) sponsored trial. This is a phase II trial which is evaluating whether there is sufficient efficacy for a Phase III trial. Sloan-Kettering Cancer Center.

- *Massage therapy for cancer-related fatigue* – patients with breast, ovarian, prostate and colorectal cancer receiving chemotherapy. Osher Center for Integrative Medicine, University of California San Francisco (UCSF).

- *Massage therapy for breast cancer treatment-related swelling of the arms and legs* – NCCAM sponsored trial. This study compares massage therapy alone to massage plus compressive bandaging; University of Arizona.

- *REST – Reducing end-of-life symptoms with touch.* Multi-centered trial with NCCAM grant to University of Colorado. This study evaluates whether physical and emotional symptoms can be relieved with massage or simple hands-on care.

SUMMARY

While treating cancer from an antineoplastic perspective is outside the scope and responsibilities of manual therapists and therapies *per se*, many patients seek the services of such practitioners for pain, anxiety and stress. Occasionally, their pain is neoplastic in origin masquerading as musculoskeletal pain. Practitioners must recognize and refer such disorders to appropriate professionals. Detection is a trained function of manual professionals, although osteopaths have the greatest exposure to clinical procedural knowledge by virtue of clinical rotations and residencies. Chiropractors acquire a great deal of declarative knowledge from classroom experience and a limited internship. Massage has the least clinical exposure to serious pathology. Appropriately trained providers may offer significant benefit in the areas of supportive cancer care and potentially through offering nutritional advice. In addition, manual medicine professionals are in a unique position to detect cancers, especially of the skin and bone. They may augment their services by managing risk for cancer-prone individuals.

GLOSSARY OF TERMS

Chiropractic   A system of healing that focuses on the adjusting of the musculoskeletal system, especially the spine, to improve the body's function. Integrative chiropractors perform physical examinations, may give nutrition advice, determine health risk, and advise on self-care. The

subluxation is reputed to be the spinal lesion responsible for health problems to greater or lesser degrees, depending upon the chiropractor.

Osteopathy   A system of healing and therapy to restore health by correcting body mechanics through various forms of manipulation. Today in the USA osteopaths practice medicine; some still practice manipulation.

Deep tissue massage   A massage that works to remove congestion in the deeper muscles, such as tissue fluid and lymph for better drainage.

Shiatsu   A type of massage from Japan which presses and holds acupuncture points to improve energy flow.

Neuromuscular therapy   A form of deep tissue massage that seeks to balance or re-establish a synergistic relationship between the nervous system and the musculoskeletal system.

RESOURCES FOR MANUAL THERAPY

American Massage Therapy Association:
www.amtamassage.org

American Osteopathic Association:
www.osteopathic.org

Osteopathy for health-care professionals:
www.do-online.org

American Chiropractic Association:
www.amerchiro.org

Foundation for Chiropractic Education and Research (FCER):
www.fcer.org

Program in Integrative Medicine, University of Arizona:
www.integrativemedicine.arizona.edu

Personal resources

Wendy Miner LMT, Memorial Sloan Kettering Cancer Center, instructor – 'Medical Massage for the Cancer Patient', a national certificate training program.

Tracy Walton LMT, MS – Cambridge, MA. Instructor and director – 'Caring for clients with cancer: simple steps to safe, effective massage therapy'.

References

1. Cherkin DC, Sherman KJ, Deyo RA, Shekelle PG. A review of the evidence for the effectiveness, safety, and cost of acupuncture, massage therapy, and spinal manipulation for back pain. Ann Intern Med 2003; 138: 898–906

2. World Health Organization. Guidelines on Developing Consumer Information on Proper Use of Traditional, Complementary and Alternative Medicine. Geneva: World Health Organization, 2004

3. Menke JM. Principles in integrative chiropractic. J Manipulative Physiol Ther 2003; 26: 254–72

4. Anonymous. How many times have you been the first health care provider to suspect or find evidence of cancer in one of your patients? Dynamic Chiropractic Chiropoll 2004; May 6: 4

5. Johnson SM, Kurtz ME. Osteopathic manipulative treatment techniques preferred by contemporary osteopathic physicians. J Am Osteopath Assoc 2003; 103: 219–24

6 Shekelle PG, Adams AH, Chassin MR, et al. Spinal manipulation for low-back pain. Ann Intern Med 1992; 117: 590-8

7 Eisenberg DM, Kessler RC, Foster C, et al. Unconventional medicine in the United States. Prevalence, costs, and patterns of use. N Engl J Med 1993; 328: 246–52

8. Eisenberg DM. Davis RB, Ettner SL, et al. Trends in alternative medicine use in the United States, 1990–1997: results of a follow-up national survey. JAMA 1998; 280: 1569–75

9. Wolsko PM, Eisenberg DM, Davis RB, et al. Patterns and perceptions of care for treatment of back and neck pain: results of a national survey. Spine 2003; 28: 292–7; discussion 298

10. Coussens LM, Werb Z. Inflammation and cancer. Nature 2002; 420: 860–7

11. Anonymous. When a rubdown requires special precautions. Johns Hopkins Medical Letter, Health After 50 2003; 15: 5

12. Anonymous. http://hip.stanford.edu/assessments/wellness.html

13. Reiser SJ. Anatomic thinking: the clinical and social consequences of health care's basic logic. Fam Community Health 1995; 18: 26–36

14. Tremblay F, Fernandes M, Habbab F, et al. Malignancy after renal transplantation: incidence and role of type of immunosuppression. Ann Surg Oncol 2002; 9: 785–8

15. Mitxelena J, Gomez-Ullate P, Aguirre A, et al. Kaposi's sarcoma in renal transplant patients: experience at the Cruces Hospital in Bilbao. Int J Dermatol 2003; 42: 18–22

16. Laube S, George SA. Adverse effects with PUVA and UVB phototherapy. J Dermatol Treat 2001; 12: 101–5

17. Bezold C. The Future of Chiropractic: Optimizing Health Gains. Alexandria, VA: Institute for Alternative Futures, 1998

18. Bezold C. The Future of Complementary and Alternative Approaches (CAAs) in US Healthcare. Alexandria, VA: Institute for Alternative Futures, 1998

19. Stephenson N. Dalton JA. Carlson J. The effect of foot reflexology on pain in patients with metastatic cancer. Appl Nurs Res 2003; 16: 284–6

20. Turner J, Hayes S, Reul-Hirche H. Improving the physical status and quality of life of women treated for breast cancer: a pilot study of a structured exercise intervention. J Surg Oncol 2004; 86: 141–6

21. Soden K, Vincent K, Craske S, et al. A randomized controlled trial of aromatherapy massage in a hospice setting. Palliative Med 2004; 18: 87–92

22. Post-White J, Kinney ME, Savik K, et al. Therapeutic massage and healing touch improve symptoms in cancer. Integrative Cancer Therapies 2003; 2: 332–44

23. McNeely ML, Parliament M, Courneya KS, et al. A pilot study of a randomized controlled trial to evaluate the effects of progressive resistance exercise training on shoulder dysfunction caused by spinal accessory neuraxpraxia/neurectomy in head and neck cancer survivors. Head Neck 2004; 26: 518–30

10f

Energy medicine

Suzanne Clewell

'The visible world is the invisible organization of Energy.' – Physicist Heinz Pagels

INTRODUCTION

The International Society for the Study of Subtle Energies and Energy Medicine (ISSSEEM) defines energy medicine as follows: '*Energy Medicine* includes all energetic and informational interactions resulting from self-regulation or brought about through other energy linkages to mind and body. In addition to various therapeutic energies that we may use, there are also energy pulses from the environment which influence humans and animals in a variety of ways. For instance, low-level changes in magnetic, electric, electromagnetic, acoustic and gravitational fields often have profound effects on both biology and psychology. In addition to energies originating in the environment, it has been documented that humans are capable of generating and controlling subtle, not-yet-measurable energies that seem to influence both physiological and physical mechanisms.'[1]

The Society goes on to describe *Subtle Energies* as 'a concept that is more difficult to define within the scientific paradigm. Ancient and modern wisdom traditions describe human bioenergies referred to by many names (e.g. Chi, Ki, Prana, etheric energy, fohat, orgone, odic force, Mana, homeopathic resonance) that is believed to move throughout the so-called *etheric* (or subtle) energy body and thus is difficult to measure using conventional instrumentation. In addition, many of the complementary and alternative therapies that are becoming increasingly popular appear to involve the flow of these subtle energies through the dense physical body. In addition, it is traditionally accepted that expansions of consciousness often are related to changes in subtle energies that cannot be quantified. These latter energies, which are said to be associated with interactions and with transcendence, may not, in fact, actually be involved with known energy fields.'[1]

The founder of the American Holistic Medical Association, C. Norman Shealy, MD, PhD, states that 'We are energetic beings. Everything in the body works both electrically and chemically. We are like a living battery. And since electricity produces magnetism, the force that attracts and repels molecules, we are electro-magnetic as well as electrochemical.'[2]

Dr Richard Gerber, in his informative text *Vibrational Medicine*, tells us that 'The future of holistic medicine will depend upon the integration of vibrational medical therapies into everyday practice. Holistic physicians accept the concept of wellness in human beings as being a function of properly integrating the physical, emotional, mental and spiritual elements of life. What needs greater clarification, however, is the true relationship of the spiritual dimension to the balance of the life-force itself.'[3] 'The ultimate approach to healing will be to remove the abnormalities at the subtle-energy level which led to the manifestation of illness in the first place. This will be the greatest difference in approach between the traditional medicine of today and the spiritual/holistic medicine of the future.'[3]

An example of a practical definition of 'energy' used in energy medicine is the concept of 'Chi' as used in Traditional Chinese Medicine. Chi is defined as life energy – the source of life. It is viewed as the vital energy that supplies nourishment and health to the body and mind. It flows through all of the organs of the body through a system of meridians upon which the acupuncture points are located. Living things extract Chi from the food that they eat and the surrounding environment.

Chi also acts as an energetic shield that provides protection against a sometimes adverse environment, be it the climate, micro-organisms, insults to the immune system or the stressors encountered daily[4]. It is believed to be the organizational and creative intelligence of the universe. This energy has long been recognized by ancient civilizations that understood that its unimpeded flow through the body supported optimal development and fulfillment. Health can be described as the harmonious flow of life energy throughout the body and in the energy field surrounding the body. However, lessening or cutting off the flow of Chi to a part of the body is thought to lead to a lowering of the circulation of the life-giving energy and may eventually cause illness or disease in that particular area.

Homeopathy, magnetic healing, acupuncture, acupressure, reflexology, Shiatzu, aromatherapy, sound healing, drumming, light therapy and flower essences are some of the modalities that fall under the heading of Energy or Vibrational Medicine. The *laying-on-of-hands* forms of energy medicine, or the biofield techniques, are those that attempt to promote healing by influencing the energy field that surrounds and penetrates the body. These include Reiki, Therapeutic Touch, Healing Touch, Qi Gong, Johrei, SHEN therapy, Pranic healing and Polarity Therapy (Table 10.3).

There is a common philosophy that runs through the practice of energy medicine. First, the energy medicine practitioner must desire to do only good. The practitioner should have the best intention directed towards the subject of their channeled energy, and be able to let go of personal ego. It is also important to know that the healing energies will flow to wherever they are most needed. The outcome of a healing is not determined by the person through whom the energy flows but rather by the intelligence of the energy itself. The energy healer must always keep in mind that *healing* does not necessarily mean *curing*. A healing will occur through energy medicine. It may manifest as a renewed ability to relax and see one's life from a different perspective. Healing may mean acceptance of a situation, a healing of a relationship, relief from pain or possibly even remission or elimination of disease. It is for the higher power and not the healer to determine the outcome. Whatever healing does occur will be that which the universal energy determines is most appropriate in that time and space (Table 10.4).

Some energy medicine modalities treat the disharmony or disease within our bodies by balancing the human energy field, which is defined

Table 10.3 Energy medicine modality chart

	Qi guided by universe	Qi guided by practitioner	Administered by others	Self-administered	Distance healing	Current research	Used in US hospitals
Acupressure		+	+	+		+	
Acupuncture		+	+			+	+
Aromatherapy	+	+	+	+		+	+
Applied kinesiology			+	+			
Network chiropractic		+	+				
Craniosacral osteopathy		+	+				
Crystal healing	+	+	+	+			+
Flower essences	+	+	+	+		+	+
Feng Shui	+		+	+		+	+
Hands of light	+	+	+	+	+		+
Healing Touch	+	+	+			+	
Herbs	+		+	+		+	
Homeopathy	+		+	+		+	
Johrei	+		+	+	+	+	+
Jin Shin Jyutsu	+	+	+			+	+
Kahuna healing		+	+			+	
Laying-on of hands	+	+	+				
Light therapy		+	+	+		+	
Magnet therapy		+	+	+			+
Massage		+	+	+		+	+
Music/drumming	+		+	+		+	+
Native American healing	+	+	+	+	+	+	
Naturopathy	+	+	+	+			
Nutrition	+					+	
Polarity	+	+	+				
Pranic healing	+	+	+	+	+	+	+
Prayer	+	+	+	+	+	+	+
Quantum touch	+		+		+	+	
T'ai Chi/Qi Gong	+		+	+		+	+
Reiki	+		+	+	+	+	+
Shamanic healing		+	+			+	
SHEN		+	+			+	
Shiatsu	+		+	+		+	+
Therapeutic touch		+	+			+	+

Table 10.4   Characteristics of energy medicine

Energy follows thought

Energy healing has its own intelligence and will migrate to where it is most needed

Living organisms posess an 'energy anatomy' as well as a physical anatomy

Flow and balance in the human energy field facilitate healing

Changes in the energy field are eventually expressed in the physical body

Human ego must move aside; it plays no part in channeling energy

Channeling or 'passing' energy should not deplete but will re-energize the provider

Energy medicine can only do good. It cannot do harm if the intention is pure

Becoming 'centered' with the Universal Life Force promotes self-healing and the healing of others

Energy medicine is non-local

by some as the *aura*. In her book *CAM Handbook: Energy Healing,* Victoria Brewer writes: 'It is hypothesized that every human being has a unique energy field that is simultaneously inside and surrounding our physical bodies. Although human energy fields have been difficult to prove scientifically, their existence does not contradict the laws of modern physics.'[5] It is this energy field that is assessed by some practitioners prior to a healing session to determine where imbalances are located. Areas of disturbance in the aura may be sensed in a variety of manners, including sight, touch, hearing and smell. Some practitioners can feel abnormalities by passing the hands over the patient and within the auric field. Areas of heat, cold, tingling or anything that differs in feel during the scanning process may be indicators of a disturbance in the aura or non-optimal energy in that area of the field. The aura is described by those who are able to see it as being luminous, as a radiating field of light that extends beyond the body to interact with our external environment. The aura itself is thought to be generated by the spinning of the chakras or smaller vortices of energy located within the body. Rosalyn Bruyere states, 'These seven chakras are what we are, what we feel, how we think and change. They are how we express ourselves and how we create.'[6] Practitioners of energy medicine may work with the chakras to help them to function optimally as vortices of energy exchange. Each of the seven major chakras is associated with specific parts of the physical body (Figures 10.1 and 10.2). A blockage of energy in a chakra can lead to health problems (e.g. cancer, heart disease) in the area that it governs. There is also a system of smaller secondary chakras whose characteristics are similar to the major chakras.

The *root* or *base chakra* is the first chakra. Located at the base of the spine and associated with the color red, it is the foundation of mental and emotional health. It is the connection to traditional beliefs and supports a sense of belonging and identity. The main function of this chakra is survival, and it governs our basic instincts and 'grounds' us with a connection to the earth's energies. The root chakra is the foundation – the higher chakras cannot function well without this fundamental groundwork in place. The areas of the body that this chakra is associated with are the base of the spine, legs and feet, bones, rectum and the immune system.

The second chakra is the *sacral chakra*. It is orange, located below the navel and governs the large intestine, lower vertebrae, pelvis, appendix, bladder, hip area and sexual organs. This is the chakra of creativity, relationships and reproduction. Blockages may be caused by issues such as blame, guilt, money or control. Physical manifestations with a blocked second chakra include: uterine problems, urinary difficulties, ovarian cysts, tumors, prostate difficulties, back and hip pain and arthritis.

The *solar plexus chakra* is the third, and it is yellow. This governs the abdomen, stomach,

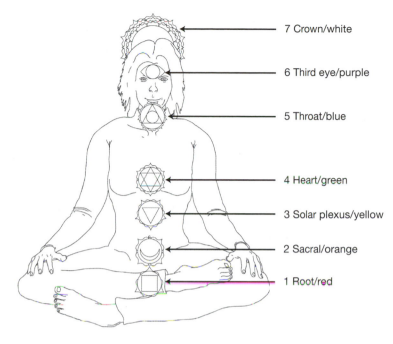

7 Crown/white

6 Third eye/purple

5 Throat/blue

4 Heart/green

3 Solar plexus/yellow

2 Sacral/orange

1 Root/red

The seven major chakras

Figure 10.1   The seven major chakras

upper intestines, liver, gallbladder, kidney, pancreas, adrenal glands, spleen and the middle spine behind the solar plexus. A poorly functioning third chakra may lead to problems associated with one or more of these areas of the body. When this chakra is flowing it provides one with personal power, a sense of self. Blockages are associated with problems such as lowered self-esteem, lack of self-respect, lack of trust, and fear. Opening of this chakra allows one to grow to respect and accept others for who they are. This chakra is responsible for the intuitive 'gut' feeling.

The *heart chakra* is the fourth and it is green. This is the power source of the human energy system. It is love, and often the focus of power for healing. This chakra is the mediator between the lower chakras and the higher ones. The first three chakras hold us securely in our human state, while the three above the heart chakra guide us toward spiritual growth. This chakra governs the heart, circulatory system and blood, rib cage, thymus, breasts, esophagus, lungs, diaphragm, shoulders, arms and hands. Holding grudges or seeking revenge will lessen the energetic flow of this vortex. Practicing forgiveness, unconditional love and compassion will strengthen it.

The fifth chakra is the *throat chakra*. Its color is blue and it allows for communication and the ability to obtain wisdom from information integration. This chakra is strengthened through speaking the truth, while lying violates the body and the spirit and weakens it. The areas of the body represented include the throat, thyroid, trachea, esophagus, neck, vertebrae, gum, teeth and mouth. A blocked chakra will often manifest as recurrent sore throats, swollen glands, colds, neck pains and dental problems.

The seventh, or *crown chakra,* is located at the top of the head. Its color is violet or white. This is the connection to healing and life force energy. With an awakened crown chakra, fulfillment, enlightenment, Divine wisdom and understanding are possible.

Here is the perfect integration of the whole being – the physical, emotional and spiritual. In their continuing education course for nurses, entitled *The Body's Energy Center (7 Major Chakras),* Joan Mazzeo-Little and Barbara Savin explain: 'The way that individuals act, think and react to life's situations plays an important part in the manifestation of good and bad health in parts of the body. As medical professionals, being in tune to this phenomenon can help us to discover what might be the underlying or root cause of a physical ailment that might otherwise remain undetected.'[5]

Dr Valerie Hunt and Rosalyn Bruyere participated in an 8-year study on the human electromagnetic field conducted at the University of California, Los Angeles (UCLA). This study, known as the Rolf Study, allowed the human energy field to be measured. It was discovered that the frequencies of the human energy field correlated with the frequencies of visible light. This led to the conclusion that the auric field that is a part of some religious traditions and what science called the human energy field were one and the same[6].

An example of a form of energy medicine that relies on the human energy field is Reiki. 'Reiki' is a Japanese word that means universal life energy. It is an ancient form of healing that was rediscovered by Mikao Usui in the mid-1800s. Reiki healing may be performed in the presence of the subject of intended healing, but it can also be transmitted across any distance. There are five principles or Ideals developed to add spiritual balance to Reiki (Table 10.5).

A necessary part of the Reiki healing experience is to help people realize that they must make a conscious decision to improve themselves in

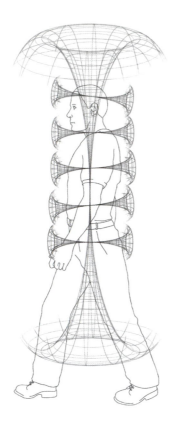

Figure 10.2 The 'chakra system'

The *third eye* or *brow chakra* is located in the middle of the forehead and is the sixth chakra. It is the chakra of inspiration, knowledge, intuition and perception. It is the area associated with the *sixth sense.* This chakra brings all chakras together to prepare for the spiritual assent to the seventh chakra. Its associated color is indigo. It governs the brain, neurological system, ears, eyes, nose, pituitary and pineal glands. Physically, it may be related to a number of problems associated with hormone and endocrine functioning. If functioning negatively on an emotional level one may see depression, stress, worry, fears and phobias. When functioning optimally, one experiences clarity of thought (learning comes easily); co-ordination is good and reflexes are working well. One feels fulfilled and at peace.

Table 10.5	The five principles of Reiki

Just for today do not worry
Just for today do not anger
Honor your parents, teachers and elders
Earn your living honestly
Show gratitude for everything

order to heal. This should not be construed as blame or cause regret but rather it is a commitment. Giving something of oneself to receive a 'gift' or blessing is a form of exchange of value, which is an integral part of many forms of energy medicine.

Therapeutic Touch, a variation of the ancient healing method of laying-on of hands, is a biofield therapy widely used in hospitals. Dr Dolores Krieger, a Professor of Nursing at New York University (NYU) School of Nursing and Dora Kunz, a well-known clairvoyant, together developed a healing curriculum for nursing students at NYU. Dr Krieger determined that one did not have to be born a healer, but that healing was a learned skill that could be taught to her nursing students[7]. The effects of Therapeutic Touch are replicable and it has developed within the context of validated teaching strategies[8]. It is being taught in respected universities and colleges and utilized in hospitals in the USA and internationally. The energy that exists in the intention to heal is thought to transcend time, space and physical barriers.

Distant healing, a non-local form of energy medicine, is a part of many energy healing modalities. Perhaps the most well-known and frequently utilized form is that of prayer. The distance that separates the person who is praying from the subject of the prayer has not been demonstrated to be a factor in its effectiveness[9]. All currently known forms of energy deteriorate with increasing distance. Healing energy, however, does not behave in the same manner as con-

ventional energy and its strength does not decrease over time or space. Distant healing and prayer have numerous research studies showing positive outcomes (reference 9, p. 61).

Healing Touch derives its methods from a variety of techniques. Healing Touch was developed by a nurse who studied Therapeutic Touch. The two forms of healing are based on much the same principle, but Healing Touch also uses methods taught by other indigenous cultures around the world. This method of biofield therapy is endorsed by the American Holistic Nurses' Association. The Healing Touch practitioner realigns the flow of energy, helping to reactivate the mind–body–spirit connection to eliminate blockages to self-healing.

Chi Kung (Qi Gong) and Tai Chi are examples of energy medicine approaches that patients can practice on their own. These ancient health-promoting practices originated in China but are now practiced by persons worldwide. They consist of moving meditative exercises with posture changes that flow from one into another, and allow for improved flow of Qi, or energy, along the meridians and through the chakras. The use of breathing techniques along with the movements balances and enhances energy resources for healing. Qi Gong is not only used for improving the flow of Qi in one's own body but also can be sent to others through the use of external Qi Gong. It is generally considered safe for the patient with cancer to participate in Qi Gong because of the slow, deliberate exercises involved.

Many Native Americans feel that healing energy is provided to us through Mother Earth. The energy resonates up through the earth and into the body. Native American healers use massage therapy to correct physical, energetic and spiritual imbalances and to increase the patient's powers of self-healing. Massage is also used in disease prevention by creating an energetic/spiritual protective field around the patient which keeps good influences in and keeps harmful forces out. Native American massage techniques incorporate different methods which include rubbing, kneading, pressing and applying pressure to specific points found to be therapeutic; laying-on of hands; removal of harmful forces energetically; and non-contact methods in which the healer holds his hands closely above but not upon the body. The Native American healings are supported with prayer, song or ceremony[10].

Polarity Therapy was created by Dr Randolph Stone. It is a holistic system that promotes deep relaxation and revitalization by balancing the body's energy. It seeks to harmonize people with the environment. In polarity therapy, in order to remain healthy a body must maintain free-flowing energy circuits. Any obstruction will result in pain and eventually illness. The entire body is seen as an energy field with specific currents and patterns. These are governed by three electromagnetic charges: positive, negative and neutral. Polarity Therapy is the science of balancing these subtle energy currents by using love, positive thoughts and attitudes, gentle manipulations, exercise and proper diet[11].

Magnet therapy is one of the most frequently used of all the energy medicine techniques[12]. Magnets are used to relieve muscle and joint pain as well as to speed healing and reduce swelling. The magnetic field is also supposed to inhibit nerve signals carrying pain messages to the brain. Despite the popularity of magnet therapy, there has been little published evidence to prove its effectiveness.

There is no dogma attached to energy medicine and nothing about this form of healing contradicts any religion in any way. During a healing, once a connection is established the flow of energy is activated. The 'healer' may envision the energy coming from an unlimited energy source that to him/her may be seen as God, Buddha, Mohammed, a white light, saints, angels or even the earth itself. The only requirement is that there is a connection between the 'source' and the one facilitating the energy flow. In his book, *A*

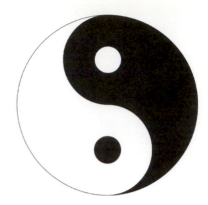

Figure 10.3   Yin and Yang

Practical Guide to Vibrational Healing, Dr Richard Gerber states that everyone is a potential healer and he likens developing the ability to heal to exercising a muscle – the more you do it the stronger your healing skills become (reference 7, p. 402).

Much of energy medicine is grounded in a philosophy of balance in all things. The concept of Yin and Yang in Chinese tradition represents balance while in constant movement. The familiar symbol of Yin and Yang is illustrated by a circle divided into tear-drop-shaped black and white halves with a dot of the color of its opposite half to indicate that these two ways are always in the process of becoming the other in a constant ebb and flow, contraction and expansion (Figure 10.3).

The objective of healing is to find the balance leading to an unimpeded flow of Chi. Treatment is not directed toward the symptoms but rather at the underlying imbalance that produces them. The definition of health then is to be in complete harmony with nature, internally as well as externally[13].

In his book, *The Four Agreements*, Don Miguel Ruiz, MD, gives us four simple 'agreements' to apply in our lives. First, is to 'Be impeccable with your word.' He explains that the human mind is a fertile ground continually being planted with seeds, which give growth to thoughts[14]. These seeds are too often those of fear or judgment either of yourself or of others. 'The word can enter our mind and change a whole belief for better or for worse' (reference 14, p. 29). This is a good reason not to tell patients that they have only a specific amount of time to live. Granted, there are those patients who will see this as a challenge and reason to strive on; others, however, may conform and succumb to the negative energy of those words.

The second agreement – 'Don't take anything personally' – tells us that what others say and do is a projection of their own reality. Do not internalize what others say about you.

Third, is 'Don't make assumptions' (reference 14, p. 68). If we make assumptions we are discouraging communication with others. We are all composed of energy and if we are in synchronization with each other, as opposed to the chaos that occurs with misunderstanding, then the energies of all involved flow optimally.

The final agreement, 'Always do your best', applies to any circumstance in your life (reference 14, p. 77). If you know that you have done your best you will not judge yourself and therefore will not suffer from guilt, blame and self-punishment – all human frailties that contribute to interference in the flow of chi. If one truly lives by these four agreements much of the stress encountered daily would be eliminated and, as we now know, stress and the chemicals that it releases in our bodies are major contributing factors in disease today.

Caroline Myss, in her book *Anatomy of the Spirit,* acknowledges that energy medicine practitioners believe that the human energy field contains and reflects each individual's energy. ' It surrounds us and carries with us the emotional energy created by our internal and external experiences – both positive and negative. This emotional force influences the physical tissue within our bodies. In this way your biography – that is the experiences that make up your life – becomes your biology.'[15] To maintain health it is necessary to clear negative energy coming from past experiences. This is integral in helping to maintain the healthy immune system that is our primary defense against disease.

One of the ways it is believed that energy medicine works is by opening the pathways of communication that enable cells in the body to 'talk to each other'. In a 2002 interview published in *Reiki News Magazine,* Dr James Oschman tells readers that energy medicine opens up the terrain through which cells are able to migrate to places where they are needed to fight disease or initiate repair. Energy medicine is also effective in calming the individual so that the immune system can operate at a more optimum level[16].

The impact of our individual energies on one another has been scientifically studied. Electrocardiographs show that the energy produced by the heart of one person has an effect upon the heart activity and brain waves of another person. This effect was measurable even when the subjects were sitting as far as three feet apart[17]. Energies from non-human sources affect us as well. Energies in our environment can be beneficial or harmful.

Individuals considered at high risk for energy disturbance which could eventually lead to disease would be those whose life experience includes emotional, mental or physical trauma. This may be attributable to multiple sources such as grief, abuse, fear, family dysfunction, physical injury or disability. One's perceptions are one's reality and adjustments may be made through the use of energy medicine to facilitate the healing of these perceptions and restore the optimal flow of Chi.

It is hypothesized that individuals exposed to 'unhealthy' environmental electromagnetic forces (EMF) may be at higher risk for developing disease. Daily use of computers, electrical equipment, cell phones, power lines or microwave towers, even the use of electric blankets or heating pads, produce electromagnetic energy. Research up to now has proved inconclusive in relating EMF to specific disease. Cognizance of the existence of EMF and attempts to lessen exposure may prove to be a reasonable means of prevention should further research show a correlation.

In her book, *Hands of Light,* Barbara Brennan tells us that energy fields are intimately associated with a person's health and well-being. If a person is unhealthy, it will show in his energy field as an unbalanced flow of energy and/or stagnated energy that has ceased to flow and appears as darkened colors. In contrast, a healthy individual will show bright colors that flow easily in a balanced field[18]. Biofield, vibrational or energy medicine therapies are generally accepted as low-risk interventions. *Do no harm* is applicable in energy medicine probably more than in any other CAM modality. The intention of the healer is to have occur only what is best for the receiver of the healing, according to the loving intelligence of the universe. Because the healer is not dictating what will occur, he can do no wrong. At the very least, energy medicine serves to provide human touch. It relaxes and calms and imparts a sense of knowing to the recipient that another human being cares about them.

Probably the only risk that could possibly be associated with energy medicine would be that of the question 'What if this is not real or does not work?' Studies using animals as well as humans have shown that energy medicine works separately from the placebo effect. Placebo, however, may also play an important part in any healing process. Although the word placebo is often thought about in a derogatory sense, the belief in the effectiveness of a placebo will often enable the patient to mobilize his own innate abilities to counter symptoms and side-effects of cancer treatment by altering the biochemical and psychosomatic responses of the body. Placebo has been shown to have a significant response in many cases, some of which include helping to adjust white blood cell values, relieve depression, and help with sleep and pain reduction[19].

In an article published in *Alternative Therapies* in 2001 entitled: "Designing clinical trials on energy healing: an ancient art encounters medical science", the authors state: 'To call an expectation-driven benefit a placebo is misleading in a therapist-involved trial, because it overlooks any benefit so created. Suppose effects of expectations and literal energy transference somehow combine in this context: a placebo effect can still be a part of the real cure of energy healing, despite its being brought about by expectations'[20].

ENERGY MEDICINE AND RESEARCH

The use of energy medicine is widespread and there is a huge amount of anecdotal level 3 evidence as to its efficacy. Because the workings of subtle energies lie beyond present technology's ability to measure consistently, biofield therapies present a special research challenge.

In addition, lack of energy medicine studies, especially in the case of cancer patients, may be occurring for a variety of reasons. Both conventional medicine practitioners and the public may lack knowledge about energy medicine modalities. Conversely, energy medicine practitioners may not have experience with research studies, contacts at research institutions, or access to grant funding. Also, those researchers who are knowledgeable about CAM practices may be hesitant to pursue CAM studies, because of the stigma attached to conducting these types of study by some of their conventional medicine colleagues. Another reason is difficulty in designing single-blind/double-blind studies and in the standardization of treatment protocols and identification of control groups. Energy medicine sessions/treatments usually are based on the clients' needs. Standardization may therefore be a problem. Reiki practitioners may also feel that the choice of the individual to participate in their healing process is lost when they commit to a randomized trial, so they may not promote study participation.

For example, there have not been many studies on Qi Gong therapy for cancer. However, findings have been consistent that cancer patients have significant improvement or better results when they received Qi Gong therapy partnered with conventional medicine than those groups who received conventional medicine alone[21]. Although the research designs may be somewhat lacking in format, the scientific studies have confirmed the inhibitory effect of external Qi therapy on cancer growth[22]. The mechanism of Qi Gong practice is that it is thought to increase Qi or the vital energy flow in the body and thus boost the immune system, or inhibit cancer growth in some other way.

The standards of replicability and generalizability so central to the scientific paradigm can be at odds with the practice of energy medicine. For example, there may be significant variations in individual practitioner effectiveness. However, the fact that so many people adopt energy medicine as a healing practice, and so many more seek treatment from providers of this modality, means that we must find ways to study its potential benefits, risks and applications[23]. Future additional research into how and who is benefited by energy medicine are necessary. Judging by the impressive list of respected medical institutions that currently incorporate energy medicine or biofield therapies into their patient care, it appears that the Western world has begun to accept that, although there has not been a long history of medical research in this field, there is an extensive history of its use throughout the world.

The University of Arizona's Program of Integrative Medicine completed two studies on biofield therapies in 2004. One examined the psychophysiological and biophysical aspects of biofield therapies such as Reiki, Qi Gong, Therapeutic Touch and Johrei.

The second study evaluated the efficacy of Healing Touch upon the stress response of neonates. Results were not available at the time of this writing. Both these studies were funded by the National Institutes of Health (NIH) and the National Center for Complementary and Alternative Medicine (NCCAM). The Program of Integrative Medicine at The University of Arizona incorporates education concerning biofield therapies into its Fellowship in Integrative Medicine curriculum for physicians.

Distant healing has received little attention from mainstream medicine; however, a substantial body of published data supports the possibility of significant effect. Over 150 formal, controlled studies have been published over the course of the past 40 years. More than two-thirds of these studies have demonstrated significant effects[24].

Although research is demonstrating that spiritual healing/energy medicine works, we still do not know how. In his book, *Healing Words: The Power of Prayer and the Practice of Medicine*, Dr Larry Dossey states: 'To acknowledge that we don't know how something works is not a particularly damaging confession in medicine.'[9] He goes on to remind us that no one knew how penicillin worked when it was discovered but, had that stopped the process, the introduction of life-saving antibiotics would have been delayed. People who are suffering from pain or infection do not first ask how a therapy works but rather, *does it work?* 'As history shows, full explanations frequently come later. So it may be for energy medicine.'[25]

CURRENT QUESTIONS

- What is the best way to study energy medicine?

- Do new devices need to be designed to measure these subtle energies of the human body?

- Can energy medicine help with cancer fatigue and other quality of life subscales such as pain, stress, anxiety, depression?

- Can energy medicine help prevent recurrence or possibly even be used as a chemopreventive strategy?

- Can energy medicine help in palliative care and in death and dying?

- What is the best way to introduce the concept of energy medicine to patients who may not have previous knowledge?

- Should there be a certification process to qualify energy healers?

- How does one identify a good energy medicine practitioner?

A SAMPLING OF CURRENT RESEARCH TRIALS

The partial list of research listed below has direct or indirect implications in the care of the oncology patient. There are many additional current studies addressing energy medicine as it relates to a variety of situations such as hypertension, cardiac patient care, stress and arthritis. A large amount of research is directed toward finding instruments that may be used to measure the energy field and document changes that occur.

Altering breast cancer cell phenotype and growth characteristics by distant healing intent[26]

G.S. Jensen, PhD, Natural Immune Systems Inc., 1437 Esplanade Ave., Klamath Falls, OR 97601

Objective

To perform pilot experiments to assess whether distant healing intent (DHI) can alter the physical, phenotypic, and growth characteristics of a breast cancer cell line *in vitro*.

Materials and methods

The researchers performing the laboratory analysis are blinded to treatment, and the healer is dissociated from data analysis. A breast cancer cell line is cultured, parallel flasks/plates are plated, and flasks are randomized to either treatment or control. At 1, 8, 24 and 48 hours after DHI, samples of cells are evaluated as described below.

Cell line   The MCF-7 breast cancer cell line was chosen based on its expression of the estrogen receptor (ER).

Healer   The person providing the DHI is selected among healers who have in the past shown reproducible results.

(1) Phenotypic changes: Two phenotypic characteristics are frequently observed on malignant cells:

　(a) increased level of hormone/growth factor receptor(s);

　(b) decreased level of MHCI antigen, reducing immune recognition.

The evaluation of phenotypic changes towards a more normal phenotype will include immunostaining for ER and MHCI and flow cytometric analysis.

(2) Proliferative rate: A lipophilic membrane dye is used for cell labeling. As cells proliferate, the fluorescent dye is shared between daughter cells. Proliferation, as loss of fluorescence intensity, is evaluated by flow cytometry.

(3) Cell death: The induction of cell death in the cultured breast cancer cells is analyzed by staining cells with annexin and propidium iodide. Flow cytometry allows evaluation of apoptotic versus necrotic cells, and of early versus late stage of apoptosis.

Results and conclusion

This pilot study distinguishes between three possible effects of DHI: normalization of phenotype, alteration of growth rate, or killing of tumor cells. This may aid future research on DHI, and assist further research into which cellular elements may be affected.

The effect of Reiki on the immune system[27]

Wendy Hodsdon, Elissa Mendenhall, Rebecca Green, Sara Kates-Chinnoy, Elizabeth Wacker and Heather Zwickey; Helfgott Research Institute at the National College of Naturopathic Medicine, Portland, OR 97201

Objectives

Although energy medicines such as Reiki have been shown to have an overall effect on health, the mechanisms by which energy medicine act are currently unknown. This study examines the effects of Reiki on cellular immunity.

Materials and methods

Two protocols have been used. The first protocol randomized subjects into three groups: Reiki, relaxation control, or neither Reiki nor relaxation control. Blood was drawn before treatment, immediately following treatment, or 4 hours after treatment. The second protocol exposed each subject to each treatment through the following process: blood draw, relaxation, blood draw, Reiki, blood draw. In both studies, white blood cells were isolated using Ficoll blood tubes and stained with markers for CD4 and CD8 T cells, B cells, NK cells and macrophages. All the cells were stained with an early activation marker (CD69) to measure activation. A flow cytometer was used to quantify the amount of activation of each cell type. In the second protocol, heart math was also used to measure general mental–emotional state.

Results

While this study is ongoing, preliminary results indicate an increase in cell activation in the group of each cell type. In the second protocol, heart math was also used to measure general mental–emotional state.

Conclusions

Our study shows a white cell activation (probably macrophages) in patients receiving Reiki. These results provide the basis for further study of the immunological effects of energy medicine.

Healing Touch and immunity in cervical cancer patients[28]

Susan Lutgendorf, PhD, Barrie Anderson, MD, Joel Sorosky, MD, David Lubaroff, PhD, John Buatti, MD, University of Iowa; and Anil Sood, MD, MD Anderson Cancer Center

Objective

Although Healing Touch (HT) is frequently used as a complementary treatment by cancer patients receiving chemotherapy and radiation, effects of this therapy during cancer treatment have been minimally investigated. Additionally, little is known about the physiological mechanisms by which HT may work. This study is designed to examine effects of HT on cellular immune function and short-term side-effects of treatment among women with advanced cervical cancer who are receiving 6 weeks of chemotherapy, external radiation and intracavitary radiation. Although combined chemotherapy and radiation is potentially curative in 69% of cases, many patients experience acute side-effects and late radiation effects. Severe immune compromise has also been reported following intensive radiation.

Materials and methods

Sixty-six cervical cancer patients are randomized to HT, relaxation, or standard care. HT or relaxation is provided 4 days a week immediately following external beam radiation in the Clinical Research Center throughout the patient's external beam radiation treatment. Standard care patients receive no additional treatment but are eligible for either HT or relaxation after their 1-month follow-up assessment. Blood draws for assessment of natural killer cell cytotoxicity and T-cell production of cytokines are taken at baseline, and weeks 4, 6, and 1 month post-radiation.

Results and significance

Data are still being collected. This study will provide preliminary data on the impact of HT on various parameters of cellular immune function and whether the magnitude of that impact is large enough to be of sufficient clinical significance to be examined in future efficacy trials.

Supported in part by the National Center for Complementary and Alternative Medicine (NCCAM:NIH) Project 4 in Exploratory Program Grant for Frontier Medicine. (Prestwood, P.I.) 1 P20 AT-756-01.

Center for Frontier Medicine in Biofield Science

Specialty: Biofield
Principal investigator: Gary E. Schwartz, PhD.

Address:
Department of Psychology
University of Arizona
PO Box 210068
Tucson, AZ 85721-0068

Description:
This center facilitates and integrates research on the effects of low energy fields. The research is focused on developing standardized bioassays (cellular biology) and psychophysiological and biophysical markers of biofield effects, and on the application of the markers developed to measure outcomes in the recovery of surgical patients.

Exploratory Program Grant for Frontier Medicine

Specialty: Touch
Principal investigator: Karen Prestwood, MD

Address:
University of Connecticut Center on Aging
MC 5215
University of Connecticut Health Center
263 Farmington Avenue
Farmington, CT 06030-5215

Description:
This center will evaluate the effects of Therapeutic Touch and healing touch on several human diseases and processes. The Center includes preclinical projects studying the effect of Therapeutic Touch on bone metabolism and on fibroblast biology, and two clinical projects, one investigating the effect of Therapeutic Touch on bone metabolism in postmenopausal women with wrist fractures and a second studying the effect of Healing Touch on immune function in advanced cervical cancer.

Prayer and breast cancer study at Johns Hopkins (subcontract with Duke)[29]

Title:
Prayer in African-American Women with Stage 1 Breast Cancer
Funding cource: NIH (NCCAM)

Objective and design

The goal is to determine the impact of a prayer intervention (in person) on neuroendocrine markers of stress and on attendant immune function in African-American women with early-stage breast cancer. The study is based on the scientific premise that the stress of having breast cancer alters natural neuroendocrine-mediated immunoprotective mechanisms and may increase the likelihood of tumor recurrence.

We propose that this cascade may be partly ameliorated by a prayer intervention in African-American women with a strong propensity to use spiritual healing. African-American women have a poor prognosis at every stage of breast cancer diagnosis and are more vulnerable to the stress associated with attended diagnosis and treatment. From a CAM perspective, strong psychosocial group support as well as mindful meditation may positively modulate the negative neuroendocrine and immune consequences of chronic stress in cancer. Prayer interventions offer both meditation-like and group supportive elements. Based on abysmal physical and psychosocial outcomes in African-American women with breast cancer and their almost 100% use of prayer for coping, we propose to determine the extent to which a personal and group prayer intervention improves neuroendocrine and immune responses in African-American women with breast cancer treated locally with surgery and irradiation. A prayer intervention ($n = 40$) will be initiated 1–2 months post-radiation and compared to a randomly assigned 'wait listed' control group ($n = 40$) 1 and 6 months after baseline. We will examine changes in (a) neuroendocrine markers of stress including plasma adrenocorticotropic hormone (ACTH) and cortisol responses to intravenous corticotropin releasing hormone, 24-hour urinary free cortisol, and the cortisol circadian rhythm using salivary cortisol; (b) parameters of immune response including CD4/CD8 T-cell subset changes in peripheral blood, NK cell activity using NK cell target K562, the total number of monocytes in the peripheral blood and peripheral blood lymphocyte proliferation and cytokine release in response to breast cancer-specific antigens including HER-2/neu, MUC-1 and MAGE 3; and (c) perceived stress, psychosocial functioning, and quality of life. We plan to establish this group as a cohort for long-term tumor surveillance to be compared with a race-, age- and stage-matched reference group.

Findings

Currently recruiting patients into this 5-year study in Baltimore (2000–2005). No study results will be available until after study completion. For more information, contact Diane Becker at Johns Hopkins Center for Health Promotion or Harold G. Koenig (koenig@geri.duke.edu).

GLOSSARY OF TERMS

Aura   Multi-layered energy field that surrounds and permeates all forms of life. The aura is continually interacting through spiritual and psychological levels by way of the chakras.

Biofield   The energy field composed of magnetic and electromagnetic energetic forces, which are created by living organisms.

Chakras   The vortices through which Chi flows in and out of the body. There are generally considered to be seven main chakras, but it is thought that hundreds exist. Each vibrates at a different rate and has a color associated with it. To maintain optimal health, the chakras should be open to the flow of energy and not blocked.

Chi   The ancient Chinese word for the subtle energy that flows throughout the body and encompasses all life forms.

Energy   The Universal Life Force, Prana, Chi, or Ki. The universe is composed of energy. All energy vibrates to a particular frequency. It is this degree of vibration that determines whether an object is animate or inanimate.

Non-local   Not confined to a specific time and place in space or to a specific moment in time. Energy may travel distances. Prayer is non-local.

Scanning   The process of 'feeling' the aura of an organism to determine areas of imbalance in the energy field.

Subtle energy The life energy, which flows through the chakras and meridians (also called Chi, Ki or Prana). This energy is affected by emotions and state of spiritual development. Difficult to measure by traditional means, it can be detected by its effects.

RESOURCES FOR ENERGY MEDICINE

www.ahna.org

www.bioelectromagnets.org

www.CCNH.edu

www.ClinicalTrials.gov

www.Healingtouch.net

www.IARP.org

www.issseem.org

www.Johrei.com

www.noetic.org

www.nursehealers.com

www.Polaritytherapy.org

www.Reiki.org

www.qigonginstitute.org

www.therapeutictouch.org

www.therapeutic-touch.org

Educational offerings

A recent study in the *Journal of the American Medical Association* reports that 64% of US medical schools offer CAM education. A sample of some that offer energy modalities is listed below.

The American Medical Student Association (AMSA)
The EDCAM Initiative: A national curriculum for medical students
www.amsa.org/humed/CAM/resources.ctm

Case Western Reserve University School of Medicine
Energy-based healing

Tanya Edwards, MD
+1-216-844-2076
http://mediswww.cwru.edu/education/catscheds.htm

Commonweal
Institute for the Study of Health and Illness
The ISHI's curriculum is offered in 35 medical schools
+1-415-868-0970

Many Streams Healing Systems
Residential retreats and workshops for cancer patients, physicians and corporate health-care workers
www.manystreamsheal.org

University of California – Los Angeles School of Medicine
Healing Touch
Susan Stangl, MD, MS, Ed.
Los Angeles, CA

University of Illinois at Chicago
Healing Touch
Dr Mary Sinclair, LAc
College of Applied Health Sciences
+1-312-996-2418

University of Minnesota School of Medicine
Center for Spirituality and Healing
Introduction to Energy Healing
Cynthia J. Satterness, MS, Reiki Master
+1-612-624-5166

Mt Sinai School of Medicine of New York University
The Power of Subtle Body: Innovative Qi Gong
Joyce Shriver, PhD
+1-212-582-0720
Qi Gong in Medicine
Warner Chen, LAc, PhD
+1-212-293-1722

Tufts University School of Medicine
Healing Connection Program at Union Hospital
Harvey Zarren, MD, FAAC
+1-781-477-3604

Yale Graduate School of Nursing
Reiki Energy Medicine I and II
Pamela Potter
+1-203-737-2230

A state-by-state listing of US medical schools offering courses in CAM can be found at www.rosenthal.hs.columbia.edu/MD-courses.html

Energy medicine may also be taught outside the university setting, as in private homes and businesses. A website that lists many schools of complementary and alternative modalities is www.naturalhealers.com

Research groups

The Center for Mind Body Medicine
Dr James S. Gordon, Director
www.cmbm.org

Institute of Frontier Science
University of Arizona

National Center for Complementary and Alternative Medicine (NCCAM)
http://nccam.nih.gov/

Touch Research Institute
University of Miami School of Medicine
www.miami.edu/touchresearch/

Physician, provider and patient retreats

The Center for Mind Body Medicine offers educational opportunities and intensive retreats during the year for healthcare professionals who wish to integrate Mind-Body Spirit Medicine into their clinical practice.

Dr James S. Gordon, Director
+1-202-966-7338
www.cmbm.org

Commonweal
Retreats for cancer patients and health
  professionals
Bolinas, CA
Michael Lerne, Founder and President
+1-415-868-0970
commonweal@commonweal.org

EcaP and the Mind–Body Wellness Center
Offers resources and training for health professionals and retreats incorporating mind–body–spirit medicine for patients with cancer and other chronic illnesses.

Meadville Medical Center Health Systems, Inc.
Barry Bittman, MD and Bernie Siegel, MD
www.e-cap-online.org/

Many Streams Healing Systems
Retreats for cancer patients and medical
  professionals
Integrative workshops and support groups.
Rome, GA
Matt Mumber, MD, Founder and CEO
+1-706-290-7700
www.manystreamsheal.org

Smith Farm Center for the Healing Arts and Cancer Care
Retreats for cancer patients and health
  professionals
Washington, DC
Michael Lerner, President and CEO
+1-202-483-8600
www.smithfarm.com/

Sunstone Healing Center
Retreats for cancer patients and their families
Retreats for medical professionals
Tucson, AZ
+1-520-749-1928
www.sunstonehealing.net

References

1. International Society for the Study of Subtle Energies and Energy Medicine, Founding Statement, 6th Annual ISSSEEM Conference Proceedings, Boulder, CO, June 1997: 2

2. Shealy CN. Electronic Newsletter, Holy Ground Farm, Vol 1, Issue 9, September 2003

3. Gerber R. Vibrational Medicine: The #1 Handbook of Subtle-Energy Therapies, 3rd edn. Rochester: Bear & Company, 2001: p. 428

4. Gordon JS, Curtin S. Comprehensive Cancer Care: Integrating Alternative, Complementary, and Conventional Therapies. Cambridge: Perseus Publishing, 2000: 113

5. Brewer VA. Cam Handbook: Energy Healing. Washington University School of Medicine. Web page http://medicine.wustl.edu/~comp med/cam_toc.htm

6. Bruyere R. Wheels of Light: Chakras, Auras, and the Healing Energy of the Body. New York: Simon and Schuster, 1994: 18–20

7. Gerber R. A Practical Guide to Vibrational Medicine: Energy Healing and Spiritual Transformation. New York: Harper Collins Publishers, 2000: 377

8. Kreiger D. Living the Therapeutic Touch: Healing as a Lifestyle. New York: Dodd, Mead and Company, 1987: 8

9. Dossy L. Healing Words: The Power of Prayer and the Practice of Medicine. New York: Harper Collins, 1997: 275–7

10. Cohen K. Honoring the Medicine: The Essential Guide to Native American Healing. New York: Random House, 2003: 261

11. Seidman M. A Guide to Polarity Therapy: The Gentle Art of Hands-On Healing. Berkeley, CA: North Atlantic Books, 1999: 1

12. Koontz K. Natural Health. October, 2003

13. Knaster M. Discovering the Body's Wisdom. New York: Bantam Books, 1996: 275

14. Ruiz DM. The Four Agreements. San Rafael, CA: Amber-Allen Publishing, 1997: 28

15. Myss C. The Anatomy of the Spirit. New York: Three Rivers Press, 1996: 34

16. Oschman JL. Interview with William Lee Rand. Reiki News Magazine, Vol. One, Issue Three, Winter 2002: 1–8

17. McCraty R. The Electricity of Touch, Paper presented at The International Society for the Study of Subtle Energies and Energy Medicine. Sixth Annual Conference, Boulder, CO, June 1996. Available through the HeartMath Institute: www.webcom/hrtmath

18. Brennan BA. Hands of Light: A Guide to Healing Through the Human Energy Field. New York: Bantam Books, 188: 7

19. Murphy M. The Body. Millennium. Boston: Houghton-Mifflin, 1981: 82

20. Ai A, Peterson C, Gillespie B, et al. Designing clinical trials on energy healing: an ancient art encounters medical science. Alternative Ther 2001; 7. 83–90

21. Cong J, Lu Z. Curative Effect on 120 Cancer Cases Treated by Chinese-Western Medicine and Qigong Therapy. 2nd World Conference Exchange Medicine Qigong; Beijing, China, 1993: 131

22. Chen XL, et al. Double-blind test of emitted Qi on tumor formation of a nasopharyngeal carcinoma cell line in nude mice. 2nd World Academic Exchange Medicine Qigong, Beijing, China, 1993: 105

23. Miles P, True G. Reiki – review of a biofield therapy history: theory, practice and research. Alternative Ther 2003; 9: 62–71

24. Benor DJ. Healing Research, Vol 1. Deddington, England: Helix Editions, 1992

25. Jonas WB, Crawford C. Healing Intention and Energy: Medicine, Science, Research Methods and Clinical Implications. London: Churchill Livingstone, 2003: 305

26. Jensen GS. Altering breast cancer cell phenotype and growth characteristics by distant healing intent. Presented at ISSSEEM conference, Colorado Springs, CO, June 2005

27. Hodson W, et al. The effect of Reiki on the immune system. J Alternative Complement Med 2004; 10: 728–33

28. www.Healingtouch.net/research/index

29. www.Dukespiritualityandhealth.org/research/ongoing/studies.html

10g

Spirituality

Howard Silverman and Toby Schneider

'Great Spirit…You have set the powers of the four quarters of the earth to cross each other. You have made me cross the good road and the road of difficulties, and where they cross, the place is holy. Day in, day out, forevermore, you are the life of things.' – Black Elk, Oglala Sioux Medicine Man

INTRODUCTION AND DEFINITIONS

In this chapter, we attempt to define spirituality and examine its role in integrative oncology from a number of perspectives. What issues does spirituality bring up for physicians and patients? How can we practically communicate about these issues? What role does an approach to spirituality have as a part of integrative oncology? These questions are addressed with the backdrop of a personal set of experiences reflecting an ongoing conversation between the authors, who are siblings. Toby was diagnosed with breast cancer 5 years ago and is now undergoing treatment for metastatic disease. Howard was trained as a family physician and is now an integrative medicine educator.

The word 'spirituality' means different things to different people and comes in an infinite variety of shapes and forms. The definition given by the Merriam-Webster online dictionary[1] defines the word 'spirit' primarily as a noun rather than a verb. The etymology is Middle English, from

Old French or Latin; Old French, from Latin *spiritus* – literally, breath, from *spirare* to blow, breathe. It then offers 11 distinct definitions, the more applicable of which are:

1: an animating or vital principle held to give life to physical organisms;

4: the immaterial intelligent or sentient part of a person;

5: the activating or essential principle influencing a person;

6: a special attitude or frame of mind;

7: a lively or brisk quality in a person or a person's actions;

9: a mental disposition characterized by firmness or assertiveness;

11: prevailing tone or tendency.

These definitions point to spirituality as somehow intimately linked to the life force within each of us and tied to our values and attitudes.

The definition of religion conveyed by the same dictionary offers four possible definitions, of which the most applicable are:

2: a personal set or institutionalized system of religious attitudes, beliefs, and practices;

3: archaic: scrupulous conformity: conscientiousness;

4: a cause, principle, or system of beliefs held to with ardor and faith.

Thus one could think of spirituality as a kind of diverging, ever-widening force and religion as a movement toward more tangible beliefs and practices. Historically, being a spiritual person was frequently associated with following a particular religious path. However, one can be highly spiritual without being religious and, conversely, one can be highly religious without being spiritual. This is one of but many paradoxes one encounters as one carefully considers the notion of spirituality. Deepak Chopra echoes the awe of these paradoxes of spirit, noting 'The spirit is a real force. It's as real as gravity, it's as real as time. It's equally abstract, equally as incomprehensible and mysterious and difficult to grasp conceptually. It's very powerful, and when we touch that spiritual core of awareness, only then can we be healed.'[2] Carl Jung phrased this slightly differently when he said 'We should not pretend to understand the world only by the intellect; we apprehend it just as much by feeling. Therefore the judgment of the intellect is, at best, only the half of truth, and must, if it be honest, also come to an understanding of its inadequacy.'[3] As noted above, since religion is generally more tangible and therefore measurable, the majority of the literature in this area will focus on religious practices such as frequency of worship, adherence to religious beliefs and practices (e.g. prayer), and similar measurable manifestations of religious adherence, such as social support.

Ultimately, spirituality is much more about presence than knowledge. A spiritual way of life is informed by experience rather than purely intellectual learning. Whereas the mind has the capacity to absorb process and store external information, the spiritual realm is experiential. This realm is based on events and interpreted from within. Not necessarily based in what we would consider rational thinking, this is the place where revelation is born.

There is no set way to be spiritual. Being spiritual has to do with being yourself, being true to yourself and coming from the heart and soul rather than the ego. The ego is that part of our psyche which defines our individuality as reflected by the Merriam-Webster online dictionary's definition of the ego as 'the self especially as contrasted with another self or the world.'[1] In a sense, it locates us as apart from others. It is necessary for our physical survival in responding to somatic functions such as hunger, thirst, temperature and the sense of danger, but it is also controlling and seeks predictable outcomes. The diagnosis of a life-threatening illness and the possibility of toxic treatments begin to undermine this sense of control and predictability. As the sense of control begins to wane, emotional states of fear, anxiety and anger may emerge as a response. However, if one chooses to respond to the situation by using cancer as a turning point, then it may be a springboard into the spiritual realm and a new perspective. This spiritual perspective honors the thought that each person is different and preciously unique.

Clinicians can open their service to a spiritual dimension by observation, sensitivity and compassion to patients' individual needs and styles. There are a number of studies that have attested to the importance of doing so[4–8]. In some cases, this can be empowered and fostered by simply including a brief spiritual assessment while taking the patient's history. It takes dedication and practice to remain open minded, non-judgmental and patient centered during this assessment process. Unless the patient's beliefs and practices are destructive, this acceptance sends a strong positive message about the importance of spiritual issues in the patient's experience, while it also becomes an opportunity for inner growth for the clinician. For some, this can bring about more openness and acceptance in the clinician's personal and professional relationships beyond their patients.

SPIRITUALITY AND CANCER RESEARCH

There is currently a paucity of high-quality research in the area of spirituality and cancer, particularly quantitative research. For example, a Pubmed search utilizing MeSH major topic headings of 'spirituality' and 'cancer' from 1960 through the present yielded 49 citations, in contrast to 1 274 902 citations for 'cancer' and, interestingly, 474 citations for 'cancer' and 'nausea'. One author laments that 'there is a paucity of published literature describing the spiritual experience of cancer care.'[9] There are several possible explanations for this small number of studies, including the difficulty in performing quantitative studies of relevance and quality; the sense of taboos regarding discussion and research regarding clinical spirituality; and the relative lack of funding and focus in this area.

Does spirituality have a role in cancer care? A recent study analyzed the spiritual dimensions of cancer care and, using qualitative methods, found that spiritual and religious concerns have a high priority among some cancer patients (reference 9, p. 92). The rank ordered themes that arose from that study were:

(1) My spirituality comforts and helps me find meaning in cancer challenges, because I place my trust in a power greater than myself.

(2) My health-care providers could provide spiritual care in ways that do not involve explicit discussions of spirituality.

(3) I would like to feel welcome to explicitly share my spiritual needs with my health-care providers.

(4) My spiritual life is enacted with a spiritual community, which provides me with valuable support during my cancer experience.

(5) My individual prayer practices comfort me and contribute to my healing.

(6) Spirituality is an important part of who I am as a person.

(7) I understand my experience of cancer is part of my spiritual life.

Whether spiritual practices have beneficial physical effects remains controversial, although there are a few interesting studies that suggest this may be the case[10–12].

Despite the fact that individuals have their own set of beliefs, preferences and concerns, the diagnosis of a potentially life-threatening disease may bring about a common set of issues. The physician can help to bring these issues to the forefront through careful history taking. Several mnemonic-based formats have been proposed for use by clinicians in soliciting a spiritual history, and these are depicted in Table 10.6. These are intended primarily as 'screening' questions. In addition to obtaining some basic information about the patient's spiritual life and preferences, it also gives the patient and family permission to bring up spiritual issues downstream.

A discussion brought about through using one of the above tools can then be framed within a series of issues that come about when dealing with any chronic illness, including cancer.

WHY (ME, THIS, NOW, FILL-IN-YOUR-OWN-QUESTION(S) HERE)

Most individuals who hear they have a potentially life-threatening illness such as cancer are

Table 10.6	Spiritual assessment tools

FICA[13]	SPIRIT[14]
F: Faith or beliefs: What is your faith or belief? Do you consider yourself spiritual or religious? What things do you believe in that give meaning to your life?	**S:** Spiritual belief system: How would you name or describe your spiritual belief system?
I: Importance or influence: Is it important in your life? What influence does it have on how you take care of yourself? How have your beliefs influenced your behavior during this illness? What role do your beliefs play in regaining your health?	**P:** Personal spirituality: What is the importance of your spirituality/religion in your daily life?
	I: Integration and involvement with others in a spiritual community: Do you belong to any spiritual or religious group or community?
C: Community: Are you part of a spiritual or religious community? Is this of support to you? If so, how? Is there a person or group of people you really love and who are really important to you?	**R:** Ritualized practices and restrictions: Are there specific practices that you carry out as part of your religion/spirituality? (e.g. prayer, meditation). Are there specific elements of medical care that you forbid on the basis of religious/spiritual grounds?
A: Address: How would you like me, your physician, to address these issues in your care?	**I:** Implications for medical care: What aspects of your religion/spirituality would you like me to keep in mind as I care for you?
	T: Terminal events planning: As we plan for your care near the end of life, how does your faith impact on your decision(s)?

jolted from their normal lives into a kind of parallel universe. This is truly an instantaneous and life-changing event. Patient and family needs must be respected with regards to education and information concerning a new set of interventions – some that fight cancer, some that are supportive in nature. Communication methods are paramount to establishing a therapeutic relationship in this time of acute need. This is how Toby experienced this:

The word 'cancer' is loaded. When I was diagnosed, the word suddenly became bigger than me – or became all of me – as though every fiber of my being was cancer. 'Hello, my name is cancer'. Even 'I have cancer' implies that I was consumed with the disease. After the initial shock of the diagnosis with all of its emotional reactions of fear, anxiety, anger – I felt the need to mobilize my resources in order to halt the immensity

of the word. The initial emotional associations were necessary to stimulate movement and action. 'Basic survival is now an issue'. After I had made the decisions of treatment and doctors, schedules and arrangements, it was then time to reduce the immensity of the word 'cancer' and put it into perspective of who I really am, where I really come from and the development of faith in my body's amazing capacity to resolve its imbalance. This doesn't happen overnight – it is an ongoing and gradual process. I believe that all people eventually find their own unique path through this process. (T. Schneider, unpublished Random Thoughts)

It is natural for one of the first responses to such news to be 'why?' – why me, why this, why now, why whatever? The intellect can occupy itself with such questions seemingly endlessly. A healthy individual will eventually let go of the need to have concrete answers to these questions, to the extent that past actions cannot be reversed. A more difficult assignment is to find a way to let go of judgments and pain for a cancer caused by smoking, environmental factors or one with a strong genetic component. This may respond to a discussion over time regarding these feelings and relevant education regarding causality. In other cases, it may require more direct intervention from a skilled counselor.

This 'Why —?' response is an activity of the ego which is looking for a reason so that it can gain control over the situation, even if this results in feelings of self-blame or guilt. It can also be part of a victim stance, where one perceives oneself to have no sense of power. If a person persistently approaches an illness in this fashion, it likely to frame how they approach their treatment as something that is being done to them, over which they have no control.

Assuming one has learned some or all of the lessons the situation may offer, letting go of the 'Why —?' can be a healthy, active and forward-looking choice. Patiently helping a patient move to this place of 'meaning making' can be both taxing and rewarding. It is, however, an important task for cancer patients and their families[15–19].

The 'Why —?' brings up a deeper reality of life, which may be that 'We don't have control anyway', at least not over the big issues in life and especially not over life and death. In hospice settings, it is quite common for clients to verbalize a desire to end their lives, yet relatively few do so. Clinical experience related personally to the author by hospice staff has shown that, when questioned later on in their course, often when close to death, almost all report that they are very glad they did not commit suicide. This may be because of additional time and closeness with family and friends, the ability to achieve some closure with important events and people in their lives, or personal evolution.

Viewed from a spiritual perspective, it may be more important to honor the question than to deify the answer, because there usually is no answer. We honor the question by stating that the unknown is part of life – as the following story shared by a friend of Howard's illustrates:

A Native American medicine man traveled to Hawaii for a conference. As he got settled into his lodgings, there was a knock at the door. Several men dressed in native garb asked if he was such-and-such, a Native American medicine man. When he responded he was, they indicated they were students of a native healer on the island, a great Kahuna. He had sent them to ask the medicine man to come to visit him on a matter of considerable importance. In such matters of the spirit, one has no choice, so the medicine man allowed the students to blindfold him and they got in a car and drove a long distance. As he emerged from the car, he was guided along a narrow trail and eventually into a cave where his blindfold was removed. After walking a short distance, the narrow cave opened into a very large natural room inside the mountain. There were many people there and it was a place that had been inhabited for a very long time. The Kahuna came forward and greeted him warmly. He pointed to a rectangular pool of water deep enough for a person to swim in with well-worn steps carved into the stone leading down to the water. The water was not still as one might suppose – rather there were waves lapping back and forth in the pool. The Kahuna explained that his people have been puzzled for centuries as to why there were waves in this water. He inquired of the medicine man – 'Do you know why?' The medicine man looked closely at the pool. There was no visible inlet or connection with the ocean outside. He could see no physical explanation for the waves. He shifted his attention inside himself to

225

meditate for a moment on the Kahuna's question. He replied that he did not know why the waves were there — only that they were very important. The Kahuna grinned widely, embraced him and motioned to him. They both took off their clothes, descended the steps and sat together in the pool and were cleansed and blessed.

Entering the realm of cancer diagnosis and treatment is like being Alice in Wonderland:

'I wonder if I've been changed in the night. Let me think: was I the same when I got up this morning? I almost think I can remember feeling a little different. But if I'm not the same, the next question is 'Who in the world am I?' Ah, that's the great puzzle!' [20]

There are a number of time-tested tools which can help patients through the transition from 'Why——?' to 'So what…'. One technique that requires relatively little expense or time is meditation. There are a growing number of centers which teach meditation and mindfulness practice. Turning one's focus temporarily from outward to inward can yield valuable and actionable insights. Over time, these can fuel the rebuilding of one's life in a way more suitably adapted for the challenges and opportunities at hand.

A simple, powerful and often challenging exercise to address some of these issues is to use meditation or other techniques to achieve a state of relative stillness of the mind and then:

(1) Carefully consider the things that you are losing as a result of the cancer (this is usually very easy). Pick the three that are the most significant for you.

(2) For each of these three losses, imagine what the gain could be. This is difficult until you are able to peer past the pain to the possibilities.

LOSS OF CONTROL

In the early stages of cancer diagnosis and treatment, almost all semblances of a normal life and control are lost. Urgent surgery changes the body landscape. The treatment itself may cause severe effects including physical debilitation, mood swings, fuzzy cognition and a lack of faith. It is like being a boxer who is knocked down and cannot get up. Sometimes it can even be somewhat comical:

The second MRI (Miraculous Reverberating Images) was ordered after I complained to my oncologist about continuous pain in my spine which had not shown up on bone scans. My understanding is that bone scans can be a crude but initial investigation concerning the appearance of tumors.

Luckily, I got in on a cancellation that afternoon. I was already used to the place and lying down on gurneys in windowless rooms where they do the most bizarre and unnatural things. The last visit was my CT scan where radioactive iodine is shot through your veins while you hold your breath. This is after a 4-hour fast of food and liquid and drinking two quarts of 'contrast' — which is coconut flavored radioactive iodine. The iodine that comes through the I-V feels hot and cold at the same time and then there is a sensation that you are peeing in your pants but you probably are not, as you are going in and out of the hole part of a large donut-shaped tube.

Being that my previous MRI was a little like being in a whirlpool with a consistent but tolerable noise, I was unprepared for this one. The set-up was the regular routine but this time the technician handed me a set of earplugs that are connected with a thin cord. I naively assumed that this was some sort of cordless earplug as part of a music system so that I can listen to music during the procedure. But noOOooo. I found out soon enough that it was to be a small protection to my eardrums in the midst of the tremendous and obnoxious noise I was about to hear. Even with loud noise that machines of various kinds can generate, there is most often to be found some sort of rhythm – a contrast in dynamics, beat and loudness. I often hear my IVs during treatment put out a rhythm in 9/8 time, and I can hear drums in my imaginary ears, sometimes I even start quietly singing. But the monotonous pounding of this MRI procedure offered nothing of the sort. This would be a quick and creative challenge of psychological survival and so I found myself getting through this procedure with cartoon-like picture frames. This is what I envisioned during the procedure.

I was placed on a gurney with some lightweight frames that smashed my nose down to assist me in remaining perfectly still. Then off goes the technician to his isolation room of control panels and pictures, and the procedure begins. Soon, the noise starts and these little earplugs, although a kind gesture, do little to mask what I am about to hear. Let's start with a submarine starting to surface when a big bomb explodes in the middle of it and now the emergency fire alarm goes off while people are attempting to evacuate. Ongoing, without missing a second, comes the overwhelming and constant pounding of the signal: Bong-Bong-Bong, etc., etc., etc. These are actually cordless alarms that are set into each mate's ears, including mine. It feels like it will never end, but it does, as it segues into a 1952 Japanese horror film sound track at maximum theater volume. This film is about giant locusts that are taking over the world (and our ears), and mass producing at accelerated rates and it is soon to be the end of the

human race and my auditory nerve endings … when I arrive in the middle of Manhattan to witness and hear a 38-foot woodpecker going to town on an 85-story steel frame and cement building in the middle of the financial district. This woodpecker is determined…. and has endless energy and strength but the building is stubborn and not a piece of rubble has given way as he goes on and on and on and on. As soon as I escape this scene, it's onto the heavy metal rock band with an electric guitarist who is at full volume playing only one single string on his guitar, accompanied by his drummer who hammers one single, solid block of steel in unison with the same rhythmless pounding as the guitarist. The nature of the noise changes in 'quality' but not in loudness and we move to a flock of Canadian geese flying directly overhead, honking and farting in unison at the same monotonous beat with small megaphones turned to full volume attached to their beaks and butts. Imagine this all…but magnify the sound by at least one hundred times… and that may give you a small taste of what this sounds like.

After this array of frames in my mind, and the sheer torture of pounding and squealing, the action stops momentarily and I hear the voice of the technician over the loudspeaker saying, 'Glkald alke mhl khgga; rmiunwi nege hselmlalmsw.' Oh boy I am thinking, I am done! But noOOOoo, he comes in makes a little adjustment, tells me I have only about 10 minutes to go and returns to the isolation booth. Godzilla Woodpecker returns again, along with the Heavy Metal Single String and Block Band, followed by another set of geese and their attached megaphones. All of this changes slightly and comes to a crescendo as I have the auditory sensation of being an ant in a toilet bowl filling with water. The noise stops. And again, the

227

announcement from the technician over the loudspeaker, 'Mefoioid, hesk ka'. He comes out and lifts the equipment off my face and tells me I am finished. At last.

A few moments later, while I am retrieving items from my locker (metal things I had to take off for the scan), I meet the technician outside of the locker room and we are conversing, when I drop my bra – prosthesis-side up on the floor between us. He doesn't seem to notice, but I suspect that, in an ancient society, this could have been considered some type of peace offering or sacrifice. Actually this whole ordeal did start almost 6 years ago with the sacrifice of one of my breasts, but at this point, that time feels like a very distant past.

Although we can complain a lot about this strange technology that so threatens our feeling or being the organic living beings we truly are, it's the best they've got for now. I don't ever want to feel ungrateful for the information it gives my doctors in monitoring the progression, or better yet, the regression of my cancer.

And so it goes, from therapeutic baths, prayer, candlelight, breathing and meditation to the world of technology and machines. In the middle of it, may we find balance, acceptance, humor and peace with it all, MRI included. (T. Schneider, unpublished Random Thoughts)

More so than any other disease, the harsh treatments with cancer are not experienced as a natural or gentle 'organic' process. It is a shock to the body, emotions, mind and spirit and an individual can respond with a fight-or-flight response to the medicine, which can feel like an assault of sorts. Consider the language: 'lost the battle with cancer' or 'war on cancer', etc. It is all about competition and opposition.

A sense of personal locus of control seems to be subverted by the fact that cancer patients must expose themselves to potentially toxic treatments. How can we find a balance where the words 'healing' and 'fight' can fit in the same space at the same time?[21]

My naturopath and others often remind me that we are all terminal, and all have the same and definite destination – death. This is so true. However, we are not all dying and being killed at the same time. I don't want to think that way but at times I do. I'm only human. On the good days, and one of them is my treatment day because I'm getting the infusion and don't feel the side-effects from the chemo right away, I can actually move myself into gratefulness and acceptance of the medicine which I am receiving. It's far from perfect, but it's better than it used to be, and it's all they've got this month. There is a great direction now in cancer research and they are really on to some things. But it takes time and one hope is that I am buying time going through these treatments to get to something less toxic in my treatment plan. It takes time.

Today I was thinking about my journey. Every week, my body is being completely poisoned, it is weakened and challenged. I am in a type of dying state. And what I have noticed happening is that my soul becomes predominant. The ego is too confused and obliterated to dominate, and the usual ways of maneuvering through life no longer work. I am given a glimpse at what I could be if I were to practice being in this state – to live, really live – through my soul's eyes. (T. Schneider, unpublished Random Thoughts)

People deal with a perceived loss of control in their own way, and at their own pace. It may take years for cancer survivors to recover and see that the process of having cancer was an opportunity for deep self-discovery. Certainly in the early days following diagnosis, such a suggestion would probably be unwelcome. However, one method of beginning to cope with the challenge of toxic treatments is to go into a place of stillness, which is like a type of sacred space. The stillness is most often imposed by the disease and/or toxic treatments such as chemotherapy or radiation. These create a physiological state of physical and cognitive disability. One who attempts to function at 'business as usual' may now find it frustrating and overwhelming. Merely accepting a decrease in physical and intellectual activity and coming to a place of rest is the first step toward stillness. The ultimate state of stillness arrives when the patient comes to accept his/her condition and value and validate rest as one of the paths to healing. One simple and ancient technique for moving into this state is the slow, deep and rhythmical breathing commonly utilized in meditation or yoga. Here is a simple technique advanced by Dr Andrew Weil[22]:

- Sit up, with your back straight (eventually you'll be able to do this exercise in any position).

- Place your tongue against the ridge of tissue just behind your upper front teeth and keep it there throughout the exercise.

- Exhale completely through your mouth, making a whoosh sound.

- Close your mouth and inhale quietly through your nose to a mental count of four.

- Hold your breath for a count of seven.

- Exhale completely through your mouth, making a whoosh sound to a count of eight.

- Repeat this cycle three more times for a total of four breaths.

- Try to do this breathing exercise at least twice a day. You can repeat the whole sequence as often as you wish, but don't do it more than four breaths at one time for the first month of practice. (This exercise is fairly intense and has a profound effect on the nervous system – more is neither necessary nor better for you.)

Becoming deeply aware of a loss of control may bring about an opportunity to let go of ego-oriented goals and activities and be in the arena of a holy or sacred time and space:

> *Through illness or oppression, since we cannot go outward or control the circumstances, we are restricted. Going inward is infinite, full of life and light. I do not find strength by overcoming my outward or physical affliction, but rather from sinking inward, by letting go to a place of peace and calm that exists within each of us. (T. Schneider, unpublished Random Thoughts)*

So, paradoxically, one may gain a locus of control by relinquishing control over outcomes. One may gain control through the active realization that it can not be given away without the fact that control is in our possession. The ultimate in control becomes a deep letting go of outcomes on multiple levels. This helps to nurture the fruits of the spirit – faith, hope and trust. It also may help those dealing with cancer to begin the process of seeing their illness as an opportunity for spiritual exploration and growth as well as reorganizing life's priorities.

SEARCH FOR MEANING

Once one because familiar and comfortable with a place of stillness and egoless connectedness, the search for meaning can emerge. This is a highly individualized issue and not everybody who finds meaning follows this path. For some, however, it may be as simple as an opening to being connected with family, with nature, or with a supportive community. For others, this may be a rough time and involve considerable wrestling within oneself. This internal wrestling has been described as far back as the Old Testament[23], where we read:

25 Jacob was left alone. And a man wrestled with him until the break of dawn. 26 When he saw that he had not prevailed against him, he wrenched Jacob's hip at its socket, so that the socket of his hip was strained as he wrestled with him. 27 Then he said, 'Let me go, for dawn is breaking.' But he answered, 'I will not let you go, unless you bless me.' 28 Said the other, 'What is your name?' He replied, 'Jacob.' 29 Said he, 'Your name shall no longer be Jacob, but Israel, for you have wrestled with beings divine and human, and have prevailed.' 30 Jacob asked, 'Pray tell me your name.' But he said, 'You must not ask my name!' And he took leave of him there. 31 So Jacob named the place Peniel, meaning, 'I have seen a divine being face to face, yet my life has been preserved.'

In this moving passage, Jacob's persistence in wrestling with his angel opens a new chapter in his life and, more importantly, in the life of his people. After this incident, he walks differently in the world – with a noticeable limp. Some might call this limp a disability or a tragedy, but for him it was the living remnant of an encounter with the divine.

This choice to continue wrestling is an essential opening and stimulus of the search for meaning and the search for a new identity in the world. Victor Frankel, noted psychiatrist and survivor of the Auschwitz concentration camp, put it this way: 'The last freedom is choosing your attitude.'

In moving through the process of living with cancer, the patient has the choice to 'switch sets' so that the disease becomes less about life and death, and more about giving and receiving. Cancer patients may be forced to receive in order to be able to heal physically. For example, cancer treatments make you sick, weak and more debilitated, and place you in a very vulnerable position. Within a close-knit family and/or community, most people want very much to aid the ailing person. It may take a variety of forms such as preparing food, running errands or just sitting with the person. It may be one's social instinct not to accept such help, as it would ordinarily be a sign of weakness. One of the opportunities is to allow the people around you to give. Thus receiving becomes as great a gift as giving.

On a deeper level, by receiving from the people around you, you can slowly learn to let go of your deep attachment to a reality based on life and death of the physical body, and thus facilitate forces that may be beyond our awareness as agents of healing for all that are involved in the process. For those who are giving, it allows them to drop the 'wall' they protect themselves behind. They reveal a side that you might not otherwise have access to – it is the side of their own spirit and heart, maybe due to the fact that they feel no threat from the person who is sick, or what they represent. That 'giving person' gets an opportunity to become better acquainted with their own heart and soul.

Physicians and other health professionals must always recognize the vulnerability of their patients. There may be some who are more open to receiving help than others. This is not a reflection of their worth as providers, but more a reflection of the patient's current status. Healthcare providers might also benefit enormously from being able to give beyond their technical abilities – to give an appropriate piece of their heart and spirit. Caregivers and health-care professionals nurture the search for meaning simply by supporting and validating the patient's choices. Ultimately it is their journey and search for meaning – no matter how incomprehensible it may be. This requires that the caregiver become a witness, sometimes giving feedback in a supportive role. It is really so simple that it is difficult for an intervention-focused mind to grasp this concept.

Sometimes receiving and the search for meaning can come from unexpected sources. The process can even go beyond our waking consciousness and come from those who are no longer physically with us.

My mother's blessing

My mother passed away about a year ago in a peaceful, progressive way. She was at Coronado House in Phoenix, a resident hospice facility. I hesitate to call it a facility because it was much too warm and full of love and tenderness for that term. The staff who worked there had one very important quality in common. They were not afraid of death and respected the process of it.

After my mother passed away, I had a difficult time feeling her presence. This has not been true with other people I have loved and been close to. Their essence was very much accessible. But not my mom. I believe that she had not yet made a complete transition to the other side that goes far enough over for souls to come back and guide and visit us. The people that we have loved who pass on drop all the human ego and material pitfalls and become wholly the true spirit of who they were while on earth. This is my belief.

One night I had my first dream in which my mother appeared and it was vivid. I dreamt that I was in a building and entered a room with lockers that were old and broken. The room looked like it had been deserted and was congested with a mess of papers and notebooks. The lockers looked like they had been slammed shut to hold in mounds of disorganized papers that were sticking out. I felt overwhelmed being there and left the room. As I walked out, I saw my mother quietly entering the room next door. This room was completely empty except for a simple reclining chair. My mother

recognized me but said nothing. I came closer to her and noticed that her skin was beautifully smooth and translucent. And around her face was an intricately painted trellis with lilacs. The top of the trellis lay on her forehead covered slightly with greenery and the lilacs were falling gracefully around her temples. I commented to her about how beautiful her skin looked and how unusual it was for her to have her face painted. She seemed to acknowledge me but, again, she said nothing.

Two days later, I was having a manicure and I suddenly realized that the first anniversary of my mother's death (known as 'yartzeit' in the Jewish tradition) had been two days earlier. I don't know why this was a catalyst because my mom and I rarely have manicures. Maybe it was the nurturing care that the manicurist had when she worked with my hands and I was sitting still for a change. Afterward, I went home and lit my mother's candle, and then I remembered that the dream had been on the night of her yartzeit two days earlier. I was touched that my mother would remind me of this milestone in this beautiful and symbolic way.

A couple of weeks later came Kol Nidre, the culmination of the Jewish New Year observances. I had received chemotherapy a few days earlier but planned to sing that evening for the service. It was not easy, physically, and I struggled to pay close attention to the order of the service. Despite my physical discomfort, I was able to use my voice with clarity and because of the toxic state of my body, I suppose much of my ego was out of the way. During the service, I had a distinct memory and connection to my childhood days in synagogue and felt many times like I was standing in the lobby of the building. The rabbi and cantor from those days were there in the rabbi's study preparing for the service and I had a fresh feeling like I often did in that spot especially in the season of fall in the Midwest. It was an eerie feeling but a positive one. Maybe that is why we light the yartzeit candles, or maybe we evoke those who have passed on when we honor their memories.

That evening I came home and lit the yartziet candles for my mom and dad and rebbe David Wolfe-Blank. After my husband and children went to bed that night, I lay down on the couch by the light of the candles. I looked out of the skylight toward the sky and the branches of giant cedars. I began to relax and breath in a deep, slow and rhythmical way and I could 'see' my parents and the rabbi and cantor, as well as my grandparents and they were all quietly looking at me. We all looked at each other for what seemed a very long time. And then my mother put the trellis with the lilacs on my head and I started to cry. I was honored because I knew I had been blessed at that moment by my mother, and all who were with her were witnesses.

I don't want to take this image for granted as it is the help I need to make my life holy. This was given to me by my mother with an immense amount of love from her and those with her. When love and blessing are simply received, fear and disbelief are removed and these, the root of almost all of our problems, disappear. More than that, it reminds us of who we really are and where we came from. (T. Schneider, unpublished Random Thoughts)

OPPORTUNITY TO MOVE FROM DOING TO BEING

How do you do? What do you do? In Western culture, there is no room or value to being ill. In order to be a successful part of society, you have to be productive. When you are ill, this is no longer a viable option. Some may force themselves to go beyond their ability to continue to do. Some may avoid or deny overt signs of disease in order to continue with business as usual. This may be a necessity of their life circumstances. Ultimately, however, there is an opportunity to begin to shift from a focus on 'doing' to a focus on 'being'. This may be one outcome of the search for meaning. For people who have an active spiritual life, this can afford them a wonderful opportunity further to deepen and develop their spirit. For those who have lived so far with little active spirituality in their lives, learning the value of being may be difficult. For example, strategies used successfully in the past involving mastery and/or control may simply not work when many things are beyond your control, including even the basic functions of your physical body.

As a cancer patient, when you are getting treatments, the majority of your life may be focused on receiving the necessary treatments. The realm of 'being' is one place where you can go to experience the inner resolve that is needed to move not only through it, but beyond it. The state of 'being' may be seen as the result of stillness, or vice versa. It is a choice, not a given on the part of the patient. Not everyone makes this choice. Their comfort level may remain in 'doing', even though it may be extremely difficult. Often, 'doing' is synonymous with 'living' and having a purpose in life. A patient may feel that if they stop 'doing', they are 'giving up'. The state of 'being' may offer something deeper – a place where one can experience, even in some small way, the interconnectedness with all living things and with 'the God force' and move beyond the realm of simple survival. This can be accomplished through the simple breathing exercise outlined above, meditation, yoga or simple quiet contemplation, but it can and must be approached in a fashion that suits the individual.

Some report achieving this state while exercising or gardening or taking a walk in the woods.

This poem, from T. Schneider, unpublished Random Thoughts, also reflects that stillness:

Old soul of memories past

look out onto the immensity of the edge of this continent
feel the surge and listen to the power of the waves.
They move in rhythm to the breath of God.
I am surrounded by ages old dead tree trunks and limbs
cradled and bathed clean in the mineral bath of the ocean
and yet they still exist.
Only the ground of the earth can offer them stillness
if they have been tossed far enough from the rush of the waves
anxious to pull them in.

For most if not all busy clinicians, 'being' is a luxury distanced by the pressures to 'do'. Yet it remains possible to achieve a significant measure of stillness in various ways. For example, you can experiment with a couple of breaths between patients, while washing your hands or preparing for a procedure. With practice, this becomes easier and feels more natural. Mindfulness training is another method[24] to expand one's capacity to bring this into even the busiest of days. In doing so, clinicians open themselves to become rebalanced, renewed and focused, even if just for a moment.

CONNECTEDNESS

Part of the experience of cancer for many people is a forced separation from body parts, from a sense of self-wholeness, and from friends, family members and often even health-care providers who may be uncomfortable with the illness. There is no way to communicate verbally how it feels to be on the firing line for one's own health. For those who do manage to find a way to break through this veil, the connections can be amazing. One can begin to focus in on those people and activities which bring light, life and connection into their lives. The other extreme is to become increasingly disconnected, which may be expressed in some self-destructive ways such as refusal of treatment or substance abuse. In some cases, this may also be associated with deterioration of relationships to family and community. These conditions should be recognized and further explored and treated following appropriate medical evaluation.

Consider the following:

How can simply feeling more connected with self and with other people lead to better health? While the exact mechanisms are still not entirely clear, some research supports this conclusion.

Women with cancer participating in support groups live longer than those without such groups; divorced and widowed people (especially men) in their twenties and thirties have much higher risk of dying than married persons of the same age; marital conflict has negative effects on the immune system; there's a link between the death of a spouse and impairment of immune function; social isolation is a major risk factor for mortality from widely varying causes and conversely social support mitigates against the harmful effects of stressful life events.[25]

By enlarging the 'frame' of our perspective, we may create an opening to see ourselves in the context of a much greater whole. We can also see that all of life exists in that way and that much of our purpose in life has to do with blending our own individuality and purpose harmoniously with this whole. This realization may foster a greater sense of inner peace through helping the person who is ill feel less isolated.

The hydrangea lady

'I know a place where dreams are born and time is never planned. It's not on any chart, you can feel it in your heart, Never Never Land…' from Peter Pan

A couple of weeks after my mother's blessing, I was leaving our town market through the floral section as I often do. It was autumn and the reality of the season was fully present. The air was cold and crisp, leaves turning color; a waning sun was low on the horizon – living things going dormant. When I look back, it's likely that the season affected my mood which was becoming dark and increasingly negative. I had hit the wall with the chemo. It had been a year of treatment every week, and I found myself fighting the enticement of being sucked into the vortex of doubt and fear.

The dried hydrangeas in the floral section caught my eye and I wanted to buy only one to place in a little hanging copper pot near our back door. As I was looking for one choice flower, a woman appeared with her shopping cart and commented on the hydrangea. We started talking about flowers and our gardens. She had a lovely, subtle Irish brogue and she was older than me, 60-ish. As we were speaking, I began to see her as a wise crone and a mother earth figure.

The woman asked the price of the hydrangea that I now held in my hand. I told her that it was $5. 'Oh no', she insisted, 'Don't pay that, it's much too expensive'. I was indefinite and she kept going on about how ridiculous that price was and don't pay it, and then went on to tell me that she had

beautiful hydrangeas in her yard, lots of them, and she would give me a bouquet. At first, I resisted. Like many chemo patients, doing anything out of the ordinary takes tremendous effort, especially when it involves social interaction. But after a while, I sensed something else going on. I knew she recognized the scarf I had tied around my head as a sign of my treatments although she didn't say a word about it. More than that, what I felt that she truly recognized was the deeply entrenched, struggling path on which I was traveling. I was moving on a path toward a higher spiritual understanding and awareness, and the pace had accelerated since my recurrence.

It felt as though we were talking in some symbolic language, but within and underneath the words, another sort of communication was taking place. Our mouths were moving and words were coming out of them about flowers and prices, but as we were blabbing about the price, flowers, whatever, I found myself being pulled back with a sort of panoramic view of the two of us in this place. We were transporting ourselves into a deeper realm. She was taking a short cut, going for it, the real deal place and that is where we connected in what seemed like an instant. This is a place of meeting that is mutually understood between human beings and you can only go there together if you give each other an invisible ticket to go inside.

So here we are in the deeper realm – in the midst of our mouths moving while we are simultaneously in the galaxy somewhere, observing ourselves. I suggested that we trade phone numbers. I sensed that she was too respectful to invade my privacy or ask my willingness for future interactions, and so I said to myself 'Ok, let's take a step in that direction'. We traded phone numbers and I agreed to come to her house for the bouquet.

Coming to her house was a part of the agreement. Before we parted that evening, she hugged me and said, several times 'Everything is going to be alright'. Her name was June.

In the darkness of the following evening, I drove to June's house. The sun was setting early now, there was no moon in the sky and it had been raining all day. I turned off the main road onto a long, narrow gravel driveway going downhill to find her house. The driveway was lined with overgrown, luscious green ferns, plants and trees, interspersed sparsely with houses. It had stopped raining by this time and the plants were glistening under a shimmering darkness. I wasn't quite sure where I was going, when I heard a voice and saw a flashlight guiding me down to her house.

It was a modest house near the water with healthy, thriving plants in pots in front. June met me and there, waiting for me, was the beautiful bouquet of flowers that she had prepared for me. The flowers were fresh and luscious like the earth on which I was standing at that moment. The bouquet consisted of about a half dozen plum and green colored hydrangeas interspersed with an equal amount of long stemmed white roses. It was exquisite.

I asked her about the white roses as it would be highly unusual for roses to still be blooming in November in the Northwest. She told me that a friend had given her a bouquet of the white roses and she wanted to give me some of them '…because you know, white roses are a sign of good things to come.' And then, she quickly went into her house and returned with a small unopened card that said 'Little Miracles'. She asked me to open it and inside it said, 'How simple it is to see that we can only be happy now and that

there will never be a time when it is not now.' Again, she hugged me and said that everything was going to be alright.

We agreed to meet again sometime for tea. And she emphasized that she would always be there for me any time that I may need anything. As I drove away with my lovely bouquet, I was overwhelmed with gratefulness for the course of these events and for the synchronistic meeting with June. The meeting, and now the flowers, helped me to regain faith and a sense of comfort. I do have to admit that I regressed momentarily to doubt – thinking that June may be a member of same strange cult that was recruiting and converting people to their fundamentalist religious sect and I looked like a vulnerable candidate. But I quickly came back to recognizing the blessing of this course of events.

When I came home that evening, I put the perfectly arranged flowers in a crystal vase on a table near our front window. About a week later, the flowers dried naturally. I placed the white rose petals in a basket near my bed to use in my salt baths. The hydrangeas dried maintaining their color, matching the plum color of our music room. Whenever I catch a glimpse of these flowers, I am reminded of June, and the fact that she must be an earth angel sent to help me in my healing process. I will call on her when I need help. That is her intent and mine. I'd like to think that this connection is also to remind me that 'On earth as in heaven.' We don't have to wait for miracles; we need only to recognize them. (T. Schneider, unpublished Random Thoughts)

One gift of the spirit, and perhaps of cancer, is to create the possibility of dissolving boundaries and beliefs which may be limiting. Even if physical cure is not realistic, another kind of healing flows from this type of connectedness. In this story, June took on the role as a silent witness with a great sense of compassion, as discussed earlier. It was a spontaneous meeting but one that could be viewed as a manifestation of Toby's intention to ask for help, all on a subconscious level. Intention is an important element in healing and seeking healers around us. Caregivers may help the patient define their intentions and reinforce them simply by talking about it and validating the power of their intentions in the form of ritual, prayer, affirmations, pictures, whatever may be the custom of the patient. One cannot predictably force these things to happen by doing something. By cultivating and practicing a state of receptivity and stillness, it is our experience that the chances are increased. Furthermore, when something remarkable does occur, you are more likely to take notice.

THE SACREDNESS OF HEALING

For many clinicians, their work with patients is like a chess game. If this happens, then you make that move. Clinicians have, by and large, lost their connection to the sacred and mysterious nature of healing work. Doctors can 'fix' many things on a physical level which might be thought of as 'curing'. 'Healing' is something more. A healer may cure the physical problem while also mobilizing inner and outer resources, teaching the participants about their place in the universe and imbuing meaning into the experience of illness. In doing so, recurrence may be more frequently prevented and the healer will often experience their own well-being as enhanced.

This is not to knock science, which has given birth to many significant and effective therapies. One major challenge for clinicians, particularly providers of integrative oncology services, is how to retain an active connection to the sacred nature of healing and thereby infuse their daily work with meaning and purpose.

Sacredness and medicine

I had my third chemo treatment of Taxotere today along with a pre-med of steroids to counteract the allergic reaction that it can cause. This came with a side order of Zometa, a bone strengthener to replenish the places that the tumor cells are eating, and Herceptin. Herceptin is a relatively newly approved genetic drug to rid my body of the Her2Nu gene that resides in some of these cells and creates more receptors on the cancer cells to glom onto weak cells and pull them in to join the tumor.

Okay, so this is my situation, as I understand it medically. But as I soaked in my bath of seaweed, lavender, rosemary and salts in silence this evening, I began to think about healing, herbs, prayer and the above mentioned drugs and to make peace with it all. How do the drugs fit into healing? How do they work with the alternative supplements and practices that I am developing for myself?

I began to ponder about indigenous people and the time before western medicine… the time before we poisoned our bodies to cure illness. Now that our health is being challenged with a physical environment of toxins in the air, water and food, all vital to our existence and stresses by living so unnaturally, being robbed of our body's natural rhythm and flow – I wonder how powerful herbs, water cures and other alternative treatments could really be. After all, cancer is an industrial strength illness. Wouldn't it take industrial strength measures to get it under control?

Tonight I re-read some writings and journaling I've been doing. The context is about revelations coming from experiences in my life and their deeper meanings or metaphors. These were mostly inspired by living with cancer and the perspective that it has given me. The writings are not about cancer, but about life and simple parts of it. It's not that I didn't have the awareness before, it's just that I didn't take the time to reflect upon these issues, and dig them out of my soul. I cried at times re-reading some of these writings this evening. I was crying because I found myself believing what I wrote. I have to say that I mostly didn't believe it after I wrote them.

While soaking in my herbal bath, I began to more truly believe that medicine of any kind will be as effective as our belief system about it. Also, that it is absolutely essential that it is received with gratefulness and with blessing. It is that sacredness which is the grace and stimulus that truly penetrates our physical and spiritual being so that we may heal.

In ancient cultures, the herbs or tinctures to address the body itself were a stimulant to healing. But around the ingestion or dressing of herbs of the earth into or onto the body, was a ritual, and a mindfulness about receiving it. The other earth elements of fire, air or water were also applied. These older cultures were so tight and the belief so clear and shared by the tribe, that the treatments were more easily absorbed by the person being treated, or tended to. This is not to say that all was perfect. I would imagine that there were also superstitions and fears of the unknown. However, are we so much more advanced on this level? Today, we maintain superstitions and fears – but without a communally held belief system. We do not trust our bodies' miraculous ability to heal over and over again. We have abandoned our own healing power and the faith that

acknowledges that God holds us in his Hand at all times and is The Healer.

Tonight, as I soaked in my bath, I put a bag of herbs on my heart and held it there. I welcomed the Taxotere into my body to do its work. I took no supplements so that it could do its own work. I will begin my supplements in a few days. After all, the Taxotere is now in there, moving and entering cancerous and healthy cells. So it is now a part of me. (T. Schneider, unpublished Random Thoughts)

Most clinicians would hardly report experiencing the sacred during their busy hectic workday. However this potential is there even in the busiest of times. Consider Howard's experience on rounds one day:

Rushing as usual to meet up with my resident and interns for morning rounds, I raced off the elevator frustrated by the delay getting to the top floor. Out of the corner of my eye I caught a glimpse of a couple walking down the hallway leading to one of the oncology units. A young woman was moving slowly accompanied by her husband who was walking both her and her IV pole. He had placed an arm around her waist and seemed endlessly patient and loving as they floated down the hall. This moment was so tender, I felt I could cry. I stood for all of two or three seconds taking in the tenderness of this scene and it felt like an eternity passed. I raced off to meet my team, strangely renewed and refreshed.

This capacity for noting the moment and experiencing awe is inherent in all of us, if we can shift our attention long enough to recognize it. What do we mean by 'awe'? Abraham Joshua Heschel once defined awe as an 'intuition for the creaturely dignity of all things and their preciousness to God.'[26] The capacity for awe, or sensing the 'dignity of all things' can be cultivated through practice and nurtured within a supportive community. Rachel Naomi Remen, a pioneer in this work, offers a number of group experiences to deepen this capacity[27] and there are a number of retreat programs throughout the country which offer similar trainings[28].

FAITH – HOPE – TRUST

Figure 10.4 depicts one way of thinking about the relationship between Faith, Hope and Trust surrounded by a permeable cloud of love which connects and supports them all. The opposite of any one direction gives that direction a groundedness. That is, it gives that direction an ability to exist and to be fully experienced by the individual.

> *Without Hope, there is no future*
> *Without Trust, there is no present*
> *Without Faith, there is no past*

The graphic also depicts the 'ever present now' as being the conduit. It is only by moving from 'doing' to 'being' in the 'ever present now' that one can come to a point where there is harmony and balance between these qualities. Let us consider each of them separately for now.

Faith

Faith can be defined as a confidence in purpose or outcome. It is the belief that all is for the good, and includes an acceptance of the mystery of life and the purpose of existence. It is what Tarzan feels when he lets go of the vine he is swinging on, just before he catches the next one. The type of faith we are talking about does not come from a mental place, but instead, is a gift of the spirit. It can be focused on many things, including faith in science and/or in the doctors and nurses who minister to them. It is truly letting go and putting yourself in the hands of God or whatever force/source of love and blessing you believe in. True faith requires a deep spiritual inner connectedness and is the bedrock that is needed to dig

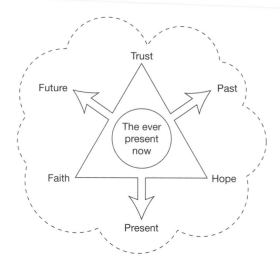

Figure 10.4   The Relationship of Faith, Hope and Trust

into when times are tough. People can be hard on themselves when they do not feel this 100% of the time. For example, people may question themselves by asking 'If I have faith, how can I have so much fear?' That is the point – it is easy to have faith when everything is great, but it is when you go through 'the valley of the shadow of death'[29] that you somehow remain connected to Faith in spite of and along with the fear, anxiety and doubt. This is where trust comes in.

> *When you have come to the edge of all the*
> *light you know*
> *And are about to step off into the darkness*
> *of the unknown*
> *FAITH is knowing one of two things will*
> *happen:*
> *There will be something solid to stand on,*
> *Or you will be taught how to fly.[30]*

Trust

The Merriam-Webster online dictionary[1] defines trust as 'assured reliance on the character, ability, strength, or truth of someone or something.' Functionally, trust is defined as a letting go of control and of the ego. The experience of illness is an opportunity to go to a different place. This is sometimes associated with the hero's journey, so well described by Joseph Campbell[31,32] – and consisting of three phases. These are (1) separation; (2) initiation and transformation; and (3) the return. During each of these phases, a great deal of trust is necessary to sustain the transition. Without this 'assured reliance', nobody would be able to continue to move through the transition to achieve the final result. It may be uncomfortable and fearful, but the only place to go is forward toward the final stage of transformation.

Hope

The Merriam-Webster online dictionary[1] offers the following definition for hope: 'to desire with expectation of obtainment.' Hope can incorporate an active component – it may include moving out of total 'being' and back into a more active mode. However, 'fulfillment' can mean many things to different people working with cancer and is certainly not the same thing as 'cure'. Hope is thus quite elastic, and may be focused on any number of human desires, including cure, relief of pain, being able to be more fully in the moment, healing, etc. Part of the art of medicine is understanding what an appropriate focus for hope is at various stages of illness and gently guiding the patient and family in that direction. In the early stages of illness, hope is often focused on cure, but this may become a dysfunctional focus should the underlying condition deteriorate significantly. In the final stages of life, it may be more appropriate for the focus of hope to be on dignity, meaning, connection, acceptance and inner peace. Of these, acceptance is perhaps the most difficult to come by.

CONCLUSION

We leave you with these writings (T. Schneider, unpublished Random Thoughts) as gifts on your journey of healing:

The healing journey

We call it a journey because it is one. It is as though one packs her/his bags with only the essential things and goes on a trip. As we move through the journey, we often dispose of many things along the way so as to lighten our load. We discover that the things we dispose of are things, things that have been unnecessary for a very long time, and will not serve a purpose in our new location.

The journey is not unlike a vacation. We may fly somewhere on an airplane to get far away, but once we are there, we move step by step throughout each day. We are sightseeing, observing and discovering new things, intellectually and esthetically. The longer we stay in this different place, the more comfortable we feel in our new surroundings. And, if we are especially open, we find ourselves moving toward scenery we had not planned on seeing but are drawn to, until, finally, the scenery does the planning and becomes the guide.

On the Healing Journey, you cannot possibly take anyone with you. You can send postcards, you can make phone calls, but it is yours alone to make the trek, step by step. Ironically, you are not alone and in some sort of abstract way, there is love and beauty all around you to give support and confidence to your steps. This is pure energy. It is the energy from which we come. It is given to us by a greater power and through those who love us. As our bodies require more rest and sleep from our illness or treatments which are causing great reorganization, another process is taking place and that is one of pure energy, pure light in the midst of whatever our human frailties and emotions may suck us into.

The pinball machine of life

And so something I've been thinking about for a while is how all of our lives are like one big pinball machine. We are launched out onto the big board, forced out with a spring lever. And then we start bumping around all over the place. Some balls gracefully go from one bumper to another, some are jaggedly moving, some bouncing on the same damn bumper over and over— but they get more points that way, and it's less work. Sometimes those bumpers light up and make a lot of noise (I think those guys get a lot of points too) and the difficult-to-get-to-ones get the most points. Sometimes if we force the whole machine around, that ball might last a little longer and get a few more points. If it goes a total straight line, it's gonna' go down that hole right away but most balls zig-zag up and down and right and left and diagonal when the people operating the ball have determination and enthusiasm.

One thing for sure is that the ball is going down that hole at the bottom no matter what. And that is life. Our destiny is going down that hole (or whole as the case may be). But in this life, maybe we are going up that hole – or maybe it isn't a hole at all. But we will find out when we get there.

RECOMMENDATIONS

Clinicians should address spirituality-related issues in patients, families, staff and self. This may include:

- Finding meaning;

- Personal and group support;

- Personal transformation;

- End-of-life transition;

- Supportive care during conventional therapy.

Further research on the role of spirituality in cancer care is necessary, especially research focused on the optimal methods of intervention. This may include:

- Role of prayer;

- Role of various modalities such as small group retreats, meditation, religious participation;

- Methods for doctor–patient communication.

- Methods of spirituality as preventive therapy for burnout of providers, or family members of cancer patients.

There is currently one clinical trial sponsored by the National Center for Complementary and Alternative Medicine which was scheduled to conclude in June of 2004. This study aims to determine whether religiosity and spirituality are related to immune functioning, as measured by interleukin-6 blood plasma level, among terminally ill cancer patients[33]. Please refer to the energy medicine section for a list of several other clinical trials investigating some aspects associated with spirituality.

RESOURCES

National Cancer Institute – Spirituality in Cancer Care PDQ
http://www.cancer.gov/cancertopics/pdq/supportive care/spirituality/patient

References

1. www.merriam-webster.com/netdict.htm

2. Chopra D. Timeless mind, ageless body. Noetic Sci Rev 1993; Winter: 17–21

3. Jung CG. Psychological Types. London: Routledge and Kegan Paul, 1923: 82

4. Levine EG, Targ E. Spiritual correlates of functional well-being in women with breast cancer. Integr Cancer Ther 2002; 1: 166–74

5. Murray SA, Kendall M, Boyd K, Worth A, Benton TF. Exploring the spiritual needs of people dying of lung cancer or heart failure: a prospective qualitative interview study of patients and their carers. Palliat Med 2004; 18: 39–45

6. Tatsumura Y, Maskarinec G, Shumay DM, Kakai H. Religious and spiritual resources, CAM, and conventional treatment in the lives of cancer patients. Altern Ther Health Med 2003; 9: 64–71

7. Schnoll RA, Harlow LL, Brower L. Spirituality, demographic and disease factors, and adjustment to cancer. Cancer Pract 2000; 8: 298–304

8. Halstead MT, Hull M. Struggling with paradoxes: the process of spiritual development in women with cancer. Oncol Nurs Forum 2001; 28: 1534–44

9. Patterson SG, Davis C, Schmitzer J, et al. Spiritual dimensions of cancer care. J Cancer Integrat Med 2004; 2: 85

10. Seeman TE, Dubin LF, Seeman M. Religiosity/spirituality and health. A critical review of the evidence for biological pathways. Am Psychol 2003; 58: 53–63

11. Sephton SE, Koopman C, Schaal M, et al. Spiritual expression and immune status in women with metastatic breast cancer: an exploratory study. Breast J 2001; 7: 345–53

12. Powell LH, Shahabi L, Thoresen CE. Religion and spirituality. Linkages to physical health. Am Psychol 2003; 58: 36–52

13. www.aafp.org/fpr/990700fr/2.html

14. Maugans TA. The SPIRITual history. Arch Fam Med 1996; 5: 11–16

15. McGrath P. Reflections on serious illness as spiritual journey by survivors of haematological malignancies. Eur J Cancer Care (Engl) 2004; 13: 227–37

16. Samson A, Zerter B. The experience of spirituality in the psycho-social adaptation of cancer survivors. J Pastoral Care Counsel 2003; 57: 329–43

17. Ferrell BR, Smith SL, Juarez G, Melancon C. Meaning of illness and spirituality in ovarian cancer survivors. Oncol Nurs Forum 2003; 30: 249–57

18. Gall TL, Cornblat MW. Breast cancer survivors give voice: a qualitative analysis of spiritual factors in long-term adjustment. Psychooncology 2002; 11: 524–35

19. Efficace F, Marrone R. Spiritual issues and quality of life assessment in cancer care. Death Stud 2002; 26: 743–56

20. Carroll L. 'Alice' from Alice's Adventure's in Wonderland. New York: Penguin Putnam, Ch 2, 28

21. Rossman ML. Fighting for health. Adv Mind – body Med 2003, 19: 6

22. www.drweil.com/u/QA/QA3677/

23. Genesis 32: 24–31. The Bible

24. Kabat-Zinn J. Wherever You Go, There You Are: Mindfulness Meditation in Everyday Life. New York: Hyperion, 1994

25. Hammerschlag CA, Silverman MD. Healing Ceremonies: Creating Personal Rituals for Spiritual, Emotional, Physical and Mental Health. New York: Perigee, 1997: 14

26. Heschel AJ. God in Search of Man. New York: Farrar, Sraus and Giroux, 1955: 75

27. www.commonweal.org/ishi/

28. www.manystreamsheal.org/, http://healingin-medicine.org/

29. Psalm 23. The Bible

30. www.patrickoverton.com/poster.html

31. Campbell J. The Hero's Journey. Joseph Campbell on His Life and Work. New York: Harper & Row, 1990

32. Campbell J. The Hero's Journey. Video cassette (VHS), Wellspring Media (3/21/2000)

33. http://clinicaltrials.gov/show/NCT00066924

10h

Alternative medical systems

Lawrence Berk

> 'For centuries knowledge meant proven knowledge—proven either by the power of the intellect or by the evidence of the senses. Wisdom and intellectual integrity demanded that one must desist from unproven utterances and minimize, even in thought, the gap between speculation and established knowledge. The proving power of the intellect or the senses was questioned by the skeptics more than two thousand years ago; but they were browbeaten into confusion by the glory of Newtonian physics. Einstein's results again turned the tables and now very few philosophers or scientists still think that scientific knowledge is, or can be, proven knowledge. But few realize that with this the whole classical structure of intellectual values falls in ruins and has to be replaced: one cannot simply water down the ideal of proving truth—as some empiricists do—to the ideal of 'probable truth' or—as some sociologists of knowledge do—to 'truth by changing consensus.' – Imre Lakatos[1]

INTRODUCTION

There are a significant number of alternative medical systems that have developed over thousands of years. Today, some remain in place in the indigenous populations in which they were developed. As a part of integrative oncology, information will be presented on how these systems work and how they address cancer. There is no attempt to present an individualized treatment recommendation using the tenets of that system as the basis for care. The majority of recommendations for alternative medical systems' use contained in the other sections of this text will include aspects of care that are a small part of the system in which they arose. It is also worthwhile to note that the general philosophy of some alternative medical systems are more in line with the 'healing oriented' philosophy of integrative oncology than the 'cure oriented' tenets typically associated with Western biomedicine.

Alternative medical systems are complete medical treatment systems based upon non-modern Western traditions. Modern Western medicine (sometimes called allopathic medicine or conventional medicine) is exemplified by the core curriculum focusing on anatomic and physiologic investigations as they apply to the clinical treatment of patients[2]. The selection of what is relevant and useful is arbitrary, based upon the biases of the medical education community[3]. Before Western physicians can understand other medical systems, it is helpful for them to recognize the philosophy underlying Western medicine. Many Western physicians envision Western medicine as the only 'scientific' medical system. Unfortunately, there is no accepted definition of 'scientific'. The meaning the Western physician and researcher perhaps have in mind is that Western medicine is inductive, based on hard facts and research. This, then, suggests that alternative medical systems are deductive, basing treatments on speculative theory rather than observation. Some alternative systems, such as ayurvedic medicine, claim divine origin. Others, including Traditional Chinese Medicine (TCM) and homeopathic medicine, claim a scientific basis. All three of these systems claim to be based on clinically proven data.

The basic principles of Western medicine are highly reductionist, whereas most alternative medical systems begin from a more holistic foundation. A reductionist system is one that holds that the sum of the system is no more than its parts[4]. In Western medicine this is a reflection of the influence of Newtonian mechanics. At the heart of Newtonian mechanics is the hypothesis that if the properties of all bodies are defined, then all future events are predictable. That is, the entire system is completely defined by the properties of the simplest components. The same principle is used in Western medicine. A complex system, such as the human body, can be explained by studying ever-smaller parts of the body. Initially the smallest parts studied were the cell, and thus this is called the Cell Theory, but now the studies are at levels down to and beyond the gene level.

The Cell Theory was developed in the mid-1800s and it has been a very successful research paradigm. Its earliest and most complete success has been in the utilization of the Germ Theory, a subset of the Cell Theory, for the classification and treatment of infectious disease. It is still the basis for studying infectious disease[5]. Many of the functions of the human body have been adequately described from Cell Theory analyses, such as the function of the kidney for excretion and the contraction of a muscle under electrical stimulation. Other aspects of human function, such as consciousness, have not yielded to the Cell Theory approach[6]. The same approach has been used to treat cancer. The current emphasis on genome research to cure cancer is the ultimate reflection of this approach[7]. So far, Cell Theory-based research has had limited success in oncology[8].

One principal weakness of the reductionist approach is in the assumption that the information gained from studying a simplified system is directly related to how the complex system functions. This exposes the philosophical basis of Western medicine, that the sum of the parts is equal to the whole. Preclinical research in Western medicine is often carried out without the recognition of this bias. The bias may be seen in the design and implementation of research. For example, a common model in cancer research is the nude mouse. This is an immunosuppressed mouse that has a human tumor implanted in its leg. Treatments are then tested using this system. It is assumed that this represents the growth of human cancer cells. What is not considered is how to reintegrate any data obtained in this model back into a human system[9]. From the reductionist vantage, holistic or emergent (non-reductionist) aspects are often dismissed as errors or a lack of understanding of the basic components. However, holistic concepts are needed to explain the functioning of the cell and the body. For example, there is nothing in the first principles of DNA to explain why certain proteins are formed. It is only when the two- and three-dimensional structures of intact DNA are analyzed that the patterns dictating protein fabrication are seen. Even then, there is no insight into the purpose and function of these proteins until the three-dimensional structure of the protein and, in the case of enzymes, the interacting molecules are known. Thus, although the pattern of research is to go to ever-smaller nodes of investigation, understanding progresses as higher-order, more holistic, patterns are discerned.

Many alternative medical systems take a different approach. They start with holistic patterns and then develop the underlying mechanism of action. They focus on the whole and worry less about the parts. There is often an extensive underlying physiology and anatomy. A common mistake is to assume that there is a direct analogy between Western terms and the alternative systems' scientific terminology. Rather, in TCM and ayurvedic medicine anatomic terms are the patterns of holistic thought interpreted through the reality of the body. Thus, the functions of the liver in TCM are only indirectly related to the Western functioning of the liver. This is not due to any Chinese anatomic ignorance. Rather, this is due to a difference in semantics. Although the word is the same, the implications are different.

Western physicians may believe that only Western medicine is scientific. In fact, most of Western medicine is based on the results of the trial-and-error method. The basis for evidence-based clinical decisions is the clinical trial[10]. Western medicine routinely tests to determine whether a proposed treatment is efficacious. It does not (in the best case) accept that a treatment will work on the basis of first principles. The same rationale underlies the practice of alternative medical systems. Treatments in Western medicine tend to approach the determination of appropriate treatments from analyses of disease-based clinical trials. The individual patient is purposefully subjugated to an impersonal amalgam within statistics. Alternative systems use the individual patient as the experimental system and base determinations of diagnoses and treatments on the patient's symptoms and signs and response to treatment. In Western medicine, the population is the level of experimentation. In alternative systems, the individual is the level of experimentation.

This chapter will give brief introductions to three widely practiced alternative medical systems: ayurvedic medicine, homeopathy and TCM. Adequate introduction to any one of these requires a book in itself, and several such books are referenced in the bibliography. The goal of this chapter is to give the general philosophical backgrounds of these traditions, and introduce how they approach cancer.

PHILOSOPHICAL AND RESEARCH BACKGROUND

Traditional Chinese Medicine

Physiology

TCM has a history extending over more than two millennia. It is a holistic system, focusing on the whole functioning of the body rather than the parts. In TCM no single part of the body can be studied in isolation.

The first theory underlying the physiology of the body in TCM is the elements. Whereas traditional Western medicine (Galenic and Hippocratic) is based on four elements (fire, water, air and earth), TCM is based on five elements: fire, water, earth, metal and wood. These five elements interact in specific ways. Water stimulates wood, wood stimulates fire, fire stimulates earth, earth stimulates metal and metal stimulates water. Further, water inhibits fire, wood inhibits earth, fire inhibits metal, earth inhibits water and metal inhibits wood. These relationships underlie the balance of nature, including those of health and illness.

Qi (Chi) is the vital energy that courses through the body. It is a physical compound and subject to physical laws. The majority of the Qi is derived from digested nutrients. Some of the Qi, the original Qi, is inherited from the parents. Yang Qi is the warming force within the body. External Qi (wei Qi) is the defensive layer of the surface of the body against external pathogens.

The second system undelying TCM physiology is the theory of opposites, Yang and Yin. Yang represents hot, rising and changing. Yin represents cold, falling and stability. Although things are classified as Yang or Yin, all things have both Yin and Yang. Thus, although, as described later, the kidney is a Yin organ, there is both Yin and Yang in the kidney. Kidney Yang would also have Yin and Yang aspects, and this dichotomy continues on indefinitely.

These physical systems are represented in the body by Chinese anatomy. Chinese anatomy is not a parallel of Western anatomy, although many of the same terms are used. The use of common terminology should not be mistaken for common meanings. The organs in TCM represent systemic aspects of the body. They are physiologic rather than anatomic. There are five zhang and five fu organs. Zhang organs are active and create or transform needed nutrients. This is a Yin function. Fu organs store the nutrients – a Yang function. The zhang organs are the liver, lung, heart, spleen and kidneys. The fu organs are the small intestine, the large intestine, the gallbladder, the stomach and the bladder. The zhang organs have an associated fu organ. For example, the large bowel is the fu organ of the lung. The organs have associated elements and the interactions between the organs tend to reflect the interactions between the elements.

There is a sixth fu organ, the Triple Burner (San Jiao). It has no corollary in Western medicine. It controls the physiologic activities of Qi within the body.

In addition to the zhang and fu organs there are the miscellaneous organs, the brain, bones, bone marrow, uterus, blood vessels and gallbladder (the gallbladder is both a fu organ and a miscellaneous organ).

The organs and the surface of the body are all interconnected through channels that carry the Qi around the body. These are the meridians, most well known for their role in acupuncture. The interference of flow through the meridians can be a cause of disease. Acupuncture is one way of stimulating flow.

There are four compounds that give life to the body. These are essence, Qi, blood and the various bodily fluids. Essence is the fundamental source of energy in the body. There is congenital essence that is inherited from the parents, and acquired essence that is obtained by conversion of food by the zhang organs. Both are stored in the kidney.

Qi is formed from essence and innervates the body. There are many types of Qi and these are stored in different locations and have different functions. For example, defensive Qi (wei Qi) circulates on the outside tissues of the body, below the skin, and protects against exogenous pathogenic factors. In general, Qi promotes growth of the body, supplies energy to the organs and protects the body against disease.

Blood is more than just the blood as defined in Western medicine, although it is associated with the red blood in the vessels. The san jiao converts essence into blood. The blood is stored in the liver. The blood nourishes the organs and supplies moisture to the organs. It is also the source of mental activities such as consciousness.

The body fluids are fluids such as the gastric and intestinal juices, saliva, tears and urine. These fluids are extracted from food and drink by the organs. The fluids moisten the various organs and tissues and also supply nutrition.

Disease

Pathogenesis Disease occurs when the body is out of balance. Many factors can contribute to this. There are two aspects in the development of a disease: the pathogenic factor and the the body's resistance due to its pathogenic Qi. It is the latter that determines the progress of the disease. If the antipathogenic Qi is strong, then the pathogenic factor (for example hot wind) will not have the ability to penetrate into the body and cause disease.

Once a pathogenic factor has penetrated the outer defenses it causes an imbalance of the physiologic factors of the body: the Yin and the Yang, the strength of the various Qis and blood and tissues, and the flow of the Qi through the meridians. This manifests with the various signs and symptoms of the Chinese disease syndromes.

Diagnosis   Diagnosis of disease in TCM uses the four methods of diagnosis to determine the underlying pathology and the needed correction. The four methods of diagnoses are looking, listening and smelling, feeling the three pulses and palpation.

The patient is first inspected for changes in the patient's mood and activity, any changes in his skin color and his appearance. The tongue's color and texture are important signs of the patient's underlying problems.

The physician listens to the patient's breathing, the sound of his voice (raspy, strong, breathless, etc.), the sound of a cough, etc. At the same time he notes any smells.

An important aspect of diagnosis is talking with the patient to assess his history and his current symptoms. This includes the time course of the illness and changes in the symptoms. The body is then palpated for abnormal masses, and the pulse is monitored. The distal radius pulse of the left hand is measured. There are three pulses which are simultaneously measured by three fingers along the radial artery. The forefinger is closest to the wrist. Each finger on each wrist measures a different organ system. The organs are reversed (right and left) for women and men. The feeling of the pulse is described in terms of its depth, frequency, rhythm, strength, smoothness and amplitude (reference 11, p. 215).

There is no standard approach to the defining of the underlying pathology. Symptoms are classified according to various pathogenic systems. As outlined by Liu[11], these include:

- The Eight Guiding Principles;

- The state of Qi and the blood;

- The theory of the zhang–fu organs;

- The theory of the Six Channels;

- The general theory of the channels;

- The theory of the wei, Qi, ying and xue system;

- The theory of the Triple Burner;

- The etiology of disease.

The Eight Guiding Principles are the pairs of extremes: Yin and Yang, interior and exterior, cold and heat, deficiency and excess.

The state of Qi and the blood is important for the treatment of cancer, which will be described later. The blood and the Qi represent the energy and nutritional state of the body.

The zhang–fu organs have been described. Each organ has a different function and different relationships with the other organs and bodily systems.

The Six Channels are the six main meridians connecting the zhang–fu organs. They are paired on each side of the body.

The wei, Qi, ying and xue system is a late addition to TCM, from the early Qing Dynasty (1644–1911). Wei is the external Qi defensive system, and is the first defense against external pathogens, such as pathogenic wind or heat. The Qi system is the deeper Qi system and represents effects of internal pathogenic factors. Attacks on the ying systems are attacks on the nutrient system (akin to ami in ayurvedic medicine). Attacks on the blood system are classified under xue.

The theory of the Triple Burner (San Jiao) also arose during the Qing Dynasty. It is useful for analyzing infectious diseases. Infectious disease arises from damp heat in one of the three parts of the Triple Burner: the upper, middle and lower parts.

The channel system supplements the Six Channels. The channels connect the zhang–fu organs and the interior of the body to the exterior. Impairment of the channels may be reflected in localized physical symptoms, such as pain or swelling.

The etiology of disease is also important. Porkert describes several agents of disease[12]. There are six climatic excesses: wind, cold, summer heat, humidity, dryness and glare (or fire). He identifies seven emotions that can cause disease: pleasure, wrath, anxiety, reflection, sorrow, fear and fright. Further agents of disease include unwholesome diet, excessive body stress and sexual excesses.

The disease is the imbalance in these various systems of the body. It may be a deficiency of Qi in one of the zhang organs, or a deficiency or excess of Yang, or excessive cold or heat. It can be a combination of different problems. Treating the disease requires the appropriate diagnosis and then choosing the appropriate remedy. The treatment will dependent on the present symptoms and the current state of the disease. The same underlying pathology will be treated differently depending on what the symptoms are and how advanced the disease is. Similarly, different diseases may be treated in the same way if the symptoms suggest analogous imbalances.

Treatment 'The ancient sages combined these various treatments for the purpose of cure, and each patient received the treatment that was most fitting for him. The treatments were so extraordinary and so different in each case that all diseases were healed. Thus the circumstances and needs of each disease were ascertained and the principle of the art of healing became known' (Yellow Emperor[13], Section 12, p. 148).

Once the patient has been examined and the problem diagnosed, a treatment must be chosen. The armamentarium of the TCM physician includes diet, herbs, acupuncture and moxibustion, among many other treatments.

Diet and herbs are used to repair the imbalances. For example, the physician recommends foods that are cooling for diseases of excessive heat, or heating foods for lack of heat. Similarly,

herbs are chosen for their ability to repair the problem. Some herbs can supply missing Qi to the deficient organ. Others strengthen the vital Qi or the blood. Some are cooling or heating. The herbs or herbal mixtures are chosen from the Chinese Medicine Materia Medica.

Acupuncture and moxibustion restore the normal flow of energy through the meridians and throughout the body. Acupuncture is the use of needles inserted intradermally at specific active points around the body. Moxibustion uses burning moxa on specific locations on the skin. Moxa is considered pure Yang and useful in conditions of cold because it is heating.

Traditional Chinese Medicine and cancer Cancer does not have a direct translation in TCM. However, there is a long history of treating swellings and ulcers. In one of the earliest TCM texts, *The Yellow Emperor's Classic of Internal Medicine*, various forms of tumor are discussed. The ancient medical dictionaries discuss both zhong and liu. Zhong are swellings whereas liu are tumors. Among other terms are yan (rock), jun (figus), sheng (substantial mass) and ji (localized mass) (reference 14, p. 1).

Zhang[14] describes eight principles currently used in the treatment of tumors:

(1) Regulating the Qi and harmonizing blood;

(2) Maintaining the unobstructed flow of the channels and collaterals;

(3) Transforming phlegm and eliminating dampness;

(4) Softening the hard and dissolving nodulation;

(5) Dissolving toxins and stopping pain;

(6) Tonifying Qi and cultivating blood;

(7) Invigorating the spleen and pacifying the stomach;

(8) Replenishing and tonifying the liver and kidneys.

How are these accomplished? The most important treatments are choosing the appropriate herbal medicines. According to Li, 'Many types of solid cancerous tumors are due to Qi stagnation and Blood stasis and can therefore be treated according to the principle of regulating Qi, invigorating the Blood and transforming Blood stasis'[15]. Surgery, chemotherapy and radiation therapy will further damage vital Qi. Because blood is derived from Qi and Qi is transformed into blood, both Qi and blood need to be supported. This lack of Qi and blood manifests as dizziness, shortness of breath, anergy, pale complexion and spontaneous sweating[15].

Acupuncture and moxibustion can also be employed. Moxibustion is useful to add warmth and break up hard nodules. It also supports vital Qi. Acupuncture can be used to support vital Qi and stimulate the spleen and kidneys.

Acupuncture is also used in conjunction with standard Western therapies. For example, the United States' National Cancer Institute concluded that sufficient evidence exists to recommend acupuncture for the treatment of nausea[16]. The use of acupuncture and TCM for cancer care is discussed in Chapter 12.

Ayurvedic medicine

The origin of ayurvedic medicine is said to be the great sages of the traditional writings of India. These writings, the vedas, are held to be several millennia old. The two classic texts of Ayurvedic medicine are the *Charaka Samhita*, reportedly from 760 BCE and the *Sushrata Samhita* from 666 BCE. Neither of the original texts are extant. They are known from commentaries on these texts, the earliest from 200 CE.

Pathogenesis

Ayurvedic medicine has a complex cosmology. It is too detailed to present in this summary. An excellent presentation is given by Ninivaggi[17].

The bases of ayurvedic medicine are the three doshas. The doshas are often considered analogous to the Hippocratic medical humors. However, the humors are physical. The doshas are a higher level of existence, both energetic and physical. The doshas are composed of the five elements (air, fire, water, earth and space or ether).

The three doshas are vata, pitta and kapha. Vata represents motion. Pitta represents change. Pitta is involved in the transformation of food into nutrients and energy. Kapha represents stability and solidity. The doshas can be viewed as representing potential energy (pitta), kinetic energy (vata) and a moderating energy (kapha). The Sanskrit term dosha is derived from the same base as the Western prefix 'dys' (reference 18, p. 73). This suggests that the doshas can be considered to be constantly out of balance and the source of disease. Almost anything can tend to put the body out of balance. Diurnal variations, seasonal changes, food, emotions and many other things can act to lead to imbalances.

When the body is out of balance, the normal digestive process is disrupted. Foods are converted to useful energy and nutrients by the internal digestive fire, the agni. When the body is in balance, there is complete or near complete conversion of the nutrients. If the doshas are not in balance, improperly digested food, ama, is formed and distributed into the tissues. Excess corrupted doshas then accumulate in the tissues, causing disease.

The pathogenesis of disease has six stages. Using the format of Singh, the first is sacaya. This is the accumulation of excessive dosha in the associated organ of the dosha. These are the small intestine for pitta, the colon for vata and the stomach for kapha.

If this imbalance is not corrected, then the accumulated dosha becomes corrupted or vitiated (prakopa). These vitiated doshas can spread (prasara). The vitiate doshas can then become fixed in other tissues (sthana sansraya). There the vitiated doshas grow and the disease becomes manifest (vyakti). These local manifestations can then spread and become widespread disease and complications (bheda).

Diagnosis

Disease is best treated with prevention. Symptomatic disease is often too advanced to be curable. Because it is so common for the there to be ama and dosha accumulation, regular removal of the toxins is needed. Daily purification techniques are incorporated into daily customs (svasthavritta). Purifications are also performed to remove the toxins from the three organs affected by vitiated doshas – the stomach, spleen and small intestine.

To diagnose the disease, the physician combines his learned knowledge, his examination and his ability to combine the two to reach the appropriate conclusion.

The examination of the patient is classically described as having ten parts. These are: to study the body constitution, the natural combination of the patient's doshas; to define the current doshic imbalances; to assess the tissue quality; to evaluate the body conformation; to measure the body proportions; to determine the patient's ability to respond to changes in diet and to herbs; to assess the mental state; to evaluate the strength of the agni (the digestive fire); to evaluate the patient's energy level; and to determine the functional age of the patient.

These can be determined using the Eightfold Examination. This includes evaluation of the pulse, tongue, eye, skin, voice, general appearance, urine and feces.

Once all of the information is gathered, the diagnosis is made. Then the appropriate treatments can be instituted.

Treatment of disease

The treatment of disease in ayurvedic medicine includes lifestyle changes and herbal medications. Panchakarma are the interventions performed to remove the vitiated doshas from the tissues. Early disease is still limited in distribution and so milder treatments can be used. More advanced disease may only be able to be palliated and more vigorous treatments are needed. The milder interventions can be started by the patient to prevent disease or treat mild problems. More advanced treatments need to be given by a trained ayurvedic physician.

There are two types of treatments: strengthening (brimhana) and detoxifying (langhana). Bimhana is used when the body is weak. This is often the result of vata disease. This approach uses rich diets and stimulating herbs. Oils and fat are taken internally by mouth or through enemas (snehana therapy). Kapha diseases (see the section on cancer, below) are exacerbated by brimhana therapy. Detoxifying therapies are designed to remove the damaged doshas from the organs and tissues. Methods include herbs that stimulate the agni and therefore improve the digestive process, fasting, yoga and sweating (swedana).

For more serious illness, a trained ayurvedic physician treats with radical purification techniques (panchakarma). The five methods used are vomiting (vamana), purgatives (virecana), herbal enemas (basti), oil enemas (sneha) and nasal treaments (nasya) (reference 19, p. 32). The intranasal and intrarectal instillations of oils are often used. The oils can be animal fats, ghee (clarified butter) or vegetable fats.

Cancer treatment

Ayurvedic medicine, as in TCM, has no direct correspondence between classical diseases and the Western medical definition of cancer. The orientation of ayurvedic medicine both encompasses and expands upon the Western approach. In Western medicine cancer starts in the tissues and then spreads (metastasizes). This is a late, and often incurable, state in ayurvedic medicine. The earliest stages are changes that occur prior to the localization in the tissues. It is these pre-symptomatic changes that are curable.

Singh reviewed the ayurvedic approach to the treatment of cancer. The earliest change which goes on to become cancer is the abnormal accumulation of doshas in their related organs. Cancer results from the accumulation of kapha. As the vitiated doshas spread, the patient will experience problems including swelling, edema and obstruction (reference 17, p. 139). The solidifying effect of kapha has the psychological manifestation of depression and slowing.

Treatment is designed to alleviate the excess accumulation of kapha. Effective kapha-relieving measures include removing obstructions in the channels in the body. Sweating and oleation help soften the hardened tissues. The goal is to drive the toxins internally and then use purgatives and enemas to flush the toxins from the system. Once the system is purified then the agni is strengthened to insure that digestion remains healthy.

Ayurvedic medicine is not as commonly used by patients as TCM. However, some ayurvedic herbs have shown *in vitro* anticancer activity. The collection of herbs was based on potential anti-kapha activity. Many of these agents showed cytostatic activity[20].

Homeopathic medicine

Introduction

Homeopathy does not have as complete a scientific scheme as either ayurvedic or Traditional Chinese Medicine. Rather, it is more an empirical approach to treatment, in which drugs are tested and entered into a materia medica. The pathophysiology of the treatments is not addressed.

Homeopathic medicine originates from the work of one physician, Samuel Hahnemann (1755–1843). Hahnemann disapproved of the harsh treatments of 18th century medicine. Through his investigations he arrived at the basis of his alternative medical system, the law of similiars. Hahnemann's law of similiars is that a medication that causes symptoms at full strength will cure those symptoms when given in diluted form. Thus, a drug that causes headaches when given at a high dose will cure headaches when given in very high dilutions (potentiations). Healthy volunteers partake in provings in which they take the medications at full dose and record their symptoms. The compilation of these provings generate the materia medica of homeopathy.

Another important concept of classical homeopathy is that the primary activity of medication is to increase the ability of the vital force within the body to heal itself. The ideal approach for a homeopathic treatment is to make the correct diagnosis and then give a single medication once. The correct diagnosis is based on the physical and mental symptoms of the patient. Diseases can be classified as acute or chronic. Acute diseases are treated according to the law of similiars.

However, some patients have continual recurrence of their acute symptoms or have symptoms that cannot be classified as acute. These patients have chronic disease. Hahnemann thought that all chronic diseases were secondary to one or more of three causes: the itch (psoric); syphilitic; and gonnorheal (sycotic). These disease states were called miasmas. Although Hahnemann's original pathogenesis for these miasmas may no longer be accepted, the susceptibilities they represent are still used. They represent emotion and physical archetypes that help to define the susceptibility to particular diseases and the appropriate treatment. All people, according to Hahnemann, are afflicted with the psoric miasms. This is the basis of chronic diseases. The treatment of chronic diseases therefore rests on curing the underlying miasma. Chronic diseases, in particular, often represent the end result of obscured problems that started in childhood.

The clinical research in support of homeopathy is ambivalent. Several analyses of available clinical trials have been published. The most widely quoted positive analysis is that of Linde *et al.*, published in *The Lancet* in 1997[21]. That analysis stated, 'The results of our meta-analysis are not compatible with the hypothesis that the clinical effects of homeopathy are completely due to placebo.' In a follow-up article in 1999 the same authors concluded, 'Since we completed our literature search in 1995, a considerable number of new homeopathy trials have been published, The fact that a number of the new high-quality trials...have negative results, and a recent update of our review for the most 'original' subtype of homeopathy (classical or individualized homeopathy), seem to confirm the finding that the more rigorous trials have less-promising results. It seems, therefore, likely that our meta-analysis at least overestimated the effects of homeopathic treatments'[22].

Cancer

Cancer is a chronic disease in the homeopathic system. The goal is the treatment of the underlying disease, not the manifest symptoms. One important aspect of classical homeopathy is that the treatment of the current symptoms does not affect a cure of the disease. In fact, treatment of these symptoms may exacerbate the disease. The appropriate treatment requires identification of the underlying disease. This may be an inherited disease or it may have been acquired early in childhood. The treatment may exacerbate the current symptoms or cause previous symptoms to recur. This is part of the cure of the deep disease.

J.T. Kent (1849–1916) was a classical homeopath of the early 20th century. He noted that by the time a malignant growth is discovered the disease is often too advanced to cure. One particular problem is that in this advanced state the original symptoms may not be discoverable. 'If the child's mental symptoms could be fully ascertained, and the symptoms from the childhood to the adult age, something might be done. Cancer generally comes on in after life, when childhood

actions have been forgotten.' He goes on to state, 'To cure any condition we must base the prescription on the totality of the signs and symptoms and not on the pathology. The cancer is the ultimate. The symptoms from the first are the outward image of the patient. If they have been suppressed or changed by drugs that are not homeopathic, there is nothing left for the homeopath to do and the surgeon can do no better. Palliation and prolonging life are not curing'[23]. If the disease is too advanced and the original signs and symptoms too suppressed, the homeopathic medications will not be effective. If the medications are effective, the current pathology will be suppressed and the original signs and symptoms will recur before they too are cured. 'When this is known, it will be easy to understand why old symptoms return, in chronic cases, after the administration of the similar remedy...' 'In patients with cancer or tuberculosis, we may be quite certain of their ultimate recovery, if old symptoms return after administration of the remedy. These patients seldom have the vital reaction strong enough to develop former symptoms, hence they are incurable'[23].

Not all modern homeopaths agree with this approach. Some recommend treatments designed to soften and alleviate the tumors. The approach is aimed at treating the current symptoms and signs.

A modern, classical homeopathic approach to cancer is presented by Master[24]. He agrees with Kent that patients with advanced cancer do not respond well to treatment. It is more effective to treat patients prophylactically. For example, he recommends treating patients with a strong family disposition but no current cancer and patients with precancerous lesions such as oral leukoplakia. Patients who have been treated with surgery, radiotherapy and/or chemotherapy with a complete response will also benefit from homeopathy. Two examples he gives are:

'A case of malignancy of the breast where the entire mass is removed, the scar has healed well, and there are no metastases detectable and no signs or symptoms.

A case of lymphoma where a complete remission has been obtained with radiotherapy and/or chemotherapy and there exist no ill-effects.'

For the side-effects of radiotherapy he recommends homeopathic preparations such as cadmium iodide, calcarea fluor and fluoric acid.

Master's book gives the cancer formularies of several homeopaths as well as his own. He reviews several case histories in which standard therapies are combined with homeopathic therapies. The results of the treatments are not given.

CONCLUSION

Alternative systems of medicine offer some effective tools for supportive care of cancer patients. However, cancer is generally seen as a late manifestation of underlying systemic problems, many of which are not considered treatable by the time that malignancy presents itself. Therefore, most alternative systems stress prevention, rather than treatment, of cancer.

RESOURCES FOR ALTERNATIVE MEDICINE SYSTEMS

Traditional Chinese Medicine

General introduction

Liu Yanchi. The Essential Book of Traditional Chinese Medicine, Vols 1 and 2. New York: Columbia University Press, 1988

Manfred Prokert. The Essentials of Chinese Diagnostics. Zurich: Chinease Medicine Publications, 1983

Traditional Chinese Medicine and cancer

Zhang Dai-Zhao. The Treatment of Cancer by Integrated Chinese–Western Medicine, trans. Zhang Ting-Liang and Bob Flaws. Boulder, CO: Blue Poppy Press, 1994

Ayurvedic medicine

General introduction

Frank John Ninivaggi. An Elementary Textbook of Ayurveda. Madison, CT: Psychosocial Press, 2001

Dominyk Wujastyk. The Roots of Ayurveda. London: Penguin Books, 1998

Ayurvedic medicine and cancer

Ram Harsh Singh. An assessment of the ayurvedic concept of cancer and a new paradigm of anticancer treatment in ayurveda. J Altern Complement Med 2002; 8: 609–14

Premalatha Balachandran, Rajgopal Govindarajan. Cancer – an ayurvedic perspective. Pharmacol Res 2005; 51: 19–30

Homeopathic medicine

General introduction

Dhawale ML. Principles and Practice of Homeopathy, 3rd edn. Bombay: Institute of Clinical Research, 2000

Homeopathy and cancer

Farokh J. Master. Tumours and Homeopathy. New Delhi: B Jain Publishers, 2002

References

1. Lakatos I. Falsification and the methodology of scientific research programmes. Lakatos I, Musgrave AE, eds. Criticism and the Growth of Knowledge. Cambridge, UK: Cambridge University Press, 1970: 91–196

2. Custers EJ, Cate OT. Medical students' attitudes towards and perception of the basic sciences: a comparison between students in the old and the new curriculum at the University Medical Center Utrecht, The Netherlands. Med Educ 2002; 36: 1142–50

3. Kemahli S, Dokmeci F, Palaoglu O, et al. How we derived a core curriculum: from institutional to national – Ankara University experience. Med Teach 2004; 26: 295–8

4. Elsasser WM. References on a Theory of Organisms: Holism in Biology. Baltimore, MD: The Johns Hopkins University Press, 1998

5. Ewald PW. Evolution of virulence. Infect Dis Clin North Am 2004; 18: 1–15

6. Hameroff S. Consciousness, the brain, and spacetime geometry. Ann NY Acad Sci 2001; 929: 74–104

7. Weir B, Zhao X, Meyerson M. Somatic alterations in the human cancer genome. Cancer Cell 2004; 6: 433–8

8. Toren A, Amariglio N, Rechavi G. Curable and non-curable malignancies: lessons from paediatric cancer. Med Oncol 1996; 13: 15–21

9. Berk LB. Reductionism and the failure of radiobiology. J Am Coll Radiol 2004; 1: 304–7

10. www.cebm.net/downloads/oxford_CEBM_Levels_5.rtf

11. Liu Y. The Essential Book of Traditional Chinese Medicine, vol 1: Theory. New York: Columbia University Press, 1988

12. Porkert M. The Essentials of Chinese Diagnositics. Zurich: Chinese Medicine Publications, 1983

13. The Yellow Emperor's Classic of Internal Medicine, trans. Veith I, new edn. Berkeley: University of California Press, 1972

14. Zhang D-Z. The Treatment of Cancer by Integrated Western–Chinese Medicine. Boulder, CO: Blue Poppy Press, 1989

15. Li P. Management of Cancer with Chinese Medicine. St Albans, UK: Donica Publishing, 2003

16. NIH Consensus Conference. Acupuncture. JAMA 1998; 280: 1518–24

17. Ninivaggi FJ. An Elementary Textbook of Aurveda. Madison, CT: Psychosocial Press, 2001

18. Svoboda R. Theory and practice of Ayurvedic medicine. In Van Alphen J, Aris, A, eds. Oriental Medicine: An Illustrated Guide to the Asian Arts of Healing. Boston: Shambhala, 1996

19. Jolly J. Indian Medicine, 3rd edn. New Delhi: Munshiram Manoharlal Publishers, 1994

20. Smit HF, Woerdenbag HJ, Singh RH, et al. Ayurvedic herbal drugs with possible cytostatic activity. J Ethnopharmacol 1995; 47: 75–84

21. Linde K, Clausius N, Ramirez G, et al. Are the clinical effects of homeopathy placebo effects? A meta-analysis of placebo-controlled trials. Lancet 1997; 350: 834–43

22. Linde K, Scholz M, Ramirez G, et al. Impact of study quality on outcome in placebo-controlled trials of homeopathy. J Clin Epidemiol 1999; 52: 631–6

23. Kent JT. Lesser Writings, 6: Why is Cancer Incurable? www.homeoint.org/books3/kentwrit/index.htm

24. Master FJ. Tumours and Homeopathy. New Dehli: B. Jain Publishers, 2002

11

Modalities – cancer prevention

PREVENTION – PRIMARY, SECONDARY, TERTIARY

Cancer prevention can be thought about as taking place on several levels. Primary prevention can be defined as the prevention of cancer in the general population. This could include individuals with a spectrum from normal to high risk for the disease, based upon family history, lifestyle practices and environmental exposures. Secondary prevention addresses individuals in whom precancerous changes have already been documented, e.g. a tobacco snuff dipper who has precancerous changes of leukoplakia. Tertiary prevention pertains to individuals who have already had a cancer diagnosis, received treatment with good results, and are interested in preventing recurrence of the disease or symptoms.

An integrative oncologist will be exposed to the full spectrum of prevention in daily practice – often all levels of prevention will be discussed during a single encounter with patients and family members. Prevention must be distinguished from early detection – both have significant importance. Any integrative plan for prevention should also take advantage of conventional screening modalities to pick up cancer at an early, treatable stage.

CANCER PREVENTION: POSSIBLE BIOLOGICAL MECHANISMS

There is no current 'magic bullet' approach that will prevent cancer. It is highly likely that multiple mechanisms of carcinogenesis exist that are embedded within an individual's specific background, including genetics, environmental exposures, lifestyle habits, current and past health status and the myriad of factors that can be included within the blanket term of 'psychosocial characterisitics'. This diversity has specific clinical implications in that it is more likely that a broad range of cancer preventive activities would have greater effect than an approach that relies on a single substance or modality[1–5]. Cessation of tobacco and alcohol consumption are two notable exceptions. The act of omitting these practices can have significant immediate health and preventive benefits (see Chapter 14).

In this section, we will discuss the effect of the various modalities concerning primary, secondary and tertiary prevention. We will also discuss the mechanisms of action by which the modality has its preventive effect.

References

1. Go VL, Wong DA, Wang Y, et al. Diet and cancer prevention: evidence-based medicine to genomic medicine. J Nutr 2004; 134: 3513S–6S

2. Heggie SJ, Wiseman MJ, Cannon GJ, et al. Defining the state of knowledge with respect to food, nutrition, physical activity, and the prevention of cancer. J Nutr 2003; 133 (Suppl 1): 3837S–42S

3. Key TJ, Schatzkin A, Willett WC, et al. Diet, nutrition and the prevention of cancer. Pub Health Nutr 2004; 7: 187–200

4. Zeegers MP, Kellen E, Buntinx F, van den Brandt PA. The association between smoking, beverage consumption, diet and bladder cancer: a systematic literature review. World J Urol 2004; 21: 392–401

5. Zochbauer-Muller S, Minna JD. The biology of lung cancer including potential clinical applications. Chest Surg Clin North Am 2000; 10: 691–708

11a

Physical activity

Robert B. Lutz

MECHANISMS OF ACTION FOR PREVENTIVE EFFECT

The biological mechanisms defining the relationship between physical activity and cancer prevention are an active area of hypothesis and research inquiry. However, many plausible explanations have been identified. It is likely that multiple mechanisms exist that demonstrate individual variability, based upon genetics, environment, cancer type and stage, and the form of physical activity performed.

IMMUNE FUNCTION

The effects of physical activity on the immune system have often been held as a primary link between physical activity and cancer, although it is believed that the majority of cancers are non-immunogenic[1]. Regular, moderate exercise and physical activity have been noted to affect a number of immune parameters, both quantitatively and functionally, to include: macrophages, natural killer cells (NK), cytotoxic T lymphocytes and lymphokine-activated killer cells (LAK)[2].

Aging-associated decreases in immune function (immune senescence) have been suggested as a possible explanation for the higher rates of cancer seen with increasing age. Conversely, regular physical activity has been noted to enhance T-cell function of elderly men and women[3]. Therefore, overall immune enhancement and slowing of immune senescence may represent the physical activity–immunity relationship.

STEROID SEX HORMONES

Steroid sex hormones are associated with the development of reproductive cancers in both women and men. Exercise affects these hormones in a variety of ways and it is believed that this relationship affects the development of these cancers.

Males

For men, it has been found that chronic endurance activities may decrease levels of testosterone, although this effect has not been reported consistently[4]. Epidemiological evidence generally supports an inverse relationship between physical activity and incidence of prostate cancer[5], although it has been noted that there is an inverse relationship between upper body mass and prostate cancer, possibly due to higher testosterone levels from increased muscularity[6]. An association has been identified between sedentary occupations and testicular cancer[7], whereas 15 or more hours of vigorous physical activity per week has been noted to decrease the risk of this cancer[8]. Concentrations of sex hormone binding globulin (SHBG) may be increased, thereby leading to depressed levels of free circulating testosterone.

Females

Likewise in women, SHBG levels may demonstrate a similar response to exercise. In premenopausal women, additional mechanisms may lead to decreases in circulating hormone levels (both estrogen and progesterone), and increased menstrual irregularities, a shortened luteal phase and increased anovulatory cycles[1]. Decreased hormone levels have also been identified in endurance-trained postmenopausal women that appear to be unrelated to body fat[9].

INSULIN, GLUCOSE AND INSULIN-LIKE GROWTH FACTOR

Elevations in insulin and insulin-like growth factor-I (IGF-I) have been associated with increased rates of many cancers[10]. IGF-I is down-regulated by increased synthesis of a binding protein (IGFBP-3) which is enhanced by physical activity. Decreased IGF-I may also lead to increases in SHBG, thereby leading to decreases in sex steroids. Finally, a strong relationship exists between physical activity and circulating levels of insulin and insulin sensitivity. This relationship may also be mediated through adiposity.

BODY COMPOSITION AND OBESITY

Obesity and fat distribution (central) have been associated with increased rates of many cancers. Abdominal fat, specifically visceral or intra-abdominal fat, is the most metabolically active fat store. This relationship is mediated through variations in hormone levels, to include sex steroid hormones, insulin and IGF-I. Physically active individuals are generally not obese and do not demonstrate central distribution of body fat[1]. Visceral fat is preferentially affected by aerobic exercise[11].

Calorie restriction has been demonstrated to have a protective effect with regards to cancer initiation[12]. Although compensatory mechanisms often exist for calorie expenditure from exercise, it is plausible that this relationship may exist to a degree in individuals who are physically active. This would suggest that, if a less fit individual burns more calories with the same level of activity than a more fit one, eating less may still be beneficial as a cancer-preventive activity for both.

MECHANICAL

It is generally noted that physical activity decreases bowel transit time, possibly mediated by increased vagal tone and increased peristalsis. This may lead to decreased exposure time of toxins within the bowel mucosa and inhibit promotion of carcinogenesis[13].

OXIDATIVE DAMAGE

Physical activity and exercise cause varying degrees of oxidative damage and generation of free radicals. Whereas moderate activity causes no to minimal damage in young and/or trained athletes[14], strenuous exercise may increase rates of oxidative stress[15]. Free radicals may adversely affect DNA and may stimulate mutagenesis and tumor proliferation[16]. Moderate physical activity and training effects may enhance the body's innate antioxidant system and scavenging of free radicals. Conversely, intense exercise may overwhelm the body's ability to manage oxidative stress, leading to increased oxidative damage.

CANCER AND SITE-SPECIFIC CANCERS

Research has provided data supporting a positive association between physical activity and overall cancer mortality and incidence with an apparent inverse dose–response relationship[17]. This has been noted for both occupational as well as leisure-time physical activity[18]. There are fewer data for women and those that exist suggest a weaker association. A meta-analysis has quantified an approximately 30% protective effect for physical activity for men, whereas no effect was identified for women[19].

GENERAL RECOMMENDATIONS FOR PRIMARY PREVENTION

The US Preventive Services Task Force recommends that health-care providers counsel all patients on performing regular physical activities appropriate for their current health status and personal lifestyle[20]. Physical activity can serve as 'first-line therapy and protection' against many chronic health conditions[21]. Physicians' recommendations have significant impact on health-related habits and yet counseling is often omitted, with time and lack of comfort with counseling often cited as reasons[22].

Current public health recommendations call for the accumulation of at least 30 minutes of moderate-intensity physical activity on most, preferably all, days of the week. This amount of activity would expend about 200 kcal/day, the equivalent of briskly walking 2 miles[23]. These emphasize that *daily* physical activity can be *accumulated* (8–10-minute periods), rather than achieved in a single episode, and accomplished by a simple activity such as walking briskly. These simple recommendations may be tailored to reflect an individual's unique situation, be it as a starting point for those who may not have been physically active in the past, but are now interested as a means for disease prevention, or for individuals who desire resuming activity after treatment for cancer. These recommendations should be advanced as individuals find themselves progressing, as there is a dose–response curve with exercise levels and disease prevention and fitness.

SECONDARY AND TERTIARY PREVENTION

Recommendations for primary prevention would intuitively seem appropriate for secondary and tertiary prevention; however, there are few data to support this conclusion. There have been six studies to date that have examined this idea. Four of the six studies reported statistically significant improvements in a number of cancer-related immune system components as a result of exercise; however, methodological considerations limit these findings[24]. With increased survivorship, this is an area of increasing future research. Until data exist, however, the above-mentioned guidelines and those forwarded by the American Cancer Society[25] should serve as the foundation upon which to provide activity recommendations for all levels of prevention (Table 11.1).

Table 11.1 American Cancer Society recommendations for physical activity and disease prevention

Adults
Engage in at least moderate activity for 30 minutes or more on 5 or more days of the week; 45 minutes or more of moderate to vigorous activity on 5 or more days of the week may further enhance reduction in the risk for breast and colon cancer

Children and adolescents
Engage in at least 60 minutes per day of age-appropriate moderate to vigorous physical activity at least 5 days per week

References

1. Westerlind KC. Physical activity and cancer prevention-mechanisms. Med Sci Sports Exerc 2003; 35: 1834–40

2. Newsholme EA, Parry-Billings M. Effects of exercise on the immune system. In Bouchard C, Shephard RJ, Stephens T, eds. Physical Activity, Fitness, and Health: International Proceedings Consensus Statement. Champaign, IL: Human Kinetics, 1994: 451

3. Mazzeo RS. The influence of exercise and aging on immune function. Med Sci Sports Exerc 1994; 26: 586–92

4. Hackney AC, Fahrner CL, Bulldege TP. Basal reproductive hormonal profiles are altered in endurance trained men. J Sports Med Phys Fitness 1998; 38: 138–41

5. Oliveria SA, Lee I-M. Is exercise beneficial in the prevention of prostate cancer? Sports Med 1997; 23: 271–8

6. Severson RK, Grove JS, Nomura AM, et al. Body mass and prostatic cancer: a prospective study. BMJ 1988; 297: 713–15

7. Coggon D, Pannett B, Osmond C, et al. A survey of cancer and occupation in young and middle-aged men: non-respiratory cancers. Br J Industr Med 1986; 40: 381–6

8. United Kingdom Testicular Cancer Study Group. Aetiology of testicular cancer: association with congenital abnormalities, age at puberty, infertility and exercise. BMJ 1994; 308: 1393–9

9. Nelson ME, Meredith CN, Dawson-Hughes B, et al. Hormone and bone mineral status in endurance-trained and sedentary postmenopausal women. J Clin Endocrinol Metab 1988; 66: 927–33

10. Leroith D, Baserga R, Helman L et al. Insulin-like growth factors and cancer. Ann Intern Med 1995; 122: 54–9

11. Schwartz RS, Shuman WP, Larson V, et al. The effect of intensive endurance training on body fat distribution in young and older men. Metabolism 1991; 40: 545–51

12. Kritchevsky D. Caloric restriction and experimental carcinogenesis. Toxicol Sci 1999; 52: 13–16

13. Moore MA, Park CB, Tsuda H. Physical exercise: a pillar for cancer prevention? Eur J Cancer Prevent 1998; 7: 177–93

14. Margaritis I, Tessier F, Richard MJ, et al. No evidence of oxidative stress after a triathlon race in highly trained competitors. Int J Sports Med 1997; 18: 186–90

15. Poulsen HE, Loft S, Vistisen K. Extreme exercise and oxidative DNA modification. J Sports Sci 1996; 14: 343–6

16. Dreher D, Junod AF. Role of oxygen free radicals in cancer development. Eur J Cancer 1996; 32A: 30–8

17. Thune I, Furberg A-S. Physical activity and cancer risk: dose-response and cancer, all sites and site-specific. Med Sci Sports Exerc 2001; 33 (Suppl): S530–S550

18. Kampert JB, Blair SN, Barlow CE, et al. Physical activity, physical fitness and all-cause and cancer mortality: a prospective study of men and women. Ann Epidemiol 1996; 6: 452–7

19. Shepard RJ, Futcher R. Physical activity and cancer: how may protection be maximized? Crit Rev Oncol 1997; 8: 219–72

20. US Preventive Services Task Force. Guide to Clinical Preventive Services, 2nd edn. Baltimore: Williams & Wilkins, 1996

21. Chakravarthy MV, Joyner MJ, Booth FW. An obligation for primary care physicians to prescribe physical activity to sedentary patients to reduce the risk of chronic health conditions. Mayo Clin Proc 2002; 77: 165–73

22. Pinto BM, Goldstein MG, Marcus BH. Activity counseling by primary care physicians. Prev Med 1998; 27: 506–13

23. Pate RR, Pratt M, Blair SN, et al. Physical activity and public health. A recommendation from the Centers for Disease Control and Prevention and the American College of Sports Medicine. JAMA 1995; 273: 402–7.

24. Fairey AS, Courneya KS, Field CJ, et al. Physical exercise and immune system function in cancer survivors: a comprehensive review and future directions. Cancer 2002; 94: 539–51

25. Brown JK, Byers T, Doyle C, et al. Nutrition and physical activity during and after cancer treatment: An American Cancer Society Guide for informed choices. CA Cancer J Clin 2000; 53: 268–91

11b

Nutrition

Cynthia Thomson and Mara Vitolins

DIET AND CANCER

Current dietary guidelines for cancer prevention

'What should I eat to prevent cancer?' When a patient asks this question, health professionals typically refer to diet guidelines established by the American Cancer Society (ACS). These recommendations are based on data that a healthy diet can reduce rates of chronic disease regardless of the type of disease.

The nutrition-based recommendations from the American Cancer Society

The ACS has historically developed dietary guidelines to reduce cancer risk. Periodically these guidelines are reviewed by leading scientists in the field. The guidelines listed below were revised in 2002 and are consistent with dietary guidelines from other lead organizations such as the World Cancer Research Fund/American Institute for Cancer Research as well as the European Guidelines from the Committee on Medical Aspects of Food Policy (COMA)[1,2].

- Eat a variety of healthful foods, with an emphasis on plant sources.

- Eat five or more servings of a variety of vegetables and fruits each day.

- Choose whole grains in preference to processed (refined) grains and sugars.

- Limit consumption of red meats, especially those high in fat and processed.

- Choose foods that help maintain a healthful weight.

- Maintain a healthful weight throughout life.

- If you drink alcoholic beverages, limit consumption.

Additional details regarding these recommendations can be reviewed on the ACS website (http://www.cancer.org).

To build on the above guidelines, several dietary components that are being investigated, and appear to have the potential for preventing cancer, are fish oils, green tea, soy protein and flax seed. These foods and beverages appear promising for imparting potential benefit and do not appear to confer harm when incorporated into a healthy diet.

Fish oils

Several studies have reported benefit between blood levels of fish oils and cancer risk. Specifically, Simonsen *et al.* reported that, in 291 women with breast cancer and 351 controls when pooling their results, women who had relatively high adipose tissue levels of eicosapentaenoic acid (EPA) and docosahexaenoic acid (DHA), and low levels of linoleic acid had lower breast cancer risk[3]. Terry *et al.* found, in a longitudinal study of 3136 pairs of male twins, that after adjusting for other known risk factors, the men who never ate fatty fish had a two- to three-fold higher risk of developing prostate cancer than men who ate moderate to high amount[4]. Norrish *et al.* showed a correlation between the presence of prostate cancer and blood level of EPA and DHA[5]. Participants with the highest quartile were found to have a 40% lower incidence than participants in the lowest quartile. The evidence for decreased risk of cancer and consumption of fish oils has been collected from populations that consume fatty fish in their diets[4,5].

The question remains, is the fish oil responsible for the risk reduction or is consumption of the entire fish necessary to impart benefit? All fish contain high-quality protein, essential fatty acids, vitamins such as niacin and B_{12}, and minerals such as heme iron and zinc, generally with fewer saturated fatty acids than meat. Therefore, until further research is conducted to elucidate this issue (food versus supplement), recommending intake of fish rather than fish oil supplements appears appropriate. Eating two servings of fish per week, especially fatty fish, has been recommended to elicit health benefits.

Soy protein

Dietary soy is widely marketed and used as both a complementary and alternative therapy for the prevention and treatment of chronic diseases. Soybeans contain a number of phytochemicals that may play a role in the chemoprevention of cancer: isoflavones, saponins, phytates, phytosterols and protease inhibitors[6]. Diet-derived soy isoflavonoids have been found to elicit anticancer activities *in vitro* and in animal models, and these isoflavones are found in serum in high concentrations after ingestion of a soy-rich meal. Owing to their estrogen antagonist and tumor growth inhibition properties, isoflavones have been proposed as protective agents against hormone-dependent cancers. Genistein, the most abudant isoflavone in soy, may act as an antiestrogen by competing for receptor binding, which may result in lowering estrogen-induced breast cell proliferation and breast tumor formation[7]. Barnes *et al.* reported a reduction in carcinogen-induced mammary tumor number and size among rats treated with soy protein isolate with the isoflavones intact compared to those fed the isolate with the isoflavones removed[8]. Lamartiniere *et al.* treated rats neonatally with genistein and found that they were protected against carcinogen-induced mammary tumors later in life[9]. Foth and Cline fed soy protein with isoflavones or a casein-based diet to non-human primates and reported no significant increases in cellular proliferation in the mammary gland and endometrium[10]. Conversely, studies of MCF-7 breast cancer cells and one human study suggest that soy isoflavones may contribute to breast cell proliferation and potentially increase breast cancer risk[11]. For endometrial tissue, Scambia *et al.* and Upmalis *et al.* reported that no effects were seen on the endometrial tissue of their soy isoflavone extract-treated participants[12,13]. Research regarding soy isoflavones is ongoing. Interestingly, in women, a soy-containing diet has been found to confer more benefit if consumed before puberty, or during adolescence[14].This is supported by conclusions of studies of immigrants and other epidemiological studies[15–18].

Experimental evidence also exists for an inhibitory effect of soy on prostate cancer, but clinical trial data are limited. Potential mechanisms of prostate cancer prevention include direct growth inhibition, induction of apoptosis and genistein-induced prostate cancer cell adhesion[19]. Genistein and other phytoestrogens have also been reported to inhibit the growth of androgen (independent and dependent) human prostate cancer cell lines.

The potential health benefits related to soy consumption have encouraged the production of a wide variety of soy dietary supplements and have led to widespread advertisement of their 'beneficial' effects. Soy isoflavone extracts/supplements in the form of pills/tablets are currently widely available and consumers are often led to believe that they will have significant health benefits, although these supplements have not been adequately studied.

Consumers should consider incorporating soy protein, a healthy source of plant-based protein, into their diets, but should be cautioned against trying to 'dose' themselves with isoflavones until more definitive data on safety and efficacy regarding their use are available.

The current recommendation for consumption of soy protein for improving cardiovascular disease risk is established at 25 g per day[20]. In Japan and some parts of China, soy food intake provides approximately 8–12 g of protein per day, which represents about 10% of adult total protein intake[21,22] As recommendations for soy protein consumption for cancer prevention have not been established, it appears warranted to emulate populations who have consumed soy protein for centuries and incorporate approximately 8–12 g of soy protein a day as a part of a healthy diet. Grams of soy protein contained in commonly consumed soy products are listed in Table 11.2.

Flax seed

Lignans and α-linolenic acid (ALA) are found abundantly in flax seed. Studies of diet and risk for chronic disease suggest a cancer-prevention role for flax seed[24,25]. There are three components in flax that may play a role in the reduction of cancer risk: ALA, which is an essential omega-3 fatty acid; dietary fiber, and the lignan secoisolariciresinol diglycoside (SDG). The actions of these constituents of flax are described in further detail below.

Study participants of the Lyon Diet Heart Study who ate a Mediterranean diet rich in ALA were reported to have a 61% reduction in their risk for developing cancer[26]. The ALA contained in flax oil has been reported to be useful for immune system function, prevention of blood clot formation and the ability to lower blood pressure. Additionally, ALA has been reported to alter the fatty acid composition of cell membranes and inhibit the release of pro-inflammatory eicosanoids which may control the growth and invasive nature of tumor cells[27]. Flax fiber contains antioxidants which may inhibit cancer processes, and the lignans have been noted to function as phytoestrogens and antioxidants.

Table 11.2 Commonly consumed soy foods, serving size and protein grams (adapted from reference 23)

Soy food	Size of serving	Soy protein (g)
Soy milk	8 ounces	7
Soy nuts	1/2 cup	34
Tofu (firm)	1/4 cup	10
Tofu (silken)	1/2 cup	9
Tempeh	1/2 cup	16
Soy burger	1 patty	10–12
Soy protein bar	1 bar	14
Cooked soybeans	1/2 cup	14

Researchers have shown that, in a mouse model, SDG decreased the number of melanoma tumors, the rate of metastasis and the size of the tumors[28].

It has been suggested that the lignans contribute to the hormone-like effects of flax seed[29]. Flax seed consumption has been found to increase the length of the luteal phase of the menstrual cycle and may therefore also alter estrogen metabolism[30,31]. Studies in mice have shown that flax seed inhibits the growth and metastasis of breast cancer and prostate cancer[32,33]. Demark-Wahnefried *et al.* demonstrated in a pilot study of men with prostate cancer that flax seed lowered prostate cancer biomarkers[34]. Like the isoflavones in soy, lignans in flax seed are classified as phytoestrogens and flax seed contains approximately 75–800 times more lignans than any other food[35,36]. Long-term studies of flax seed effects in breast and prostate cancer are currently under way, as researchers recognize that it is important to further characterize its physiological effects. Like soy, intake of lignans, especially in large amounts, by survivors of estrogen-driven tumors, is discouraged simply because data regarding their safety are lacking. Flax oil, however, is devoid of lignans and is a good source of n-3 fatty acids that can be incorporated into the diets of survivors of estrogen-positive cancers.

The recommended level of intake of ALA for men is 1.6 g and for women 1.1 g per day. A daily intake of approximately 1 tablespoon of ground flax seed will provide 1.8 g of ALA, more than enough to obtain the recommended intake for both men and women. Consumption of the entire flax seed appears to be the most efficacious way to reap the health-related benefits.

Tea

Antioxidants called catechins found in tea appear to inhibit enzyme activities that lead to cancer. These catechins may also be able to target and repair DNA abnormalities caused by oxidants[37]. Studies have reported that tea catechins inhibit cancer growth by several mechanisms, including: (1) stopping oxidation before cell damage can occur; (2) reducing the incidence and size of chemically induced tumors; and (3) inhibiting the growth of tumor cells. In mouse models of liver, skin and stomach cancer, mice fed green and black tea were noted to develop smaller chemically induced tumors than control mice[37].

Two studies conducted in China have reported encouraging findings regarding tea consumption. One study in males reported that tea drinkers were about half as likely to develop stomach or esophageal cancer as men who drank very little tea[38]. A second study in males found that consuming about two cups of tea along with the application of a tea extract packet placed on the oral lesions (precancerous) reduced the proliferation and size of those lesions[39].

Recommendations for consumption have yet to be established. Green tea has been noted to contain higher levels of antioxidants than black tea, potentially because it is less processed. It appears that, in general, allowing tea to steep in hot water for 5 minutes will release approximately 80% of the catechins and the total amount of polyphenols in 600 ml or 20 ounces of tea has been reported to provide a significant protective effect[40,41]

These foods and beverages appear promising for imparting potential benefit and do not appear to confer harm. However, there may be specific situations in which they must be carefully monitored. For example, fish oils can cause an increase in bleeding time – this may be especially pertinent for patients already taking blood thinners.

EVIDENCE FOR A CANCER-PROTECTIVE EFFECT OF A PLANT-BASED DIET

The relationship between eating a plant-based, or vegetarian, diet and decreased risk of disease is well documented. Many studies from around the world have established that diets high in plant foods are associated with lower rates of heart disease as well as cancer. Block *et al.* reviewed a large number of studies of cancer and fruit and vegetable intake. A protective effect was found (statistically significant) for fruits and vegetables in 128 of 156 studies that gave relative risks[42].

Typically a vegetarian diet is high in fiber, fruit and vegetables, and low in fat. It is important to note, however, that one dietary component cannot change without affecting other dietary components. For example, eating a great deal of fiber impacts the ability to consume other foods. Additionally, it is assumed that many vegetarians consume plant-based diets because they are aware of the health benefits of doing so. This makes measuring the health benefits of a plant-based diet alone difficult, because it is impossible to remove the effect of dietary intake from the other beneficial health behaviors shown to be associated with those who consume vegetarian diets. Following this line of reasoning – this may provide further support to a multidimensional recommendation for integrative care that includes multiple modalities with a focus on the whole person to reduce cancer risk.

VEGETABLE AND FRUIT INTAKE AND CANCER

Numerous studies have shown an inverse relationship between vegetable intake, and to a lesser extent fruit intake, and cancer occurrence[42]. These foods contain biologically active compounds – non-nutrients such as vitamins C and E, carotenoids, phenols and other phytochemicals. By reducing reactive oxygen species, including free radicals that cause cellular damage, antioxidants are likely to protect against cancer. Experimental evidence also suggests that markers of cellular oxidative damage to cells and DNA are lowered when fruit and vegetable consumption is increased[43].

Research supports the finding that diets high in fruits and vegetables reduce the risk of cancer. Although a single fruit or vegetable may contain many nutrients and beneficial chemicals, eating a wide variety of both fruits and vegetables is where the best protection is afforded. For example, diets containing dark green and yellow vegetables have been shown to protect against stomach and lung cancers[44,45]. Consuming allium vegetables and tomatoes have been shown to protect against stomach cancer[46]. Cruciferous vegetables are noted for potentially protecting against colorectal cancers[47]. High carrot consumption has been suggested to protect against lung, bladder and stomach cancers[45].

Evidence continues to mount regarding the beneficial compounds within fruits and vegetables. Although there are no exact recommendations for the type to consume, the National Cancer Institute recommends increasing intake of dietary fiber from grains, fruits and vegetables of 15–20 g/day[1]. This is the equivalent of 4–7 servings of fruits and vegetables of a variety of colours daily (Table 11.3).

Dietary fiber and cancer

Dietary fiber has been central to our study of cancer prevention. Table 11.4 lists food sources of both soluble and insoluble fiber. In recent years much attention has been focused on the possible protective role of fiber in the prevention of cancer of the colon and rectum. Historically, this concept stemmed from the observations that the incidence of colon cancer was lower among Africans, who consumed a diet high in insoluble fiber, than among African-Americans who consumed diets low in fiber[48]. However, once again, other dietary factors cannot be ignored. Consuming high amounts of dietary fiber requires a person to eat many fruits, vegetables, grains, beans and other unrefined foods. Typically this means that a person has less appetite for high-fat meats and refined foods.

Table 11.3 Fiber content of commonly consumed vegetables and fruit

Vegetables	Dietary fiber content (g)
Artichoke	16.2
Asparagus	1.4
Black beans	15.0
Broccoli	1.3
Brussels sprouts	2.0
Carrots	2.2
Cauliflower	1.3
Celery	0.7
Corn (maize)	2.3
Cucumber	0.4
Green beans	2.0
Kidney beans	13.1
Lettuce, iceberg	0.3
Peas	4.4
Potato	4.6
Spinach	2.2
Squash, summer	1.3
Tomato	1.4
Yam	2.7

Table 11.4 Dietary sources high in soluble and insoluble fiber

Soluble	Insoluble
Apples	Fresh fruit
Barley	Legumes
Citrus fruits	Nuts
Oats and oat bran	Raw vegetables
Strawberries	Root vegetables
	Seeds
	Wheat bran
	Whole grain breads and cereals

Fiber has multiple biological mechanisms by which it may be cancer preventive. When consumed as part of a healthy diet, fiber stimulates colon muscle activity and supports beneficial microflora activity. Dietary fiber (water insoluble) provides bulk that decreases the transit time through the colon and reduces the risk of constipation. The quantity of dietary fiber also affects bile salt metabolism and fecal bulk – all of which may be involved in colon cancer. This provides biologic plausibility to the hypothesis that a high-fiber diet would be associated with a lower incidence of colorectal cancers. Fiber can also favorably affect the balance of steroid hormones by lowering levels of the precursor molecule cholesterol, which impacts levels of sex hormones including estrogen and testosterone.

Investigators recently reported that higher intakes of plant foods or fiber did not lower the risk of colon cancer. However, the data suggested that very low intakes of plant foods may increase the risk[49].

Bonithon-Kopp *et al.* provide intervention study evidence that fiber supplements might have a detrimental effect on colon health, suggesting that fiber should be consumed as part of a healthy diet rather than in the form of fiber supplements[50].

Phytochemicals

Scientists are learning more about the role of plant phytochemicals (from fruits, vegetables, whole grains and legumes) for preventing various chronic diseases. The term 'phytochemical' is used only for those plant chemicals that may have effects on health, but are not considered essential nutrients. These non-nutritive substances include capsaicin, catechins, coumesterol, genestein, indole, lycopene and saponins – all of which are being further studied regarding their role in human health.

Knowledge regarding the existence of phytochemicals has helped health professionals consider not only prevention of deficiency diseases through diet, but also what should be consumed to support optimal health. The ACS has recognized the importance of the benefits of plant-based foods by having the first recommendation in their nutrition guidelines read 'Eat MOST of your foods from plant sources.' Additional research in this area is certainly warranted. Table 11.5 describes common phytochemicals and their mechanisms of biological action.

OBESITY AND WEIGHT CONTROL

Excess weight is estimated to contribute to 400 000 deaths each year in the USA. Being overweight or obese is associated with a greater prevalence of chronic disease conditions including cancer. Several large-scale prospective studies that evaluated the long-term effects of obesity have noted that being obese increases a person's risk of developing some form of cancer. The pattern of mortality versus relative weight for 900 000 subjects followed for 12 years was described by the American Cancer Society Study, which found that being overweight or obese may account for 20% of cancer deaths in women and 14% of cancer deaths in men[51].

The hormonal profile associated with obesity, including alterations in estradiol and insulin-like growth factor, and their binding proteins, is thought to promote the growth of tumors[52–54]. Excess abdominal fat increases insulin resistance, predisposing to hyperinsulinemia, glucose intolerance, dyslipidemia and hypertension. Hyperinsulinemia raises plasma levels of the free form of insulin-like growth factor (IGF-I), a stimulatory hormone of cancerous cell growth[52]. Treatment of obesity with calorie restriction, physical activity and weight loss has been shown to decrease levels of insulin and IGF-I[55].

The ACS guidelines appropriately recommend maintaining healthy weight in their cancer-prevention guidelines[1].

INSULIN CONTROL

In the past several years there has been increased recognition that certain types of cancer may be promoted by hyperinsulinemia, characterized by raised plasma insulin levels and an exaggerated insulin response to increases in plasma glucose concentrations. Hyperinsulinemia is a compensatory response that maintains glucose homeostasis in patients who become resistant to insulin action. IGF-I is a potent mitogen whose proteins play an important role in tumorigenesis and the inhibition of apoptosis[56,57]. Increasing levels of IGF-I increase the risk of malignant disease, specifically that of breast, prostate, lung and colorectum, and subsequently a decrease in serum IGF-I decreases this risk[58–62]. We know that the insulin-like growth factor-I receptor (IGF-IR) regulates normal cell growth and development, but abnormal stimulation can contribute to the development of the above-listed cancers[63]. In estrogen receptor-positive breast cancer, the IGF-IR is significantly overexpressed and hyperphosphorylated in comparison to normal mammary epithelium or benign mammary tumors[64,65]. Furthermore, overexpression of IGF-IR correlates with resistance to anticancer treatments, leading to recurrence at the primary site[65].

Dietary modification of total energy and protein has been shown to decrease IGF-I, lowering cancer risk and inhibiting tumor growth. A study by Dunn et al. found that when diet-restricted mice (with low circulating IGF-I levels) were supplemented with IGF-I, the effect of the dietary restriction on the cancer growth disappeared and the tumor growth rate became the same as in the animals not on the food restriction; thus, the effect of the energy restriction on cancer was mediated by IGF-I[66]. IGF-I will also be decreased in response to protein–calorie malnutrition and fasting. However, this response is smaller in obese individuals, demonstrating less dependency on energy intake to maintain IGF-I[67–69]. As one might suppose, overnutrition

Table 11.5   Phytochemicals and their proposed biological mechanisms

Class	Most common phytochemicals	Specific foods	Biological properties
Capsaicin	capsaicin	chillies	antibacterial, promotes intestinal activity; preliminary evidence of healing effect on oral ulcerations
Carotenoids	β-carotene	apricots, cantaloupe, carrots, collard greens, fennel, kale, mustard greens, peaches, pumpkin, red pepper, romaine lettuce, spinach, sweet potatoes, Swiss chard, winter squash	may modulate mutagenesis, cell differentiation, and proliferation; excess supplemental β-carotene may be pro-oxidant
	lycopene	tomato, grapefruit, watermelon, guava, apricots, mango, oranges, peaches, papaya	free radical scavenging protects against oxidative damage and lipid peroxidation
	lutein zeaxanthin canthaxanthin	kale, broccoli, spinach, winter squash, Brussels sprouts, celery, dill, leeks, mustard greens, peas, green onions, summer squash	inhibit macrophage-mediated LDL oxidation; reduced oxidative damage
Glucosinolates	dithiolthiones sulfuraphane isothiocyanates indoles	cruciferous vegetables: cabbage, kale, broccoli, cauliflower, Brussels sprouts, watercress, radish	activates detoxifying enzymes, anticancerous, induction of phase II detoxifying enzymes
Flavanol	catechin epicatechin epigallocatechin epicatechin gallate epigallocatechin gallate	tea plant, Camellia sinensis. cocoa, black and green tea	suppress cancer promotion, antibacterial and antiviral, antioxidant, potentiate insulin action, protect cells against oxidative stress
Isoflavones/ phytoestrogens	daidzein genistein luteolin coumesterol glycitein	legumes and soy	estrogen modulator, cancer enzyme inhibitors, antioxidant, immune system enhancers and stimulants inhibit α-amylase activity, protect against gastric cancer
Flavonol	kaempferol	endive, leek, broccoli, radish, grapefruit, black tea, onion, lettuce, cranberry, apple skin, berries, olive, tea, red wine	antioxidant and antiproliferative activities

Continued

Table 11.5 *Continued*

Class	Most common phytochemicals	Specific foods	Biological properties
Flavonol	quercetin	red and yellow onions, kale, broccoli, red grapes, cherries, French beans, apples and cereals	prevents the cytotoxicity of oxidized LDL, protect cells against oxidative stress, inhibited TNF-α production
	myricetin	cranberry, grapes, red wine	induce secretion of TNF-α, antioxidant
Flavone	chrysin	fruit skin	protect cells against oxidative stress, hypoglycemic effect
Proantho-cyanidins/ tannins	procyanidin prodelphinidin propelargonidin	pine bark, hawthorn berries, bilberry, green tea, black tea, lemon tree bark, hazel nut tree leaves, blueberries, cherries, cranberries, black currants	free radical scavengers, antiproliferation, insulin-like biological activity
Anthocyanidins	malvadin cyanidin delphinidin pelargonidin peonidin petunidin	red grapes, red wine, cherries, raspberries, strawberries, grapes	induced TNF-α production and acted as modulators of the immune response in activated macrophages
Other polyphenoic compounds or phenyl propanoids	ferulic acid	corn, rice, tomatoes, prunes, spinach, cabbage, asparagus	induce apoptosis, protection of LDL against oxidation
	chlorogenic acid	apple, pears, cherries, prunes, plums, peaches, apricots, berries, tomatoes, anise, coffee	antioxidant and antiproliferative activities, inhibit LDL oxidation
	gallic acid	cranberries, wine	TNF-α production decrease, inhibit oxidative modification of LDL particles, antiproliferative activities
	caffeic acid	white grapes, olives, spinach, cabbage, asparagus, coffee	protect cells against oxidative stress, antiproliferative activities
	cinnamic acids	cranberries, wine	antioxidants, potentiate insulin action, and lessen effect on oxidation of lipoproteins
	coumarins	white grapes, wine, cranberries, tomatoes, spinach, cabbage, asparagus, carrots, caraway, celery	antioxidant and antiproliferative activities, induce a multiplicity of phase II enzymes

Continued

Table 11.5 *Continued*

Class	Most common phytochemicals	Specific foods	Biological properties
Other polyphenoic compounds or phenyl propanoids	ellagic acid	strawberries, raspberries	antioxidant, anti-inflammatory, and anti-tumor
	curcumin	turmeric, ginger	anticarcinogenic, scavenge oxygen radicals
	resveratrol	wine and peanuts	antioxidant inhibitor of cancer cell growth, antiproliferative activities
	benzoic acid	berries	antiproliferative, protection against oxidation of LDL
Lipoic acid	lipoic acid	dark leafy greens: spinach and broccoli	suppression of malignant cell growth, block release of oxygen radicals
Protease inhibitors	protease inhibitors	soy bean, potato, corn	reduces tumors, inhibits carcinogenesis
Monoterpenes	mycrene D-limonene carvone	citrus fruit, peppers, basil, thyme, caraway, whole grains	
Diterpenes	carnosol, rosmarinic acid	oregano, rosemary	
Triterpenes	glycyrrhizin saponin	citrus fruit, peas, soy-beans, herb, licorice root, legumes	antifungal, antibacterial, inhibit cancer growth and tumor, HMACoA-reductase activity
Sulfides	allyl sulfur/ajoene	garlic, leek, chives, onions, shallots, cabbage	antimicrobial activity, induce apoptosis

Adapted from reference 97

will increase IGF-I levels[70]. A diet high in fat and refined carbohydrates, and a lifestyle low in physical activity, leads to insulin resistance and compensatory hyperinsulinemia. Recommendations for decreasing serum levels of IGF-I include a low-fat diet high in complex carbohydrates and daily aerobic activity. Bernard *et al.* used these recommendations in prostate cancer patients to decrease serum insulin levels, which *in vivo* led to decrease in prostate tumor cell growth *in vitro* and induced apoptosis in cancer cells[71].

MICRONUTRIENTS AND CANCER PREVENTION

Apart from food and its role in cancer prevention, dietary supplementation with micronutrients has also been a focus of research. The general assumption is that the cancer-protective benefits of a specific food or food group are due substantially to one or a select few micronutrients or phytochemicals contained within the food or food group that can be isolated in pill form. This reductionistic approach, while attractive (because of the assumed ease of behavior change), has not generally been proved scientifically. In fact, in the early 1990s, supplemental β-carotene was associated with increased lung cancer rates among Finnish male smokers and was also shown to increase cancer in the Carotene And Retinol Efficacy Trial (CARET)[72]. Dietary β-carotene had shown strong potential as a cancer-preventive strategy in animal and case–control studies; however, isolation of a given nutrient or carotenoid and the higher dosage levels achievable by supplementation appeared to result in negative biological effects.

It is of interest that mounting evidence has shown that long-term (more than 10 years) supplementation with a multivitamin–mineral product may protect against cancer. In 1998, data from the Nurse's Health Study demonstrated that regular multivitamin users showed a 20% reduction in colon cancer incidence as compared to non-users, but the benefit was not demonstrated until after 5 years of supplementation[73]. Jacobs et al. showed a similar reduction in risk for colorectal cancer of 29% after 10 years of supplementation[74]. Both studies suggested that folic acid played a key role, potentially through epigenetic modulation of disease, including alteration of methylation at the molecular level[75]. These data suggest that even mild inadequacies in micronutrient status over time may contribute to the development of cancer, although this hypothesis needs to be tested more fully[76].

Micronutrient supplementation may also play a role in reducing oxidative damage, damage that can contribute to carcinogenesis. In a study by Atamna et al., adequate iron–sulfur nutrition was shown to protect the mitochondria against damage[77]. Low folate intake has been associated with suboptimal DNA repair, which is responsive to folic acid supplementation[78]. While the mechanism has not been clearly defined, selenium supplementation, probably through antioxidation potential, is associated with reduced risks for

several cancers including prostate and colon cancer[79]. The role of supplementation with vitamin C in cancer prevention is an area of active scientific debate, with some suggesting that high levels of supplementation increase DNA damage and thus cancer risk, and others supporting a role of vitamin C supplementation in modulating cancer initiation and promotion[80].

The same study that showed an increased risk for lung cancer related to β-carotene supplementation also demonstrated a significant reduction in risk for prostate cancer with α-tocopherol supplementation[81]. Evidence that calcium supplementation may reduce colon cancer risk is also emerging and there is mixed evidence that zinc supplementation, while reducing oxidative stress and modulating immune response, may reduce or increase cancer risk[82,83].

Currently the multicenter SELECT trial is being conducted across the USA to evaluate the role of vitamin E and/or selenium supplementation in the primary prevention of prostate cancer. In the future, the Vitamins and Lifestyle cohort study and the Physician's Health Study II will provide prospective, hypothesis-driven, longitudinal study of the effects of micronutrient supplementation on cancer outcomes[84,85]. In 2003, the US Preventive Services Task Force (USPSTF) reviewed the available evidence that supplementation with vitamins A, C or E, and multivitamins with folic acid or antioxidants reduced cancer risk. The USPSTF found insufficient evidence of a protective effect. They also cautioned against the use of β-carotene supplements (www.preventiveservices.ahrq.gov).

IMMUNE ENHANCEMENT

Current evidence suggests that immune dysfunction may be an underlying factor in the majority of cancers diagnosed. Immune function is significantly reduced in populations where

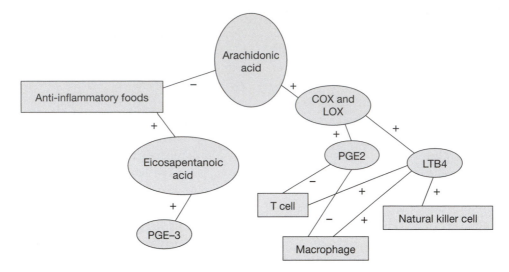

Figure 11.1 Role of anti-inflammatory foods in modulation of immune inflammatory response pathways

micronutrient deficiencies are common. Even in the USA, where food is in abundance, intake of select micronutrients that have key roles in optimizing our immune status is often inadequate. For example, NHANES III data suggest that 24% of adults between the ages of 31 and 50 years are not meeting the estimated adequate requirement (EAR) for vitamin C, and 51% of males and 93% of females are not meeting the EAR for vitamin E. Intake of zinc, another nutrient essential to optimal immune health is insufficient in 9% of adult males and 16% of adult females. To support self-report data, NHANES has also measured micronutrient levels in plasma. As an example, 5% of Whites and 15% of Blacks aged 20–39 have plasma vitamin C levels below 0.3 mg/dl. Thus, ethnicity is associated with an even higher potential for inadequate intake as is aging, with almost 30% of Blacks over age 55 years demonstrating depleted plasma levels of vitamin C. These data and data from Chandra reported over the past 15–20 years suggest that daily use of a multivitamin mineral supplement may be warranted not only to improve immune function but also potentially to reduce cancer risk[86].

A second area where diet may play a critical role in modulating the immune response toward reduced cancer risk is the association between dietary intake of select foods and modulation of the inflammatory response. Growing evidence suggests that, in the multi-stage process of carcinogenesis, even subclinical levels of inflammation may significantly increase cancer risk over time. Of primary importance is the role of fatty acids. Figure 11.1 illustrates the interaction between food constituents and the inflammatory or anti-inflammatory response.

Thus, food selections can directly affect the presence and degree of inflammation present. Making food selections that enhance omega-3 fatty acids and antioxidant vitamin and phytochemical intake (Table 11.6) may reduce inflammation at the cellular level, indirectly reducing cancer risk.

Food preparation

Several highly mutagenic heterocyclic amines (HCAs) are produced during the cooking of meats[87]. Many of these have been shown to be carcinogenic in rats and mice[87]. HCA formation

Table 11.6 Foods and nutrients to increase immunity and decrease inflammation

Nutrients to increase immunity
Vitamin A
Vitamin C
Vitamin E
Selenium
Zinc
Copper

Foods to be eliminated from the diet because of the inflammatory response
Polyunsaturated fats
Partially hydrogenated fats
Hydrogenated fats
Trans fatty acids

Foods to be promoted in the diet to reduce the inflammatory response
Fruits and vegetables
Citrus fruit
Monounsaturated oils such as olive oil
Salmon and sardines
Flax seed
Walnuts
Turmeric

centers on four factors: temperature, cooking method, type of food and time. HCAs are found in cooked muscle meats; other sources of protein (eggs, organ meats, tofu) have very little or no HCA content naturally or when cooked. The most important factor in the formation of HCAs is the temperature of cooking. Barbecuing, broiling and frying cooking methods create the greatest amounts of HCAs because they are high-temperature cooking methods. One study conducted by researchers showed a three-fold increase in the content of HCAs when the cooking temperature was increased from 200° to 250°C (392° to 482°F)[88]. Foods cooked over a long period of time (well-done versus medium) will also form slightly more HCAs[87]. Exposure to HCAs can be reduced by varying methods of cooking meats – microwaving meats more often, especially prior to barbecuing, broiling, or frying[89].

As recommendations have been made regarding limiting one's exposure to HCAs via reduced consumption of charred meat, this also provides support for increased consumption of a diet high in vegetable protein.

General recommendations

The value of food and nutrition in the primary, secondary and tertiary prevention of cancer is being widely studied. The take-home message appears to be that the diet that prevents cancer may also prevent recurrence of cancer, although data confirming this hypothesis are limited. General recommendations for dietary intake should follow the diet guidelines established by the ACS. The recommendations are based on studies which demonstrate that a healthy diet can reduce rates of chronic disease regardless of the type of disease.

PRIMARY PREVENTION

Typically it is less expensive to prevent disease than it is to treat it. As diet is a modifiable environmental exposure, more emphasis is being placed on evaluating the role of diet and nutrient intake in the prevention of disease and enhancement of health. A diet high in plant foods is naturally unrefined, high in antioxidants, fiber and other beneficial phytochemicals and is typically lower in fat. Dietary recommendations from the ACS support high consumption of plant-based foods for prevention of cancer.

SECONDARY PREVENTION

Dietary guidelines for secondary prevention of cancer should be personalized to the patient. Once diagnosed with pre-cancerous changes, the patient should have a care plan that includes a dietary assessment component to evaluate whether he is consuming a healthy diet; if not, dietary counseling should follow. Data showing that a healthy diet can reverse precancerous lesions are limited. Should the patient progress to frank malignancy, a healthy diet may enable him to heal more quickly and be more tolerant of treatment and treatment side-effects (see Chapter 12).

TERTIARY PREVENTION

Data regarding the nutritional factors that influence cancer recurrence are also lacking. However, it seems reasonable that cancer survivors should follow the nutrition guidelines for prevention of cancer, as it is believed that the same factors that increase cancer incidence might also be important in cancer recurrence. This is illustrated by data that prostate cancer recurrence may be increased by high saturated fat consumption and low levels of micronutrients[90-92]. For breast cancer, the risk of recurrence may be increased by diets high in fat and low in fruits and vegetables, and by being obese[93-96]. Survivors need a nutritionally balanced diet that is varied and adequate in calories and provides sufficient amounts of micronutrients (as detailed in the ACS Guidelines for Diet, Nutrition and Cancer Prevention)[1].

There are particular foods that cancer survivors of estrogen-positive tumors might consider limiting or avoiding, specifically: isoflavone-enhanced soy products and high levels of flax seed consumption, as the phytoestrogens contained in these foods have not been adequately tested for safety in populations of estrogen-positive cancer surviors. Previous research using animal models suggest that isoflavones might have the ability to act as an antagonist when estrogen concentrations are high, as in premenopausal women, and act as estrogen agonists when estrogen concentrations are low, as they are in postmenopausal women. It is speculated that isoflavones may bind estrogen receptors, which then stops the more potent form of estrogen (human) from binding, thus functioning as an overall antiestrogen. However, until further clinical trial evidence is available regarding their safety profile, survivors should err on the side of being cautious and limit their consumption of these foods.

References

1. Byers T, Nestle M, McTiernan A, et al. American Cancer Society guidelines on nutrition and physical activity for cancer prevention: reducing the risk of cancer with healthy food choices and physical activity. CA Cancer J Clin 2002; 52: 92-11

2. European Commission. Nutrient and Energy Intakes for the European Community. Report of the Scientific Committee for Food (Thirty-first series). Luxembourg: Office for Official Publications of the European Communitites, 1993.

3. Simonsen NR, Navajas JFC, Moreno-Martin JM, et al. Tissue stores of individual monounsaturated fatty acids and breast cancer: the EUR-MIC study. Am J Clin Nutr 1998; 68: 134-41

4. Terry P, Lichtenstein P, Feychting M, et al. Fatty fish consumption and risk of prostate cancer. Lancet 2001; 357: 1764-66

5. Norrish AE, Skeaff CM, Arribas GL, et al. Prostate cancer risk and consumption of fish oils: a dietary biomarker-based case–control study. B J Cancer 1999; 7: 1238-42

6. Hasler CM, Finn SC. Soy: just a hill of beans? J Wom Health 1998; 7: 519–23

7. Messina M, Barnes S. The role of soy products in reducing risk of cancer. J Natl Cancer Inst 1991; 83: 541–6

8. Barnes S, Peterson G, Grubbs C, et al. Potential role of dietary isoflavones in the prevention of cancer. Adv Exp Med Biol 1994; 354: 135–47

9. Lamartiniere CA, Moore J, Holland M, et al. Neonatal genistein chemoprevents mammary cancer. Proc Soc Exp Biol Med 1995; 208: 120–3

10. Foth D, Cline JM. Effects of mammalian and plant estogens on mammary glands and uteri of macaques. Am J Clin Nutr 1998; (Suppl): 1413S–1417S

11. Petrakis NL, Barnes L, King EB, et al. Stimulatory influence of soy protein isolate on breast secretion in pre- and postmenopausal women. Cancer Epidemiol Biomarkers Prev 1996; 5: 785–94

12. Scambia G, Mango D, Signorile PG, et al. Clinical effects of a standardized soy extract in postmenopausal women: a pilot study. Menopause 2000; 7: 71–5

13 Upmalis DH, Lobo R, Bradley L, et al. Vasomotor symptom relief by soy isoflavone extract tablets in postmenopausal women: a multicenter, double-blind, randomized, placebo-controlled study. Menopause 2000; 7: 236–42

14. Shu XO, Jin F, Dai Q, et al. Soyfood intake during adolescence and subsequent risk of breast cancer among Chinese women. Cancer Epidemiol Biomarkers Prev 2001; 10: 483–8

15. Wu AH, Yu MC, Tseng CC, et al. Plasma isoflavone levels versus self-reported soy isoflavone levels in Asian-American women in Los Angeles County. Carcinogenesis 2004; 25: 77–81

16. Zheng W, Dai Q, Custer LJ, et al.Urinary excretion of isoflavonoids and the risk of breast cancer. Cancer Epidemiol Biomarkers Prev 1999; 8: 35–40

17. Ingram D, Sanders K, Kolybaba M, et al. Case–control study of phyto-oestrogens on breast cancer. Lancet 1997; 350: 990–9

18. Wu AH, Ziegler RG, Horn-Ross PL, et al. Tofu and risk of breast cancer in Asian-Americans. Cancer Epidemiol Biomarkers Prev 1996; 5: 901–6

19. Moyad MA. Soy, disease prevention, and prostate cancer. Semin Urol Oncol 1999; 17: 97–102

20. United States Food and Drug Administration. Food labeling, health claims, soy protein, and coronary heart disease. Fed Reg 1999; 57: 699–733

21. Messina M, Messina V. Provisional recommended soy protein and isoflavone intakes for healthy adults: rationale. Nutr Today 2003; 38: 100–9

22. Nagata C, Takatsuka N, Kurisu Y, et al. Decreased serum total cholesterol concentration is associated with high intake of soy products in Japanese men and women. J Nutr 1998; 128: 209-13

23. US Department of Agriculture, Agricultural Research Service. 2004. USDA Nutrient Database for Standard Reference, Release 17. Nutrient Data Laboratory Home Page http://www.nal.usda.gov/fnic/foodcomp

24. de Lorgeril M, Renaud S, Mamelle N, et al. Mediterranean alpha-linolenic acid-rich diet in secondary prevention of coronary heart disease. Lancet 1994; 343: 1454–9

25. Meydani SN. Interaction of omega 3 polyunsaturated fatty acids and vitamin E on the immune response. World Rev Nutr Diet 1994; 75: 155–61

26. de Lorgeril M, Salen P, Martin JL, et al. Mediterranean dietary pattern in a randomized trial: prolonged survival and possible reduced cancer rate. Arch Intern Med 1998; 158: 1181–7

27. Zhou JR, Blackburn GL. Bridging animal and human studies: what are the missing segments in dietary fat and prostate cancer? Am J Clin Nutr 1997; 66: 1572S–80S

28. Li D, Yee JA, Thompson LU, Yan L. Dietary supplementation with secoisolariciresinol diglycoside (SDG) reduces experimental metastasis of melanoma cells in mice. Cancer Lett 1999; 142: 91–6

29. Hutchins AM, Martini MC, Olson BA, et al. Flaxseed influences urinary lignan excretion in a dose-dependent manner in postmenopausal women. Cancer Epidemiol Biomarkers Prevention 2000; 9: 1113–18

30. Phipps WR, Martini MC, Lampe JW, et al. Effect of flax seed ingestion on the menstrual cycle. J Clin Endocrinol Metab 1993; 77: 1215–19

31. Haggans CJ, Hutchins AM, Olson BA, et al. Effect of flaxseed consumption on urinary estrogen metabolites in postmenopausal women. Nutr Cancer 1999; 33: 188–95

32. Lin X, Gingrich JR, Bao W, et al. Effect of flaxseed supplementation on prostatic carcinoma in transgenic mice. Urology 2002; 60: 919–24

33. Chen J, Stavro PM, Thompson LU. Dietary flaxseed inhibits human breast cancer growth and metastasis and downregulates expression of insulin-like growth factor and epidermal growth factor receptor. Nutr Cancer 2002; 43: 187–92

34. Demark-Wahnefried W, Price DT, Polascik TJ, et al. Pilot study of dietary fat restriction and flaxseed supplementation in men with prostate cancer before surgery: exploring the effects on hormonal levels, prostate-specific antigen, and histopathologic features. Urology 2001; 58: 47–52

35. Adlercreutz H, Mousavi Y, Clark J, et al. Dietary phytoestrogens and cancer: in vitro and in vivo studies. J Steroid Biochem Mol Biol 1997; 41: 331

36. Thompson LU. Experimental studies on lignans and cancer. Baillière's Clin Endocrinol Metab 1998; 12: 691–705

37. Dufresne CJ, Farnworth ER. A review of latest research findings on the health promotion properties of tea. J Nutr Biochem 2001; 12: 404–21

38. Sun CL, Yuan JM, Lee MJ, et al. Urinary tea polyphenols in relation to gastric and esophageal cancers: a prospective study of men in Shanghai, China. Carcinogenesis 2002; 23: 1497–503

39. Hakim IA, Harris RB. Joint effects of citrus peel use and black tea intake on risk of squamous cell carcinoma of the skin. BMC Derm 2001; 1: 3

40. Weisburger JH, Chung FL. Mechanisms of chronic disease causation by nutritional factors and tobacco products and their prevention by tea polyphenols. Food Chem Toxicol 2002; 40: 1145–54

41. Hakim IA, Weisgerber UM, Harris RB, et al. Preparation, composition and consumption patterns of tea-based beverages in Arizona. Nutr Res 2000; 20: 1715–24

42. Block G, Patterson B, Subar A. Fruit, vegetables, and cancer prevention: a review of the epidemiological evidence. Nutr Cancer 1992; 18: 1–29

43. Thompson HJ, Heimendinger J, Haegele A, et al. Effect of increased vegetable and fruit consumption on markers of oxidative cellular damage. Carcinogenesis 1999; 20: 2261–6

44. Ngoan LT, Mizoue T, Fujino Y, et al. Dietary factors and stomach cancer mortality. Br J Cancer 2002; 87: 37–42

45. Kvale G, Bjelke E, Gart JJ. Dietary habits and lung cancer risk. Int J Cancer 1983; 31: 397–405

46. Gao CM, Takezaki T, Ding JH, et al. Protective effect of allium vegetables against both esophageal and stomach cancer: a simultaneous case-referent study of a high-epidemic area in Jiangsu Province, China. Jpn J Cancer Res 1999; 90: 614–21

47. Turner F, Smith G, Sachse C, et al. Vegetable, fruit and meat consumption and potential risk modifying genes in relation to colorectal cancer. Int J Cancer 2004; 112: 259–64

48. Levy RD, Segal I, Hassan H, Saadia R. Stool weight and faecal pH in two South African populations with a dissimilar colon cancer risk. S Afr J Surg 1994; 32: 127–8

49. McCullough ML, Robertson AS, Chao A, et al. A prospective study of whole grains, fruits, vegetables and colon cancer risk. Cancer Causes Control 2003; 14: 959–70

50. Bonithon-Kopp C, Kronborg O, Giacosa A, et al. Calcium and fibre supplementation in prevention of colorectal adenoma recurrence: a randomised intervention trial. European Cancer Prevention Organisation Study Group. Lancet 2000; 356: 1300–6

51. Calle EE, Rodriguez C, Walker-Thurmond K, Thun MJ. Overweight, obesity, and mortality from cancer in a prospectively studied cohort of U.S. adults. N Engl J Med 2003; 348: 1625–38

52. Ng EH, Ji CY, Tan PH, et al. Altered serum levels of insulin-like growth-factor binding proteins in breast cancer patients. Ann Surg Oncol 1998; 5: 194–201

53. Kaye SA, Folsom AR, Soler JT, et al. Associations of body mass and fat distribution with sex hormone concentrations in postmenopausal women. Int J Epidemiol 1991; 20: 151–6

54. Yu H, Rohan T. Role of the insulin-like growth factor family in cancer development and progression. J Natl Cancer Inst 2000; 92: 1472–89

55. Thissen JP, Ketelslegers JM, Underwood LE. Nutritional regulation of the insulin-like growth factors. Endocr Rev 1994; 15: 80–101

56. Romano G, Prisco M, Zanocco-Marani T, et al. Dissociation between resistance to apoptosis and the transformed phenotype in IGF-I receptor signaling. J Cell Biochem 1999; 72: 294

57. Pash J, Delani A, Adamo M, et al. Regulation of IGF-I transcription by prostaglandin E2 in osteoblast cells. Endocrinology 1995; 136: 33

58. Hankinson S, Willet W, Colditz G, et al. Circulating concentrations of insulin-like growth factor-1 and risk of breast cancer. Lancet 1998; 351: 1393–6

59. Chan J, Stampfer M, Giovannucci E, et al. Plasma insulin-like growth factor-I and prostate cancer risk: a prospective study. Science 1998; 279: 563–6

60. Yu H, Spitz M, Mistry J, et al. Plasma levels of insulin-like growth factor-I and lung cancer risk: a case–control study. J Natl Cancer Inst 1999; 91: 151–6

61. Ma J, Pollak M, Giovannucci E, et al. Prospective study of colorectal cancer risk in men and plasma levels of insulin-like growth factor (IGF)-I and IGF-binding protein-3. J Natl Cancer Inst 1999; 91: 620–5

62. Furstenberger G, Senn H. Insulin-like growth factors and cancer. Lancet Oncol 2002; 3: 298

63. Mauro L, Salerno M, Morelli C, et al. Role of the IGF-I receptor in the regulation of cell–cell adhesion: implications in cancer development and progression. J Cell Physiol 2002; 194: 108–16

64. Resnik J, Reichart D, Huey K, et al. Elevated insulin-like growth factor I receptor autophosphorylation and kinase activity in human breast cancer. Cancer Res 1998; 58: 1159–64.

65. Surmacz E. Function of the IGF-IR in breast cancer. J Mammary Gland Biol Neopl 2000; 5: 95–105

66. Dunn S, Kari F, French J, et al. Dietary restriction reduces insulin-like growth factor I levels, which modulates apoptosis, cell proliferation, and tumor progression in p53-deficient mice. Cancer Res 1997; 57: 4667–72

67. Soliman A, Hassan A, Aref M, et al. Serum insulin-like growth factors I and II concentrations and growth hormone in response to arginine infusion in children with protein–energy malnutrition before and after nutritional rehabilitation. Pediatr Res 1986; 20: 1122–30

68. Clemmons D, Klibanski A, Underwood L, et al. Reduction of plasma immunoreactive somatomedin C during fasting in humans. J Clin Endocrinol Metab 1981; 53: 1247–50

69. Snyder D, Clemmons D, Underwood L. Treatment of obese, diet-restricted subjects with growth hormone for 11 weeks: effects of anabolism, lipolysis, and body composition. J Clin Endocrinol Metab 1988; 67: 54–61.

70. Forbes G, Brown M, Welle S. Hormonal response to overfeeding. Am J Clin Nutr 1989; 49: 608–11

71. Bernard R, Aronson W, Tymchuk C, et al. Prostate cancer: another aspect of the insulin-resistance syndrome? Obesity Res 2002; 3: 303–8.

72. Beta Carotene Cancer Prevention Study Group. The effect of vitamin E and beta carotene on the incidence of lung cancer and other cancers in male smokers. N Engl J Med 1994; 330: 1029–35

73. Giovannucci E, Stampfer MJ, Colditz GA, et al. Multivitamin use, folate, and colon cancer in women in the Nurses' Health Study. Ann Intern Med 1998; 129: 517–24

74. Jacobs EJ, Connell CJ, Patel AV, et al. Multivitamin use and colon cancer mortality in the Cancer Prevention Study II cohort (United States). Cancer Causes Control 2001; 10: 927–34

75. Piyathilake CJ, Johanning GL. Cellular vitamins, DNA methylation and cancer risk. J Nutr 2002; 132 (Suppl): 2340S–2344S

76. Ames BN. Micronutrient deficiencies. A major cause of DNA damage. Ann NY Acad Sci 1999; 889: 87–106

77. Atamna H, Walter PB, Ames BN. The role of heme and iron–sulfur clusters in mitochondrial biogenesis, maintenance, and decay with age. Arch Biochem Biophys 2002; 397: 345–53

78. Wei Q, Shen H, Wang LE, et al. Association between low dietary folate intake and suboptimal cellular DNA repair capacity. Cancer Epidemiol Biomarkers Prev 2003; 12: 963–9

79. Clark LC, Dalkin B, Krongrad A, et al. Decreased incidence of prostate cancer with selenium supplementation: results of a double-blind cancer prevention trial. Br J Urol 1998; 81: 730–4

80. Lee KW, Lee HJ, Surh YJ, Lee CY. Vitamin C and cancer chemoprevention: reappraisal. Am J Clin Nutr 2003; 78: 1074–8

81. Virtamo J, Pietinen P, Huttunen JK, et al. ATBC Study Group. Incidence of cancer and mortality following alpha-tocopherol and beta-carotene supplementation: a postintervention follow-up. JAMA 2003; 290: 476–85

82. Prasad AS, Kucuk O. Zinc in cancer prevention. Cancer Metastasis Rev 2002; 21: 291–5

83. Leitzmann MF, Stampfer MJ, Wu K, et al. Zinc supplementation use and risk of prostate cancer. J Natl Cancer Inst 2003; 95: 1004–7

84. White E, Patterson RE, Kristal AR, et al. VITamins And Lifestyle cohort study: study design and characteristics of supplement users. Am J Epidemiol 2004; 159: 83–93

85. Christen WG, Gaziano JM, Hennekens CH. Design of Physicians' Health Study II – a randomized trial of beta-carotene, vitamins E and C, and multivitamins, in prevention of cancer, cardiovascular disease, and eye disease, and review of results of completed trials. Ann Epidemiol 2000; 10: 125–34

86. Chandra RK. Nutrition and the immune system from birth to old age. Eur J Clin Nutr 2002; 56 (Suppl 3): S73–6

87. Overvik E, Gustafsson J-A. Cooked-food mutagens: current knowledge of formation and biological significance [review]. Mutagenesis 1990; 5: 437–46

88. Chen BH, Meng CN. Formation of heterocyclic amines in a model system during heating. J Food Prot 1999; 62: 1445–50

89. Felton JS, Fultz E, Dolbeare FA, Knize MG. Effect of microwave pretreatment on heterocyclic aromatic amine mutagens/carcinogens in fried beef patties. Food Chem Toxicol 1994; 32: 897–903

90. Kolonel LN, Nomura AM, Cooney RV. Dietary fat and prostate cancer: Current status. J Natl Cancer Inst 1999; 91: 414–28

91. Yoshizawa K, Willet WC, Morris SJ, et al. Study of prediagnostic selenium level in toenails and the risk of advanced prostate cancer. J Natl Cancer Inst 1998; 90:1219–24

92. Heinonen OP, Albanes D, Virtamo J, et al. Prostate cancer and supplementation with alpha-tocoperol and betacarotene: incidence and mortality in a controlled trial. J Natl Cancer Inst 1998; 90: 440–4

93. Jain M, Miller AB. Tumor characteristics and survival of breast cancer patients in relation to premorbid diet and body size. Breast Cancer Res Treat 1997; 42: 43–55

94. Zhang S, Folsom A, Sellers TA, et al. Better breast cancer survival for postmenopausal women who are less overweight and eat less fat. The Iowa Women's Health Study. Cancer 1995; 76: 275–83.

95. Hebert JR, Toporoff E. Dietary exposures and other factors of possible prognostic significance in relation to tumour size and nodal involvement in early-stage breast cancer. Int J Epidemiol 1989; 18: 518–52

96. Newman SC, Miller AB, Howe GR. A study of the effect of weight and dietary fat on breast cancer survival time. Am J Epidemiol 1986; 123: 767–74

97. Gregory-Mercado KY. Predictors of fruit and vegetable consumption in older mostly Hispanic women in Arizona. Dissertation, University of Arizona, Department of Nutritional Sciences. Tucson, Arizona, 2004

11c

Mind–body interventions

Linda E. Carlson and Shauna L. Shapiro

PREVENTION

Primary and secondary prevention

There has been very little research investigating the possibility that mind–body interventions could prevent the onset of cancer. Partially this has been due to the immense methodological challenges faced in this type of research. Sound epidemiological evidence of this kind requires recruitment of a very large cohort of individuals prior to the onset of disease, determining exposure to different interventions, following participants for many years and finally comparing the incidence of cancer. At the same time, other potentially confounding factors that co-occur with the exposures of interest need to be statistically controlled. To our knowledge this has never been done for any of the interventions of interest.

However, there has been carefully conducted research investigating the role of psychological factors such as major life events (a proxy measure of stress), depression and personality characteristics on cancer onset[1–5]. The idea of a cancer-prone personality (dubbed 'type C' personality) was introduced based on observations that cancer patients tended to be 'nice' and deny their own needs[6]. When this concept failed to provide consistent empirical associations with cancer incidence, additional factors such as repression of negative emotions and a helpless/hopeless coping style were suggested as useful markers[7]. The most rigorous recent review concluded that the evidence overall for psychological factors, including the type C personality, is weak, once methodological considerations are taken into account[1]. However, the review did report that support for depression as a risk factor is compelling[1].

In terms of breast cancer, an epidemiologic review concluded that emotional repression and severe life events showed the strongest association with the development of breast cancer[5]. Thus, mind–body interventions that have proven efficacy in decreasing symptoms of depression and enhancing emotional expression may provide some prevention against the development of cancer, although this has not been specifically demonstrated.

Such interventions primarily include cognitive behavioral therapy (CBT), which is a well-validated treatment for major depression[8], and supportive–expressive therapy, which is commonly used with persons diagnosed with cancer[9].

Hence, in terms of prevention, if CBT is effective in treating depression this may also lower the chances of developing cancer in the future. Other treatments, such as mindfulness-based stress reduction (MBSR), have also been documented to decrease depressive symptoms in students and the general population[10–12]. In addition, mindfulness-based cognitive therapy (MBCT) has been demonstrated to decrease rates of relapse in patients with three or more episodes of major depressive disorder[13]. Thus, any mind–body intervention that has documented effects in treating depressive symptoms and encouraging emotional expression may have the potential to protect against the development of cancer.

The mechanisms behind the association between depression and cancer incidence are speculative at present. However, depression is associated with increased levels of circulating glucocorticoids (cortisol) known to have suppressive effects on some aspects of immune functioning, and decreased levels of melatonin, speculated to be oncostatic[14]. This in turn could result in increased susceptibility to the unchecked cell growth characteristic of carcinogenesis.

Alternatively, depression may operate to increase risk indirectly, through health behaviors known to affect cancer incidence or immune function. The most obvious example is smoking, which has been implicated in the etiology of at least 30% of all cancers and which is much more common in depressed individuals. Other health behaviors that are compromised in depressed individuals compared to the general public include sleep patterns and nutrition. Depressed people are also more likely to abuse alcohol and other substances, all of which may contribute to an environment of increased susceptibility to disease. It has even been observed in animal models that the use of antidepressant medication can promote tumor growth. Hence, the observed associations between depression and cancer incidence could arise from any combination of these factors.

Tertiary prevention

The area of tertiary prevention, preventing disease progression after initial diagnosis, is similar in the context of mind–body interventions to that of antineoplastic care. The majority of studies in this area have investigated whether different mind–body interventions are capable of affecting either survival time after diagnosis, or intermediary moderators that are thought to be prognostic of survival, such as immune system functioning.

This area of tertiary prevention, or antineoplastic care, is best illustrated indirectly by the research into psychoneuroimmunology (PNI). PNI research generally measures the effects of psychosocial interventions on indicators that are considered to be potentially important mediators of disease outcomes such as progression and survival. Few studies in the area of PNI have demonstrated direct links between mind–body interventions and disease course, but those few have garnered a great deal of attention and excited the imaginations of a generation of researchers. The most well-known of these is the Stanford study of supportive–expressive therapy conducted by Spiegel et al.[15]. This study demonstrated with a randomized design an increase in survival of an average of 18 months in women with metastatic breast cancer who participated in a year of supportive-expressive therapy, compared to a control condition. Around the same time, Fawzy et al. showed a survival advantage in patients with melanoma who participated in a 6-week psychoeducational intervention, which was associated with increases in natural killer cell function as well as 5–6 year survival[16,17]. Interestingly, the survival advantage was weaker, but was still upheld at 10-year follow-up[18]. Other studies over the years have also investigated survival – the most recent review tallied a significant effect on survival in four of the eight randomized controlled trials in which survival was assessed[19]. Other reviews have drawn similar conclusions [20–22]. The types of interventions that appear to hold the most promise in terms of promoting survival are those that include social support and emotional expression, as well as components of stress reduction and/or relaxation.

A novel approach to the investigation of the effects of psychosocial work on survival in metastatic cancer patients has been undertaken by Cunningham and colleagues [23,24]. They have employed a correlational design in order to be able to look at the amount of psychological work that each patient engages in, and compare subsequent survival outcomes to those predicted by experts, based upon disease characteristics alone. They have consistently found that patients who participated in psychological work and outlived their medical prognoses were characterized by three features: authenticity – a clear understanding of life values; autonomy – the perceived freedom to shape life around these values; and acceptance – a perceived change towards greater tolerance for emotional closeness to others, and an affective experience described as more peaceful and joyous[23] (Table 11.7). The biological correlates of such psychological features have yet to be explored, but possible explanations for the impact on survival in these metastatic cancer patients include neuroendocrine, neuroimmune and health behavior pathways[25].

Other studies in cancer have investigated the effects of psychosocial interventions on intermediary mechanisms such as immune cell counts and function, and stress hormones. MBSR was shown to engender changes in hormone and endocrine profiles of breast and prostate cancer patients towards patterns more characteristic of healthy individuals, suggesting a process of normalization of these systems[26,27]. Another interesting study combining MBSR and dietary changes for men with prostate cancer investigated the effects of the program on

Table 11.7 Characteristics of cancer patients who outlived expectations (from reference 25)

Authenticity	– a clear understanding of life's values
Autonomy	– the perceived ability to shape life around these values
Acceptance	– greater tolerance for emotional closeness with others and an affective experience described as peaceful and joyous

prostate-specific antigen (PSA) levels, an indicator of tumor activity. In a pilot study of ten men and their partners, the rate of PSA rise decreased in eight of the ten men, while three had a decrease in absolute PSA. Doubling time increased from 6.5 months before to 17.7 months after the intervention, indicating a possible slowing of the rate of tumor progression in cases of biochemically recurrent prostate cancer[28].

Other interventions such as experiential–existential group psychotherapy for breast cancer have also shown changes in immune and hormone profiles, again suggesting a trend towards normalization of cortisol levels[29] and less reactivity to stress as a consequence of enhanced emotional expression abilities[30]. The thorny issue of whether these types of change are relevant or important to cancer progression have been addressed recently in a special issue of the journal *Brain, Behavior and Immunity* entitled 'Biological mechanisms of psychosocial effects on disease: implications for cancer control'[31]. The volume was dedicated to addressing issues of possible pathways by which psychosocial factors and interventions could affect the incidence and progression of general and specific cancer-related disease processes. This area of research remains a hotbed of interest and innovation.

References

1. Dalton SO, Boesen EH, Ross L, et al. Mind and cancer. Do psychological factors cause cancer? Eur J Cancer 2002; 38: 1313–23

2. Fox BH. The role of psychological factors in cancer incidence and prognosis. Oncology 1995; 9: 245–53

3. Hilakivi-Clarke L, Rowland J, Clarke R, Lippman ME. Psychosocial factors in the development and progression of breast cancer. Cancer Res Treat 1993; 29: 141–60

4. Levenson JL, Bemis C. The role of psychological factors in cancer onset and progression. Psychosomatics 1991; 32: 124–32

5. Butow PN, Hiller JE, Price MA, et al. Epidemiological evidence for a relationship between life events, coping style, and personality factors in the development of breast cancer. J Psychosom Res 2000; 49(3): 169-181

6. Greer S, Watson M. Towards a psychobiological model of cancer: psychological considerations. Soc Sci Med 1985; 20(8): 773-777

7. Temoshok L. Personality, coping style, emotion and cancer: towards an integrative model. Cancer Surv 1987; 6(3): 545-567

8. Bergen AE, Garfield SL. Handbook of Psychotherapy and Behavior Change, 4th edn. New York: Wiley, 1994

9. Spiegel D, Classen C. Group Psychotherapy for Cancer Patients: A Research-based Handbook of Psycosocial Care. New York: Basic Books, 2000

10. Bishop SR. What do we really know about mindfulness-based stress reduction? Psychosom Med 2002; 64: 71–83

11. Williams KA, Kolar MM, Reger BE, Pearson JC. Evaluation of a wellness-based mindfulness stress reduction intervention: a controlled trial. Am J Health Promot 2001; 15(6): 422-432

12. Shapiro SL. Effects of mindfulness-based stress reduction on medical and premedical students. J Behav Med 1998; 21: 581–99

13. Teasdale JD, Segal ZV, Williams JM, et al. Prevention of relapse/recurrence in major depression by mindfulness-based cognitive therapy. J Consult Clin Psychol 2000; 68: 615–23

14. Spiegel D, Giese-Davis J. Depression and cancer: mechanisms and disease progression. Biol Psychiatry 2003; 54: 269–82

15. Spiegel D, Bloom JR, Draemer HC, Gottheil E. Effect of psychosocial treatment on survival of patients with breast cancer. Lancet 1989; 2: 888–91

16. Fawzy FI, Fawzy NW, Hyun CS, et al. Malignant melanoma. Effects of an early structured psychiatric intervention, coping, and affective state on recurrence and survival 6 years later. Arch Gen Psychiatry 1993; 50: 681–9

17. Fawzy FI, Kemeny ME, Fawzy NW, et al. A structured psychiatric intervention for cancer patients. II. Changes over time in immunological measures. Arch Gen Psychiatry 1990; 47: 729–35

18. Fawzy FI, Canada AL, Fawzy NW. Malignant melanoma: effects of a brief, structured psychiatric intervention on survival and recurrence at 10-year follow-up. Arch Gen Psychiatry 2003; 60: 100–3

19. Ross L, Boesen EH, Dalton SO, Johansen C. Mind and cancer: does psychosocial intervention improve survival and psychological well-being? Eur J Cancer 2002; 38: 1447–57

20. Cwikel JG, Behar LC, Zabora JR. Psychosocial factors that affect the survival of adult cancer patients: a review of research. J Psychosoc Oncol 1997; 15: 1–34

21. Edelman S, Craig A, Kidman AD. Can psychotherapy increase the survival time of cancer patients? J Psychosom Res 2000; 49: 149–56

22. Newell SA, Sanson-Fisher RW, Savolainen NJ. Systematic review of psychological therapies for cancer patients: overview and recommendations for future research. J Natl Cancer Inst 2002; 94: 558–84

23. Cunningham AJ, Watson K. How psychological therapy may prolong survival in cancer patients: new evidence and a simple theory. Integr Cancer Ther 2004; 3: 214–29

24. Cunningham AJ. A new approach to testing the effects of group psychological therapy on length of life in patients with metastatic cancers. Adv Mind Body Med 2002; 18: 5–9

25. Spiegel D, Sephton SE. Psychoneuroimmune and endocrine pathways in cancer: effects of stress and support. Semin Clin Neuropsychiatry 2001; 6: 252–65

26. Carlson LE, Speca M, Patel KD, Goodey E. Mindfulness-based stress reduction in relation to quality of life, mood, symptoms of stress and levels of cortisol, dehydroepiandrostrone-sulfate (DHEAS) and melatonin in breast and prostate cancer outpatients. Psychoneuroendocrinology 2004; 29: 448–74

27. Carlson LE, Speca M, Patel KD, Goodey E. Mindfulness-based stress reduction in relation to quality of life, mood, symptoms of stress, and immune parameters in breast and prostate cancer outpatients. Psychosom Med 2003; 65: 571–81

28. Saxe GA, Hebert JR, Carmody JF, et al. Can diet in conjunction with stress reduction affect the rate of increase in prostate specific antigen after biochemical recurrence of prostate cancer? J Urol 2001; 166: 2202–7

29. van der Pompe G, Duivenvoorden HJ, Antoni MH, et al. Effectiveness of a short-term group psychotherapy program on endocrine and immune function in breast cancer patients: An exploratory study. J Psychosom Res 1997; 42: 453–66

30. van der Pompe G, Antoni MH, Duivenvoorden HJ, et al. An exploratory study into the effect of group psychotherapy on cardiovascular and immunoreactivity to acute stress in breast cancer patients. Psychother Psychosom 2001; 70: 307–18

31. Biological mechanisms of psychosocial effects on disease: implications for cancer control. Brain Behav Immun 2003; 17 (Suppl 1): S1–S134

11d

Botanicals

Lise Alschuler

GENERAL CANCER PREVENTION

The use of botanicals in the prevention of cancer is alluring, given the relative ease of consumption, the generally excellent tolerability and the traditional health benefits associated with the use of medicinal herbs. Over the past several decades, epidemiological and investigational studies have elucidated both how certain botanicals prevent carcinogenesis and also which cancer types may be most preventable by botanicals. Several herbs have been identified as having the ability to prevent carcinogenesis in a wide variety of tumor types and are thus considered to be applicable as general cancer-prevention agents. Notable among these herbs are: *Allium sativum* (garlic), *Camellia sinensis* (green tea), *Silymarin marianum* (milk thistle), *Panax* spp. (ginseng), resveratrol from *Vitis vinifera* (grape), polysaccharides from mushrooms such as *Lentinus edodes* (shitake), *Ganoderma lucidum* (maitake) and *Coreolus versicolor* (Yun zhi), and soy (also covered in Chapter 11b).

Cancer chemoprevention encompasses the idea that regularly ingested substances can inhibit or delay the process of cancer development. The preventive effects derived from herbal compounds are determined from large epidemiological studies as well as from investigational studies into the mechanisms of cancer chemoprevention. Herbal compounds may prevent the activation of pro-carcinogens, may support the inactivation of carcinogens, may prevent the DNA damage caused by carcinogens, may interfere with tumor initiation, may delay or suppress tumor promotion and may reduce tumor progression. As botanicals contain numerous phytochemicals, one herb may exert chemopreventive effects in a variety of ways. The more points of interference, along with the strength of the interference, together determine the chemoprevention potential of a botanical agent (Table 11.8). The botanicals described below are promising chemopreventive substances.

Garlic

Humankind has used *Allium sativum,* or garlic, as a medicinal food for thousands of years. In the early 1980s, researchers began to discover various ways in which garlic inhibits tumor formation. In 1988, a large epidemiologic study published by You *et al.*[1] piqued the interest of investigators into the chemoprevention properties of garlic.

Table 11.8   Botanical interference with carcinogenesis

	Inactivate pro-carcinogens and carcinogens	Prevent/repair DNA damage	Interfere with tumor initiation (induction of apoptosis)	Delay or suppress tumor promotion	Reduce tumor progression
Garlic	•	•	•		
Green tea (equivalent to ≥ 10 cups daily)	•	•	•	•	•
Milk thistle			•	•	
Soy isoflavones			•	•	•
Curcumin	•	•	•		
Scutellaria baicalensis	•				
Ganodermai			•	•	•
Resveratrol	•			•	
Flax					•
Glycyrrhiza			•		

This study used a structured questionnaire to assess the frequency of intake of *Allium* spp. vegetables. The study subjects were grouped into tertiles or quartiles of intake, based on their intake of *Allium* spp. vegetables. Intake of *Allium* spp. vegetables was inversely correlated with death from gastric carcinoma. The highest tertile of garlic intake (more than two cloves of garlic/day) had the lowest gastric cancer death rate (3.45/100 000) compared to the lowest tertile of garlic consumers with the highest cancer death rate (40/100 000). Despite the significance of these trends, it is worth noting that only 50% of the gastric cancers were confirmed histopathologically. Nonetheless, these compelling epidemiological data have spurred continued investigation into the general cancer-preventive properties of garlic.

It is now generally accepted that garlic inhibits the early stages of tumor promotion[2]. This activity is thought to be the result of the organosulfur compounds in garlic, particularly ajoene, which is the natural breakdown product from allicin. Ajoene inhibits experimental mutagenesis and inhibits DNA binding and adduct formation[3]. Additionally, garlic grown in selenium-enriched soil blocks mammary carcinogenesis in both the initiation and post-initiation phases by suppressing dimethylbenz[a]anthracene – DNA adducts[4]. High-selenium garlic demonstrates greater protection against tumorigenesis than does regular garlic, suggesting that selenium enhances the cancer-prevention potential of garlic.

Green tea

In addition to garlic, green tea has been extensively studied for its chemoprevention effects. After water, tea is the most commonly consumed beverage in the world. Over two-thirds of the world's population consumes tea regularly. The general cancer-chemoprevention actions of green tea have been demonstrated in epidemiological studies as well as experimental studies. A 1998 review of the epidemiological studies demonstrated a chemopreventive effect of green tea for several common cancers, although this effect was not unequivocally evident[5]. In this review, two of the three published studies on green tea and pancreatic cancer reported an inverse association. The largest of these studies showed a significant inverse relationship between green tea consumption and pancreatic cancer. However, one study showed an increased risk of pancreatic cancer with daily consumption of ≥ 5 cups of green tea[6]. Of five studies[7–11] on the relationship of green tea consumption and colorectal cancer, three studies found an inverse association. Of ten studies[12–21] on the association between green tea and stomach cancer, six suggested an inverse relationship, three reported a positive association and one concluded that there was no association. Of these studies, the most comprehensive study[15] supported an inverse association of green tea and stomach cancer. Studies of the association between green tea and esophageal cancer are more difficult to interpret. The majority of these studies found the strongest association between hot beverages, green tea included, and esophageal cancer. Research on other cancers, namely pancreatic[22] and urinary bladder[23] cancers, is more limited but is suggestive of an inverse relationship between green tea consumption and cancer incidence. Other epidemiological studies have attempted to clarify the effect of green tea consumption on cancer incidence. A recent prospective study in Japan by Nagano *et al.*[24] followed 58 540 people for 15 years. A self-administered questionnaire ascertained the consumption of green tea (never, once daily, 2–4 times daily, and 5 or more times daily). The incidence of solid cancers, hematopoietic cancers and cancers of all sites combined were noted. The study concluded that green tea consumption was unrelated to the incidence of the cancers under study. However, the authors noted that this study may not have evaluated a minimum effective dose. The maximum studied dose in this study was 5 cups daily, far below the effective concentration of green tea extract used in animal experiments – an amount equivalent to 10 cups of green tea per day in humans. In fact, another large prospective cohort study[25] of individuals consuming 10 cups of green tea daily did show a chemopreventive effect. This 10-year study was conducted in Japan with 8552 male and female participants, all of whom were over the age of 40. During the study, 153 men and 109 women died of cancer. Male patients who consumed over 10 cups of green tea daily died 3.6 years later than did their male counterparts who drank less than 3 cups daily. Female patients who consumed over 10 cups of green tea daily died 7.8 years later than did their female counterparts who drank less than 3 cups daily. In addition, the age at onset of cancer was 3.0 years later in men and 8.7 years later among women who drank over 10 cups of green tea daily than those drinking less than 3 cups of green tea daily. The difference between male and females was explained by the higher tobacco use by men. Finally, in an extension of this same study, the researchers determined that women who drank over 10 cups of green tea daily showed a lower relative risk of cancers of the lung, colon and liver[25]. While this quantity of green tea may seem to be high, it appears to be well tolerated. Of note is a phase I trial of oral green tea extract in adult patients with solid tumors that determined that a dose of $1.0\,g/m^2$ three times daily (equivalent to 20–25 Japanese cups (120 ml) daily) was well tolerated with only caffeine-related side-effects[26].

The mechanisms of cancer chemoprevention by green tea have been well studied. The polyphenols in green tea have been shown to interfere with almost every identified step in carcinogenesis[27]. These actions are summarized in Figure 11.2. Tea extract inhibits mutagens and carcinogens extracellularly (desmutagenesis). Green tea catechins, namely epicatechin (EC), epicatechin-3-gallate (ECG), epigallocatechin-3-gallate (EGCG) and gallocatechin (GC), inhibit mutagens intracellularly (bio-antimutagenesis).

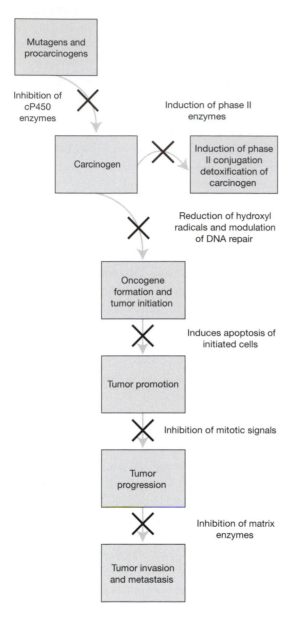

Figure 11.2 Tumor inhibition by green tea polyphenols

tea theaflavins exert antioxidant effects by scavenging free radicals to inhibit oncogene mutations, or tumor initiation. EGCG and ECG increase DNA repair and the fidelity of DNA replication. EGCG also inhibits telomerase, leading to suppression of cell viability and induction of apoptosis. This effect does not occur in normal cells[28]. EGCG inhibits the replication of neoplastic cells, thus interfering with tumor promotion. Largely owing to the work of Fujiki, the role of tumor necrosis factor-α (TNFα) as an endogenous tumor promoter and a central mediator of cancer development has emerged. Fujiki *et al.* have further discovered that EGC, EGCG and GC inhibit TNFα release from neoplastic cells[29]. This action is considered to be one of the most important mechanisms of the anti-tumor promotion activity of green tea[30]. Green tea catechins and EGCG inhibit matrix enzymes (urokinase), thus inhibiting tumor invasion and metastasis. Finally, EGC and EGCG induce apoptosis by inhibition of telomerase. These mechanisms of antimutagenesis and anticarcinogenesis by tea polyphenols indicate the chemopreventive potential of green tea[31]. The systemic concentrations required to produce these actions typically require oral doses 100-fold higher than intravenous doses. This is due to the fact that bioavailability of orally consumed green tea polyphenols is low, because of the first-pass effect, wide tissue distribution and incomplete absorption[32]. This may explain the apparent need for the ingestion of 10 cups daily to produce the chemoprevention effects noted in human studies.

Milk thistle

Another herb with significant experimental evidence as a general chemopreventive agent is *Silybum marianum*, or milk thistle. Milk thistle has been used for hundreds of years by European herbalists for the treatment of liver diseases, specifically alcoholic liver disease. Milk thistle

This is accomplished by inhibition of P450-dependent metabolic activation of promutagens and induction of detoxification of mutagens via induction of glutathione and other phase II enzymes. Additionally, EC, ECG, EGCG and contains a polyphenoloic flavonoid antioxidant, silymarin. Using the SENCAR mouse skin tumorigenesis model, silymarin has been discovered to be a highly effective inhibitor of stage I tumor promotion[33]. Stage I tumor promotion is characterized by the conversion of the initiated cell to a dormant tumor cell, which then proliferates to tumors in the propagation stage, or stage II, of tumor promotion. Silymarin and its main flavonoid, silybinin, inhibit the conversion of initiated cells to dormant tumor cells. This growth inhibition has been further noted in human prostate, breast and cervical carcinoma cells *in vitro*[34]. This effect is mediated via impairment of receptor and non-receptor tyrosine kinase signaling pathways along with inhibition of TNFα release[35] and associated changes in cell cycle progression. These effects are also seen in bladder transitional cancer cell lines. Silybinin treatment of these cells results in a significant dose- and time-dependent growth inhibition and cell arrest. These effects appear to be due to silybinin's modulation of the cyclin cascade and specific activation of capase-3, leading to growth inhibition and apoptosis[36].

Soy

Although soy has been identified as an important chemopreventive agent in breast and prostate cancers, the accumulating evidence suggests a wider chemopreventive effect. Soy isoflavones, namely genistein, have been shown, through a variety of mechanisms, to inhibit the growth of breast, prostate, leukemia, lymphoma, lung and head and neck cancer cells[37]. Soy isoflavones and their metabolites have been found in the plasma, prostatic fluid, breast aspirate and cyst fluid, urine and feces in individuals on a soy-rich diet. Genistein and daidzein bind to estrogen receptors and, at low concentrations (≤ 1 μmol/l in an estrogen-free condition) act as agonists, stimulating estrogen-dependent cell proliferation. In concentrations over 5 μmol/l, genistein and daidzein inhibit

estradiol-stimulated cell division[38]. This has potential clinical relevance for patients with cancers that are hormonally responsive. For example, small amounts of soy may stimulate the growth of estrogen-sensitive breast cancer cells, while larger concentrations may inhibit growth. It is also important to remember that genestein alters the expression of 6–8 times as many genes as does a physiological estrogen such as 17β-estradiol[39]. Thus, the cellular and biological targets of isoflavones and the mechanisms they influence are manifold and largely unknown. What is known begins to build a compelling story of chemoprevention, albeit an unfinished one.

In addition to being both an estrogen agonist and an antagonist, genistein inhibits the protein-tyrosine kinase-mediated signaling pathway[40]. Genistein also inhibits topoisomerase I and II[41] and inhibits NF-κB DNA-binding activity[42], and the Akt signaling pathway[43], all of which increase apoptotic processes. Genistein inhibits prostate-specific antigen (PSA) synthesis in prostate cancer cells through both androgen-dependent and androgen-indpendent pathways[44]. Additionally, genistein down-regulates the expression of *c-erb*B-2-induced and MMP-induced invasive and metastatic properties of breast cancer cells[45] and head and neck cancer cells[46], respectively. These mechanisms underlie the evidenced chemopreventive effect of soy, which will be further elucidated in the discussion of chemoprevention of specific cancers.

RECOMMENDATIONS

The botanicals listed below have at least preliminary data which support their use for the specified aspects of prevention. Further research is necessary concerning amounts necessary for an effect, and situations in which maximal benefit is derived. Please see Table 11.9 for specific malignancies and appropriate botanicals, as well as current levels of evidence.

> **Table 11.9** Evidence for botanical chemoprevention. Level IV evidence includes *in vitro* studies, *in vivo* studies and traditional use. Level II evidence includes level IV and prospective trials, cohort trials and epidemiological studies. Level I evidence includes level II and randomized controlled trials

Level of evidence	General cancer prevention	Breast cancer	Prostate cancer	Gastrointestinal cancers (including oral)	Lung cancer	Skin cancer
IV	*Silybum marianum*	Flax Curcumin	Green tea Soy *Scutellaria baicalensis* Milk thistle			*Silybum marianum* Resveratrol
II	Garlic Green tea Soy	Soy Green tea		Green tea	Green tea	
I						

Primary prevention

- *Allium sativum* (garlic)
- *Camellia sinensis* (green tea)
- *Glycine max* (soy)

Secondary prevention

- *Silymarin marianum* (milk thistle)
- *Glycine max* (soy)

Tertiary prevention

- *Camellia sinensis* (green tea) (evidence strongest for breast cancer)

References

1. You WC, Blot WJ, Change YS, et al. Diet and high risk of stomach cancer in Shandong, China. Cancer Res 1988; 48: 3518–23
2. Nishino H, Iwashima A, Itakura Y, et al. Anti-tumor-promoting activity of garlic extracts. Oncology 1989; 46: 277–80
3. Dorant E, van den Brandt PA, Goldbohm RA, et al. Garlic and its significance for the prevention of cancer in humans: a critical view. Br J Cancer 1993; 67: 424–9
4. Ip C, Lisk DJ. Efficacy of cancer prevention by high-selenium garlic is primarily dependent on

the action of selenium. Carcinogenesis 1995; 16: 2649–52

5. Bushman JL. Green tea and cancer in humans: a review of the literature. Nutr Cancer 1998; 31: 151–9

6. Mizuno S. Watanabe S, Nakamura K, et al. A multi-institute case-control study on the risk factors of developing pancreatic cancer. Jpn J Clin Oncol 1992; 22: 286–91

7. Kono S, Shinchi K, Ikeda N, et al. Physical activity, dietary habits and adenomatous polyps of the sigmoid colon: a study of self-defense officials in Japan. J Clin Epidemiol 1991; 44: 1255–61

8. Blot WJ, Chow WH, McLaughlin JK. Tea and cancer: a review of the epidemiological evidence. Eur J Cancer Prev 1996; 5: 425–38

9. Watanabe Y, Tada M, Kawamoto K, et al. A case-control study of cancer of the rectum and the colon. Nippon Shokakibyo Gakkai Zasshi 1984; 81: 185–93

10. Ji BT, Chow WH, Hsing AW, et al. Green tea consumption and the risk of pancreatic and colorectal cancers. Int J Cancer 1997; 70: 255–8

11. Kato I, Tominaga S, Matsuura A, et al. A comparative case-control study of colorectal cancer and adenoma. Jpn J Cancer Res 1990; 81: 1101–8

12. Oguni I, Cheng SJ, Lin PZ, Hara Y. Protection against cancer risk by Japanese green tea [Abstr]. Jpn J Cancer Res 1985; 76: 705–16

13. Tajima K, Tominaga S. Dietary habits and gastro-intestinal cancers: a comparative case-control study of stomach and large intestinal cancers in Nagoya, Japan. Jpn J Cancer Res 1985; 76: 705–16

14. Yu G, Hseih C. Risk factors for stomach cancer: a population-based control study in Shanghai, China. Cancer Causes Control 1991; 2: 169–74

15. Yu G, Hsieh C, Wang L, Yu S, et al. Green tea consumption and risk of stomach cancer: a population-based case-control study in Shanghai, China. Cancer Causes Control 1995; 6: 532–8

16. Ji BT, Chow WH, Yang G, et al. The influence of cigarette smoking, alcohol, and green tea consumption on the risk of carcinoma of the cardia and distal stomach in Shanghai, China. Cancer 1996; 77: 2449–57

17. Kono S, Ikeda M, Tokudome S, Kuratsune M. A case-control study of gastric cancer and diet in Norther Kyushu, Japan. Jpn J Cancer Res 1988; 79: 1067–74

18. Hoshiyama Y, Sasaba T. A case-control study of stomach cancer and its relation to diet, cigarettes, and alcohol consumption in Saitama Prefecture, Japan. Cancer Causes Control 1992; 3: 441–8

19. Lee HH, Wu HY, Chuang YC, et al. Epidemiologic characteristics and multiple risk factors of stomach cancers in Taiwan. Anticancer Res 1990; 10: 875–82

20. Galanis DJ, Lee J, Kolonel LN. The influence of cigarette smoking, alcohol and green tea consumption on the risk of carcinoma of the cardia and distal stomach in Shanghai, China. Cancer 1997; 79: 1840–1

21. Inoue M, Tajima K, Hirose K, et al. Life-style and subsite of gastric cancer - joint effect of smoking and drinking habits. Int J Cancer 1994; 56: 494–9

22. Ji BT, Chow WH, Hsing AW, et al. Green tea consumption and the risk of pancreatic and colorectal cancers. Int J Cancer 1997; 70: 255–8

23. Wakai K, Ohno Y, Obata K, Aoki K. Prognostic significance of selected lifestyle factors in urinary bladder cancer. Jpn J Cancer Res 1993; 84: 1223–9

24. Nagano J, Kono S, Preston DL, Mabucki K. A prospective study of green tea consumption and cancer incidence, Hiroshima and Nagasaki (Japan). Cancer Causes Control 2001; 12: 501–8

25. Imai K, Suga K, Nakachi K. Cancer-preventive effects of drinking green tea among a Japanese population. Prev Med 1997; 26: 769–75

26. Pisters KM, Newman RA, Coldman B, et al. Phase I trial of oral green tea extract in adult patients with solid tumors. J Clin Oncol 2001; 19: 1830–8

27. Lin JK, Liang YC, Lin-Shiau SY. Cancer chemoprevention by tea polyphenols through mitotic signal transduction blockade. Biochem Pharmacol 1999; 58: 911–15

28. Mittal A, Pate MS, Wylie RC, et al. EGCG down-regulates telomerase in human breast carcinoma MCF-7 cells, leading to suppression of cell viability and induction of apoptosis. Int J Oncol 2004; 24: 703–10

29. Fujiki H, Suganuma M, Okabe S, et al. A new concept of tumor promotion by tumor necrosis

factor-alpha, and cancer preventive agents (-)-epigallocatechin gallate and green tea – a review. Cancer Detect Prev 2000; 24: 91–9

30. Fujiki H. Two stages of cancer prevention with green tea. J Cancer Res Clin Oncol 1999; 125: 589–97

31. Kuroda Y, Hara Y. Antimutagenic and anticarcinogenic activity of tea polyphenols. Mutat Res 1999; 436: 69–97

32. Zhu M, Chen Y, Li R. Oral absorption and bioavailability of tea catechins. Planta Med 2000; 66: 444–7

33. Lahiri-Chatterjee M, Katiyar S, Mohan R, Agarwal R. A flavonoid antioxidant, silymarin, affords exceptionally high protection against tumor promotion in the SENCAR mouse skin tumorigenesis model. Cancer Res 1999; 59: 622–32

34. Bhatia N, Zhao J, Wolf D, Agarwal R. Inhibition of human carcinoma cell growth and DNA synthesis by silibinin, an active constituent of milk thistle: comparison with silymarin. Cancer Lett 1999; 147: 77–84

35. Zi X, Mukhtar H, Agarwal R. Novel cancer chemopreventive effects of a flavonoid antioxidant silymarin: inhibition of mRNA expression of an endogenous tumor promoter TNFα. Biochem Biophys Res Commun 1997; 239: 334–9

36. Tyagi A, Agarwal C, Harrison G, et al. Silibinin causes cell cycle arrest and apoptosis in human bladder transitional cell carcinoma cells by regulating CDKI-CDK-cyclin cascade, and caspase 3 and PARP cleavages. Carcinogenesis 2004; 25: 1711–20

37. Sarkar FH, Li Y. Soy isoflavones and cancer prevention. Cancer Invest 2003; 21: 744–57

38. Martin P, Horwitz K, Ryan D, McGuire W. Phytoestrogen interaction with estrogen receptors in human breast cancer cells. Endocrinology 1978; 103: 1860–67

39. Barnes S. Soy isoflavones – phytoestrogens and what else? J Nutr 2004; 134: 1225S–1228S

40. Akiyama T, Ishida J, Nakagawa S, et al. Genistein, a specific inhibitor of tyrosine-specific protein kinases. J Biol Chem 1987; 262: 5592–5

41. Okura A, Arakawa H, Oka H, et al. Effect of genistein on topoisomerase activity and on the growth of [Val 12] Ha-ras-transformed NIH 3T3 cells. Biochem Biophys Res Commun 1988; 157: 183–9

42. Davis J, Kucuk O, Sarkar F. Genistein inhibits NF-kappa B activation in prostate cancer cells. Nutr Cancer 1999; 35: 167–74

43. Li Y, Sarker F. Inhibition of NF-kB activation in PC3 cells by genistein is mediated via Akt signaling pathway. Clin Cancer Res 2002; 8: 2369–71

44. Davis J, Muqim N, Bhuiyan M, et al. Inhibition of prostate specific antigen expression by genistein in prostate cancer cells. Int J Cancer 2000; 16: 1091–97

45. Tan M, Yao J, Yu D. Overexpression of the c-erbB-2 gene enhanced intrinsic metastasis potential in human breast cancer cells without increasing their transformation abilities. Cancer Res 1997; 57: 1199–205

46. Alhasan S, Aranha O, Sarkar F. Genistein elicits pleiotropic molecular effects on head and neck cancer cells. Cancer Res 2001; 7: 4174–81

11e

Energy medicine

Suzanne Clewell

GENERAL CANCER PREVENTION

There are numerous physical factors that may contribute to someone either remaining healthy throughout their life or contracting a disease such as cancer. Heredity, environmental exposures and lifestyle choices are all accepted as factors that can predispose an individual to getting cancer at some point.

From an energy medicine perspective, however, we have access to a power that can place a variable in the midst of those factors. The practice of energy medicine subscribes to the belief that the prevention of cancer is accomplished by maintaining an optimal flow of Qi throughout the body. This involves a commitment to taking care of our body, mind and spirit.

Cancer or disease will eventually present itself if there is a blockage of the life force energy that is ignored and not dealt with. It is compared to a cutting off of the circulation of blood to an organ; eventually it will suffer and die. These blockages may have a number of causes, but trauma, either physical or emotional, is often the culprit. Trauma may be the result of issues from one's childhood that have been carried along through life. The practice of forgiveness is one of the primary ways we can get our life energy flowing again.

Practitioners of the biofield techniques, or energy medicine, work with the chakras to help them to function optimally as vortices of energy exchange. Each of the seven major chakras is associated with specific parts of the physical body. A blockage of energy in a chakra can lead to health problems (e.g. cancer, heart disease) in the area that it governs. Being in tune with this phenomenon can help us discover the underlying or root cause of a physical ailment that might otherwise remain undetected. Awareness of the chakras, their functions and effects on the physical body can be beneficial to us as well as our patients.

There is some research to support the finding that energy medicine boosts the immune system. The relaxation component reduces stress, and stress reduction is important in preventing illness. When Qi flows smoothly throughout the meridians of the body, good health is maintained. Research on prevention, however, is difficult to validate.

PRIMARY PREVENTION

The North American Nursing Diagnosis Association in 1995–1996 classified energy disturbance as a professional nursing diagnosis. It is defined as 'a disruption of the flow of energy surrounding a person's being which results in disharmony of the body, mind, and/or spirit.'[1]

Vibrational, biofield or energy medicine views the body as an integrated life–energy system that provides a vehicle for human consciousness. In the world of vibrational medicine illness is thought to be caused not only by exposure to germs, toxins and physical trauma but also by chronic dysfunctional emotion-energy patterns and unhealthy ways of relating to ourselves and others[2].

In his book *A Practical Guide to Vibrational Medicine,* Richard Gerber explains that, although we may inherit a tendency toward a particular disease, there must be numerous other factors working together to allow that disease to manifest. Diet, genetics and environmental exposures are all measurable physical factors included in the human equation of who becomes ill and who does not. However, often two individuals who have these same factors operating in unison will have very different outcomes – one becoming ill while the other remains healthy. Gerber states that, along with the growing body of evidence that points to the importance of psychosomatic medicine and psychoneuroimmunology in showing us that our emotions can play an extremely important role in disease causation, the physiology of the mind–body connection has more facets to it than just the problems caused by the stress-induced neurochemical imbalance. The vibrational–medical model teaches us that our mind–body–spirit complex is positively or negatively impacted upon by the health of our thoughts and our emotions and the amount of love that we allow to flow through our hearts (reference 2, p. 404). Gerber states 'Our reactions to life are recorded not only in the biochemical patterns of memory storage in the brain but also in the seven major life centers (chakras) of the body' (reference 2, p. 10).

It would certainly be preferable to treat the imbalance while it is still only a disturbance in the energy field rather than waiting until it has progressed into a physical symptom that is more difficult to reverse or treat. Maintaining the flow of Qi in and around us is accomplished in various ways, and it should be a natural occurrence. Probably the most effective way to maintain our flow of life-giving energy is not to subscribe to lifestyle choices that impede the flow. Letting go of anger, grief, hatred, envy, ego and anything that our body tells us is detrimental is the most important step. Practicing unconditional love and forgiveness, although admittedly very difficult at first for most of us, is the most rewarding and effective method for surrounding ourselves with healing energy and not cutting off the vital force. Dismissing unhealthy habits such as smoking, unhealthy eating and sedentary lifestyles in favor of proper diet and exercise will supply our bodies with additional sources of positive energy vital for maintaining health. Listening to the messages that our body sends to us is basic to being able to supply what may be needed or has been depleted.

To maintain health it is necessary to clear negative energy coming from past experiences. This is integral in helping to maintain the healthy immune system that is our primary defense against disease.

Recommendations for primary prevention

One of the ways it is believed that energy medicine works is to open the pathways of communication that enable cells in the body to 'talk to each other'. It opens up the terrain through which cells are able to migrate to places where they are needed to fight disease or initiate repair. Energy medicine is also effective in calming the individual so that the immune system can operate at an optimum level[3].

The impact of one individual's energies on another has been scientifically studied.

Electrocardiographs showed that the energy produced by the heart of one person would have an effect upon the heart activity and brain waves of another person. This effect was measurable even when the subjects were sitting as far apart as 3 feet[4]. Energies from non-human sources affect us as well. Energies in our environment can be beneficial or harmful.

Individuals considered at high risk for energy disturbance, which could eventually lead to disease, would be those whose life experience includes emotional, mental or physical trauma. This may be attributable to multiple sources such as grief, abuse, fear, family dysfunction, physical injury or disability. One's perceptions are one's reality. Adjustments may be made through the use of energy medicine to facilitate the healing of these perceptions and restore the optimal flow of Qi.

It is hypothesized that unhealthy electromagnetic fields (EMF) may potentially lead to a higher risk of developing certain cancers and disorders. Daily computer use or exposure to other electrical equipment, living in close proximity to power lines or microwave towers, even the use of electric blankets or heating pads may be the source of unhealthy exposures. The research in this area is still inconclusive and additional studies are needed.

In her book *Hands of Light,* Barbara Brennan tells us that energy fields are intimately associated with a person's health and well-being. If a person is unhealthy, it will show in his energy field as an unbalanced flow of energy and/or stagnated energy that has ceased to flow and appears as darkened colors. In contrast, a healthy individual will show bright colors that flow easily in a balanced field[5].

SECONDARY PREVENTION

Energy medicine has a multi-faceted role to play in secondary prevention of cancer.

Detection and screening for disease (or energy disturbance) is an integral part of the energy medicine practitioner's initial assessment prior to a full body treatment. Subtle changes in the energy field surrounding all living things can be detected through the hands of the energy worker. Some who work with these subtle energies are also medical intuitives and can sense what may be happening inside the body. If an anomaly is located, further investigation in the form of more medically traditional screening and diagnostic tests can be ordered.

Cessation of exposure to carcinogenic agents is a major component of secondary prevention. The fabric of energy medicine is about love and respect for ourselves and appreciation of life. Receiving healing energy can provide the strength needed for an individual to stop smoking cigarettes or using drugs or alcohol inappropriately.

TERTIARY PREVENTION

Quite often we hear the person who has had cancer state that it has changed their lives. They appreciate each new day as a gift and live more 'mindfully'. To have gleaned this message from having experienced cancer can lead to a life-altering attitude and a search for more knowledge on the part of the survivor. This search often leads them to complementary medicine.

Ideally, guidance and information regarding integrative options would be provided to the patient in the oncologist's office some time during the course of the treatment regimen. There is a plethora of 'new age' practitioners today and the cancer patient, desperate to attain optimum health, may be taken in by individuals who may not be of the purest intention. The ideal situation would be one in which the oncologist was the hub of the wheel with spokes from whose direction the patient would be sent to the appropriate complementary practitioners.

In the process of healing it is essential that the patient contemplate the deeper meaning of his illness. Individuals who live long past the expected survival times for their prognosis appear to have reversed the kind of adaptation to life that has been shown to be associated with the onset of some types of cancer[6]. 'There is a mirrored symmetry between the psychological patterns possibly promoting disease and the changed adaptations that may lead to a longer survival in some cases.'[7] Is there something that this illness is telling the patient, something to be learned? To quote Barbara Brennan 'The source of the illness needs to be searched for in this way. A return to health requires much more personal work and change than simply taking pills. Without personal change you will eventually create another problem to lead you back to the source that caused the disease in the first place' (reference 5, p. 7). An obvious example would be the patient presenting with lung cancer with a long history of tobacco use. Continuing this habit after receiving treatment for his illness rejects the possibility of life change, or the opportunity of learning from the experience, and eventually the pattern is repeated. On a deeper level, the tobacco use may be used as a crutch to conceal some traumatic life event that is unresolved. The source of illness is not always in plain sight. People unknowingly may resist healing because the illness benefits them in some way. A decisive choice to heal must be made by the client.

Eric Pearl states that it is not the disease that is healed, it is the human being. 'Resistance to a healing can take many forms, some of them so thoroughly linked to other aspects of a patient's life that you can only see them with a lot of perspective'.[8] In her book *Why People Don't Heal and How They Can*, Caroline Myss addresses this issue when she explains how we are ultimately responsible for our own health. She states that our 'biography becomes our biology' and that forgiveness is the single most important thing one can do for one's 'biology'. She believes that many people practice what she has termed 'woundology'. This is the language of past traumas and resentments that enable those who use it to manipulate or legitimize otherwise unethical behavior. It provides a surrounding comfort zone while at the same time giving one permission to resist change in their lives. Through 'woundology' unhealthy relationships may be created in which each person's wounds are honored. One may even become addicted to the power the wound may supply. The person entrenched in his wounds may feel that others 'owe' him. His requirement may be sympathy, certain privileges (such as sick days off from work), support from family and friends which may be in the form of financial or emotional. This is a handicap to healing. Often those who care for this person will feed into the language of the wounded and misconstrue this as nurturing. By subscribing to woundology one's energy is focused in the past. For healing to occur it is necessary to bring one's energy out of the past, release the wounds we carry with us, embrace the present and practice forgiveness'[9].

Rosalyn Bruyere feels that 'Cancer, perhaps more than any other disease, represents a misuse of power.' In cancer, the body believes that the tumor that has been created must be nourished and protected in the same manner as an injury. So, using the wrong kind of power for the wrong thing, the body sends a blood supply and feeds the tumor. Bruyere states that often cancer patients have had lives filled with crises and loss and consider themselves undeserving. 'They have difficulty accepting and using power properly. Inappropriate use of power, as well as grief and fear, is connected to the body's inability to produce white blood cells to fight off malignancy. When cancer patients reorder their psychological inventories, their bodies can, and will fight the disease.'[10]

Energy healing is successful if the client is receptive to it and a connection is made with the universal energies available to all. The healing is magnified by the healer or practitioner, who has honed the ability to focus this available energy. The intention is to have healing occur in whatever manner is deemed by the creative intelligence to be most appropriate for this person at this particular time. A healing will occur; exactly what that healing may entail is not up to the discretion of the healer.

Recommendations for tertiary prevention

The objective of tertiary prevention in oncology is to prevent further disability and restore a higher level of functioning to the patient. Treatment, rehabilitation and pain control are areas in which energy medicine may hold promise.

One of the most common complaints cancer patients have is that of fatigue. Energy medicine by its very nature can assist in replenishing some of this vital energy.

'The application of external Qi has been reported to protect *normal* cells from harmful assaults, increase anti-tumor immunity, reduce tumor metastases, promote cell death of tumor cells, and increase survival time of tumor-embedded animals.'[11]

Qi Gong has been reported in both *in vitro* and *in vivo* studies to have all the positive effects of external Qi as well as the ability to produce analgesic effects and increase blood flow to vital organs (reference 11, pp. 115–116).

The subject of energy medicine as it relates to pain is frequently studied. In a double-blind crossover study in which the treatment group consisted of 21 patients having surgery for an impacted third molar, distance healing was used (Reiki and LeShan). No placebo was necessary as patients were unaware of whether they were being prayed for or not. The treatment group showed a decrease in the intensity of pain and greater relief of pain postoperatively[12]. A study to determine whether Healing Touch could be clinically effective[13] concluded that its data supported Healing Touch as an effective modality for health enhancement in raising secretory immunoglobulin A concentrations, reducing stress and relieving pain[13].

Music therapy is used to promote relaxation, reduce anxiety and supplement other pain control methods[14]. A study[15] concluded that listening to music along with a positive suggestion of pain reduction had an effect on the pain level of cancer patients. 'Given the initial effectiveness of music, its availability, and low risks, future research is needed to help identify the specific parameters of its usefulness.'[15]

Wound healing is a concern for the patient who has had surgery or may be experiencing skin irritation from radiation therapy. Wirth carried out a study in 1990 in which 44 volunteers received a punch biopsy in the arm, some received a 5-minute non-contact Therapeutic Touch healing and the rest received no treatment. Treatments were administered daily for 16 days. On the eighth day the Therapeutic Touch group had significantly smaller wounds and by day 16 the number of wounds differed significantly[16]. According to the text *Healing Intention and Energy Medicine*[11], the three best-designed reported studies demonstrated statistically significant positive effects of non-contact Therapeutic Touch on anxiety, pain control and wound healing (reference 11, p. 97).

Research has not given definitive answers in the field of energy medicine. The difficulties in setting controls and defining measurements go with the territory of spirituality and subtle energies. This has not discouraged respected hospitals and medical facilities throughout the world from offering energetic healing to their patients for relief of stress and anxiety and reduction of pain.

References

1. Dossy BM, Keegan L, Guzzetta CE. Holistic Nursing: A Handbook for Practice, 3rd edn. Gaithersburg, MD: Aspen Publishers, 2000: 621

2. Gerber R. A Practical Guide to Vibrational Medicine: Energy Healing and Spiritual Transformation. New York: HarperCollins Publishers, 2000: 3–6

3. Oschman JL. Interview with William Lee Rand. Reiki News Magazine, vol. one, issue three, Winter 2002: 1–8

4. McCraty R. The Electricity of Touch. Paper presented at The International Society for the Study of Subtle Energies and Energy Medicine. Sixth Annual Conference, Boulder, CO, June 1996. Available through the HeartMath Institute. www.webcom/hrtmath

5. Brennan BA. Hands of Light: A Guide to Healing Through the Human Energy Field. New York: Bantam Books, 1988: 7

6. Temoshok L, Dreher H. The Type C Connection: The Behavioral Links to Cancer and Your Health. New York: Random House, 1992

7. Cunningham AJ, Watson Kimberely MA. How Psychological Therapy May Prolong Survival in Cancer Patients: New Evidence and a Simple Theory. Integrat Cancer Ther 2004; 3: 214–29

8. Pearl E. The Reconnection: Heal Others Heal Yourself. Carlsbad, CA: Hay House, 2001: 143

9. Myss C. Why People Don't Heal and How They Can. Audiocassette. Boulder, CO: Sounds True, 1997

10. Bruyere RL. Wheels of Light: Chakras, Auras, and the Healing Energy of the Body. New York: Fireside, 1994: 190

11. Jonas WB, Crawford CC. Healing Intention and Energy Medicine: Science, Research Methods and Clinical Applications. London, UK: Churchill Livingstone, 2003: 105

12. Wirth DP, Brenlan DR, Levine RJ, Rodriguez CM. The effect of complementary healing therapy on postoperative pain after surgical removal of impacted third molar teeth. Complement Ther Med 1993; 1: 133–8

13. Wilkerson DS, Knox PL, Chatman JE, et al. The clinical effectiveness of Healing Touch. J Alternative Complement Medicine 2002; 8: 33–47

14. Bailey LM. The use of songs with cancer patients and their families. Music Ther 1984; 4: 5–17

15. Zimmerman L, Pozehl B, Duncan K, Schmitz R. Effects of music in patients who had chronic cancer pain. Western J Nurs Res 1989; 11: 298–309

16. Wirth DP. The effect of non-contact Therapeutic Touch on the healing rate of full-thickness dermal wounds. Subtle Energies 1990; 1: 1–20

12

Modalities – supportive care

The field of supportive care in oncology is rapidly growing. This is evidenced by the wide range of experiences that individuals can face during the process of cancer prevention, diagnosis, treatment and after-care. There is at least one journal dedicated to the subject – *The Journal of Supportive Oncology* (www.SupportiveOncology.net) – and entire meetings are dedicated to the field (1st Chicago Supportive Oncology Conference, September, 2005 (CSOC@SupportiveOncology. net)). The American Society of Clinical Oncology (ASCO) states as its policy that 'it is the oncologists' responsibility to care for their patients in a continuum that extends from the moment of diagnosis throughout the course of illness.' Further, ASCO emphasizes that 'cancer care optimizes quality of life throughout the course of an illness through meticulous attention to the myriad physical, spiritual, and psychosocial needs of the patient and family.' (http://www.asco.org).

This chapter will explore supportive care measures in general oncology care. This will include managing both cancer and treatment-related symptoms. A broad range of symptoms can occur, including sleep changes, pain, depression, anxiety, weight gain/loss, changes related to sexuality, fatigue, mucositis, nausea and diarrhea. An integrative oncology addresses these situations for all involved in cancer care.

12a

Physical activity

Robert B. Lutz

The overwhelming evidence supporting the health benefits of physical activity has been well noted[1]. In addition to its role in preventing many chronic diseases (e.g. cardiovascular disease, type 2 diabetes mellitus, overweight and obesity), it also serves to lessen many symptoms of illness that individuals experience, such as sleep disturbances, depression and anxiety, muscle and joint stiffness/inflexibility and imbalance. Regular physical activity promotes general well-being, alleviation of stress and improved self-esteem. Although documentation of these benefits has primarily been seen in non-cancer patients, it is reasonable to believe that they would be experienced by patients with cancer as well[2].

Fatigue is a common symptom of patients with cancer at all stages in their course. The exact mechanism for this is not known, but it is probably multifactorial (e.g. impaired nutritional status, metabolic disturbances, pain, medications). Additionally, depression may accompany this symptom as well as playing a causative role. It is interesting that, historically, physicians have recommended that their patients 'rest' in response to this fatigue. Although appropriate rest is a necessary component of any set of recommendations, inappropriate rest may establish

a self-reciprocating cycle of increasing muscle weakness, leading to greater fatigue. Physical activity and exercise may break this cycle by re-establishing more normal cardiorespiratory and musculoskeletal fitness. Additionally, individuals may gain a sense of mastery and personal control over their illness, leading to improved mood[3].

The first such report presented in the early 1980s found that women with breast cancer undergoing chemotherapy, who were enrolled in a bicycle ergometer training program of 30 minutes, three times per week for 10 weeks, demonstrated improved physical performance compared to controls[4]. Subsequent research found that individuals also experienced improved mood and anthropometric parameters (i.e. body weight and per cent body fat)[5]. Exercise may also address chronic anemia, a common finding in patients with cancer-related fatigue. Sixteen patients enrolled in an aerobic exercise program following high-dose chemotherapy and stem cell transplantation were compared to controls. Physical performance (maximum speed on the treadmill test), cardiac function and hemoglobin concentration were compared at baseline and 7 weeks later. Fatigue and limitations in daily activities due to impaired endurance were assessed during personal interviews. At follow-up, individuals in the training group demonstrated improved physical performance, increased hemoglobin and less fatigue than controls. The results of this study suggested that physical activity, rather than rest, should be encouraged[6]. The research therefore suggests that the effects of physical activity on cancer-related fatigue are both physiologic and psychologic.

RECOMMENDATIONS

It is important for clinicians to tailor their physical activity and exercise recommendations as determined by the unique situation of the individual patient with cancer. An emphasis should be placed upon getting all individuals to limit their sedentary behavior and increase their activity as tolerated. The recommendations below are those provided to the general population and should be seen as a goal rather than an absolute.

Adopt a physically active lifestyle.

Adults:

- Engage in at least moderate aerobic physical activity for ≥ 30 minutes on most, preferably all days of the week.

- Engage in resistance training 2–3 days per week. A minimum of 8-10 exercises involving the major muscle groups should be performed that incorporate a minimum of one set of 8–15 repetitions[7].

Youths:

- Accumulate at least 60 minutes, and up to several hours, of age-appropriate moderate-to-vigorous physical activity on most, preferably all, days of the week[8].

All individuals should look to incorporate more physical activity into their daily lives. Simple measures such as the following can enhance regular activity and improve overall health.

- Wear a pedometer to gauge daily activity levels.

- Engage in moderate housework and/or yard-work where and when available.

- 'Actively commute' by walking or bicycling where and when appropriate.

- Take walk breaks at work.

- Take the stairs rather than the elevator or escalator.

- Schedule 'activity-focused' family outings and vacations, such as skiing, hiking or rafting.

- Get together regularly with friends and/or family members for activity outings.

- Walk the dog.

- Take the first available parking space and walk to the store entrance.

- Carry bags of groceries in from the car one at a time.

The American Cancer Society identifies specific issues for cancer survivors that may prevent or limit their physical activity[9].

- Individuals with anemia should refrain from activity, other than those of daily living (ADL), until anemia improves.

- Individuals with compromised immune systems should avoid public gyms and other public venues; survivors after bone marrow transplantation should avoid these spaces for 1 year following transplant.

- Persons experiencing significant fatigue should listen to their bodies and do as much as they feel able to do, and are encouraged to do 10 minutes of stretching daily.

- Individuals should avoid chlorinated pools if undergoing radiation therapy.

- Persons with indwelling catheters should avoid water or other microbial exposures that may result in infections. They should also avoid resistance training that may cause dislodgement of the catheter.

- Persons who are experiencing significant peripheral neuropathy that may impede their ability to perform exercises and activities that make use of the affected limbs may consider using a recumbent bicycle or similar exercise equipment in controlled settings rather than performing activities outdoors.

References

1. Physical Activity and Health: A Report of the Surgeon General. Atlanta, GA: US Department of Health and Human Services, Centers for Disease Control, National Center for Chronic Disease Prevention and Health Promotion, 1996

2. Physical Activity Fundamental to Preventing Disease. US Department of Health and Human Services. Office of the Assistant Secretary for Planning and Evaluation, 20 June 2002

3. Dimeo FC. Effects of exercise on cancer-related fatigue. Cancer 2001; 92: 1689–93

4. Winningham ML. Effects of a bicycle ergometry program on functional capacity and feelings of control of patient with breast cancer (dissertation). Columbus, OH: Ohio State University, 1983

5. MacVicar MG, Winningham ML, Nickel JL. Effects of aerobic interval training on cancer patients' functional capacity. Nurs Res 1989; 38: 348–51

6. Dimeo FC, Tilmann MH, Bertz H, et al. Aerobic exercise in the rehabilitation of cancer patients after high dose chemotherapy and autologous peripheral stem cell transplantation. Cancer 1997; 79: 1717–22

7. Pollock ML, Gaesser GA, Butcher JD, et al. American College of Sports Medicine Position Stand: The recommended quantity and quality of exercise for developing and maintaining cardiorespiratory and muscular fitness, and flexibility in healthy adults. Med Sci Sports Exerc 1998; 30: 975–91

8. Physical Activity for Children: A Statement of Guidelines for Children Ages 5–12. Reston, VA: NASPE, 2003

9. Brown JK, Byers T, Doyle C, et al. Nutrition and physical activity during and after cancer treatment: an American Cancer Society guide for informed choices. CA Cancer J Clin 2003; 53: 268–91

12b

Nutrition

Mara Vitolins and Cynthia Thomson

THE ROLE OF DIET DURING CANCER THERAPY

Nutrition recommendations for cancer patients may be very different from the usual nutrition-related guidelines. In some cases, the recommendations given to cancer patients may be completely opposite to what they have heard, which may cause the patient to be confused about who and what to believe. For example, patients may be given instructions to consume more high-calorie foods, and to eat less of certain high-fiber foods, since these may exacerbate problems such as a sore mouth or diarrhea. Additionally dietitians may suggest that a patient eat more fats such as oil, margarine and butter, and to put high-fat gravies and sauces on their foods – advice that certainly is not on any healthy eating guidelines. These recommendations, however, are typically given to help cancer patients build strength and better tolerate the effects of the cancer and the prescribed cancer treatment. See Tables 12.1 and 12.2 for guidelines concerning disease-specific recommendations and a low-residue diet.

Weight management

Patients may not experience changes in weight during their cancer treatment. However, some may gain weight. Typically these patients include those being treated for breast, prostate and ovarian cancer and are using hormone therapy or chemotherapy. Patients should be encouraged to discuss weight gain with their physician in order to evaluate the cause. If the patient is found to be edematous, a lower sodium diet might be suggested and a prescription diuretic may be in order.

Cancer survivors who may benefit from modest weight loss should be encouraged to lose no more than two pounds per week during treatment[1,2]. Weight loss should be closely monitored and should be discontinued if it has the potential to interfere with treatment. Weight loss should be accomplished by consuming a well-balanced diet and participating in moderate physical activity tailored to the needs of the particular patient[3].

Unintentional weight loss

Among patients with non-hormone-related cancers, and particularly those with advanced

Table 12.1 Web-based tips for coping with treatment-related symptoms that alter diet

Treatment	Nutrition problem	Symptom management
Radiation therapy		
Head and neck	lack of smell	add spices, heat food
	xerostomia	soften foods with gravy, sauces; liquids with meals; energy-dense beverages (e.g. Ensure®, Boost®)
	loss of teeth	soft diet, ground meat, energy-dense beverages
	dysphagia	upright sitting position during and after meals; caution with thin liquids; use of food-thickening agents, such as corn starch
Abdomen/pelvis	diarrhea	fluids such as Pedialyte®, avoid lactose-containing foods (milk, ice cream); trial probiotic foods such as yogurt (live cultures)
	nausea/vomiting	small, frequent meals; cold foods; bland foods – avoid spicy food; hydrate
	stenosis/obstruction	caution with fiber; adequate fluids; low residue diet (see Table 12.2)
Surgical therapy		
Radical head/neck	chewing/swallowing difficulties	see 'dysphagia' above
	gastric stasis	higher carbohydrate/simple sugar with meals, such as table sugar; liquid-rich meals
Esophagectomy	steatorrhea: symptom in which fecal matter is frothy, foul-smelling and floats because of a high fat content. It is common in malabsorption syndromes	Low-fat diet; supplemental water-soluble/fat-soluble vitamin supplement to replace nutrients lost in fecal matter
	diarrhea	as above
Gastrectomy	early satiety	small, frequent meals; liquids between meals; energy-dense food and beverage selections
	dumping syndrome: gastro-intestinal symptoms resulting from rapid gastric emptying. usually occurs following gastric surgery	fiber; low-carbohydrate diet; avoidance of simple sugars, such as table sugar, and consuming complex carbohydrates such as pectins and guar, is encouraged because these compounds slow gastric emptying and diminish symptoms
	vitamin B_{12} deficiency	vitamin B_{12} supplementation
Intestinal resection	early satiety	see above
	diarrhea	see above

Continued

Table 12.1   Continued

Treatment	Nutrition problem	Symptom management
Intestinal resection	malabsorption of most B vitamins	supplementation of B vitamins (marketed as B-complex vitamin supplements)
	dehydration	fluids and electrolytes, Pedialyte®, Gatorade®
Drug treatment		
Corticosteroids	nitrogen, calcium losses	calcium supplementation, amount and type (suggest high-protein foods)
	hyperglycemia	modified sugar/carbohydrate diet; lower glycemic index eating plan; increase fiber
Sex hormone analogs	nausea, emesis	see above
Immunotherapy	fluid retention	reduce salt intake; monitor fluid intake
General chemotherapeutic agents	nausea, emesis	see above
	fluid retention	see above
	oral/gastrointestinal ulcerations	liquid diet; citrus avoidance

Table 12.2   Low-residue diet recommendations

Group	Recommendations
Milk and milk products (2 or more cups daily)	low-residue diet only 2 cups daily of all milk products
Starches – bread and grains (4 or more servings/day)	bread, cereals, pasta made from refined flours, white rice
Fruits (2 or more servings/day)	fruit juices without pulp, canned fruit except melons, pineapple, ripe bananas
Vegetables (3 or more servings/day)	lettuce; vegetable juice without pulp; the following cooked vegetables: carrots, yellow squash (without seeds), green beans, wax beans, eggplant, potatoes (without skin), asparagus, beets
Meat or meat substitutes (5 to 6 oz daily)	meat, poultry, eggs, seafood (do not contain fiber)
Fats and oils (servings depend on caloric needs)	all oils, margarine, butter
Desserts and candy (amount depends on caloric needs)	all without fiber, avoid coconut
Miscellaneous	avoid popcorn, pickles, horseradish, relish

309

disease, weight loss becomes the norm. Cancer patients frequently become malnourished. This is often due not only to biochemical changes related to cancer cachexia, but also to poor dietary intake. It is widely accepted that malnutrition impairs immune function, is associated with cancer-related fatigue, depression, impaired wound healing and decreased quality of life. It is very important to encourage patients being treated for cancer to eat better overall (e.g. nutrient-dense foods – foods that are low in calories although high in nutrients) but compliance is often a problem as the side-effects of the treatment may cause food aversions. The patient should be encouraged to relate any food-related complications to the health care team immediately. The American Cancer Society has a section of their website devoted to cancer and nutrition during and after treatment that provides excellent information which patients can easily access at http://www.cancer.org.

Pretreatment weight loss has been found to be a major indicator of poor survival and response to cancer therapies[4]. Early and ongoing assessment of nutritional status, perhaps followed by an immediate intervention with nutritional support, is strongly recommended. The goals of this intervention are to avoid marked deterioration of the patient, improve nutritional and immunological measures, avoid complications, and potentially improve quality of life. The nutrition 'therapy' should be based on the knowledge of the specific situation of each patient (e.g. ability to consume food orally), assessment of his or her nutritional status using standard clinical nutrition assessment forms, response to treatment (e.g. magnitude of side-effects: nausea, vomiting), and the availability of social support (to assist in obtaining and preparing food).

The route of the nutritional support may be oral, enteral or parenteral, depending on the clinical situation. The oral route, supervised by the health-care team, is the safest and most effective, but the patient must be capable of maintaining adequate caloric intake and have a functioning digestive system.

It is critical that a dietitian be involved in evaluating each patient and be able to provide information for how best to provide nutrition support to the patient.

Antioxidant/micronutrient supplements during treatment

Patients may be anxious to try alternative and complementary therapies to feel more in control of their cancer treatment. It is very common for patients to try vitamin–mineral supplements and non-nutritive supplements. Supplements are considered to cause few, if any, side-effects and, because they can be purchased without a prescription, are thought to be non-toxic. Many supplements have undefined biologic impact on tumor activity, and also could potentially interfere with treatment regimens. The blood levels of conventional medications may be altered by over-the-counter supplements. For example, St John's wort may decrease the effectiveness of various medications including digoxin (for heart disease), statin drugs and chemotherapy drugs[5–7]. Particularly during treatment, cancer patients should be encouraged to discuss their use of supplements with their health-care team.

It has been reported that antioxidants may reduce adverse effects of radiation and chemotherapy; however, it has also been reported that they could diminish the therapeutic efficacy of these treatment regimens[8]. As free radical formation is central to the cytotoxic effects of radiation and some chemotherapy agents, the use of antioxidant vitamins may lower their effectiveness. Evidence for the ability of antioxidants to inhibit effectiveness of radiation treatment has been reported in animal trials[9]. Studies conducted in humans that have evaluated the combination of non-prescription antioxidants with chemotherapy and radiation have reported mixed results. Most studies have not reported differences in efficacy with antioxidant use, although one study did report inhibition of a chemotherapy agent by vitamin B_6[10]. These are issues of concern with regards to antioxidant use during treatment: (1) individual antioxidants have functional properties beyond their antioxidant activity and there is uncertainty regarding their effect on treatment regimens; (2) antioxidant activity may vary among cancer cell types; and (3) cancer patients may respond differently (e.g. body size, gender) to the dose of the antioxidant consumed. Owing to the lack of data regarding the use of antioxidants and their effect on treatment efficacy, it seems the safest approach for cancer patients to avoid the use of high-dose antioxidant supplements during treatment until convincing data advocating their use are made available.

Assessment of supplement use

It is important that dietary supplement use, including micronutrients and antioxidants, be routinely assessed during cancer treatment. Figure 1 is a sample dietary supplement intake form that can be used to assess intake, with an emphasis on supplements that are more commonly used by cancer patients and survivors.

Glutamine and arginine

The amino acids L-glutamine and L-arginine have been utilized as a therapeutic approach to the maintenance of the gastrointestinal (GI) tract by some providers of complementary and alternative medicine. Although neither is essential to the body, during times of stress they both can enhance the immune response[11]. In the body, L-glutamine is the preferred substrate for enterocytes and lymphocytes and increases nitrogen retention. It decreases the incidence of infection, has been shown in laboratory studies to decrease tumor growth, and may decrease toxicity due to chemotherapy[12–16]. L-Arginine stimulates the immune system, enhances the immune response in patients with malignancies, and also influences tumor latency, size and regression[17–19].

Although they have well-documented *in vitro* and *in vivo* effects, arginine and glutamine supplements are not yet considered as standard of care for either supportive or antineoplastic care. Increasingly, however, supplementation has been considered, in particular for patients undergoing bone marrow transplant chemotherapies[20,21]. In addition, select enteral formulas developed for use in clinical oncology also contain glutamine and/or arginine. Basic science research focused on glutamine supplementation during cancer has been conflicting, in that early *in vitro* work showed a proliferative effect of glutamine supplementation on tumor growth[22]. However, these findings were later dismissed with *in vivo* modeling by Bartlet *et al.*[23]. Of interest, Scott *et al.* demonstrated a reduction in malignant cell line survival when cells were deprived of arginine, suggesting that arginine may be utilitzed as a nutrient source by select cancer cells[24]. Data from a clinical trial conducted by Johnson *et al.*[25] found that oral glutamine supplementation restored the GI production of glutathione, thus reversing the block of glutathione transport from the GI tract to the liver associated with a specific type of breast cancer (7,12-dimethylbenz[a] antracene). In this animal model, 1 g/kg of glutamine was administered per day for 14 days. The effect was maintenance of GI glutathione production even in the presence of breast cancer cells, possibly representing one mechanism by which glutamine blocks carcinogenesis[25].

There is some compelling data for recommending supplementation during chemotherapy treatment. May *et al.* found that stage IV cancer patients with $\geq 5\%$ weight loss from a soild tumor had both increased fat-free mass and body weight when given an oral supplement containing 14 g L-glutamine, 14 g L-arginine and 3 g β-hydroxy-β-methylbutyrate for 4 weeks during treatment[26]. More randomized controlled clinical trials involving glutamine and arginine are needed, but the preliminary data presented here suggest that supplementing with glutamine

Dietary Supplement Intake Form for Oncology Care					
Supplement	Type	Dose	Frequency	Length of use	Reason for use
Multi-nutrient supplements					
Multivitamin					
Multivitamin-mineral					
Antioxidant vitamin complex					
B complex vitamin					
Single nutrients					
Vitamin A					
Vitamin C					
Vitamin D					
Vitamin E					
Folic acid					
Niacin					
B6					
B12					
Mineral/mineral combinations/trace elements					
Calcium					
Calcium with vitamin D					
Calcium with vitamin D and magnesium					
Magnesium					
Iron					
Selenium					
Zinc					
Food constituents or herbals					
Co-enzyme Q10					
Echinacea					
Evening primrose oil					
Fish oil					
Garlic					
Ginger					
Ginkgo					
Ginseng					
Grape seed					
Green tea					
Lycopene					
Maitake mushroom					
Milk thistle					
PC-SPES					
Red clover					
Reishi mushroom					
Saw palmetto					
Shark cartilage					
Soy					
Other not listed					

Figure 12.1   Sample dietary supplement intake form

during treatment may be of therapeutic benefit[27,28]. Supplementation could ameliorate cancer weight loss and increase tolerability to chemotherapeutic agents. Specific dosage levels for glutamine may vary across studies, ranging from 1.5 to 20 g/day.

DIETARY INTERVENTION IN THE SUPPORTIVE CARE SETTING

Meal supplements can be provided to minimize weight loss, prevent nutrition deficiencies and support the immune system response.

Cancer patients must consume adequate amounts of calories, protein, vitamins and minerals to avoid becoming malnourished, as this would adversely affect their immune systems, which could result in increased risk of infection and reduced treatment efficacy and tolerance. Malnutrition can range from slight weight loss (decreased appetite) to metabolic disturbances resulting in cancer cachexia.

Meal replacements/supplements

For cancer patients who are unable to consume an adequate diet, specific formulas can be used as a source of nutrition, or as supplements to meals. The health-care team should discuss which oral supplement would best suit the patient's needs (such as higher protein, or perhaps, lower fat meal replacement products). Enteral nutritional support can help normalize body protein levels, support immune function and assist in weight gain. The goal of nutritional support should be to improve survival, promote tolerance to therapy, maintain functional status and improve nutritional status[28]. Giving nutrition support for supplemental protein and energy (oral or enteral route) not only improves nutrition status, but has been reported to enhance survival in a wide range of adult patients[29].

Potter and colleagues[30] conducted a systematic review of randomized controlled trials comparing oral or enteral protein supplementation with no routine supplementation. All trials of adult subjects were included, except those addressing nutrition in pregnancy, in a wide range of clinical states and age groups. The study populations varied from chronically ill to relatively 'healthy', and included elderly and younger subjects. The 30 trials they analyzed, in total, involved more than 2000 patients. The results showed that patient groups that received routine nutrition support had consistent benefits. The treatment groups receiving routine nutritional supplementation showed consistently improved changes in body weight and anthropometry compared with controls. The benefits were similar statistically, regardless of the type of patient, illness and duration of treatment[30]. This evidence supports the use of routine nutrition support to elicit improvements in body weight.

Appetite enhancement

Loss of appetite due to altered taste, mouth sores, xerostomia, nausea and vomiting are common symptoms in patients undergoing cancer therapy. These nutritional problems have been addressed in Table 12.1. There are times when pharmacologic intervention is necessary. There are several pharmacologic agents that can be administered to improve saliva production and appetite in oncology patients (Table 12.3).

In addition to medications there are several dietary approaches which can be employed to enhance appetite. For example, many patients have improved appetite if they share meals with friends, have a *small* amount of alcohol with the meal, enhance the meal setting with candles, consider an outside venue for meals (picnic, patio), etc. Others will need to 'eat-by-the-clock', not waiting for their appetite to improve, but rather eating small amounts of energy-dense foods every 1–2 hours. To avoid nausea which may reduce appetite, nutrition practitioners

Table 12.3 Methods of appetite enhancement

Possible appetite-stimulating agents	Dose	Mechanism of action
Saliva stimulant		
Pilocarpine (*Salagen*®)	5 mg tablet TID	stimulates cholinergic receptors in the mouth to produce saliva
Appetite stimulant		*Side-effects:*
Megestrol (*Megace*®)	800 mg qd	edema, break-through bleeding and amenorrhea, headache, rash, weight gain
Dronabinol (*Marinol*®)	2.5 mg tablet BID	mood changes, increased appetite, hypotension, tachycardia, blurred vision
Metoclopramide (*Reglan*®) Cisapride (*Propulsid*®)	10 mg tablet four times per day	weakness, restlessness, drowsiness, diarrhea, insomnia, rash, dry mouth, extrapyramidal reactions (rare)

suggest eating small, frequent meals, avoiding foods with a strong smell such as fish or cruciferous vegetables, or snacking on dry, salted crackers. In addition, several websites have been developed to provide additional suggestions to enhance intake during cancer treatment, including websites of the American Cancer Society, the American Institute for Cancer Research and the Arizona Cancer Center Nutrition Ways.

Maintaining visceral protein stores

There are several mechanisms by which cancer patients can become protein deficient. Protein deficiency can result in an impaired immune response and generalized weakness which reduces the patient's ability to perform activities of daily living. Tumor necrosis factor-α is a substance that is produced by cancer cells. It can promote catabolic processes that result in protein degradation and suppression of protein synthesis as well as inducing anorexia. C-reactive protein (CRP) is a positive acute-phase respondent protein used to monitor stress reaction and as a potential indicator of the need for more aggressive nutrition

intervention. High levels of CRP are associated with suppression of albumin synthesis and are commonly seen during the initial phase of acute stress. If patients demonstrate increases in CRP concurrent with a reduction in prealbumin and/or albumin levels, efforts to initiate more substantial nutrition support should be employed. For example, patients who are on an oral diet may require supplemental protein-dense snacks or oral beverage supplements, while patients already receiving such supplementation may require enteral support to meet the increasing demand for protein. Daily monitoring of both protein and energy intake from all sources (oral, enteral and/or parenteral) is critical to ensuring either that the patient achieves positive nitrogen balance or that protein losses are minimized when positive nitrogen balance cannot be achieved.

Nutrition therapy in palliative care

Palliative care can be defined as the active total care of a patient when curative measures are no longer considered an option by either the medical team or the patient. The goals of nutritional therapy during this time could include: (1) managing symptoms of the disease or side-effects of treatment; (2) preventing further morbidity; and (3) maintaining an optimal quality of life through the provision of sufficient dietary intake to sustain energy and strength. As with all clinical situations in oncology care, the wishes of the patient and family must be taken into account during this period.

Hydration

Adequate hydration should be provided to maintain blood pressure, avoid electrolyte disturbance, combat constipation and minimize nephrotoxic effects of medications. If intravenous administration of fluids is necessary in order to accomplish these goals, the wishes of the patient and family members should be identified before administration. The American Medical Association's code of ethics views dehydration as appropriate when death is imminent and the patient does not want artificial hydration or nutrition. Generally in the terminal stages of disease, fluid requirements will need to be met using intravenous glucose/electrolyte solutions. Oral liquids may pose a risk for aspiration if the patient is not coherent. If the patient is able to swallow oral beverages safely, the choice of beverage should be first and foremost the beverage the patient selects. If there is a risk for aspiration, thicker liquids such as the 2.0 kcal/ml canned nutritional supplements may be more safely swallowed. Those who can tolerate thinner liquids should be encouraged to consume beverages that provide some nutrients, including electrolytes. Fluid can also be consumed in the form of foods such as flavored gelatins, popsicles, Italian ice, sorbet, etc., which are sometimes more palatable for the patient. Estimates of fluid requirements are generally based on the patient's body weight.

A good rule of practice is to provide 30 ml/kg body weight daily. Additional replacement will be necessary if the patient experiences fever, excess perspiration, diarrhea and/or losses through open wounds or ostomy sites.

Food as comfort/end-of-life care

Food can serve as a great source of comfort. During palliative care, patients should have the ability to decide what and when they are going to eat, with few exceptions. Feeding the terminally ill patient can be challenging, but it affords family members and significant others an opportunity actively to participate in the care process. Patients should be offered old favorites as well as foods associated with improved health, an indication that the family holds hope for the patient's well-being.

Risk of aspiration is a possible exception to the patient-dictated menu. In this situation the medical professional should do their best to get an appropriate substitution that is as close as possible to the original item selected. Certainly thin liquids or 'slippery' foods such as gelatin, custards or even oysters are of potential concern. Thickening agents are available to reduce the risk for aspiration. In addition, adding banana flakes or other dehydrated infant food can help to thicken the foods served.

During the advanced stages of disease many patients also experience anxiety and sleeplessness. Food can play a role in reducing these symptoms as well. In particular it is important to avoid foods containing caffeine, which can disturb sleep and increase anxiety. Highly spiced foods are also to be avoided. Alcohol can also contribute to sleeplessness and even depression. The folkore surrounding the use of warm milk actually does have merit, in that the amino acids in milk can promote serotonin production and induce sleep.

References

1. Expert Panel on the Identification, Evaluation, and Treatment of Overweight in Adults. Clinical guidelines on the identification, evaluation, and treatment of overweight and obesity in adults: executive summary. Am J Clin Nutr 1998; 68: 899–917

2. Cummings S, Parham ES, Strain GW. Position of the American Dietetic Association: Weight management. J Am Diet Assoc 2002; 102: 1145–1155

3. Brown JK, Byers T, Doyle C, et al. American Cancer Society. Nutrition and physical activity during and after cancer treatment: an American Cancer Society guide for informed choices. CA Cancer J Clin 2003; 53: 268–91

4. Ross PJ, Ashley S, Norton A, et al. Do patients with weight loss have a worse outcome when undergoing chemotherapy for lung cancers? Br J Cancer 2004; 90: 1905–11

5. Jobst KA, McIntyre M, St George D, et al. Safety of St John's wort (*Hypericum perforatum*). Lancet 2000; 355: 575

6. Sugimoto KK, Ohmori M, Tsuruoka S, et al. Different effects of St John's wort on the pharmacokinetics of simvastatin and pravastatin. Clin Pharmacol Ther 2001; 70: 518–24

7. Mathijssen RH, Verweij J, de Bruijn P, et al. Effects of St. John's wort on irinotecan metabolism. J Natl Cancer Inst 2002; 94: 1247–9

8. Lamson DW, Brignall MS. Antioxidants in cancer therapy; their actions and interactions with oncologic therapies. Altern Med Rev 1999; 4: 304–29

9. Sakamoto K, Sakka M. Reduced effect of irradiation on normal and malignant cells irradiated in vivo in mice pretreated with vitamin E. Br J Radiol 1973; 46: 538–40

10. Wiernik PH, Yeap B, Vogl SE, et al. Hexamethylmelamine and low or moderate dose cisplatin with or without pyridoxine for treatment of advanced ovarian carcinoma: a study of the Eastern Cooperative Oncology Group. Cancer Invest 1992; 10: 1–9

11. Field CJ, Johnson L, Pratt VC. Glutamine and arginine: immnuonutrients for improved health.

12. Anderson P, Schroeder G, Skubitz K. Oral glutamine reduces the duration and severity of stomatitis after cytotoxic cancer chemotherapy. Cancer 1998; 83: 1433–9

13. Yoshida S, Matsui M, Shirouzu Y, et al. Effects of glutamine supplements and radiochemotherapy on systemic immune and gut barrier function in patients with advanced esophageal cancer. Ann Surg 1998; 227: 485–91

14. Klimberg V, McClellan J, Claude H, et al. Glutamine, cancer, and its therapy. Am J Surg 1996; 172: 418–24

15. Klimberg V, Kornbluth J, Cao Y, et al. Glutamine suppresses PGE2 synthesis and breast cancer growth. J Surg Res 1996; 63: 293–7

16. Ziegler T, Young L, Benfell K, et al. Clinical and metabolic efficacy of glutamine-supplemented parenteral nutrition after bone marrow transplantation. A randomized, double-blind, controlled study. Ann Intern Med 1992; 116: 821–8

17. Ma J, Pollak M, Giovannucci E, et al. Prospective study of colorectal cancer risk in men and plasma levels of insulin-like growth factor (IGF)-I and IGF-binding protein-3. J Natl Cancer Inst 1999; 91: 620–5

18. Gurbuz A, Kunzelman J, Ratzer E. Supplemental dietary arginine accelerates intestinal mucosal regeneration and enhances bacterial clearance following radiation enteritis in rats. J Surg Res 1998; 74: 149–54

19. Barbul A. Arginine: biochemistry, physiology, and therapeutic implications. J Parenter Enteral Nutr 1986; 10: 227–38

20. Savarese DM, Savy G, Vahdat L, et al. Prevention of chemotherapy and radiation toxicity with glutamine. Cancer Treat Rev 2003; 29: 501–13

21. Muscaritoli M, Grieco G, Capria S, et al. Nutritional and metabolic support in patients undergoing bone marrow transplnatation. Am J Clin Nutr 2002; 75: 183–90

22. Kang Y, Feng Y, Hatcher E. Glutathione stimulates A549 cell proliferation in glutamine-defi-

Med Sci Sports Exerc 2000; 32 (Suppl 7): S377–88

cient culture: The effect of glutamine supplementation. J Cell Phys 1994; 161: 589–96

23. Bartlett D, Charland S, Torosian M. Effect of glutamine on tumor and host growth. Ann Surg Oncol 1995; 2: 71–6

24. Scott L, Lamb J, Smith S, Wheatley DN. Single amino acid (arginine) deprivation: rapid and selective death of cultures transformed and malignant cells. Br J Cancer 2000; 83: 800–10

25. Johnson A, Kaufmann Y, Luo S, et al. Effect of glutamine on glutathione, IGF-I, and TGF-β_1. J Surg Res 2003; 111: 222–8

26. May P, Barber A, D'Olimpio J, et al. Reversal of cancer-related wasting using oral supplementation with a combination of β-hydroxy-β-methylbutyrate, arginine, and glutamine. Am J Surg 2002; 183: 471–9

27. Decker GM. Glutamine: indicated in cancer care? Clin J Oncol Nurs 2002; 6: 112–15

28. Ziegler TR. Glutamine supplementation in cancer patients receiving bone marrow transplantation and high dose chemotherapy. J Nutr 2001; 131 (Suppl 9): 2578S–84S

29. Wong PW, Enriquez A, Barrera R. Nutritional support in critically ill patients with cancer. Crit Care Clin 2001; 17: 743–67

30. Potter J, Langhorne P, Roberts M. Routine protein energy supplementation in adults: systematic review. BMJ 1998; 317: 495–501

12c

Mind–body interventions

Linda E. Carlson and Shauna L. Shapiro

SUPPORTIVE CARE

Symptom management and enhancing vitality

There is substantial evidence demonstrating the efficacy of several mind–body interventions in the management of symptoms related to cancer and cancer treatments. Below we highlight hypnosis, guided imagery/relaxation, meditation, yoga, psychotherapy and creative therapies.

Hypnosis

Hypnosis has proved effective for pain reduction, treating dyspnea, and anxiety reduction in cancer patients[1,2]. Hypnosis has been defined as a natural state of aroused, attentive focal concentration coupled with a relative suspension of peripheral awareness[2]. It involves three main factors: absorption, dissociation and suggestibility. Techniques most often used for symptom reduction involve physical relaxation coupled with imagery that redirects attention from the distressing symptoms. In this sense, it is sometimes difficult to distinguish, methodologically, hypnosis from imagery and/or relaxation, although hypnosis typically includes more attention regulation. Mechanisms of action are suggested to be through physical relaxation and attention control[2].

Much of the hypnosis research in cancer has been in the form of case studies, but one interesting trial compared oral mucositis pain levels in four groups of bone marrow transplant patients: (1) traditional control; (2) therapist support; (3) hypnotic relaxation; and (4) hypnotic relaxation plus cognitive–behavioral therapy (CBT)[3]. The patients who received hypnosis alone or in combination with CBT reported less pain than the two other groups. Similarly, hypnosis combined with supportive–expressive therapy resulted in a 50% reduction in pain experiences of women with metastatic breast cancer compared to a no-treatment control[4]. Surgical and procedural pain, too, can be effectively controlled by hypnosis. Studies have shown superior analgesia when using hypnosis compared to control conditions of sympathetic attention in children undergoing painful procedures[5,6]. A randomized controlled trial compared patients who received either standard care, structured attention, or self-hypnotic relaxation during surgery. Hypnosis was found to have more pronounced effects on pain and anxiety reduction, and also improved hemodynamic stability[7]. Further, hypnosis in children with cancer is effective in controlling anticipatory nausea and vomiting, which is a conditioned response that often occurs well before administration of chemotherapy agents[8]. Overall, hypnosis has demonstrated efficacy for decreasing pain from surgical procedures and during end-of-life care, as well as in areas of anxiety reduction in oncology populations.

Imagery/relaxation

Guided imagery is defined as using the imagination to create sensory experiences through any of the sense modalities (vision, olfaction, taste, touch, hearing), for a particular purpose. These purposes may range from the specific (slowing the heart rate, stimulating the immune system, reducing pain, or reducing stress symptoms) to the general (such as accessing inner resources for healing, promoting physical, emotional, and spiritual well-being, or training the mind to create a physiological or psychological effect). Imagery is often combined with either progressive or passive muscle relaxation. Progressive muscle relaxation involves successively tensing and then relaxing major muscle groups of the body, while passive relaxation uses the same process, but without inducing muscle tension. Passive relaxation is useful in any case where active tensing of muscles may be difficult or painful. The advantages to progressive relaxation with inexperienced patients is in learning what each state actually feels like subjectively, as people are often unaware of holding muscle tension. Relaxation of this nature triggers what has been termed the 'relaxation response' by Herbert Benson[9,10], defined as a cascade of physiological events resulting in decreased heart rate, respiration and blood pressure, accompanied by systemic muscle relaxation. This occurs in response to disengaging the fight or flight (arousal) system through the use of relaxation techniques.

Early studies[11] reported that relaxation and guided imagery are useful ways to help control the nausea and vomiting associated with chemotherapy treatment. The techniques can also help patients decrease the use of pain medications[12]. The National Comprehensive Cancer Network (NCCN) guidelines for the treatment of nausea and vomiting include self-hypnosis, progressive muscle relaxation, biofeedback, guided imagery and systematic desensitization. (www.nccn.org/patient_gls/_english/_nausea_and_vomiting/index.htm). Not only has imagery been successful in treating nausea and vomiting caused as a result of chemotherapy drugs, but it has also been effective in the treatment of the conditioned anticipatory nausea that many patients develop even at the sight of the treatment center[8].

In other research, a guided imagery program combined with music was successful in decreasing mood disturbance and improving quality of life (QOL) in cancer survivors[13]. Another study investigating the effect of progressive muscle relaxation on anxiety and QOL after stoma surgery in colorectal cancer patients found significant decreases in state anxiety, and improved QOL in the domains of physical and psychological health and social concerns in the experimental group[14]. Similarly, in a group of 96 women randomly assigned to either progressive relaxation and imagery treatments during chemotherapy or usual care, mood and QOL improved significantly in the treatment group as compared to controls[15].

Relaxation and imagery appear to reduce the sensory experience of pain, and have equivocal effects on affective measures. However, these results are preliminary and need support from more experimental studies, which should include more complete descriptions of pain, improved statistical reporting, controls over adequacy of and compliance with the interventions, use of single interventions and use of more complex measures of affective outcomes[16].

Meditation

Meditation, previously viewed by Western science as an esoteric Eastern novelty, has become a worldwide practice, therapy and research topic. 'Meditation is now not only one of the world's oldest and most widely practiced therapies, but also the second most researched'[17]. Meditation can broadly be defined as a family of techniques that involve intentionally training the mind in awareness and attention. Despite common features, there are many varieties of meditation. For simplicity, 'the family' of techniques has commonly been classified under two categories: concentration meditation and mindfulness meditation[18,19]. Concentration meditation attempts to restrict awareness to focus on a single object of attention. Mindfulness meditation, by contrast, involves attending non-judgmentally to all stimuli in the internal and external environment.

Although the research on meditation over the past four decades has yielded significant effects on both psychological and physical well-being[17,20], very little research has examined the effects of meditation in cancer patients. In fact, there have been only two published randomized controlled trials of meditation-based interventions for cancer patients[21,22], both of which applied the mindfulness-based stress reduction (MBSR) program of Jon Kabat-Zinn and colleagues[23]. Kabat-Zinn describes the MBSR program as, 'A well-defined and systematic patient-centered educational approach which uses relatively intensive training in mindfulness meditation as the core of a program to teach people how to take better care of themselves and live healthier, more adaptive lives'[24]. The program consists of eight weekly group meetings with components of didactic and experiential learning, consisting of gentle hatha yoga stretches and mindfulness meditation. Daily home practice is also strongly encouraged. In the first cancer MBSR study, heterogeneous outpatients ($n = 109$) were randomly assigned to a meditation-based condition (MBSR) or a wait-list control group. Results demonstrated that participants in the experimental group had significantly lower scores on total mood disturbance, depression, anxiety, anger and confusion as well as increased vigor as compared to the control group. Further, participants in the experimental group showed a significant decrease in stress symptoms (e.g. fewer cardiopulmonary and gastrointestinal symptoms)[21]. These benefits of the program persisted at a 6-month follow-up assessment[25].

The other study focused specifically on women with stage II breast cancer who had recently completed treatment. The study used a 2 (intervention vs. wait-list control) by 4 (baseline, post-treatment, 3-month follow-up, 9-month follow-up) study design. A total of 63 participants were randomized into a MBSR condition or a self-monitoring control group. The treatment consisted of a 6-week group intervention focusing on training participants in mindfulness meditation and its application to daily life. Participants in the control group were given stress management and support resources and self-monitored the stress management activities they chose to engage in each day. Results indicated that over time *all* participants' psychological well-being improved, regardless of the experimental condition. The MBSR condition did not improve significantly more than the control condition. Within the MBSR group, however, those participants reporting greater mindfulness practice demonstrated decreased feelings of hopelessness/helplessness and anxiety and increased sleep quality relative to those who practiced less[22].

Non-randomized studies have also reported positive benefits associated with meditation. For example, Meares[26] reported that 73 patients with advanced cancer who attended at least 20 sessions of meditation experienced a significant reduction of anxiety and depression. Single case studies also have proven promising[27–29]. Recent studies focusing on immune and hormonal changes associated with MBSR have also replicated the positive effects of meditation-based interventions for persons with breast and prostate cancer in terms of improved quality of life, enhanced positive mood states and fewer stress symptoms, as well as improved subjective sleep quality[30,31].

In addition, it is important to note that many of the psychosocial and mind–body interventions share components similar to meditation. For example, Fawzy and colleagues[32] randomly assigned participants with malignant melanoma to a psychoeducational treatment group or a control group. The psychoeducational group included a stress management component comprising several attentional techniques sharing commonalities with meditation. Results from the 6-month follow-up demonstrated that the intervention group had significantly decreased negative mood states and immune function changes (summarized in the next section).

Another example is the landmark psychosocial intervention study for women with metastatic breast cancer, which included components similar to meditation[33]. The psychosocial intervention, 'supportive/expressive group therapy', included parallels with mindfulness meditation. It included a self-hypnosis exercise and a stress management technique called 'simple breath awareness exercise' which is very similar to the breathing techniques in mindfulness meditation. Findings demonstrated that the year-long weekly psychosocial intervention enhanced patients' psychosocial functioning and reduced pain as compared to a standard care treatment control group.

The research clearly supports meditation as a potentially effective intervention for persons with cancer. However, future research, with a more sophisticated methodological design, must continue to explore the specific benefits of meditation for persons with cancer. It will be important to address the role that type of cancer, stage of cancer, and phase of treatment play in the efficacy of meditation-based interventions. Further,

it will be important to expand the paradigm of meditation research, exploring it not merely as a symptom-reduction technique, but in terms of prevention, as well as positive development and growth[34]. It is hoped that the many questions that remain will be thoroughly explored, so that the potential healing effects of this 2500-year-old practice can be realized.

Yoga

'Yoga' is derived from the Sanskrit word *yug*, meaning 'to yoke' or 'union'[35]. This, according to traditional yoga philosophy, is the ultimate intent of a yoga practice – to yoke or unite the individual with the totality of the universe – giving the yoga student a deeper awareness of life, one where the student no longer experiences living as separate, but instead as part of the larger whole, both with the universe and with oneself[35]. The techniques of yoga include ethical practice (do's and don'ts of daily living), physical exercise (*asanas*), breathing techniques (*pranayama*) and meditation training[36]. Over the centuries, the practice of yoga *asanas* or postures, has evolved to exercise every muscle, nerve and gland in the body[35]. They provide a combination of static and active stretching, and isometric and dynamic strengthening which enables a student to gain flexibility, and develop stability, strength and balance[37].

Traditionally, most yoga practiced and studied in behavioral medicine has focused on learning the *asanas*, or postures. Much of the intervention work in cancer that has incorporated yoga, as in the MBSR paradigm, rarely separates the different components of the intervention when measuring outcomes, so it is impossible to know the degree of contribution of the yoga component alone versus the combination of a number of useful modalities. However, two recent reports support the possibility that yoga itself may be helpful for patients. A Tibetan yoga intervention incorporating controlled breathing and visualization, mindfulness techniques and low-impact postures in patients with lymphoma was evaluated using a randomized controlled trial (RCT) design. Patients in the yoga group reported significantly lower sleep disturbance scores during follow-up compared with patients in the wait-list control group including better subjective sleep quality, faster sleep latency, longer sleep duration and less use of sleep medications[38]. This finding is significant in the context of the high prevalence of sleep disturbance and its undesirable consequences in cancer patients, including fatigue, inability to tolerate treatment regimes, mood disturbances and immune system alterations[39].

Another study used a similar wait-list RCT design to evaluate a 7-week yoga program in groups of mixed-diagnosis patients. In this study, the style of yoga used was a modified version of *hatha* yoga called yoga therapy. Influenced by the Iyengar tradition of yoga and the study of kinesiology, the yoga *asanas* (or postures) are modified for people who are particularly stiff, immobile, injured, ill or under extreme stress. Yoga therapy enables the student to move slowly and safely into the modified *asana* concentrating initially on relaxing their body, breathing fully and developing awareness of the sensations in their body and thoughts in their mind. As the sessions progressed, the student moved from the modified version toward the full version of the *asanas*, building flexibility, strength and balance while maintaining that initial understanding of being relaxed and aware. As a result, the student was always moving mindfully and in their pain-free range of motion while improving at their optimum speed. The practice utilized small groups with individualized attention. The yoga participants had scores indicating more improvement than the controls post-intervention on global QOL, stress symptoms, emotional function, emotional irritability, tension, depression, anger and confusion. They also had greater cardiovascular endurance and lower resting heart rates[40].

Thus, although the literature is still nascent in this area, yoga interventions do hold potential for overall symptom reduction, as well as physical rehabilitation promise.

Psychotherapy

There has been a proliferation of research examining psychotherapeutic interventions designed to help people cope with cancer across the entire spectrum of the disease trajectory. Outcomes generally assessed include psychological functioning, primarily anxiety and depression, and overall QOL. These interventions have been thoroughly reviewed several times over the past decade[41–55]. Most reviews have concluded that psychosocial interventions are often efficacious in decreasing distress and improving QOL. These findings have been robust and cover a number of different interventions and outcomes.

Interventions usually assume one of four common forms: psychoeducation, cognitive–behavioral training (group or individual), group supportive therapy and individual supportive therapy. The psychotherapeutic interventions are usually targeted to one of three points on the illness trajectory: diagnosis/pre-treatment, immediately post-treatment or during extended treatment (such as radiotherapy or chemotherapy), and disseminated disease or death[55]. Certain modalities of treatment have been shown to be more efficacious at one or more of these periods. For example, psychoeducation may be most effective during the diagnosis/pre-treatment period, when patient information needs are high. However, for later-stage adjustment with more advanced disease, group support may be more effective[53]. Cognitive–behavioral techniques such as relaxation, stress management and cognitive coping may be most useful during extended treatments[49,56]. Cunningham has identified a hierarchy of different types of therapy, based on increasingly active participation by the recipient. These five types are: information, emotional support, behavioral training in coping skills,

Table 12.4   Hierarchy of psychosocial needs and suggested interventions across the disease trajectory

Clinical stage	Psychosocial picture	Suggested psychosocial intervention	Patient level of involvement
Diagnosis	anxiety, information seeking, depression	psychoeducation information provision emotional support	low low medium
Treatment	anxiety, treatment side-effects	coping skills training emotional support	medium medium
Recovery	reintegration, depression	emotional support psychotherapy	medium high
Recurrence	depression, death and dying	psychotherapy spiritual/existential therapy	high high

psychotherapy and finally spiritual/existential therapy[43]. All five levels of therapy are supported by research demonstrating their efficacy, although the majority of research is in the area of supportive and cognitive–behavioral interventions, such as supportive–expressive therapy and coping skills training (Table 12.4).

Creative therapies

Creative therapies for cancer patients are generally intended to integrate physical, emotional and spiritual care by facilitating creative ways for patients to respond to their cancer experience[57]. Creative therapies include some of the following techniques: drawing, painting, writing, sculpting, music, photography and dance. It has been suggested that, by offering opportunities to engage in the arts and creative expression, persons with cancer can be enabled to mourn, grieve, celebrate life, be empowered to endure their situation, and find healing and meaning[58].

The overall mission of one program was stated as the identification and development of connections between the creative arts and the healing arts to improve the physical, mental, emotional and spiritual health within the community[59]. The basic assumption underlying this program is that every individual can be a natural artist. The program posited that creating opportunities for everyone to explore the possibilities of artistic expression without judgment or criticism can lead to greater self-awareness and self-esteem and can release innate creative energy. Further, this energy can then be directed as a potent force into our physical, mental and spiritual healing[59]. Similarly, the stated goals of another program developed co-operatively by artists and health-care professionals were: (1) to provide an environment that develops into a nurturing community; (2) to create opportunities for emotional healing; (3) to help participants to find meaning in their experiences; and (4) to promote creativity as a vehicle for self-knowledge through the creation of a piece of artwork[60].

Benefits that have been reported from creative therapy programs include support, psychological strength, and new insights about the cancer experience[61]. However, although there are many descriptions of different programs in the literature, with content ranging from the visual arts[62] to dance[63], music therapy[64], creative writing[62] and mixed-modality programs[59,60], few have included rigorous evaluation components. Most reports of programs have been before-and-after research designs demonstrating that patients felt they had received benefit from the interventions.

The most carefully evaluated therapies may be the music therapy interventions, many of which have reported improvements in mood and QOL[13]. In addition, music therapy interventions have been effective in alleviating pain perception and nausea in cancer patients[65–67]. In one RCT of 80 palliative-care patients, routine hospice services and clinical music therapy were compared to routine hospice services only. QOL was higher for those patients receiving music therapy, and their QOL increased over time as they received more music therapy sessions. Subjects in the control group, however, experienced a lower QOL than those in the experimental group, and without music, their QOL decreased over time[68].

Interest and research on expressive writing as an intervention has recently flourished as a consequence of Pennebaker's work demonstrating the efficacy of expressive writing about traumatic experiences for dealing with upsetting life events, in terms of both physical and mental health[69,70]. One pilot study of 30 prostate cancer patients randomized participants into experimental (expressive writing) and control (factual writing) groups. Compared to controls, patients in the expressive disclosure condition showed improvements in the domains of physical symptoms and health-care utilization, but not in psychological variables nor in disease-relevant aspects of immunocompetence[71]. Another small study of expressive writing assigned 42 patients with metastatic renal cell carcinoma to either expressive writing about their cancer, or neutral writing about health behaviors. Patients in the expressive group reported significantly less sleep disturbance, better sleep quality and sleep duration, and less daytime dysfunction compared with patients in the neutral group[72]. A study of early-stage breast cancer patients randomly assigned women to write over four sessions about: (1) their deepest thoughts and feelings regarding breast cancer; (2) positive thoughts and feelings regarding their experience with breast cancer; or (3) facts of their breast cancer experience[73]. The emotional writing was relatively effective for women low in avoidance, but positive writing was more useful for women high in avoidance. Compared with neutral writing participants, the emotional writing group reported significantly decreased physical symptoms and had significantly fewer medical appointments for cancer-related morbidities, suggesting significant benefit of the intervention.

In summary, creative therapies that incorporate music and expressive writing have the most evidential support, but other modalities such as visual art and dance are also commonly practiced in oncology settings and patients report benefit from participation in these programs. These types of creative therapy have great potential for positive growth in the periods following active cancer treatment (Table 12.5).

Table 12.5   Mind–body interventions and supportive care: applications and IO level of evidence

Symptom	Modality(ies)	Level of evidence
Sleep enhancement	Hypnosis	II
	Guided imagery/relaxation	II
	Meditation	I, II
	Psychotherapy	I
	Yoga	I
	Creative arts	II (writing)
Fatigue	Hypnosis	
	Guided imagery/relaxation	
	Meditation	I, II
	Psychotherapy	
	Yoga	I
	Creative arts	
Anxiety relief	Hypnosis	I, II
	Guided imagery/relaxation	II
	Meditation	I, II
	Psychotherapy	I
	Yoga	I
	Creative arts	I
Pain	Hypnosis	I, II
	Guided imagery/relaxation	I
	Meditation	II
	Psychotherapy	I
	Yoga	I
	Creative arts	I, II (music), II (writing)
Nausea	Hypnosis	I, II
	Guided imagery/relaxation	II
	Meditation	
	Psychotherapy	
	Yoga	
	Creative arts	II (various)
Improved self-esteem	Hypnosis	II
	Guided imagery/relaxation	II
	Meditation	II
	Psychotherapy	I
	Yoga	III
	Creative arts	II
Improved coping with cancer and conventional therapies in general	Hypnosis	I
	Guided imagery/relaxation	II
	Meditation	II
	Psychotherapy	II
	Yoga	III
	Creative arts	II (various)

Continued

Table 12.5 *Continued*

Symptom	Modality(ies)	Level of evidence
Improved depression	Hypnosis	II
	Guided imagery/relaxation	I, II
	Meditation	I
	Psychotherapy	I
	Yoga	I
	Creative arts	II (various)
Finding meaning	Hypnosis	
	Guided imagery/relaxation	
	Meditation	II
	Psychotherapy	II
	Yoga	II
	Creative arts	II (various)
General quality of life	Hypnosis	II (dyspnea)
	Guided imagery/relaxation	II
	Meditation	I, II
	Psychotherapy	I, II
	Yoga	I
	Creative arts	I (hospice; music), II (various)

References

1. Marcus J, Elkins G, Mott F. The integration of hypnosis into a model of palliative care. Integr Cancer Ther 2003; 2: 365–70

2. Spiegel D, Moore R. Imagery and hypnosis in the treatment of cancer patients. Oncology (Huntingt) 1997; 11: 1179–89

3. Syrjala KL, Donaldson GW, Davis MW, Kippes ME, Carr JE. Relaxation and imagery and cognitive–behavioral training reduce pain during cancer treatment: a controlled clinical trial. Pain 1995; 63: 189–98

4. Spiegel D, Bloom JR. Group therapy and hypnosis reduce metastatic breast carcinoma pain. Psychosom Med 1983; 45: 333–9

5. Zeltzer LK, Jay SM, Fisher DM. The management of pain associated with pediatric procedures. Pediatr Clin North Am 1989; 36: 941–64

6. Zeltzer L, LeBaron S. Hypnosis and nonhypnotic techniques for reduction of pain and anxiety during painful procedures in children and adolescents with cancer. J Pediatr 1982; 101: 1032–5

7. Lang EV, Benotsch EG, Fick LJ, et al. Adjunctive non-pharmacological analgesia for invasive medical procedures: a randomised trial. Lancet 2000; 355: 1486–90

8. Newell SA, Sanson-Fisher RW, Savolainen NJ. Systematic review of psychological therapies for cancer patients: overview and recommendations for future research. J Natl Cancer Inst 2002; 94: 558–84

9. Benson H. The relaxation response: therapeutic effect. Science 1997; 278: 1694–5

10. Benson H. The relaxation response: history, physiological basis and clinical usefulness. Acta Med Scand Suppl 1982; 660: 231–7

11. Burish TG, Snyder SL, Jenkins RA. Preparing patients for cancer chemotherapy: Effects of coping preparation and relaxation interventions. J Consult Clin Psychol 1991; 59: 518–25

12. Sloman R, Brown P, Aldama E, Chu E. The use of relaxation for the promotion of comfort and pain relief in persons with advanced cancer. Contemp Nurs 1994; 3: 6–12

13. Burns DS. The effect of the bonny method of guided imagery and music on the mood and life quality of cancer patients. J Music Ther 2001; 38: 51–65

14. Cheung YL, Molassiotis A, Chang AM. The effect of progressive muscle relaxation training on anxiety and quality of life after stoma surgery in colorectal cancer patients. Psychooncology 2003; 12: 254–66

15. Walker LG, Walker MB, Ogston K, et al. Psychological, clinical and pathological effects of relaxation training and guided imagery during primary chemotherapy. Br J Cancer 1999; 80: 262–8

16. Wallace KG. Analysis of recent literature concerning relaxation and imagery interventions for cancer pain [Review]. Cancer Nurs 1997; 20: 79–87

17. Walsh R, Shapiro SL. The art and science of meditation: implications of classic claims and recent research. Am Psychol 2005; in press

18. Goleman D. The Buddha on meditation and states of consciousness. Part 1: The teaching. J Transpers Psychol 1972; 4: 1–44

19. Goleman D. The Buddha on meditation and states of consciousness. Part II: A typology of meditation techniques. J Transpers Psychol 1972; 4: 151–210

20. Murphy M, Donovan S. The Physical and Psychological Effects of Meditation, 2nd edn. Sausalito, CA: Institute of Noetic Sciences, 1997

21. Speca M, Carlson LE, Goodey E, Angen M. A randomized, wait-list controlled clinical trial: the effect of a mindfulness meditation-based stress reduction program on mood and symptoms of stress in cancer outpatients. Psychosom Med 2000; 62: 613–22

22. Shapiro SL, Bootzin RR, Figueredo AJ, et al. The efficacy of mindfulness-based stress reduction in the treatment of sleep disturbance in women with breast cancer: an exploratory study. J Psychosom Res 2003; 54: 85–91

23. Kabat-Zinn J. Full Catastrophe Living: Using the Wisdom of Your Body and Mind to Face Stress, Pain and Illness. New York: Delacourt, 1990

24. Kabat-Zinn J. Mindfulness meditation. What it is, what it isn't and its role in health care and medicine. In: Haruki Y, Suzuki M, eds. Comparative and Psychological Study on Meditation. Delft, Netherlands: Erubon, 1996: 161–70

25. Carlson LE, Ursuliak Z, Goodey E, et al. The effects of a mindfulness meditation based stress reduction program on mood and symptoms of stress in cancer outpatients: Six month follow-up. Support Care Cancer 2001; 9: 112–23

26. Meares A. What can the cancer patient expect from intensive meditation? Aust Fam Physician 1980; 9: 322–5

27. Meares A. Regression of recurrent carcinoma of the breast at mastectomy site associated with intensive meditation. Aust Fam Physician 1981; 10: 218–19

28. Meares A. Psychological mechanisms in the regression of cancer. Med J Aust 1983; 1: 583–4

29. Gersten DJ. Meditation as an adjunct to medical and psychiatric treatment. Am Psychiat Assoc J 1978; 135: 598–9

30. Carlson LE, Speca M, Patel KD, Goodey E. Mindfulness-based stress reduction in relation to quality of life, mood, symptoms of stress and levels of cortisol, dehydroepiandrosterone-sulfate (DHEAS) and melatonin in breast and prostate cancer outpatients. Psychoneuro-endocrinology 2004; 29: 448–74

31. Carlson LE, Speca M, Patel KD, Goodey E. Mindfulness-based stress reduction in relation to quality of life, mood, symptoms of stress, and immune parameters in breast and prostate cancer outpatients. Psychosom Med 2003; 65: 571–81

32. Fawzy FI, Fawzy NW, Hyun CS, et al. Malignant melanoma. Effects of an early structured psychiatric intervention, coping, and affective state on recurrence and survival 6 years later. Arch Gen Psychiatry 1993; 50: 681–9

33. Spiegel D, Bloom JR, Draemer HC, Gottheil E. Effect of psychosocial treatment on survival of patients with breast cancer. Lancet 1989; 2: 888–91

34. Shapiro SL, Schwartz GE, Santerre C. Meditation and positive psychology. In: Snyder CR, Lopez S, eds. Handbook of Positive Psychology. New York: Oxford University Press, 2002: 632–45

35. Iyengar BKS. Light on Yoga. New York: Allen and Irwin, 1976

36. Christensen A. The American Yoga Association's Beginners Manual: The Definitive Guide from the Nation's Preeminent Yoga Centre. New York: Fireside, 2002

37. Raub JA. Psycho-physiologic effects of Hatha Yoga on musculo-skeletal and cardiopulmonary function: a literature review. J Complement Med 2002; 8: 7–12

38. Cohen L, Warneke C, Fouladi RT, et al. Psychological adjustment and sleep quality in a randomized trial of the effects of a Tibetan yoga intervention in patients with lymphoma. Cancer 2004; 100: 2253–60

39. Savard J, Morin CM. Insomnia in the context of cancer: a review of a neglected problem. J Clin Oncol 2001; 19: 895–908

40. Culos-Reed S, Carlson LE, Daroux LM, Hately-Aldous S. Discovering the physical and psychological benefits of yoga for cancer survivors. Int J Yoga Ther 2004; 14: 45–52

41. Andersen B. Psychological interventions for cancer patients to enhance the quality of life. J Consult Clin Psychol 1992; 60: 552–68

42. Trijsburg RW, van Knippenberg FC, Rijpma SE. Effects of psychological treatment on cancer patients: a critical review. Psychosom Med 1992; 54: 489–517

43. Cunningham AJ. Group psychological therapy for cancer patients. A brief discussion of indications for its use, and the range of interventions available. Support Care Cancer 1995; 3: 244–7

44. Fawzy FI, Fawzy NW, Arndt LA, Pasnau RO. Critical review of psychosocial interventions in cancer care. Arch Gen Psychiatry 1995; 52: 100–13

45. Meyer TJ, Mark MM. Effects of psychosocial interventions with adult cancer patients: A meta-analysis of randomized experiments. Health Psychol 1995; 14: 101–8

46. Greer S. Improving quality of life: adjuvant psychological therapy for patients with cancer. Support Care Cancer 1995; 3: 248–51

47. Bottomley A. Group cognitive behavioural therapy interventions with cancer patients: a review of the literature. Eur J Cancer Care [English Language Edn] 1996; 5: 143–6

48. Iacovino V, Reesor K. Literature on interventions to address cancer patients' psychosocial needs: What does it tell us? J Psychosoc Oncol 1997; 15: 47–71

49. Bottomley A. Where are we now? Evaluating two decades of group interventions with adult cancer patients. J Psychiat Mental Health Nurs 1997; 4: 251–65

50. Fobair P. Cancer support groups and group therapies: Part I. Historical and theoretical background and research on effectiveness. J Psychosoc Oncol 1997; 15: 63–81

51. Fawzy FI, Fawzy NW, Canada AL. Psychosocial treatment of cancer: an update. Curr Opin Psychiatry 1998; 11: 601–5

52. Fawzy FI. Psychosocial interventions for patients with cancer: what works and what doesn't. Eur J Cancer 1999; 35: 1559–64

53. Blake-Mortimer J, Gore-Felton C, Kimerling R, et al. Improving the quality and quantity of life among patients with cancer: a review of the effectiveness of group psychotherapy. Eur J Cancer 1999; 35: 1581–6

54. Cunningham AJ. Adjuvant psychological therapy for cancer patients: putting it on the same footing as adjunctive medical therapies. Psychooncology 2000; 9: 367–71

55. Schneiderman N, Antoni MH, Saab PG, Ironson G. Health psychology: psychosocial and biobehavioral aspects of chronic disease management. Annu Rev Psychol 2001; 52: 555–80

56. Fawzy FI. A short-term psychoeducational intervention for patients newly diagnosed with cancer. Support Care Cancer 1995; 3: 235–8

57. Deane K, Fitch M, Carman M. An innovative art therapy program for cancer patients. Can Oncol Nurs J 2000; 10: 147

58. Bailey SS. The arts in spiritual care. Semin Oncol Nurs 1997; 13: 242–7

59. Lane MT, Graham-Pole J. Development of an art program on a bone marrow transplant unit. Cancer Nurs 1994; 17: 192

60. Heiney SP, Darr-Hope H. Healing icons: art support program for patients with cancer. Cancer Pract 1999; 7: 183–9

61. Tedeschi RG, Calhoun LG. The posttraumatic growth inventory: measuring the positive legacy of trauma. J Trauma Stress 1996; 9: 455–71

62. Gabriel B, Bromberg E, Vandenbovenkamp J, Walka P, Kornblith AB, Luzzatto P. Art therapy with adult bone marrow transplant patients in isolation: a pilot study. Psychooncology 2001; 10: 114–23

63. Molinaro J, Kleinfeld M, Lebed S. Physical therapy and dance in the surgical management of breast cancer. A clinical report. Phys Ther 1986; 66: 967–9

64. Trauger-Querry B, Haghighi KR. Balancing the focus: art and music therapy for pain control and symptom management in hospice care. Hosp J 1999; 14: 25–38

65. Sabo CE, Michael SR. The influence of personal message with music on anxiety and side effects associated with chemotherapy. Cancer Nurs 1996; 19: 283–9

66. Standley J. Clinical applications of music and chemotherapy: The effects on nausea and emesis. Music Ther Perspect 1992; 10: 35

67. Curtis S. The effect of music on pain relief and relaxation of the terminally ill. J Music Ther 1986; 23: 10–24

68. Hilliard RE. The effects of music therapy on the quality and length of life of people diagnosed with terminal cancer. J Music Ther 2003; 40: 113–37

69. Pennebaker JW. Telling stories: the health benefits of narrative. Lit Med 2000; 19: 3–18

70. Pennebaker JW. The effects of traumatic disclosure on physical and mental health: the values of writing and talking about upsetting events. Int J Emerg Ment Health 1999; 1: 9–18

71. Rosenberg HJ, Rosenberg SD, Ernstoff MS, et al. Expressive disclosure and health outcomes in a prostate cancer population. Int J Psychiatry Med 2002; 32: 37–53

72. de Moor C, Sterner J, Hall M, et al. A pilot study of the effects of expressive writing on psychological and behavioral adjustment in patients enrolled in a Phase II trial of vaccine therapy for metastatic renal cell carcinoma. Health Psychol 2002; 21: 615–19

73. Stanton AL, Danoff-Burg S, Sworowski LA, et al. Randomized, controlled trial of written emotional expression and benefit finding in breast cancer patients. J Clin Oncol 2002; 20: 4160–8

12d

Botanicals

Lise Alschuler

SUPPORTIVE CARE WITH BOTANICALS

Managing cancer-related symptoms

Many people with cancer turn to botanical remedies in an effort to manage side-effects from their conventional treatment and/or from the malignancy itself. There are numerous anecdotal reports of beneficial side-effect management; unfortunately, the majority of these reports are not supported by scientific evidence in the form of controlled clinical trials. There may be botanical remedies that successfully reduce cancer-related and cancer treatment-caused symptoms. However, without scientific evidence of their safety in the context of malignancy, these substances should be approached cautiously. It is entirely possible that an herb that relieves symptoms associated with cancer or its treatment could also promote tumor growth or interfere with conventional treatment. While this area of scientific investigation is still largely unexplored, there are a few examples that illustrate this concern.

Many women with tamoxifen-induced hot flushes use *Cimicifuga racemosa* (black cohosh).

Black cohosh is an effective way to reduce hot flushes in these women[1]. However, a recent presentation at the American Association for Cancer Research Annual Meeting (13 July 2003) described a 12-month study of mice with mammary tumors that were given black cohosh extract. The oral administration of black cohosh in a dose comparable to 40 mg a day in humans (the most commonly used dose) increased the number of metastatic tumors in the lungs of these mice (27.1% of treated mice compared to 10.9% of mice on the control diet)[2]. Whether this tumor-promoting effect occurs in women taking black cohosh is unknown. Of note is the fact that the length of administration was equivalent to supplementing with black cohosh from the time of puberty through menopause. It is also important to note that this presentation has yet to be published. These considerations warrant significant concern regarding the validity and applicability of these data. Nonetheless, until this effect is proved not to occur in women, a cautious approach merits the discontinuance of long-term use of black cohosh for the management of tamoxifen-induced hot flushes.

Another area of possible interaction with herbal remedies and chemotherapeutic agents is at the level of metabolism. Botanical agents can cause significant activation or inhibition of cytochrome P450 enzymes. These enzymes are prominent in the metabolic pathway of many chemotherapeutic drugs. Thus, the concurrent use of these botanicals with drugs that are metabolized by these same enzymes could affect the efficacy of these drugs. This interaction has been aptly illustrated in the case of St John's wort (*Hypericum perforatum*). St John's wort induces CYP 3A4, which results in increased metabolism of drugs that use CYP 3A4, such as cyclosporine, taxol (minor pathway)[3], indinavir, digoxin and others[4]. Another example of this interaction is between quercetin, a flavonoid extracted from onions, and taxanes. The principal taxol biotransformation reaction of humans is 6α-hydroxylation via P450 2C8. Quercetin competitively inhibits P450 2C8 hydroxylation of taxol[5]. Therefore, although quercetin has extensive, preclinical experimental evidence as a potent antineoplastic agent, its use is theoretically contraindicated in patients receiving taxol chemotherapy. Many other chemotherapeutic agents are metabolized by cytochrome P450 enzymes (see Table 12.6)[6–13]. For these botanicals, their concurrent use with chemotherapeutic agents may pose the risk of interaction and altered efficacy of the chemotherapeutics. Unfortunately, the degree to which some botanical agents affect cytochrome P450 enzyme activity is often not known. This is particularly so, as the vast majority of data on the influence of botanicals on cytochrome activity is *in vitro*. Human trials on the botanical effects on cytochrome enzyme activity, while few in number, tend to show a negligible effect of herbal extracts on drug metabolism. This is the case, for instance with ginkgo, which has 3A4 inhibitory activity documented in a number of *in vitro* trials[14,15], but two human studies failed to demonstrate this inhibition[16,17]. The concurrent use of these herbs may be a risk worth taking, but should always be evaluated in the context of the overall therapeutic intent.

These interactions are covered in the section on antineoplastic therapies and botanicals.

Given the fact that botanicals could negatively influence known antineoplastic mechanisms of action for conventional agents, and coupled with the fact that information about the possible interactions of botanical agents with chemotherapeutic agents is generally lacking, a conservative botanical approach to management of side-effects during active chemotherapy delivery includes very few botanical remedies. There are, however, some botanicals that have been studied in this regard with encouraging results.

Nausea and vomiting

One of the most common side-effects of chemotherapy and radiation treatment is nausea and vomiting. An herb that has shown efficacy in reducing nausea and vomiting is *Zingiber officinale*, or ginger root. Although antiemetic 5-HT$_3$ receptor antagonists are highly effective against chemotherapy-induced emesis, they are ineffective in 10–30% of patients[18]. A meta-analysis conducted in 2000 of randomized controlled trials regarding the efficacy of ginger for nausea and vomiting collectively favored ginger over placebo[19]. Six studies met the inclusion criteria. Of these studies three looked at postoperative nausea and vomiting, one studied seasickness, one studied morning sickness and one studied chemotherapy-induced nausea. There are no reported side-effects associated with ginger use. The mechanism of ginger's anti-emetic action is not entirely understood. One of the constituent groups in ginger, gingerols, particularly gingerol-6, may increase gastric motility, absorb neutralizing toxins and acids and block nausea feedback[20]. Galanolactone, another constituent of ginger, is a competitive antagonist at ileal 5-HT$_3$ receptors[21]. Ginger root has demonstrated anti-emetic effects in cisplatin-induced nausea in both rats[22] and dogs[23]. Cisplatin inhibits gastric emptying

Table 12.6 Possible herbal–chemotherapeutic interactions mediated through cytochrome activites. From references 6–13

Botanicals	Chemotherapy drugs	Cytochrome enzymes	Expected effect on drug
Echinacea purpurea (coneflower)			
Ginkgo biloba (ginkgo)	Cyclophosphamide	2C8, 2C9, 2C19	increased exposure
Harpagophytum procumbens (Devil's claw)	Ifosfamide	3A4	decreased exposure
	Dacarbazine	1A2	increased exposure
Hypericum perforatum (St John's wort)	Paclitaxol	2C8, 3A4	decreased exposure
	Docetaxel	3A4	decreased exposure
Mentha piperita (peppermint)	Vinblastine	3A4	decreased exposure
	Vincristine	3A4	decreased exposure
Piper methysticum (kava-kava)	Navelbine	3A4	decreased exposure
	Etoposide	3A4	decreased exposure
Polygonum multiflorum (Fo-ti root)	Irinotecan	3A4, 3A5	decreased exposure
	Topotecan	3A4	decreased exposure
Tanacetum parthenium (feverfew)	Tamoxifen	3A4, 1A2	decreased exposure
	Armidex	3A4, 1A2, 2C8-9, 2C19	decreased exposure
Trifolium pretense (red clover)	Aromasin	3A4, 1A2, 2C8-9, 2C19	decreased exposure
	Femara	3A4, 1A2, 2C8-9, 2C19	decreased exposure
Schisandra chinensis (wu wei)	Iressa	3A4	decreased exposure
Valeriana officinalis (valerian)			

which is thought to be one of the main reasons it causes nausea. The effectiveness of ginger may, therefore, be due to its ability to increase gastric motility. While more studies are needed regarding the interaction of ginger with specific chemotherapeutic agents, it is a viable alternative treatment for chemotherapy-induced nausea that deserves further clinical oncology research.

Immunosuppression

Another consequence of many chemotherapeutic and therapeutic radiation treatments is immunosuppression. Chemotherapy can also induce defects in the function of leukocytes and platelets, and suppress cellular and humoral immunity in addition to causing myelosuppression. While botanical agents are unlikely to counteract the myelosuppressive effects of chemotherapeutic agents and radiation therapy, they may mobilize and activate the immune cells in circulation, thus helping to prevent opportunistic infections. There have been no large randomized clinical trials conducted to study the effect of herbs on the immune function in oncology patients. There is, however, a growing body of experimental data that support future clinical study of selected immunopotentiating herbs.

Astragalus membranaceus (astragalus) has been studied for its immune-potentiating activity. One model looked at the effects of various fractions of astragalus on mononuclear cells derived from healthy normal donors and from colon cancer patients using the local xenogeneic graft-versus-host reaction. The astragalus extracts exhibited remarkable immunopotentiating activity and one fraction was capable of fully correcting *in vitro* T-cell function deficiency[24]. Further research in mice immunosuppressed by cyclophosphamide or radiation treatment demonstrated that astragalus extracts enhanced antibody production and this effect was shown to be associated with increased Th cell activity[25]. Another *in vitro* study demonstrated that urological neoplasms (murine renal cell carcinoma and murine bladder tumor) suppressed macrophage function. This suppression was reversed by astragalus extract[26].

Similar immunostimulatory effects have been experimentally demonstrated with extracts from *Coriolus versicolor*, a mushroom traditionally used in China for its immune-stimulating properties. A small polypeptide from *C. versicolor* was given to mice for 2 weeks prior to inoculation with leukemic, colon, hepatoma and stomach tumor cells. The *C. versicolor*-treated mice had decreased incidences of tumor mass and increased white blood cell counts than did the untreated mice[27]. The polysaccharides from *C. versicolor* have also been shown to activate peritoneal macrophages in tumor-bearing mice by activating the transcription of the tumor necrosis factor gene in these cells[28].

In another study, the immunopotentiating effect of *Uncaria tomentosa* (cat's claw) was studied in rats. Doxorubicin was administered to rats and caused the predicted myelosuppression with resultant leukopenia. Co-administration with *U. tomentosa* extract shortened the leukocyte recovery time and, unlike Neupogen®, which recovers non-lymphocytic fractions, *U. tomentosa* extract recovered all fractions of white blood cells. The immunostimulatory effect of *U. tomentosa* was postulated to be the result of repair of DNA strand breaks, which normally occur from doxorubicin administration[29].

Finally, *Withania somnifera* (ashwagandha) has demonstrated immunostimulatory effects in chemotherapy-induced immunosuppression. Ashwagandha was fed to mice at a dose that corresponds to 4–6 g a day in humans. When ashwagandha was combined with cyclophosphamide, it prevented myelosuppression, and resulted in a significant increase in hemoglobin concentration, red blood cell count, white blood cell count, platelet count and body weight as compared with untreated (cyclophosphamide only) mice[30]. While this study does not rule out the possibility that ashwagandha could interfere with the activity of cyclophosphamide, the cytotoxic effects of cyclophosphamide on target tissues remained intact in the ashwagandha-treated mice. This suggests that the immunostimulatory actions of ashwagandha are the result of direct effects on the immune system. Thus, this preliminary study suggests that ashwagandha may have beneficial and non-competitive immunostimulatory effects in chemotherapy-induced immunosuppression.

BOTANICAL MEDICINE AND CHEMOTHERAPY-RELATED SYMPTOMS

Cisplatin

Several preliminary studies and a few clinical trials have investigated the effects of concurrent administration of botanical agents with chemotherapeutic agents. Several botanicals have been investigated for their combined effects with cisplatin. Cisplatin exerts cytotoxic effects on a multitude of cell types. However, it also produces adverse effects on normal kidney cells, which can limit its use. The cytotoxicity of cisplatin is closely related to increases in lipid peroxide content due to damage to superoxide dismutase (SOD) catalase and glutathione-related enzymes. In rats, co-administration of protein-bound polysaccharide (PS-K), a constituent of *Coriolus versicolor*, partially prevented this decrease in SOD activity in normal kidney cells. At the same time, the PS-K did not appear to be incorporated into rat hepatoma cells or human ovarian cancer cells, and therefore did not interfere with cytotoxicity to those cells[31]. Silybin, a constituent of *Silybum marianum* (milk thistle) has also been studied for its protective activity against cisplatin toxicity in an animal model of testicular cancer. When silybin was infused into rats prior to infusion with cisplatin, there was a significant reduction in glomerular and tubular kidney toxicity. Dose–response curves of human testicular cell lines for cisplatin combined with silybin did not deviate significantly from those of cisplatin alone[32].

Cyclophosphamide

Cyclophosphamide (CPA) is an alkylating agent that is cytotoxic, particularly against rapidly dividing cells. The tolerance to CPA can be limited by the immunosuppression that this drug may cause. CPA reduces leukocyte counts and suppresses both humoral and cellular immune responses. Several botanicals have been studied in animal models for their ability to reverse CPA-induced immunosuppression. An aqueous extract of an isolated fraction from *Astragalus membranaceus* was given intravenously to rats for 8 days. The study rats that also received immunosuppressive CPA experienced almost complete restoration of immune function, as evidenced by their increasing ability to reject grafted human tissue[33]. This same pattern of immunorestoration by astragalus from CPA-induced immunosuppression was seen in an earlier *in vivo* animal study, although the results did not approach statistical significance[34]. The apparent

weak effect noted in this earlier study could be due to the fact that a different form of astragalus was used. This form was not concentrated to the same fraction as the astragalus used in the later study.

Withania somnifera, ashwagandha, has also been studied *in vivo* for its immunological potentiation in mice treated with CPA[35]. Over a 10-day course of CPA, the group of mice that also received intraperitoneal ashwagandha extract demonstrated a significantly higher white blood cell count than did the CPA-only mice. The ashwagandha mice regained a normal white blood cell count at the end of treatment, whereas the CPA-only mice did not regain a normal white blood cell count until 30 days after treatment. In addition, the ashwagandha mice had almost twice the number of bone marrow cells on the 11th day than did the CPA-only mice. Mice that did not receive the CPA, but did receive ashwagandha, had the highest bone marrow cellularity, indicating the ability of ashwagandha to stimulate stem cells, when given via an intraperitoneal route in mice. A protein-bound polysaccharide (PSP) extracted from *Coriolus versicolor*, an edible mushroom, has also been studied in rats as an immunostimulatory agent in CPA-induced immunosuppression. The group of rats that were fed PSP along with CPA experienced an increased lymphocyte proliferation rate over controls and CPA-only rats[36].

Although the data on the immunopotentiating effect of these herbs are preliminary and do not address any potential adverse interactions, they are, nonetheless, indicative of a potential role for these botanicals in co-management of cyclophosphamide-induced immunosuppression.

Radiation therapy

Aloe vera has been investigated to determine whether its anti-inflammatory and wound-healing properties would be beneficial with radiation therapy. A phase III study was carried out to determine the efficacy of topical aloe vera gel on irradiated breast tissue[37]. This trial involved 225 patients with breast cancer after lumpectomy or partial mastectomy, who required a 2-week course of radiation therapy using tangential fields, a relatively unusual treatment course relative to the average of 5–6 weeks usually prescribed in the USA. The patients were randomized to either topical aloe vera gel or topical aqueous cream. Both creams were applied three times daily throughout the treatment. In this study, the aqueous cream was significantly better than aloe vera gel in terms of controlling dry desquamation, erythema, pruritis and pain. The authors concluded that aloe vera was not effective in reducing radiation-induced skin side-effects. The results of this study are somewhat disappointing, given earlier *in vivo* evidence[38] that was suggestive of a radioprotective effect of aloe vera extract. This relatively short course of radiation therapy is atypical and may have been too toxic to demonstrate a therapeutic effect of aloe vera.

In contrast, a phase III trial of 254 patients receiving a postoperative standard course of radiation therapy demonstrated a significant reduction in acute dermatitis and radiation-induced pain with the application of calendula ointment. Women were randomized to apply a *Calendula officinalis* petrolatum ointment (Bioron Ltd, Levallois-Perret France) or trolamine ointment to the irradiated area after each 2-Gy irradiation (5 days weekly). The calendula group experienced a significantly lower incidence of acute dermatitis grade 2 or higher (41% vs. 63% in the placebo group; $p < 0.001$). In addition, the calendula group had less frequent interruption of radiotherapy and significantly reduced radiation-induced pain[39].

The concurrent use of botanicals with chemotherapy and/or radiation therapy is summarized in Table 12.7.

RECOMMENDATIONS

Botanicals deserve further study as they may be useful to help manage some of the toxicities associated with chemotherapy and radiation. If a patient is experiencing side-effects that are unresponsive to conventional treatment, or if the person cannot, or will not, tolerate the conventional treatment, botanicals may become an

Table 12.7 Evidence for co-management of selected adverse effects with botanicals. Level IV of evidence includes *in vitro* studies, *in vivo* studies, and traditional use. Level II of evidence includes level IV and prospective trials, cohort trials and epidemiological studies. Level I of evidence includes level II and randomized controlled trials. The symbol '(-)' denotes evidence against the use of the therapy

Condition or therapy	Level of evidence IV	Level of evidence II	Level of evidence I
Hot flushes	(-) Black cohosh		
Nausea/vomiting			Ginger
Immunosuppression	*Astragalus membranaceus* *Coriolus versicolor* *Uncaria tomentosa* (cats claw) *Withania somnifera* (ashwagandha)		
Multidrug resistance	*Panax ginseng*		
Radiation therapy	*Aloe vera* *Withania somnifera* (ashwagandha)		(-) Aloe vera *Calendula officinalis* (calendula ointment)

important option, given the caveats previously noted. However, owing to the many possible interactions and interference of several botanicals with chemotherapy agents (see Table 12.6), it is generally advisable to administer these herbs after the terminal half-life of the chemotherapeutics has elapsed. This will minimize interference, while still providing therapeutic value. In cases where this interference is not theorized to occur, simultaneous administration of the herb with the chemotherapy may be acceptable, and in many cases preferred (e.g. using ginger as an anti-emetic). Overall, the role of botanicals in the co-management of symptoms is a promising arena which deserves further study in human trials, and careful application.

References

1. Hernandez M, Pluchino S. Cimicifuga racemosa for the treatment of hot flushes in women surviving breast cancer. Maturitas 2003; 14 (Suppl 1): S59–65
2. Davis V. Black cohosh and breast cancer a dangerous mix. American Association for Cancer Research news release, 12 July, 2003
3. Harris JW, Rahman A, Kim BR, et al. Metabolism of taxol by human hepatic microsomes and liver slices: participation of cytochrome P450 3A4 and an unknown P450 enzyme. Cancer Res 1994; 54: 4026–35
4. Markowitz JS, Donovan JL, DeVane CL, et al. Effect of St John's wort on drug metabolism by induction of cytochrome P450 3A4 enzyme. JAMA 2003; 290: 1500–4
5. Rahman A, Korzekwa KR, Grogen J, et al. Selective biotransformation of taxol to 6 alpha-hydroxytaxol by human cytochrome P450 2C8. Cancer Res 1994; 54: 5543–6
6. Gorski JC, Huang SM, Pinto A, et al. The effect of echinacea (Echinacea purpurea root) on cytochrome P450 activity in vivo. Clin Pharmacol Ther 2004; 75: 89–100
7. Iwata H, Tezuka Y, Kadota S, et al. Identification and characterization of potent CYP3A4 inhibitors in schisandra fruit extract. Drug Metab Dispos 2004; 32: 1351–8
8. Jang EH, Park YC, Chung WG, et al. Effects of dietary supplements on induction and inhibition of cytochrome P450s protein expression in rats. Food Chem Toxicol 2004; 42: 1749–56
9. Lefebvre T, Foster BC, Drouin CE, et al. In vitro activity of commercial valerian root extracts against human cytochrome P450 3A4. J Pharm Pharm Sci 2004; 7: 265–73
10. Mannel M. Drug interactions with St John's wort: mechanisms and clinical implications. Drug Saf 2004; 27: 773–97
11. Sparreboom A, Cox MC, Acharya MR, Figg WD. Herbal remedies in the United States: potential adverse interactions with anticancer agents. J Clin Oncol 2004; 22: 2489–503
12. Unger, M, Frank A. Simultaneous determination of the inhibitory potency of herbal extracts on the activity of six major cytochrome P450 enzymes using liquid chromatography/mass spectrometry and automated online extraction. Rapid Commun Mass Spectrom 2004; 18: 2273–81
13. Zhou S, Gao Y, Jiang W, et al. Interactions of herbs with cytochrome P450. Drug Metab Rev 2003; 35: 35–98
14. von Moltke LL, Weemhoff JL, Bedir E, et al. Inhibition of human cytochromes P450 by components of Ginkgo biloba. J Pharm Pharmacol 2004; 56: 1039–44
15. Gaudineau C, Beckerman R, Welbourn S, Auclair K. Inhibition of human P450 enzymes by multiple constituents of the Ginkgo biloba extract. Biochem Biophys Res Commun 2004; 318: 1072–8
16. Markowitz JS, Donovan JL, Liindsay De Vane C, et al. Multiple-dose administration of Ginkgo biloba did not affect cytochrome P-450

2D6 or 3A4 activity in normal volunteers. J Clin Psychopharmacol 2003; 23: 576–81

17. Gurley BJ, Gardner SF, Hubbard MA, et al. Cytochrome P450 phenotypic ratios for predicting herb–drug interactions in humans. Clin Pharmacol Ther 2002; 72: 276–87

18. Cubeddu L. Mechanism of cancer chemotherapeutic agents. Semin Oncol 1992; 19: 2

19. Ernst E, Pittler MH. Efficacy of ginger for nausea and vomiting: a systematic review of randomized clinical trials. Br J Anaesth 2000; 84: 367–71

20. Bone ME, Wilkinson DJ, Young JR, et al. Ginger root – a new antiemetic. The effect of ginger root on postoperative nausea and vomiting after major gynaecological surgery. Anaesthesia 1990; 45: 669–71

21. Huang Q, Iwamoto M, Aoki S, et al. Anti-5-hydroxytryptamine$_3$ effect of galanolactone, diterpenoid isolated from ginger. Chem Pharm Bull (Tokyo) 1991; 39: 397–9

22. Sharma, S, Gupta Y. Reversal of cisplatin-induced delay in gastric emptying in rats by ginger (Zingiber officinale). J Ethnopharmacol 1998; 62: 49–55

23. Sharma S, Kochupillai V, Gupta SK, et al. Antiemetic efficacy of ginger (Zingiber officinale) against cisplatin-induced emesis in dogs. J Ethnopharmacol 1997; 57: 93–6

24. Chu D-T, Wong W, Mavligit GM, et al. Immunotherapy with Chinese medicinal herbs I. Immune restoration of local xenogeneic graft-versus-host reaction in cancer patients by fractionated Astragalus membranaceus in vitro. J Clin Lab Immunol 1988; 25: 119–23

25. Zhao K, Mancini C, Doria G. Enhancement of the immune response in mice by Astragalus membranaceus extracts. Immunopharmacol 1990; 20: 225–34

26. Rittenhouse J, Lui P, Lau P, et al. Chinese medicinal herbs reverse macrophage suppression induced by urological tumors. J Urol 1991; 146: 486–90

27. Yang M, Chen Z, Kwok JS, et al. The anti-tumor effect of a small polypeptide from coriolus versicolor (SPCV). Am J Chin Med 1992; XX: 221–32

28. Liu WK, Ng TB, Sze SF, Tsui KW, et al. Activation of peritoneal macrophages by polysaccharopeptide from the mushroom, Coriolus versicolor. Immunopharmacology 1993; 26: 139–46

29. Sheng Y, Pero R, Wagner H, et al. Treatment of chemotherapy-indcued leukopenia in a rat model with aqueous extract from Uncaria tomentosa. Phytomedicine 2000; 7: 137–43

30. Ziauddin M. Phansalkar N, Patki P, et al. Studies on the immunomodulatory effects of Ashwagandha. J Ethnopharmacol 1996; 50: 69–76

31. Kobayashi Y, Kariya K, Saigeni K, Nakamura K. Enhancement of anti-cancer activity of cis-diaminedichloroplatinum by the protein-bound polysaccharide of Coriolus versicolor QUEL (PS-K) in vitro. Cancer Biother 1994; 9: 351–8

32. Bokemeyer C, Fels L, Dunn T, et al. Silibinin protects against cisplatin-induced nephrotoxicity without compromising cisplatin or ifosfamide anti-tumour activity. Br J Cancer 1996; 74: 2036–41

33. Chu D-T, Wong WL, Mavligit GM, et al. Immunotherapy with Chinese medicinal herbs. II. Reversal of cyclophosphamide-induced immune suppression by administration of fractionated Astragalus membranaceus in vivo. J Clin Lab Immunol 1988; 25: 125–9

34. Khoo KS, Ang PT. Extract of Astragalusmembranaceus and Ligustrum lucidum does not prevent cyclophosphamide-induced myelosuppression. Singapore Med J 1995; 36: 387–90

35. Davis L, Kuttan G. Suppressive effect of cyclophosphamide-induced toxicity by Withania somnifera extract in mice. J Ethnopharmacol 1998; 62: 209–14

36. Qian ZM, Xu MF, Tang PL. Polysaccharide peptide (PSP) restores immunosuppression induced by cyclophosphamide in rats. Am J Chin Med 1997; XXV: 27–35

37. Heggie S, Bryant GP, Tripcony L, et al. A Phase III study on the efficacy of topical aloe vera gel on irradiated breast tissue. Cancer Nurs 2002; 25: 442–51

38. Pande S, Kumar M, Kumar A, et al. Radioprotective efficacy of aloe vera leaf extract. Pharm Bio 1998; 36: 227–32

39. Pommier P, Gomez F, Sunyach MP, et al. Phase III randomized trial of Calendula officinalis compared with trolamine for the prevention of acute dermatitis during irradiation for breast cancer. J Clin Oncol 2004; 22: 1447–53

12e

Manual therapy

J. Michael Menke

There are significant benefits of massage therapy concerning symptom control, with various studies showing a benefit in cancer patients with regards to pain, anxiety, nausea and fatigue[1–4]. There are some caveats to the use of manual therapies in cancer patients. Manipulation of bones with cancer may cause pathologic fractures; manipulation of soft tissue could theoretically facilitate tumor growth with increased blood supply, or possibly spread the disease. To date, there is no evidence for the latter phenomenon, although the conjectured mechanisms are plausible and must be considered in the cancer patient, especially with regards to future research. Some massage interventions have an especially low impact, and have only preliminary evidence concerning efficacy (as in foot massage)[3].

In cases where a joint dysfunction is co-morbid but non-contiguous with a cancer, the joint may be carefully manipulated or mobilized to address painful joint dysfunction. In an interesting case study by Polkinghorn[5], a patient with breast cancer metastases also injured her shoulder. Polkinghorn, a chiropractor, used an Activator adjusting instrument to focus the force of the manipulation and minimize impact on the surrounding tissue. A few treatments gave the patient mobility and reduced the pain due to the co-morbid mechanical shoulder problem.

After axillary dissection from breast cancer, lymphedema can occur in the upper extremity. Massage, with or without compressive bandaging, can help to reduce this lymphedema once it occurs. Massage as a part of complete decongestive therapy is the current standard of care in this situation[6].

All such manipulation is done with the utmost care, only after careful study of images, physical diagnosis and concomitant physician consultation. Manual therapies may be carefully used for co-morbid musculoskeletal events such as a sprain or strain. Foot and shoulder massage, for example, may help cancer patients rest, sleep better and lower hypertension associated with anxiety and tension[7].

The greatest contributions of manual medicines to cancer care are probably in the area of supportive care. It is also a reasonable hypothesis that manual medicine providers could help in monitoring adherence, progress and side-effects of conventional cancer care.

References

1. Ahles TA, Tope DM, Pinkson B, et al. Massage therapy for patients undergoing autologous bone marrow transplantation. J Pain Symptom Manage 1999; 18: 157–63

2. Cassileth BR, Vickers AJ. Massage therapy for symptom control: outcome study at a major cancer center. J Pain Symptom Manage 2004; 28: 244–9

3. Grealish L, Lomasney A, Whiteman B. Foot massage. A nursing intervention to modify the distressing symptoms of pain and nausea in patients hospitalized with cancer. Cancer Nurs 2000; 23: 237–43

4. Post-White J, Kinney ME, Savik K, et al. Therapeutic massage and healing touch improve symptoms in cancer. Integr Cancer Ther 2003; 2: 332–44

5. Polkinghorn BS. Instrumental chiropractic treatment of frozen shoulder associated with mixed metastatic carcinoma. Chiropr Tech 1995; 7: 98–102

6. Williams AF, Vadgama A, Franks PJ, Mortimer PS. A randomized controlled crossover study of manual lymphatic drainage therapy in women with breast cancer-related lymphoedema. Eur J Cancer Care (Engl) 2002; 11: 254–61

7. Soden K, Vincent K, Craske S, et al. A randomized controlled trial of aromatherapy massage in a hospice setting. Palliat Med 2004; 18: 87–92

12f

Energy medicine

Suzanne Clewell

PREVENTION OF SYMPTOMS FROM CANCER TREATMENTS

Many hospitals around the USA support the use of energy medicine in helping oncology patients improve their quality of life through reduction of pain and alleviation of the side-effects associated with radiation and chemotherapy treatment.

In a randomized, prospective, 2-period, crossover intervention study at the University of Minneapolis, Healing Touch and therapeutic massage were compared to presence alone or standard care in the reduction of side-effects of cancer treatments. The study consisted of 230 cancer patients, and determined that Healing Touch and massage therapy lowered blood pressure, respiratory rate and heart rate. Healing Touch lowered fatigue, and both modalities lowered total mood disturbance. Ratings showed reduced pain and less use of non-steroidal anti-inflammatory drugs[1].

A 2003 study representing the largest sample size of Therapeutic Touch (TT) outcomes to date suggests that TT promotes calmness, comfort and well-being among hospitalized patients. There was also found to be increased patient satisfaction among this same population[2].

There are data to suggest that Qi Gong may reduce the dosages of certain prescribed medications and reduce the side-effects of some cancer therapies[3].

Pain

Energy practitioners generally do not align themselves to outcome. However, when treating an individual in pain, the result is often pain relief. There are many possible explanations for this, including the fact that energy medicine relaxes and calms the treated individual and this could assist with pain control. Another reason is that, although there may be lessons to learn from a disease process, pain, once it has alerted a person to a problem to be addressed, does not serve a positive function and may often be reduced or eliminated.

The Memorial Sloan-Kettering Hospital conducted a pilot program in the summer of 1998 that incorporated the use of Reiki and Healing Touch treatments. Pain assessment data for patients who received these modalities showed an average pain reduction of 48%[4]. In 1997, Olsen and Hansen investigated the impact of Reiki on chronic pain. Twenty volunteers who were experiencing chronic pain due to cancer and other causes demonstrated a significant decrease in pain after a single 75-minute Reiki healing session[5].

Breath moves energy. Focusing the breath may help the patient gain some control over their pain. Much as Lamaze breathing is used to help women through the pain of childbirth, the Chi we gain through the breath is believed to ease pain. One mantra taught to guide people through an acute episode of pain is a method of pursed-lipped breathing also used to help patients with asthma and chronic obstructive pulmonary disease (COPD) to move air in and out of the lungs in a more efficient manner. Breathe in through the nose and blow out through the mouth while remembering the phrase: *smell the rose, blow out the candle.* This visualization helps to keep the person who may be having acute pain focused upon the breath.

By bringing balance back into the energy field, energy medicine may assist the patient by mobilizing biological healing resources. In their book *Reiki Energy Medicine*, Barnett et al. cite anecdotal experiences that have led them to conclude that Reiki can reduce the need for pharmacologic intervention with respect to both dosage and administration[6]. The process of relaxation that Reiki and other forms of energy medicine facilitate may allow pain medication to work faster and more effectively while using smaller dosages. A Canadian study explored the usefulness of Reiki as an adjunct to opioid therapy in the management of pain. Both a visual analog scale and a Likert scale demonstrated significant reduction in pain following the Reiki treatment[7].

German scientists investigated the influence of music therapy upon the heart in cancer patients with chronic pain. It was found that the music had a profound effect. The patients in the study group showed increasing synchronization and co-ordination of heart rate and musical beat.

The patients reporting the best relaxation and relief of pain were the ones showing the most synchronization. Music therapy led to an improvement in falling asleep and a decrease in consumption of analgesics[8].

Depression/anxiety

Anxiety is commonplace in individuals who have recently been diagnosed with a life-altering disease such as cancer. It does not matter what stage their cancer is in – it is still *cancer*. Life will present the newly diagnosed individual with new challenges daily. Potentially toxic treatments on a routine basis may be scheduled for many months. The process of treatment itself often causes anxieties to multiply. Patients sitting in the waiting room may overhear others discussing their cancer experiences. This may give the new patient additional, inappropriate anxieties that he had not even imagined previously. There is a litany of stress-producing situations: the unavoidable wait for the nurse to call the patient's turn, watching others go first, worrying about whether or not their boss will be understanding regarding all the time missed from work, financial fears, never-ending scans, tests and treatments. When a patient is initially seen by the oncologist in consultation, there can be many additional causes of anxiety. The examination itself may be painful or embarrassing. In a radiation oncology practice, the machines themselves are very frightening to a patient. The word 'radiation' may strike fear into someone who remembers when his grandmother was treated many years ago and was 'burnt-up'. 'Chemotherapy' may bring to mind frightening images of weight loss, nausea and alopecia, even if their specific treatment course will cause none of these symptoms.

Fear of the unknown may lead to panic. Educators have known for many years that people experiencing a high level of stress do not retain information well. It is thought that providing healing energy along with patient education may help the patient to remember more of the information given to him in the office.

In our radiation oncology office there are a number of clinical staff members attuned to Reiki. The nurses channel energy to the patient as soon as he is escorted from the waiting room to the consultation room. An arm around the shoulder not only imparts the warmth of touch, it also sends healing energy for relaxation. The initial introduction and information gathering that is performed by the nurse is a time to offer presence and energy.

The physician may use the initial consultation as an opportunity to pass energy to the patient as he is obtaining the history and conducting the physical examination. The physician might also use this time to gain an overview of not only the diagnosis of cancer and treatment options, but also the energetic diagnosis that will also need to be addressed. Watson's transpersonal caring–healing model expands the view of the person to one that embodies energy and is composed of spirit, a universal mind and consciousness[9]. The North American Nurses' Diagnosis Association (NANDA) recognizes energy therapy intervention related to the approved nursing diagnosis of energy field disturbance (no. 1.8)[10].

Many of the radiation therapists in our facility are also attuned to Reiki; as they are positioning the patient on the treatment table they send energy to help the patient to remain calm and relax. Even the financial office has staff who are able to help patients be less anxious by passing energy. When the intention is present, healing energy flows. Touch is not necessary, as energy travels through space and distance.

There are a number of common-sense, practical modalities that can be optimized in order to lessen patient anxiety through the process of cancer diagnosis, treatment and after-care. These include optimal use of the environment, music, color and therapeutic presence.

The environment

Environment is an extremely important factor and can either create or dispel anxiety. Music, color, light, plants and water (fountains or aquaria) may help to diminish patient anxiety upon entering the office building. The purpose of Feng Shui is to create environments in which Chi flows smoothly to achieve physical and mental health[11]. Even without having a professional come to the office to create correct Feng Shui, one can get a 'feel' for a room. Does traffic flow smoothly through the room (consider walkers and wheelchairs and heavy doors)? Are the five elements of wood, fire, earth, metal and water represented? These elements do not actually have to be physically in the room; a framed painting or photograph of water in any form will suffice, candles or the color red can symbolize fire, etc. Living plants have energy and impart a relaxing dimension as well as beauty to the environment. There are many options available to the medical practitioner. Healing gardens, use of color, well-placed windows, music, art and design arrangement are all possible ways of providing a calming atmosphere in the home or office setting.

Color and light therapy

The practice of color therapy is based upon the hypothesis that different colors represent specific levels of vibrations that are believed to have an effect on certain parts of the body. Specific colors may help to regenerate and re-energize areas that are diseased or have blocked energy. Proponents feel that this system is effective in removing toxins from the body, and will stimulate the immune system to reverse any disease processes[12]. It is hypothesized that each color has specific vibrations associated with it and that the vibrations of the body may be influenced by the colors one consumes (food or breath) or comes in contact with (clothes, room color, seasons, etc.).

It is estimated that approximately 25 million people in the USA are affected by the disorder known as seasonal affective disorder (SAD). This condition is described by the National Institute of Mental Health as an emotional disorder characterized by drastic mood swings and depression that arrives in the winter and leaves in the spring[13]. Those with this disorder suffer from sunlight starvation. Radiation oncology departments have historically been located in the lower, underground levels of hospitals where there is a lack of natural light.

In his book *Light: Medicine of the Future*, Jacob Liberman explains that the pineal gland induces sleep and influences our moods by its secretion of melatonin in a cyclic rhythm. The pineal gland is primarily regulated by environmental light[14]. Long hours spent indoors with artificial lighting and shorter daylight hours in the wintertime predispose those at risk to develop SAD.

In 1980, a double-blind controlled study by Thomas Wehr and Norman Rosenthal established the existence of SAD and its treatment and greatly expanded the approach to treatment beyond the field of psychiatry[15]. Although the exact mechanism of action is not known, bright light treatment via the eyes has been found to have significant anti-depressant effects on more than 80% of SAD sufferers[16].

Some psychiatrists are reporting good results in treating what they call 'seasonal energy syndrome' with colored glasses. Red glasses are used for fall/winter depression and blue/green lenses for spring and summer agitation[17]. The majority of research attempting to determine what colors are most effective has proved inconclusive and sometimes contradictory. Workplaces are, however, increasingly incorporating the use of full-spectrum lighting on the assumption that it may help reduce anxiety and depression in those exposed.

In his book *A Practical Guide to Vibrational Medicine*, Richard Gerber writes that the use of color and light in healing was used by many ancient civilizations. He names some traditional therapies in use today that incorporate light and color, such as ultraviolet phototherapy in combination with psoralen-containing creams for psoriasis and the increasing use of lasers in medicine and surgery. Dr Gerber states that 'In order to better understand the varied applications of light therapy, or phototherapy, as it is sometimes called, we need to examine how light affects the physical body, as well as how it may affect the spiritual bodies and subtle-energy systems that make up the multidimensional human being'[18].

Art

Art speaks in ways that transcend words. Art has been used since ancient times as a method of communication and expression; however, formal art therapy is a relatively recent introduction into the medical field.

Cathy Malchiodi, art therapist and author of the book *The Art Therapy Sourcebook* states: 'Art therapy is based on the belief that images can help us understand who we are and enhance life through self-expression.'[19] Art can communicate powerful messages about our bodies and our minds and the creative process, it is effective therapy for those confronting serious illnesses. Malchiodi goes on to explain that 'It helps individuals cope with pain and other debilitating symptoms to identify feelings and physical symptoms and to become active participants in their medical care.' (reference 19, p. 165).

Research scientist Jeanne Achterburg has concluded from her studies that imagery in the form of visualization or drawings can be highly predictive of whether those with certain illnesses will improve or deteriorate. Her research with cancer patients indicates that the clarity of images may be related to recovery, and that the specific images which patients include in their drawings may reflect either healing or remission of their illness[20].

'People who are seriously ill often have two explanations for their condition, one spoken and one unspoken. The spoken one is a rational description of their condition based on medical knowledge. The other, the unspoken one, is a more personal and often private perception of their illness. This personal explanation may or may not be conscious, and may involve apprehension, confusion, misunderstanding, fear, or anxiety. It is also more likely to be revealed through art rather than communicated with words.' (reference 19, p. 176).

Bernie Siegel has used drawings for many years and believes that art is a reliable way to reveal his patient's feelings and perceptions that otherwise might remain unexpressed. Siegel states that: 'Drawings can be powerful tools for helping us deal with the important issues in our lives. Like dreams, they speak in the language of symbols, of metaphors. If we are willing to listen to that language and allow it to help us confront our fears, revelation will occur. We will be directed with all the energy and knowledge needed, and love and peace of mind will enter our lives. I wish all physicians would add a box of crayons to their diagnostic and therapeutic tools.'[21]

Music

Music is a type of vibrational energy whose effects can often be felt immediately. The medical office may take advantage of this fact through the use of appropriate, soothing music throughout, including the waiting room, examination and dressing rooms, and especially the treatment rooms. When receiving radiation, for example, the patient is often extremely anxious while lying completely still on a very hard table with thousands of pounds of machinery rotating around their body. From a medical oncology perspective, this translates into long hours in a chair receiving chemotherapy.

Music therapy is the application of music to produce relaxation and desired changes in emotions, behaviors and physiology[22]. In her book, *Tune Your Brain: Using Music to Manage Your Mind, Body and Mood*, Elizabeth Miles states that

a large body of clinical evidence has shown that music can counteract stress both physically and psychologically. She cites research that has demonstrated music to lower blood pressure, heart rate and respirations, and to relax tense muscles[23]. Music has also been shown to reduce levels of serum stress hormone levels[24].

Musical selections have been created by companies for use in various medical settings. The *Music Rx* system was tested on a population of patients in an intensive care unit (ICU) and post-surgical units at two hospitals. The studies, published in *ICM West Newsletter*, showed that patients who listened to this music had reduced heart rates, positive psychologic ratings and greater relief from pain[25].

Interestingly, in a study by Bailey[26] it was discovered that there was a significant improvement in the mood of cancer patients when live music was played as compared to previously taped music. The human element was attributed to contributing to the difference.

Patients may want to create a tape of music that they particularly enjoy listening to while using a portable player with head phones, as long as this does not interfere with their specific treatment. It is hypothesized that, as we learn more about how vibratory frequencies and patterns affect our body/mind, healing music will be composed to realign our altered vibratory patterns and bring them back to balance[22].

Music is used at Sloan-Kettering Cancer Center as part of a supportive care program to promote relaxation and reduce anxiety, supplement other methods of pain control and enhance communication between patient and family[27].

Drumming is increasingly being used to heal. The mechanism is thought to be the process of entrainment which is the tendency of people and objects to synchronize to a dominant rhythm. Michael Thaut, Neuroscientist and Director of the Center for Biomedical Research in Music at the Colorado State University, describes entrainment as 'the frequency of a moving system being determined by the frequency of another moving system.'[28] Entrainment provides us with the clearest explanation as to how drumming may aid in the healing of various maladies[29]. It is believed that drumming can synchronize the right and left hemispheres of the brain. Layne Redmond, author of *When Drummers Were Women*, explains that 'One of the most powerful aspects of drumming and the reason that people have done it since the beginning of being human is that it changes people's consciousness. Through rhythmic repetition of ritual sounds, the body, the brain and the nervous system are energized and transformed.'[30]

For a further discussion of supportive care uses of music therapy, please see the 'Mind–body' sections of this text.

Presence

Presence is a form of energy exchange. It can be thought of in a therapeutic sense as the physician or nurse relating to the client as one whole being to another whole being, using all the resources of mind, body, emotions and spirit. This can be experienced as a form of unconditional acceptance that requires the letting go of judgment and believing that a person is doing his or her best in this situation. The cancer care provider has the opportunity to be in the room with a patient who is experiencing great anxiety and to look into their eyes, listen and really *be there* attuned to what they are saying (spoken or unspoken). This interaction may allow the client to gain access to their own innate healing abilities and, thus, gain insights into self-healing[30]. Healing, in this sense, requires looking at parts of one's life that have been previously ignored or dismissed.

In an article published in *Nursing Forum*, Osterman and Schwartz-Barcott define 'Transcendent presence' as being 'physically, psychosocially, and spiritually in a relationship that is transforming (energy centered) and illuminates the oneness of the physician, and patient. It is felt as peaceful, comforting and harmonious. The outcome is a positive change in the affective state, such as diminished anxiety, and a feeling of being connected to another and not being alone.'[31] The supportive energy provided by having loved ones accompany the patient whenever possible cannot be overemphasized. The family will often experience even more anxiety than the patient, and efforts will be required to minimize the stress they feel. If the patient is agreeable, significant others should be included in the initial consultation so that all questions may be answered, and information given by the physician may be assimilated by all. However, if the patient is reluctant to have family/friends join him when he sees the physician, these wishes, as well as any confidentiality issues, should be respected. The power of open and honest communication in healthy therapeutic relationships has added to our resources for healing.

MANAGING TREATMENT-RELATED SYMPTOMS

General oncology

Fatigue

Fatigue in cancer patients is commonly related to radiation, chemotherapy, low blood component values and the cancer diagnosis itself. Cancer-related fatigue may linger long after treatments have ended. Fatigue may lead to depression as the patient questions: What is wrong? When will my energy will return? Cancer fatigue has been described as being devastating, unlike fatigue experienced by otherwise healthy persons. Cancer patients may literally feel unable to place one foot in front of another. Mental fatigue and an inability to focus one's thinking may also be present. According to Jane Poulson, in her article 'Not just tired' published in *The Journal of Clinical Oncology*, fatigue in patients with cancer deserves the same attention as pain, nausea and other well-recognized complications. While exercising or taking a nap may be helpful for fatigue associated with other conditions, it has variable effects upon cancer fatigue[32].

One of the most appropriate applications of energy medicine is in the treatment of fatigue. Fatigue can be seen as a depletion of vital energy. Energy medicine theorizes that receiving energy back into the body will often demonstrate improvement beyond anything that medical science has to offer.

In a randomized clinical trial conducted at Barnes-Jewish Hospital in St Louis, MO, 62 women who were receiving radiation for breast and gynecologic cancer were found to experience proportionately larger reductions in fatigue when given Healing Touch than those in the control group[33]. There is a need for more research to verify these important findings.

Therapies which focus on the breath may provide another avenue for fatigue related research. 'Improper breathing can lead to deficits in metabolic energy' according to Andrew Weil in his book *Spontaneous Healing*. Poor breathing can limit metabolism and the amount of energy available for healing.'[34] Weil goes on to say that if breath is the movement of spirit in the body, then working with the breath is a form of spiritual practice. The breath impacts health and healing and reflects the state of the nervous system. Heart rate, circulation, blood pressure and digestion can be regulated by conscious control of the breath[34]. There are many exercises described in Weil's books, as well as other publications to optimize the way we breathe for health.

Breath is Qi, or energy, in the vocabulary of energy medicine. To breathe correctly is to bring Qi into the body which is believed to increase energy and may help decrease fatigue. Please see the chapter on spirituality for a presentation of the 4-7-8 breath technique.

Weight gain/loss

In the cancer patient, weight loss or weight gain may be caused by medications, changes in activity, location of the cancer itself, anorexia due to nausea from treatment, as well as a number of other potential etiologies. From an energetic perspective, this makes it extremely important that food that is taken in be appropriate and high in nutritional value. Refined foods and foods that contain empty calories do not provide the vitamins, minerals and other ingredients so important to give the body the best possible chance to heal itself. Elimination of chemicals, sugar and other additives that are potentially detrimental, while choosing the foods that provide the optimum amount of nutritional content, demonstrates a respect for one's body and life, and so is said to impart a higher vibrational level.

Living foods are foods that have not been altered by any processes that may change its biochemical structure, therefore they are commonly raw and unprocessed. These foods are usually organically grown and are considered 'whole foods' in that they are considered to have their 'life force', or energy-giving qualities, intact.

It is hypothesized that foods carry with them vibrational energy that is related to their color, purity, the conditions surrounding harvesting, and even how they were handled and by whom prior to being eaten. Gabriel Cousens is a holistic physician and author. In his book *Spiritual Nutrition and the Rainbow Diet* Dr Cousens tells us that the colors of the foods we eat resonate with and feed color energy to the chakras[35].

Appetite is affected by color. Dining establishments have known for years that blue and violet tend to decrease appetite while yellow and orange will stimulate it. This information could be researched in more depth to discover ways in which to make food more appealing to the cancer patient with loss of appetite.

Exercise is a critical factor in maintaining optimum health and weight. Physical activity appropriate to the individual will help to increase appetite, raise beneficial (high-density lipoprotein (HDL)) cholesterol and increase bone density. Walking for a few minutes a day and working up to at least 20 to 30 is minutes as long as it remains within the individual's range of comfort is valuable on many levels: physical, emotional and spiritual.

Depression and anxiety

When one experiences anxiety one may buy into the perception that all that exists is anxiety, and it becomes a part of oneself. It becomes real and all-encompassing. When such an energetic pattern is maintained in one's mental and emotional body for a length of time, illness such as colitis or an ulcer may manifest. Redirecting one's thought patterns and energy away from a negative pattern and focusing on accessing the intrinsic wholeness and harmony of the body may give the patient a sense of empowerment and a rekindled knowledge that he has some control over the healing process. Increased perception of control will also help to decrease anxiety and depression. The fatigue study using Healing Touch at Barnes-Jewish Hospital also demonstrated more pronounced improvements in patients' levels of depression, anxiety and anger compared to the control group.

In a study published in the *ISSSEEM Journal*, it was found that Reiki was an effective modality for reducing pain, depression and anxiety[36].

Another study, published in the journal *Holistic Nursing Practice: The Science of Health and Healing* in October 2004, found that the experimental group had lower states of anxiety and depression and a higher state of self-esteem after the meridian exercise intervention than did the control group[37]. This was a double-blind study of a population of female college students, who were randomly assigned: 26 to the experimental group and 28 to the control group. The experimental treatment – meridian exercise – was led by a meridian exercise instructor for a total of 30 minutes per session for 12 sessions. Results showed that the experimental group had statistically significantly lower anxiety scores than those of the control group ($t = -7.982$, $p = 0.000$). The

depression scores of the experimental group were lower than the scores of the control group, and the difference was significant ($t = -8.814$, $p = 0.000$). The experimental group's self-esteem scores were higher than those of the control group, and the difference was significant ($t = 9.649$, $p = 0.000$).

Drum circles and drumming are being studied for stress and anxiety management. Barry Quinn, a licensed clinical psychologist, has found that alpha waves (the brain waves that occur when the brain relaxes into a cyclic pattern of 8–12 waves/second) increased in 50% of the patients he studied after a session of drumming. The drumming was more effective in producing alpha waves than biofeedback had been[38].

Sleep changes

In a 2003 study published in a journal for critical care nurses, the use of Therapeutic Touch, along with music and environmental interventions, was recommended to promote sleep in critically ill patients[39]. The hypothesis regarding the use of energy medicine such as Reiki to assist in induction of sleep is that the muscle relaxation and calming of the mind that accompanies this type of therapy allows the individual to slip into sleep with less effort. This has been noted in numerous anecdotal and personal experiences, although the hard science is lacking with regards to research studies.

Melatonin is the hormone produced by the pineal gland that is being studied because of the role it appears to play in sleep as well as in other functions of the body. Melatonin has been found to have a natural sedative quality and its production has been found to be directly linked to the amount and timing of exposure to light[18].

The use of lavender essential oil is beginning to be investigated to determine its potential in promoting relaxation. Participants at Oldham Cottage Hospital were monitored for 7 days. During this time their sleep, dozing and alert patterns were recorded. The following 7 days, one drop of *Lavandula augustfolia* was put on each patient's pillow at night. No other changes were made to their daily routine or medications. At the conclusion of the study the researchers observed increased daytime alertness, improved sleep patterns and as much as a 50% decrease in those patients who were previously experiencing confusion[40].

Sexuality

Feelings of undesirability related to change in body image perception, such as loss of a body part (mastectomy, orchiectomy), weight gain or hair loss – in addition to the myriad of symptoms associated with hormone manipulation and other therapies – may cause problems with sexuality in both the male and female cancer patient.

Reiki in particular is a form of energy healing that its practitioners believe is able to address relationships specifically. The outcome, whatever it may be, is understood to be in the best interests of all concerned. Therefore, it may be incorporated not only for the individual but also for couples. The hypothesis is that in this way there may be a healing of the relationship (which in Reiki is considered a third entity), and a greater empathy and stronger bond between all involved may ensue. The research in this area is lacking but it is thought that an improvement in the flow of Qi may assist in healing on many levels.

Other

Along with energy medicine, placebo may play a very important part in the healing process. Although the word 'placebo' is often thought about in a derogatory sense, the belief in the effectiveness of a placebo enables the patient to mobilize his own innate abilities to counter the symptoms and side-effects of cancer treatment by altering the biochemical and psychosomatic responses of the body. Placebo has been shown to have a significant response in many cases, some of which include helping to adjust white blood cell values, relieve depression, help with

sleep, and reduce pain[41]. In the book *Healing Intention and Energy Medicine*, placebo is described as a force for healing that is so varied it defies classification. The authors go on to describe placebo as being the effect of one's expectation, varying among individuals, seeming to be partially heritable, being diluted over a predictable period of time and able to be blocked by endorphin antagonists[42]. Non-local effects may occur from the interaction of a healer's conscious activity, which may possibly influence the physiology of the patient. 'This may be one mechanism for healing which occurs during the placebo effect, spiritual and mental healing and in all medical care.'[42]

Recommendations

Rosalyn Bruyere, a prominent energy medicine practitioner, recommends receiving energy medicine immediately after a course of radiation or chemotherapy. 'While retarding the growth of malignancy, radiation and chemotherapy also lower the basic vibration of the body. That lowered vibration may cause more malignant growth later on.'[43] She states that, because of the reduced vibrational level of the body, the new group of cells growing after treatment are not receiving enough energy and, as a result, cancerous cells may again be produced.

CHEMOTHERAPY-RELATED SYMPTOMS

General chemotherapy

'Chemotherapy clogs the whole auric field, but especially the liver', according to Barbara Brennan, an energy medicine researcher and practitioner[44]. The hypothesis would then be that energy medicine would be an appropriate concurrent modality when a patient is receiving a regimen of chemotherapy, due to its reported success in reduction of pain, nausea, nervousness and ability to improve blood laboratory values. It is also the contention of energy medicine practitioners that this modality assists medications (chemotherapy) to be optimally effective with minimal toxicity.

Qi Qong therapy may help patients to tolerate chemotherapy better. A case report published in 1999 described a patient with metastatic colon cancer who wanted to stop his chemotherapy. He was given external Qi Gong and then taught to practice at home. He finished his chemotherapy, and 3 years after his diagnosis is alive and in good health. He continues to practice Qi Gong for 4 hours a day[45].

The application of external Qi emitted from Qi Gong specialists (*in vivo* studies) has been reported to protect normal cells from harmful assaults, increase anti-tumor immunity, reduce tumor metastases, promote cell death of tumor cells and increase survival time of tumor-embedded animals. Some studies have proved inconclusive or had negative results due to the inconsistent effectiveness of Qi emitted by each practitioner.

The therapeutic claims of Qi Gong are vast, and there are extensive reports of research both clinical and in the laboratory; however, this literature is mostly in Chinese and not easily obtained. Most Chinese research accepts Qi as a given and is carried out from that perception rather than attempting to prove its existence… as is the case in the Western world[42].

Myelosuppression

Myelosuppression is the most common, and can be the most lethal, dose-limiting toxicity of chemotherapy[46]. This may take the form of neutropenia, anemia or thrombocytopenia.

Energy medicine, specifically Therapeutic Touch, has been proven to be highly effective in improving blood values.

In the 1960s, Delores Kreiger developed a research study that looked at the effect that laying-on-of-hands healing would have upon hemoglobin values. She chose to study hemoglobin because it is basic to oxygen transport in the body, and oxygen transport is central to the physical healing process. She found that, in the experimental group, both the hemoglobin values and the hematocrit showed significant changes. Both indicators increased consistently following the healing treatment, and always remained within normal limits. The control group did not receive laying-on-of-hands treatment, and both their hemoglobin and hematocrit values remained unchanged. These results have been replicated in later studies[47].

Richard Gerber states that 'The tendency for healing energy to increase hemoglobin has been found to be so strong that cancer patients who have undergone laying-on-of-hands healing have occasionally shown rises in hemoglobin levels in spite of treatment with bone marrow suppressive agents which predictably induce anemias.'[48]

Anticipatory nausea and/or vomiting may occur before chemotherapy and may last several hours to days. It may affect 25% of patients receiving chemotherapy and is usually not observed in infants and small children – leading researchers to conclude that it is an effect of classical conditioning[46]. Hypothetically, this would be very amenable to healing energy and could be given by the health-care provider, family member or the patient himself. Theoretically, as the patient is in the process of receiving the chemotherapy drugs he could self-treat and pass Qi throughout his body and even send it to the hanging chemotherapy bag.

Acute nausea occurs shortly after administration of the chemotherapy agent and may last 24–48 hours. Delayed nausea occurs at least 24 hours after the chemotherapy infusion and may continue for several days. If energy medicine is helpful in assisting in relaxation and sleep for these patients, it may potentially be able to assist in the effectiveness of prescribed antiemetics.

In a study funded by the National Cancer Institute and located at the University of Rochester Cancer Center it was found that those who wore motion sickness wrist bands, which incorporate acupressure to reduce nausea and vomiting, were reported to have 15% less nausea than those who did not apply acupressure[49]. Acupressure has been found to be effective in relief of chemotherapy-induced nausea. Additional studies are currently ongoing[50].

ENHANCING VITALITY

There are many ways the cancer patient can be proactive in getting the Chi flowing more optimally, thus enhancing vitality and healing. Many of the energy medicine modalities are available to be applied for self-healing and are constantly and inexpensively available to the patient. In her book *Living the Therapeutic Touch*, Delores Kreiger explains: 'The more thoroughly and consciously healing becomes a part of one's lifestyle, the more clearly it is perceived that in the last analysis it is the patient who heals him- or herself.' She goes on to say that once patients are able to accept responsibility for healing, they may realize that they have the ability to bolster their immune system for self-protection, and to support the natural intelligence of the body for self-healing. Patients can then be educated in preventative techniques that will assist them in maintaining a state of vibrant well-being (reference 47, p. 122).

Data support the clinical effectiveness of Healing Touch in health enhancement. In one study, themes reported by clients were increased relaxation, connection and enhanced awareness[51].

The physician

In their book *Reiki: Energy Medicine*, Reiki Masters Libby Barnett and Maggie Chambers write that Reiki not only enhances the healing skills of the physician or health-care provider, it is also a rejuvenating practice of self-care. It is a method for health-care professionals to augment their ability to heal, while also receiving an invaluable tool for attending to their own health maintenance, personal growth and self-renewal[6].

'We are capable of healing through more than just touch', writes Richard Gerber in *A Practical Guide to Vibrational Medicine*. He states that we can heal through the energy of our voice, the soft and caring tones, the content of our speech. Through our intention to bring healing, comfort and love, we have the ability to tap into the healing powers of the higher spiritual energies[18].

The office or hospital where the physician practices may itself be a place of healing energy. Conversely, it could be an environment of stagnated Chi. Sometimes only minor changes in the placement of items can make a difference. Gill Hale, author of *A Practical Encyclopedia of Feng Shui*, writes: 'In an office where chi flows freely, employees will be happy and supportive, projects will be completed on time and stress levels will be low. Where the chi is stuck, there will be disharmony and the business will not flourish.'[11]

Reiki can be used to facilitate communication and well-being among staff. According to Reiki practitioners and the authors of the book *Reiki: Energy Medicine*, nurses who practice Reiki report that it helps to harmonize personalities and builds a sense of co-operation among workers[6]. Providers of Reiki, as well as of many forms of energy medicine, are believed to receive the life force while offering it to others. The theory is that, as they channel the energy from the universal source, they are energized as the energy moves through them and into the receiver. Therefore, they do not have to sacrifice their own life force but actually receive increased physical stamina[6]. Reiki is also believed to assist in maintaining mental clarity and emotional stability in a profession that is emotionally demanding to the health-care provider.

In *Hands of Light* Barbara Brennan writes that 'In healing, you do not generate the energy you transmit, but you must first raise your frequency to that needed by the patient in order to entrain the energy from the universal energy field.'[44] The theory is that the energy of the one transmitting the healing needs to be higher than that of the patient receiving the healing.

Time for meditation and centering is necessary in the self-care regimen for all healers. The hypothesis is that, in this way, the connection to the energy source is more readily facilitated. Intuition and intention are said to be important components of energy medicine, and centering the self reduces the stresses and confusion of daily life, clears the mind and revitalizes the body. It is assumed to be difficult for healing to take place when the mind is cluttered by anxieties and distractions. The breath is all-important when channeling energy and also will assist in the process of relaxation and grounding. The process of centering itself brings one back to calmness, back to a state of mind wherein the healer reminds himself that he is part of a universal whole, and as such has universal support as an instrument of healing. If he has been questioning his ability because of an unexpected outcome, he will remember that, as long as he did his best and with healing intention, the outcome of any individual is ultimately in the hands of the Universal Power and will always be in the best interest for that individual patient.

Andrew Weil, in his book *Spontaneous Healing*, speaks of the breath as the movement of spirit in the body that connects us to all creation. It impacts health and healing. How we breathe reflects the condition of the nervous system as well as influencing it. We are able to regulate blood pressure, heart rate, circulation and digestion by adjusting the rhythm and depth of the breath. Weil explains that the healing system may be affected by the breath also. The energy felt in the body after doing certain breathing exercises is 'Qi'. It may be felt as warmth or tingling or a subtle vibration. It can be felt more easily with practice. Weil states that 'The more one can experience yourself as energy, the easier it is not to identify yourself with your physical body.' (reference 34, p. 259).

In a 2001 article in the *Journal of Clinical Oncology*, Matt Mumber states that mindful meditation techniques have been used successfully to help medical students cope with anxiety[52]. A deep cleansing breath can bring back the focus of the present moment. The physician must practice what he preaches in integrative medicine. Mumber explains that 'In order to be effective guides, we must be natives to the territory of effective self-care. We must walk the talk.'[52] Those physicians who do are more effective in helping patients to make appropriate changes regarding lifestyle and health[53]. All the nutritional and lifestyle advice applies to the healer as much as to the patient. The higher vibrational frequencies that one's body attains through physical care and respect carries through to the healing he passes to the patient.

The family

Day-to-day observation would seem to imply that one of the most frustrating issues for those close to the individual with cancer is the feeling of helplessness. To be able to help in some way, other than with just the physical, supportive care that may be required, lends a positive aspect to the experience of all involved. For a friend or loved one simply to give the gift of touch imparts a feeling of worth and caring to both parties. To focus positive energy, to cleanse a room of previous negativity, and ask loving, healing energies to surround the practitioner and the client, in theory, creates an environment conducive to relaxation, openness and communication. Some of the stress the family has been experiencing may subside, and exhaustion may give way to renewed strength and hope. Energy medicine is not only for the patient; caregivers benefit as well.

Hope

Experiencing integrative modalities such as energy medicine also may provide hope to the person with cancer. Hope may give patients who have a potentially terminal diagnosis the ability to maintain their spirits and continue on. It would stand to reason that patients have the greatest confidence in physicians who, while continuing to be open and honest, do not take away hope.

According to Bernie Siegel in his book *Peace, Love and Healing*, 'Anything that offers hope has the potential to heal, including thoughts, suggestions, symbols and placebos'[21]. He goes on to say (p. 155) that 'Perhaps more powerful than any visualization or other specific technique you can use to alter the inner environment of your body are feelings of hope and love.'[21]

Burkhardt and Jacobson in *Holistic Nursing: A Handbook for Practice* state that 'Hope is a desire accompanied by an expectation of fulfillment, hope goes beyond believing or wishing. Hope is future oriented.'[54] Physician and psychiatrist Victor Frankel wrote: 'Hope is a significant factor in overcoming illness and living through difficult situations.'[55] Hope helps people cope with uncertainty and fear and helps them to visualize a positive outcome.[54]

Meaning

The search for meaning in one's life is a universal quest. An introduction to the concept of energy medicine may assist in this endeavor. Delores Kreiger states that 'Research is but one basis for reality. Life itself provides an irrefutable experiential base to our concepts of reality. In the relationship we call the healing act, it is obvious from the powerful changes that frequently occur in the experienced healer's life that deep, core structures of the self may be stimulated to enter into and affect everyday life activities. The transfer of the locus of control of personal behavior to the inner core of being is important to the well-being of a society that values actualization of the potential of the self. The persistent reality of the healing act can activate compelling life-affirmative drives in those who heal. Surely it is worth the attention of our most astute minds, as well as those who are merely compassionate.'[47] Kreiger goes on to say that the committed healer experiences values of self-actualization as described by Maslow[56,57]. Self-actualized persons share many characteristics if they are not blocked by society[58]:

(1) Perceive reality accurately;

(2) Are accepting of themselves and others;

(3) Live their lives with spontaneity, simplicity and naturalness;

(4) Believe their lives are meaningful (they have a mission to fulfill);

(5) Enjoy privacy, time alone to reflect and contemplate;

(6) Do not take life for granted;

(7) Experience times when they are so involved in what they are doing that sense of time and self-awareness are forgotten;

(8) Take a social interest;

(9) Have profound interpersonal relationships;

(10) Have little religious, social or racial prejudice (democratic character structure);

(11) Are creative;

(12) Are autonomous, independent, self-sufficient.

See comparison between Maslow's hierarchy of needs (Table 12.8) and the seven chakras (Table 12.9).

Healers have reported critical changes in self-image and in the way they relate to others in the world. They have a more acute appreciation for creativity, spontaneity, expressiveness and idiosyncrasy. 'They [healers] sense meaningfulness in life because they have touched the more subtle reaches of its nature during their peak experiences of helping others' states Kreiger[47].

Connection

The hypothesis that energy exists in the connections we have with everything that surrounds us is strengthened by numerous studies on the subject. Relationships with other humans, and the energy bonds that are formed, are believed to be a major influence upon our energetic environment. The need for love and intimacy are powerful determinants of our health and survival[59]. Dean Ornish, in his book *Love and Survival* states: 'Anything that promotes love and intimacy is healing: Anything that promotes isolation, separation and loneliness, loss, hostility, anger, cynicism, depression, alienation, and related feelings often leads to suffering, disease and premature death from all causes. While the evidence on the relationship of psychosocial factors to illness is controversial[60], most scientific studies have demonstrated the extraordinarily powerful role of love and relationships'[59].

Two studies which look at the importance of relationships and interaction that have withstood the test of time are the Alameda County Study and the Tecumseh Study.

The Alameda County Study was conducted in 1965 by Lisa Berkman and her colleagues at the California Health Services. They studied almost 7000 men and women living in Alameda County, California. It was found that the participants who lacked social or community ties were 1.9 to 3.1 times more likely to die during the 9-year follow-up period[61]. The association between social and community ties and premature death was found to be independent of and a more powerful predictor of health and longevity than age, gender, race, socioeconomic status, smoking, alcohol consumption or numerous other lifestyle

Table 12.8   Maslow's hierarchy of needs (references 56 and 57)
Asthetic needs
Need to know and understand
Need for self-actualization
Need for esteem
Need for love and belonging
Need for safety/security
Psychologic survival needs

Table 12.9   The chakra system
7th – Crown   Spiritual
6th –Third eye   Intuition/understanding
5th – Throat   Expression
4th – Heart   Love/compassion
3rd – Solar plexus   Power/control
2nd – Sacral   Emotions/self-worth
1st – Root   Survival/security

and health practices. Berkman was quoted in an article in *Psychosomatic Medicine* as saying: 'Those who lacked social ties were at increased risk of dying from coronary heart disease, cancer, stroke, respiratory diseases, GI disease and all other causes of death.'[62]

The Tecumseh Study looked at almost 3000 men and women who were studied for 9–12 years. The researchers found that men who reported higher levels of social relationships and activities were significantly less likely to die during the follow-up period. 'When these social relationships were broken or decreased, disease rates increased two to three times as much during the succeeding ten to twelve year period.'[63]

Ornish writes: 'Love and intimacy are at the root of what makes us sick and what makes us well, what causes sadness and what brings happiness, what makes us suffer and what leads to healing.'[59]

Animal/pet therapy

The 'healthy connection' of love and relationships is not limited to human–human. Animals and pets can be extremely important in facilitating communication and connection, and are spiritually uplifting. In the text *Animal-Assisted Therapy* the authors write that: 'Companion animals offer seemingly unlimited opportunities for affection and unconditional love, both of which are key elements in the development of attachment relationships.'[64] In his book *The Healing Power of Pets*, Becker states that 'Part of the healing power of pets is their capacity to make the atmosphere safe for emotions, the spiritual side of healing.'[65]

Although animal-assisted activities have been documented as therapeutic for various populations, there has been little study in the cancer population. A pilot study entitled *Animal Assisted Activity and Anxiety Among Radiation Therapy Patients: A [University of Missouri] MU Interdisciplinary Randomized Clinical Trial* represents an initial investigation of the potential benefit of animal-assisted activity for cancer patients. This study had a quasi-experimental design, involved 30 hospitalized patients over age 18 who were randomly assigned to a visit in one of three 15-minute sessions: (1) a certified visitor dog and its handler; (2) a friendly human visitor; or (3) no visitor, for a quiet reading time. At the end of each session an intervention questionnaire (IQ) was completed. Internal consistency for IQs was demonstrated by Cronbach alpha coefficients: 0.87 for dog visit, 0.86 for friendly human visit and 0.81 for quiet reading.

Statistically significant differences (Stdiff) between item mean scores for the dog and the reading group (Stdiff 3.94, $p = 0.00008$), and for the visitor and reading group (Stdiff 2.54, $p = 0.011$) were identified. Statistically significant differences between the dog and the visitor group were not identified (Stdiff 1.397, $p = 0.1624$). However, more participants in the dog group reported that the dog comforted them, made them feel happy and gave them more energy than participants with the human visitor[66].

Edward T. Creagan, an oncologist at the Mayo Clinic, believes that pets offer such benefit to patients that he prescribes them as part of the treatment for approximately one-third of his cancer patients. He feels that pets provide purpose and meaning to patients during difficult times (reference 66, p. 220). When cancer and chemotherapy have compromised the immune system, being happy and at peace may stimulate natural cancer-killing cells. Pets have been shown to bring about these qualities when interacting with humans. Animals intuitively know when and where someone hurts. The importance of touch in humans has been documented but, when someone has a disease that friends and family may not understand, often there is a fear of coming too close or touching. Even the most well-meaning friends will sometimes avoid contact as if they were afraid that the cancer were contagious. This presents a trauma to the person with cancer who may require touch more now than at any other time of his life. Animals, however, give unconditional permission to touch, pet and hug, and they give back (reference 66, p. 97). Evidence supports the theory that animals provide definite health benefits. Documentation of the positive impact of animals on human health comes from epidemiologic studies that support long-term health effects of pet ownership[67].

Horses are becoming very popular as therapeutic animals for emotional as well as physical difficulties. Horses provide honest feedback and have been found to help with a multitude of issues such as self-confidence, anger management, depression and communication, among others. All of these may be applicable to the needs of cancer patients or their families. Sunstone Healing Center in Tucson, AZ, under the direction of University of Arizona neurosurgeon and horseman Allen Hamilton, uses horses in retreat settings to enable cancer patients and their children to 'learn different psychological and spiritual strategies to assist in restoring themselves to empowerment, health and harmony.'[68] Horses have the ability to mirror what human body language says to them and can provide insight in situations where a human therapist alone may not succeed.

Nature therapy

The importance of connection with nature is becoming accepted as having therapeutic value in reducing stress and enhancing positive attitudes. In one hospital study, patients who had a window with a natural view of trees had shorter postoperative stays, slightly fewer postoperative complications and took fewer moderate and strong analgesic medications than those with a window that looked out onto a wall[69].

Nature therapy, ecotherapy, or environmental therapies represent a variety of entities now being used. 'Nature is more than an intimate part of each individual', writes Linda Nebbe, 'and we are part of nature. Nature therapy is human interaction with all facets of nature as well as the human's part in and connection to the entire biosphere. The connection can be as simple as food to eat or a complex philosophical or spiritual, guiding connection'[70].

Kreiger tells us that one's sense of connection with the environment can be an important source of comfort and strength. To feel the wind, see the stars, smell the flowers and feel that energetic connection with nature can be a very important aspect in one's healing journey (reference 47, p. 112).

It is hypothesized that the use of subtle energies in healing appears to help in forming a connection between both the person channeling and the one receiving. Connectedness continues to grow and envelopes relationships with others and relationships with the entire natural world on all levels.

Spirituality

It is believed that a deepened awareness of spiritual connection is among the many benefits attributed to both practicing and receiving energy medicine. The very essence of energy medicine is the act of making a connection with an infinite source of energy, power, intelligence and benevolence. This source may be envisioned differently by each individual. It may be thought of as emitting from above. Some feel that it originates from the earth, or that it is all-encompassing and surrounds everything at all times. It may be felt as warmth, white or colored light, angels or spirits; there is no limit to the variety of perceptions possible. There is commonality, however, in the fact that the practice of all forms of energy medicine provides one with an opportunity to take time out from their busy lives, and connect with the energy within and without all of us. Energy medicine joins human being to human being on a level far deeper than the superficial interactions we have become used to in our daily lives.

In his book *Honoring the Medicine*, Kenneth Cohen tells readers that in Native American tradition the healer is a hollow tube through which the power of the Great Spirit flows. The healer must remain in a state of prayer to maintain the link to that power. Healers who are connected to this life current are never in danger of losing personal energy when they interact with a patient. They are not in danger of having negative energies or evil spirits connect with them because, during the healing, they no longer exist as separate individuals, they are in a state of spiritual unity with life[71].

Larry Dossey, when differentiating between a 'cure' that may be expected for the presenting disease process, and a 'cure' for the human spirit, states that, there is comfort in the realization that 'physical illness, no matter how painful or grotesque, is at some level of secondary importance in the total scheme of our existence'[72]. He goes on to tell us that sometimes the disease will regress or disappear when one attains this realization, but that the true 'cure' is in knowing that we are all spirits whose essential energy cannot be touched by the ravages of disease and death.

Eliminating toxins

The hypothesis in energy medicine is that purification – or the elimination of toxins – may sometimes manifest itself as an illness. Maintaining our body/mind/spirit with only that which is nourishing and positive will assist in elimination of the toxins that we are bombarded with daily. Chi is everything, it is the vital energy of life. If the flow of Chi is obstructed, toxins will collect; however, having Chi flow optimally will assist the body in continually eliminating the toxins we are subjected to. Living our lives in this manner may greatly reduce or eliminate the need for future illnesses.

Treatment related

Energy medicine can be used to help the body rid itself of toxins received from the cancer treatment itself. While surgery, chemotherapy and radiation may be life-saving treatments, they also leave toxins in their wake. Toxins or byproducts from anesthesia, narcotics or other medication, chemotherapeutic drugs, or even tumor kill as a result of conventional therapy are all potentially toxic or undesirable substances that, when there is no use for them in the body, would be best removed. Hypothetically, energy medicine can be used to enable the body to cleanse and work towards elimination of these toxins, initially on an energetic or spiritual level, and eventually resulting in a physical cleansing.

ENVIRONMENTAL

The energetic environment

A basic tenet of energy medicine is that the aura, or etheric body, is the higher-energy template of the physical body. It is able to sense itself in space and time, and may become unbalanced by less than beneficial influences in our environment (food, thoughts or emotions). The aura is normally able to rebalance itself naturally. Under adverse conditions the imbalances may become longstanding or chronic, and finally lead to disease. Exposure to certain toxic energies (radiation, pesticides, herbicides and other toxic substances) may not produce results for many years, but the aura will change long before any signs of disease in the physical body become apparent.

In Richard Gerber's *Vibrational Medicine* one theory holds that the energy characteristics of the earth's electromagnetic, gravitational and subtle energetic fields vary with geographic location. The presence of large underground mineral deposits or water sources can affect the electromagnetic fields in the overlying regions and have been detected by satellite. There is evidence to suggest that the earth has its own meridian system made up of subtle energies. Man-made metallic structures can disrupt this pattern of energy flow (reference 48, p. 460). If we, as vibrational beings, become entrained to the planetary fields that surround us, the various energy patterns and fields probably cause both beneficial and detrimental effects. The Chinese have been aware of these energy patterns since ancient times and the practice of Feng Shui selects the most favorable energetic sites for the need at hand. Stressful effects upon human health, caused by abnormal fields associated with a particular geographical region, are referred to as 'geopathic stress'.

In his book *Spontaneous Healing*, Andrew Weil addresses the problem of energy pollution in our environment. 'I am concerned about toxic forms of energy as well as matter; electromagnetic pollution may be the most significant form of pollution human activity has produced in this century, all the more dangerous because it is invisible and insensible.'[34] Weil goes on to explain that toxins, either energetic or material, can potentially damage DNA, disrupt the process of biological healing, weaken our immune system and promote cancer and other diseases[34]. He warns against the use of electric blankets and heating pads as they generate large electrical fields and are used close to the body. Another practical recommendation is that placement of electric clock radios should not be near one's head while sleeping. Studies have been inconclusive for the most part regarding electromagnetic field pollution as it relates to disease, but it may be reasonable to be aware of the simple recommendations for preventive avoidance of overexposure.

Natural environment

Spirituality and an appreciation for the power and the energy available to us cannot be separated from a true respect and love of nature and the earth. Many energy medicine practitioners feel that the energy they facilitate comes from the earth itself. It does not matter where the source is, but in the opinion of many, it does matter that we take care of the earth. It is becoming all too clear that when we waste and pollute, we destroy beauty and health, and leave ourselves vulnerable to disease and discord. The devastating results of irresponsible individuals and corporations leaving a legacy of hazardous waste behind have been shown to us repeatedly. Chemical dumps, air pollution, filthy living conditions, pesticides and additives in our food, growing landfills, etc. all serve to clog the earth's energies and, as a result, our energy.

Healing and caring apply to our earth, as well as to one another. Responsibility and love for nature is an integral part of change that needs to occur in concert with spiritual growth for true healing to manifest in each of us. Involvement in one or more of the many environmentally conscious groups can be a healing experience both for ourselves and for our planet. These organizations strive to protect the air, water, animals, old growth forests, and other sources of beauty and irreplaceable natural resources that otherwise run the risk of being destroyed forever and, along with them, the demise of life as we know it. The earth and its gifts must be appreciated and revered for its energy to endure. Even if we take responsibility only for ourselves and our families, living our lives practicing respect for the earth, being conscious of energy and conservation, and recycling, we will remember that each one of us as inhabitants of planet earth make a huge difference collectively. It should also be remembered that many of the most active and promising chemotherapy agents in existence and under study today come from natural sources.

Local grassroots organizations are always in need of volunteers in many capacities.

A sampling of respected national and international environmental protection groups, many of which have local chapters, are listed below:

- Greenpeace
  702 H Street, NW,
  Suite 300, Washington, DC 20001
  www.greenpeaceusa.org

- The Natural Resources Defense Council
  40 W. 20th St., New York, NY 10011
  www.nrdc.org

- Environmental Defense
  257 Park Ave. West, New York, NY 10010
  www.environmentaldefense.org

- National Wildlife Federation
  11100 Wildlife Center Drive, Reston, VA
  20190-5362
  www.nwf.org

- The Nature Conservancy
  4245 N. Fairfax Drive, Suite 100
  Arlington, VA 22203-1606
  www.nature.org

- The Sierra Club
  85 Second St., 2nd Floor
  San Francisco, CA 94105
  www.sierraclub.org

Family environment

Theoretically, the energies that we are surrounded with on a daily basis can affect our energy fields (auras) tremendously. Ideally, the family environment is one of love and unconditional acceptance. This is often not the case, however, and in order to avoid any detrimental effects to one's health it would be wise to be aware of the potential that may exist either for health or for harm.

The Harvard Mastery of Stress Study, a study of Harvard students in the early 1950s, became a powerful example of how loving relationships may affect susceptibility to disease[73,74]. In this study 126 healthy men were chosen from the Harvard classes of 1952–1954. They were given questionnaires to measure their perceived relationship with their parents. Students were asked to rate the descriptions from one (1) to four (4), with the number 4 meaning a 'very close' relationship and the number 1 representing a 'strained and cold' relationship. Thirty-five years later, medical records were obtained and detailed histories were taken. Researchers found that 91% of participants who did not believe that they had had a warm relationship with their mothers 35 years previously had been diagnosed with some form of serious disease in midlife compared to

45% of the participants who perceived that they had had a warm relationship with their mothers. The measurements of low warmth with fathers concluded that 82% were diagnosed with disease compared to 50% of the study group who had high warmth and closeness scores with their fathers. These effects appeared to be additive in that 100% of all participants who rated relationships with both the mother and father to be low were diagnosed with disease. Only 47% of those who believed that they had had a warm relationship with both parents had diagnosed diseases in midlife[59]. The researchers then looked at this study in a different way and asked participants to describe their parents with questions such as: 'What kind of person is your father?' The relationship of these descriptions was independent of family history of disease or other stressors. It was found that students who described their parent(s) with more negative statements had more diagnosed disease in midlife. When these researchers combined these two measures they found that '95% of subjects who used few positive words and rated their relationship low in caring had diseases diagnosed in midlife, whereas only 29% of subjects who used many positive words and rated their parents high in caring had disease'[73].

In the 1950s another study, The Scotland Study, looked at men who were admitted to the hospital with chest discomfort prior to learning they had cancer. They found that men who were diagnosed with lung cancer had experienced significantly more difficulties earlier in life (these included traumas such as death of a parent) than those whose etiology was benign[75]. They were also found to have more disturbed interpersonal relationships, and difficulty in expressing their emotions[76].

Numerous studies have come to similar conclusions. There is hope, however, according to Dean Ornish: 'We can't change what happened to us in our childhood or adolescence, but we do not need to do so. I believe that it is the ongoing pattern of relating to others that is most important, not a particular event that happened much earlier in life'[59]. Ornish goes on to say that an important reason that early relationships are such good predictors of illness in later life is that these patterns of relating usually do not change. Everyone is aware of how difficult it is to modify behaviors such as diet, smoking or other lifestyle habits, and changing our ongoing pattern of relating to others is even more difficult[59].

Gary Schwartz, director of the University of Arizona's Human Energy Systems Laboratory, believes that love is measurable. He states that, when people use the word 'love', and this may be in many different contexts, they all refer to a strong attraction or force. There is some sort of reception, a deep wishing to connect and to receive, when we love something,' states Schwartz in a discussion with Ornish (reference 59, p. 189). He describes love as the fundamental attractive process through which we receive information. 'Love and loving are the back-and-fourth relationship that takes place in all systems. Love affects us via the direct transmission or reception of energy' (reference 59, p. 190). Schwartz believes that someone who is feeling isolated, lonely or depressed is metaphorically cutting himself off from the energy source of life and wellness and after a time this may lead to illness.

Doctor–patient relationship

According to Richard Gerber, in *A Practical Guide to Vibrational Medicine* (reference 18, p. 399), the physician is capable of healing through more than just touch. He can heal through the energy of his voice, the soft and caring tones, the content of his speech. Through his intention to bring healing, comfort and love, he has the ability to tap into higher energies that have healing powers. When physicians bring the intention to work with their patients on an energetic level, the doctor and patient can learn methods for changing dysfunctional behavior patterns in order to create an inner and outer environment more conducive to wellness. Gerber goes on to say: Enlightened physicians will be able to work with patients to try to alter dysfunctional patterns of emotion via counseling, vitamins, stress reduction techniques and meditation. Patients will modify the higher elements of their consciousness using flower essences, gem elixirs, homeopathic remedies, and various other subtle-energy modalities. However, it will still be important that people use these therapies adjunctively while they are implementing other changes in their modes of thinking, feeling, nutritional habits and general lifestyle, if a more lasting healing and inner balance is to occur. Once we have learned the real reasons for feeling ill, we must begin to make lasting changes that will result in a healing on many simultaneous levels. We must learn to accept responsibility for our own lives.' (reference 48, p. 478).

Community environment: emotional/mental/societal

Ease of access to reliable information regarding integrative modalities that may be appropriate for each individual's cancer or concern is a major priority. It has been found to be beneficial for people to gather with others who may share a life-altering experience (such as a diagnosis of cancer). In our society people who are living with a cancer diagnosis often experience strained relationships with friends and family who may have difficulty knowing what to say or do. What may be perceived as an act of kindness by a well-meaning individual may be seen by the person with cancer as pity or over-concern. Many patients have told me that they feel better, and more in control, if they continue to adhere to most of their normal daily activities. The well-intentioned family member who wants to place limits on what they should and should not do serves as an unwelcome message to the patient that somehow he is different now that he has cancer. Access to integrative modalities may assist patients in regaining a sense of control. Patients are able to make informed decisions as to which modality they wish to incorporate into their healing plan. Experiencing integrative modalities, such as energy medicine, also may provide hope to the person with cancer.

Energy medicine is offered in the majority of integrative medicine clinics and educational groups for cancer patients. A small sampling of some of the most recognizable institutions in the USA which provide integrative medicine supportive care and information to cancer patients include:

- Beth Israel Medical Center's Continuum Center for Health and Healing, New York;

- The Dana-Farber Cancer Institute's Zakim Center for Integrated Therapies, Boston, MA;

- Memorial Sloan-Kettering Cancer Center, New York;

- Stanford Hospital and Clinic's Stanford Center for Integrative Medicine, Stanford Cancer Supportive Care Program, Stanford, CA;

- Thomas Jefferson University, Myrna Brind Center of Integrative Medicine, Philadelphia, PA;

- University of Pittsburgh Medical Center, UPMC Cancer Center Integrative Medicine Program, Pittsburgh, PA;

- University of Texas, MD Anderson Cancer Center, Huston, TX;

- Scripps Health Care Network, Scripps Center for Integrative Medicine, San Diego, CA;

- Yale-Griffin Hospital, Integrative Medicine Center at Griffin Hospital, New Haven, CT.

END-OF-LIFE CARE

The hypothesis that energy medicine not only addresses symptoms, but can directly improve quality of life was tested in a 1998 study in Canada entitled 'Effect of Therapeutic Touch on the Well-Being of Persons with Terminal Cancer'. The results supported the hypothesis that even as few as three non-contact energy sessions would increase the sensation of well-being in persons with terminal cancer[77]. This was a small, randomized controlled trial set in a palliative care unit of a university-affiliated hospital. Twenty patients with terminal cancer between the ages of 38 and 68 were randomized. The majority of these patients were diagnosed with lung cancer. Ten patients were assigned to the control group and ten to the experimental group. The well-being scale evaluates pain, nausea, depression, anxiety, shortness of breath, activity, appetite, relaxation and inner peace. A significant difference was observed in the mean progression of well-being between the experimental group and the control group ($t = -3.73$; $p = 0.0015$). The experimental group showed a mean increase of 1.70 (SD 1.28) in sensation of well-being, whereas the control group showed a decrease of 0.31 (SD 1.12). Sensation of well-being for only the experimental group improved significantly over time ($f = 17.56$, d.f. (1,9), $p < 0.025$). The conclusion was that patients with terminal cancer receiving Therapeutic Touch treatments had a higher sensation of well-being than did those who simply rested, and these sensations of well-being increased following three Therapeutic Touch interventions[77].

Reiki provides deep relaxation and pain reduction. Severe pain or fear can be managed using less medication without sacrificing consciousness[4–7]. This, in turn, leaves the client more alert to deal with the emotional issues of closure with loved ones[6].

Reiki is supportive therapy for hospice and palliative care, as demonstrated in a 1997 study of Reiki in a hospice setting. This article[6] describes the treatment of a 70-year-old man who had an aggressive cancer. He was receiving palliative radiation and medication and Reiki. Through her hospice experiences the author concluded that: 'Some general trends seen with Reiki use include: periods of stabilization in which there is time to enjoy the last days of one's life, a peaceful, calm passing if death is imminent; and relief from pain, anxiety, dyspnea, and edema. Reiki is a valuable complement in supporting patients in their end-of-life journey, enhancing the quality of their remaining days.'[6]

In a noteworthy, randomized double-blind study of distant healing, Elizabeth Targ and colleagues studied a population of people with advanced AIDS. They chose this group for three reasons. First, at the time of this research there was little that could be done for these people (this meant that it was not likely that a positive outcome would be due to the result of expectation or psychological input). Second, this group obviously needed *something*. Third, often people with an advanced illness have little money available, and distant healing would be a modality that could be offered for a low fee or free, if given by friends or family members. Researchers looked at 27 different baseline variables, and the treatment group was scored as being a little more ill than the control group at the beginning of the study. Targ chose healers who met specific criteria for experience and reputation. Included in her healing group was a Qi Gong healer, a Native American healer, a kabalistic healer, and many from other energy modalities, such as prayer and Reiki healing. Each healer had information sheets on the patients which included a photograph, the patient's first name and T-cell count, and two sentences describing their condition. Eleven outcome variables were measured.

The final results showed that there was a significant difference between the number of acquired illnesses in the groups, with the treatment group contracting fewer and less severe illnesses. There were no deaths in the treatment group, while there was one death in the control group. The treatment group had significantly fewer hospitalizations and shorter hospital stays. The Profile of Mood States instrument revealed a statistically significant difference, in that the treatment group went down in their distress points by 25, and the control group increased in their distress by 14 points. When the Profile of Mood States was broken down into its subscales, the treatment group had less confusion, tension, depression and fatigue. Differences in vigor and anger were not significant, and there was no correlation between the Profile of Mood scores and medical outcome. The data suggest that the control group was more ill at the conclusion of the study[78]. This would point to prayer, or distant healing, as being an extremely important energy modality for patients and their loved ones for supportive and end-of-life care.

Animals, with their unconditional acceptance, have been found to be useful in helping people work through their feelings. In a 1984 study looking at patients with terminal cancer it was found that those who were able to care for an animal were more in control[79]. 'When patients have another living creature to care for, they are able to shift some of the focus from their own illness'[80].

A randomized clinical controlled trial at Florida State University sought to evaluate the effects of music therapy upon quality of life, length of life in care, physical states and relationship of death occurence to final music interactions of hospice patients diagnosed with terminal cancer. The 80 subjects were randomized to one of two groups: hospice care and clinical music therapy or hospice care alone. The outcome revealed that quality of life showed a significant increase over time in the group receiving music therapy. No significant differences were found, however, between groups in the categories of physical states, length of life or time of death in relation to the last scheduled visit by the music therapist or counselor[81].

Energy medicine is extremely valuable as it relates to end-of-life issues. It may provide the spiritual connection necessary to accept physical death as a positive experience. It is used by a growing number of hospices in the USA (hospices in Europe have been using energy medicine along with other complementary medicine modalities for many years) to relieve pain and to give dying patients the ability to relax.

A few of the many hospice and palliative care programs successfully incorporating integrative modalities are listed below. This serves only as a sampling; the modalities listed may not be complete.

- Casa de la Luz Hospice
  400 West Magee Rd, Tucson, AZ 85704
  www.casahospice.com
  Therapeutic animal visitation, energy therapies, music therapy, meditation, guided imagery and massage

- Hospice of Cincinnati
  4310 Cooper Road, Cincinnati, Ohio 45242
  www.hospiceofcincinnati.org

Art therapy, aromatherapy, healing touch, massage, Reiki, reflexology, relaxation breathing, visualization

- The Community Hospice
  295 Valley View Boulevard, Rensselaer, NY 12144
  www.stpetershealthcare.org/hospice/
  Art therapy, massage, music therapy, Reiki

- Mercy Health Partners
  Palliative Care Demonstration Project
  Ohio, Kentucky and Indiana
  www.careofding.org
  Healing touch, massage therapy, music therapy, Reiki

- NCJW/Montefiore Hospice Program
  One David N. Myers Parkway, Beachwood, Ohio 44122
  www.montefiorecare.org
  Massage therapy, music therapy, Reiki

- San Diego Hospice
  4311 Third Ave., San Diego, CA 92103
  www.sdhospice.org
  Healing touch, Teiki, Therapeutic Touch

References

1. Post-White J. Kinney ME, Savik K, et al. Therapeutic touch and healing touch improve symptoms in cancer. Integrat Cancer Ther 2003; 2: 332–44
2. Newshan G, Schuller-Civitella D. Large clinical study shows value of Therapeutic Touch program. Holistic Nurs Pract 2003; 17: 189–92
3. Sancier KM. Therapeutic benefits of QiGong exercises in combination with drugs. J Altern Complement Med 1999; 5: 383–9
4. Merritt P, Randall D. The Effect of Healing Touch and Other Forms of Energy Work on Cancer Pain. St. Clare's Center for Complementary Medicine, Memorial Sloan-Kettering

Oncology Complementary Medicine Pilot Program, New York, 1998

5. Olsen K, Hanson J. Using Reiki to manage pain: a preliminary report. Cancer Prev Control 1997; 1: 108–13

6. Barnett L, Chambers M, Davidson S. Reiki Energy Medicine: Bringing the Healing Touch into Home, Hospital and Hospice. Rochester, VT: Healing Arts Press, 1996: 57

7. Edmonton, Alberta, Canada: Olson and Hanson Cross Center Institute, June 1997

8. Reinhart U. Investigation into synchronisation of heart rate and music rhythm in relaxation therapy in patients with cancer pain. Forschende Komplementaermedizen 1999; 6: 135–41

9. Watson J. Postmodern Nursing. London: Churchill Livingstone, 2000

10. North American Nurses' Diagnosis Association. Nursing Diagnosis: Definitions and Classification. Philadelphia: NANDA, 2001–2002

11. Hale G. A Practical Encyclopedia of Feng Shui. London: Arness Publishing, 2002: 13

12. Klotsche C. Color Medicine: The Secrets of Color/Vibrational Healing. Sedona, AZ: Light Technology Publishing, 1993

13. Rovner S. Treating SADness with Light. Washington Post, Health Section, 19 September 1989

14. Liberman J. Light: Medicine of the Future. Rochester, VT: Bear and Company, 1991: 22

15. Lewy AJ, Wehr T, Goodwin FK, et al. Light suppresses melatonin secretion in humans. Science 1980; 210: 1267–9

16. Rosenthal NE. Seasons of the Mind. New York: Bantam, 1989

17. Mueller P, Davies R. Seasonal affective disorder: seasonal energy syndrome. Brain/Mind Bull No.11, 6 June 1986: 2

18. Gerber R. A Practical Guide to Vibrational Medicine: Energy Healing and Spiritual Transformation. New York: Harper Collins, 2000; 220–2

19. Malchiodi CA. The Art Therapy Sourcebook. Los Angeles, CA: Lowell House, 1998

20. Achterburg J. Imagery in Healing. New York: Random House, 1985

21. Siegel BS. Peace, Love and Healing: Bodymind Communication and the Path to Self-Healing: An Exploration. New York: Harper Collins, 1989: 81

22. Guzzetta C, Dossy B, Keegan LS. Music therapy: healing the melody of the soul. In: Holistic Nursing: A Handbook for Practice, 3rd edn. Gaithersburg, MD: Aspen Publishers, 2000: 585

23. Miles E. Tune Your Brain: Using Music to Manage Your Mind, Body and Mood. New York: Berkley Publishing Group, 1997; 58

24. Mockler M, Stork T, Rocker J, et al. Stress reduction through listening to music: effect on mental state in patients with arterial hypertension and in healthy persons. Deutsch Med Wochenschrift 1995; 120/21: 745–52

25. Bonny H. Sound spaces: Music Rx is proven in the ICU. ICM West Newsletter 1982; 2: 1–2

26. Bailey LM. The effects of live musicversus tape-recorded music on hospitalized cancer patients. Music Ther 1986; 3: 17–28

27. Coyle N. A model of continuity of care for cancer patients with chronic pain. Med Clin North Am 1987; 7: 259–70

28. Thaut M. The use of auditory rhythm and rhythmic speech to aid temporal muscular control with gross motor dysfunction. J Music Ther 1985; 22: 108–28

29. Friedman RL. The Healing Power of the Drum: A Psychotherapist Explores the Healing Power of Rhythm. Reno, NV: White Cliffs Media, 2000: 43

30. Redmond L. When Drummers Were Women: The Spiritual History of Rhythm. New York: Crown Publishing, 1997

31. Osterman P, Schwartz-Barcott D. Presence: four ways of being there. Nurs Forum 1996; 31: 28

32. Poulson MJ. Not just tired. J Clin Oncol 2001; 19: 4180–1

33. Guerrerio J, Slater V, Cook C. The effect of Healing Touch on radiation-induced fatigue in women receiving radiation therapy for gynecological or breast cancer. Healing Touch Newslett 2001(3): 5

34. Weil A. Spontaneous Healing: How to Discover and Embrace Your Body's Natural Ability to Maintain and Heal Itself. New York: Ballantine Books, 1995: 162–3

35. Cousens G. Spiritual Nutrition and the Rainbow Diet. Boulder, CO: Cassandra Press, 1987

36. Dressen LJ, Singg S. Effects of Reiki on pain and selected affective and personality variables of chronically ill patients. ISSSEEM J 1998; 9(1)

37. Kim KB, Cohen SM, Oh HK, et al. The effects of meridian exercise on anxiety, depression and

self esteem of female college students in Korea. Holistic Nurs Pract: Sci Health Healing 2004; 8(5)

38. Quinn B. Interview with Friedman, Robert L., The Healing Power of the Drum: A Psychotherapist Explores the Healing Power of Rhythm. Reno, NV: White Cliffs Media, 2000: 88

39. Richards K, Nagel C, Markie M, et al. Critical care nursing. Clin North Am 2003; 15: 329–40

40. Hudson R. The value of lavender for rest and activity in the elderly patient. Complement Ther Med 1996: 4; 52–7

41. Murphy M. The body. In: Millennium. Boston: Houghton-Mifflin, 1981: 82

42. Jonas WB, Crawford CC. Healing Intention and Energy Medicine: Science, Research Methods and Clinical Implications. Churchill Livingstone, 2003: 302

43. Bruyere RL. Wheels of Light: Chakras, Auras, and the Healing Energy of the Body. New York: Fireside, 1994: 195

44. Brennan BA. Hands of Light: A Guide to Healing Through the Human Energy Field. New York: Bantam Books, 1988: 143

45. Loh S-H. Qigong therapy in the treatment of metastatic colon cancer. Altern Ther Health Med 1999; 5: 111–12

46. Brown KA, Esper P, Kellerher LO, et al. Chemotherapy and Biotherapy: Guidelines and Recommendations for Practice. Pittsburgh, PA: ONS Publishing Division, 2001; 88

47. Kreiger D. Living the Therapeutic Touch: Healing as a Lifestyle. New York: Dodd, Mead & Co., 1987: 13–16

48. Gerber R. Vibrational medicine: In: The #1 Handbook of Subtle-Energy Therapies. 3rd edn. Rochester, VT: Bear & Company, 2001: 308

49. Roscoe J, Morrow G, Brushunow P, et al. Wristbands can ease cancer nausea especially in those who expect them to work. James P. Wilmont Cancer Center, University of Rochester Medical Center, 2003

50. Wright LD. Complementary and alternative medicine for hospice and palliative care. J Cancer Integrat Med 2004; 2: 58

51. Wilkinson DS, Knox PL, Chatman JE, et al. The clinical effectiveness of healing touch. J Alternat Complement Med 2002; 8: 33–47

52. Mumber MP. Full-impact medicine. J Clin Oncol 2001; 19: 3793–4

53. Frank E, Breyan J, Elon L. Physician disclosure of healthy personal behaviors improves credibility and ability to motivate. Arch Fam Med 2000; 9: 287–90

54. Dossy BM, Keegan L, Guzzetta CE. Holistic Nursing: A Handbook for Practice, 3rd edn. Gaithersburg, MD: Aspen Publishers, 2000: 98

55. Frankel V. Man's Search for Meaning. New York: Washington Square Press, 1984

56. Maslow AH. A theory of human motivation. Psychol Rev 1943; 50: 370–96

57. Maslow AH. Motivation and Personality. New York: Harper and Row, 1954

58. Bischof LJ. Adult Psychology, 2nd edn. New York: Harper and Row, 1976

59. Ornish D. Love and Survival: The Scientific Basis for the Healing Power of Intimacy. New York: Harper-Collins, 1997; 22

60. Cassileth BR, Lusk EJ, Miller DS, et al. Psychosocial correlates of survival in advanced malignant disease. N Engl J Med 1985, 312: 1551–5

61. Berkman LF. Syme SL. Social networks, lost resistance and mortality: A nine-year follow-up study of Alameda County residents. Am J Epidemiol 1979; 109: 186–204

62. Berkman LF. The role of social relations in health promotion. Psychosom Med 1995; 57: 245–54

63. House JS, Robbins C, Metzner HL. The association of social relationships and activities with mortality: Prospective evidence from the Tecumseh Community Health Study. Am J Epidemiol 1982; 116: 123–40

64. Triebenbacher S. Psychosocial benefits of animal companionship. In: Fine AH, ed. Handbook on Animal-Assisted Therapy: Theoretical Foundations and Guidelines for Practice. San Diego, CA: Academic Press, 2000: 373

65. Becker M. The Healing Power of Pets: Harnessing the Amazing Ability of Pets to Make and Keep People Happy and Healthy. New York: Hyperion, 2002: 80

66. Haubner J, Johnson R. Animal Assisted Activity and Anxiety Among Radiation Therapy Patients: A MU Interdisciplinary Randomized Clinical Trial. Columbia, MO: University of Missouri Sinclair School of Nursing, 2000

67. Friedmann E. The animal–human bond: health and wellness. In: Fine A, ed. Handbook on

Animal-Assisted Therapy: Theoretical Foundations and Guidelines for Practice. San Diego, CA: Academic Press, 2000: 53

68. Sunstone Healing Center. Tucson, AZ. www.sunstonehealing.net

69. Ulrich RS. View through a window may influence recovery from surgery. Science 224, 420–1. In: Fine A, ed. Handbook on Animal-Assisted Therapy: Theoretical Foundations and Guidelines for Practice. San Diego, CA: Academic Press, 2000: 35

70. Nebbe L. Nature Therapy. In: Fine A, ed. The Handbook on Animal Assisted Therapy. San Diego, CA: Academic Press, 2000: 385–6

71. Cohen K. Honoring the Medicine: The Essential Guide to Native American Healing. New York: Ballantine Books, 2003: 239

72. Dossy L. Healing Words: The Power of Prayer and the Practice of Medicine. New York: Harper-Collins, 1997: 49

73. Russek LG, Schwartz GE. Perceptions of parental caring predict health status in midlife: a 35-year follow-up of the Harvard Mastery of Stress Study. Psychosom Med 1997; 59: 144–9

74. Funkenstein D, King S, Drolette M. Mastery of Stress. Cambridge, MA: Harvard University Press, 1957

75. Kissen DM. The significance of personality in lung cancer in men. Ann NY Acad Sci 1966; 125: 820–6

76. Kissen DM, Brown RI, Kissen M. A further report on personality and psychosocial factors in lung cancer. Ann NY Acad Sci 1969; 164: 535–45

77. Giasson M, Bouchard L. Effect of therapeutic touch on the well-being of persons with terminal cancer. J Holistic Nurs 1998; 16: 383–98

78. Targ E, Hendler S. Distant Healing Aids. www.cmbm.org/conferences/ccc99/transcripts99/su1.html

79. Muschel IJ. Pet therapy with terminal cancer patients. Social Casework 1993; 65: 451–8

80. Fine AH, ed. Handbook on Animal-Assisted Therapy: Theoretical Foundations and Guidelines for Practice. San Diego, CA: Academic Press, 2000: 222

81. Hilliard RE. The effects of music therapy on the quality and length of life in people diagnosed with terminal cancer. J Music Ther 2003; 40: 113–37

12g

Alternative medical systems

Lawrence Berk

TRADITIONAL CHINESE MEDICINE

The majority of research in Traditional Chinese Medicine (TCM) is in acupuncture. Studies have also been carried out in Qi Gong exercises and in Chinese herbal medicine. Although there are many retrospective studies and prospective studies in the literature, the focus of this section is on randomized trials.

ACUPUNCTURE

Nausea

Patient-individualized acupuncture, as a traditional Chinese physician would practice, has not been evaluated in randomized clinical trials of treatment for nausea. Various Western adaptations, such as acupressure and acustimulation, have been tested. They are based on TCM principles, particularly the activity of the P6 point, for prevention of nausea. However, a particular point is used for all patients. This limits the strength of these studies, and prohibits any conclusion about the use of classical TCM-based acupuncture in the treatment of nausea.

Roscoe et al. studied the use of acupressure (Sea-Bands®) and acustimulation (ReliefBand®) on the wrist to manage chemotherapy-induced nausea[1]. This was based on a smaller trial of acustimulation by Roscoe *et al*[2]. No specific acupuncture point was targeted. A total of 731 patients receiving cisplatin or doxorubicin were randomized to an acupressure wrist band, acustimulation wrist band or no band. For men, the acustimulation decreased nausea ($p < 0.05$ vs. no treatment). For women, acupressure tended to decrease nausea ($p = 0.052$ vs. no treatment).

Shen and colleagues randomized 104 women receiving high-dose chemotherapy for high-risk breast cancer to one of three treatments: antiemetics and electroacupuncture at the P6 point and the ST36 point, antiemetics and minimal needling but no manipulation or stimulation at the nearby but inactive LU7 and GB34 points, or antiemetics only[3]. The protocol was designed to detect a difference in emesis events in any of the three pairwise comparisons. There was a significant decrease in median number of emesis events with the electroacupuncture during the 5-day evaluation period when compared to antiemetics only (5 vs. 15 events during the 5-day evaluation period), between the electroacupuncture arm and sham acupuncture arm (5 vs. 10 events in the 5-day period) and the sham acupuncture and the anti-emetic-only group (10 vs. 15 events). There was no difference in the number of emetic events between the three arms in the 6–14 day follow-up period (4, 7 and 8 events, respectively).

Dibble *et al.* evaluated acupressure at the P6 and ST 36 points to decrease nausea during breast cancer chemotherapy[4]. Seventeen patients were randomized to finger acupressure at the above points and standard of care or just standard of care. The patient's symptoms were measured using the Chemotherapy Problem Checklist[5] asking the patient's perception of 21 side-effects on a 6-point scale and with a daily log containing the Rhodes Index of Nausea, Vomiting and Retching (INVR)[6] and the maximum nausea intensity over the previous 24 hours (0–10 scale). Both scales showed a statistically significant decrease in nausea among patients in the acupressure arm.

Noga *et al.* evaluated acupressure for nausea during bone marrow transplantation. This has only been presented in abstract form[7]. A total of 120 patients were randomized either to acupressure bands on the P6 point or to acupressure on an inactive point. Nausea was measured with the Rhodes Index (INVR). The active acupressure group had higher nausea levels ($p = 0.001$) and required more antinausea medications than the control group ($p < 0.10$). Thus, in this trial, the use of acupressure increased patient symptoms.

Pearl et al. studied the use of transcutaneous nerve stimulaion at the P6 point with the commercially available Relief Band[8]. Forty-two patients were randomized to either an active ReliefBand or an identical but inactive ReliefBand. Ten patients were not evaluable. Further, six received the device but did not use it. Four could not use the device despite instructions, and two devices stopped working and could not be replaced. Overall, 32 patients were evaluable, 16 in each group. The severity of nausea was similar for both groups. A subgroup of patients having more than two cycles of chemotherapy crossed over to the alternative treatment (18 patients). The authors called the overall result 'indeterminate' because the high rate of patient loss negated the power in the trial design. However, the nausea results in the two arms are so similar (absent or minimal nausea were 56% in the active arm and 62% in the placebo arm) that it is unlikely that increased accrual would have rendered the results significantly different. Fifty per cent of the patients in each arm felt that the device decreased their nausea and vomiting. In the crossover section of the trial, a subgroup analysis (whether planned or unplanned is unclear) showed that there was less nausea in the active group during days 2–4 but not on days 1 or 5–7. More patients thought the device was helpful during the active cycle than during the placebo cycle (71% vs. 21%).

A second study of the ReliefBand was among 25 patients receiving platinum-based chemotherapy – 14 patients with testicular and 11 with bladder cancer[9]. During the first three cycles of chemotherapy the patients randomly received each of three treatments: odansetron, ReliefBand, or the combination of odansetron and ReliefBand. The primary endpoint was patient-reported nausea (0–10 scale) during the administration of the platinum chemotherapy. The mean nausea scores for ReliefBand alone, odansetron alone and ReliefBand and odansetron were 5, 3 and 1, respectively. The combination of odansetron and the ReliefBand resulted in statistically significantly less nausea than odansetron alone ($p = 0.000$).

Finally, Treish *et al.* also studied transcutaneous nerve stimulation at the P6 point with ReliefBand[10]. Forty-nine patients receiving emetogenic chemotherapy were randomized to either electrical stimulation at the P6 point with a ReliefBand or an inactive device. Patients reported nausea and vomiting in a daily diary. Patients wearing the active ReliefBand experienced statistically significantly less vomiting (1.9 vs. 4.6 mean episodes) and less severe nausea (0.91 vs. 1.65 cm on a visual analog scale (VAS)).

In conclusion, there are significant level 1 data concerning the use of acupressure, acupuncture and electroacupuncture using the Relief-Band device for the relief of chemotherapy-associated nausea and vomiting. Some of these data are conflicting; however, the majority of studies show a positive benefit when used as a complementary addition to standard antiemetics.

Cancer pain

The literature on acupuncture for cancer pain is much less substantial than that for its use for nausea or its use for chronic pain. Two studies evaluating acupuncture for cancer pain are reviewed.

Alimi *et al.* reported on the use of auricular acupuncture for cancer pain[11]. Ninety patients with pain from advanced cancer underwent electrodermal response evaluation of the anticipated areas on the ear corresponding to the clinical pain syndromes. The active sites were recorded. The patients were then randomized to one of three groups: permanent auricular acupuncture using 0.7 mm long steel implants inserted into the active sites; permanent insertion into inactive sites; or placement of dummy seeds without the underlying needle at placebo points. Patients maintained a pain log. They were seen 1 month after the initial treatment; the ear was remapped and a second course of treatment was given at the same sites as the first course. A final evaluation with a VAS pain measurement was conducted 1 month later. Analgesic use was recorded by the patient in a daily log. A total of 102 patients were randomized and 99 were evaluable. Seventy-nine patients completed the primary endpoint, the day-60 pain assessment. All of the patients had neuropathic pain. The results at day 60 showed a statistically significant difference in pain on a

0–100 VAS score of 37 in the true acupuncture group, 55 in the placebo acupuncture group and 58 in the placebo seeds group. Day-30 pain scores were also statistically significantly lower in the true acupuncture group (44 vs. 54 vs. 56, respectively). The pain intensity at day 0 correlated with the average electric potential measured on the ear at day 0, and the pain response also correlated with the decrease in auricular electric potential.

Priess and Meisel presented the results of a prospective trial of 'auricular neural therapy' for neuropathic pain among cancer patients[12]. Twenty-two patients with neuropathic pain from oxaliplatin received 0.5% procaine injected into auricular acupuncture points which correlate with the projections of the paravertebral sympathetic ganglion of the cervical and lumbar spine and the projections of the skeleton of hands and feet (and if necessary the forearms and lower legs). In 20 of 22 patients the neuropathic pain was reduced from grade 1–3 to grade 1 or 0. The response correlated with an increase in blood flow in the hands and feet as measured with an infrared camera.

Acupuncture as delivered in these two trials appears efficacious, though further research is needed. It is especially interesting that acupuncture appeared to help with chemotherapy-associated neuropathy – a treatment-related morbidity for which little therapy is available other than narcotic pain relievers.

Fatigue

No randomized trials of acupuncture for fatigue have been published. Vickers *et al.* reported a prospective study of 37 patients treated with acupuncture for fatigue without anemia after chemotherapy[13]. Thirty-seven patients were treated with acupuncture either twice a week (25 patients) or once a week (12 patients). The twice weekly patients received bilateral treatment given at ST36, SP8 and SP9, and unilateral needling at

CV6 and CV4. LI11 was treated bilaterally unless the patient had had an axillary dissection, in which case only the contralateral arm was treated. The once weekly treated patients were treated at ST36, SP6, CV6, CV4, KI3 and KI27. The authors stated that these are traditional acupuncture points for fatigue. Patient response was monitored with the Brief Fatigue Inventory (BFI) and the Hospital Anxiety and Depression Scale (HADS). The mean improvement in fatigue was 31% with a 95% confidence interval of 21–41%. The authors concluded that randomized trials of acupuncture for fatigue are warranted.

Radiation therapy-induced salivary dysfunction

There have been several prospective and retrospective studies of acupuncture for xerostomia[14–19]. However, the absence of a control arm makes it difficult to know whether any effects seen are more than placebo effects. The only randomized trial is from Blom and colleagues in Sweden[20]. In this small trial, 38 patients with radiation-induced xerostomia were randomized to active acupuncture (20 patients) or sham acupuncture (18 patients). The acupuncture and sham treatments were given in two series of 12 treatments twice a week for 6 weeks with a 2-week break in between. Active body and auricular points were chosen based upon the clinical evaluation of the patient by the acupuncturist. In the control group the acupuncture was done with only superficial insertion (no Qi activation) at points about 1 cm from the active sites. The stimulated and unstimulated salivary volumes were measured prior to any treatment, after the first series of treatments, after the 2-week break, at the end of the second series and then at 3, 6 and 12 months. The active group's baseline salivary function appeared to be higher than that of the control group (Table 12.10). This would predict that the active group could have a superior response, because response correlates with the initial salivary flow[21]. There was an equivalent increase in salivary flow in both arms of the trial. The authors concluded that this may have represented the failure of the sham acupuncture to be truly inactive. An alternative conclusion is that the increase was secondary to a placebo effect.

Results from prospective non-randomized trials are encouraging. There is no general agreement as to the specific points to be used, the method of stimulation or the best method of producing a placebo.

Hot flushes and menopausal symptoms

Tukmachi reported on 22 consecutive breast cancer patients having had both chemotherapy and tamoxifen and suffering from hot flushes[22]. Patients were treated with two 20–30-minute sessions weekly for up to 7 weeks. The acupuncture was given at specific points based on the physical status of the patient. The daytime hot flushes fell from 315 (total of all of the patients)

Table 12.10 Salivary flow (g/min) adapted from reference 20							
Unstimulated saliva				Stimulated saliva			
Active		Sham		Active		Sham	
Median	Range	Median	Range	Median	Range	Median	Range
0.000	0.00–0.16	0.00	0.00–0.08	0.125	0.00–1.01	0.000	0.00–0.18

to 31 at the end of treatment and 33 at the 3–5-week follow-up. The nighttime hot flushes fell from 153 to 19 at the end of treatment and 26 at follow-up.

Hammar *et al.* reported on seven men with hot flushes due to castration therapy for prostate cancer[23]. Treatments were given for 30 minutes twice weekly for 2 weeks and then once a week for 10 weeks. The same points were used for all patients. There was an average of 70% reduction in hot flushes at the end of treatment and a 50% decrease at the 3-month follow-up.

The only randomized trial of acupuncture for hot flushes is that of Wyon *et al.*[24] Forty-five women were randomized to either electoacupuncture, sham electroacupuncture or estradiol. The electroacupuncture used superficial needle insertion twice a week for 30 minutes for 2 weeks then once a week for 10 weeks. The active acupuncture points were BL15, BL23, BL32 bilaterally, and HT7, SP6, SP9, LR3, PC6 and GV20 unilaterally. In the sham group, the needles were placed 1–15 cm away from these active points. The estradiol group recieved 2 mg of 17-β-estradiol orally for 12 weeks. At 12 weeks (the end of treatment) the hot flushes in the acupuncture, sham and estradiol groups had fallen from 7.3 to 3.5, 8.1 to 3.8 and 8.4 to 0.8, respectively. As in the Blom trial of acupuncture for xerostomia[20], the authors concluded that superficial needle insertion is an inappropriate control.

Acupuncture as a supportive care option for patients with hot flushes has some preliminary evidence base; however, no definitive conclusions can be made based on the current literature.

Cancer-related breathlessness

There has been a single trial of acupuncture for cancer-related breathlessness[25]. Twenty patients with breathlessness from advanced malignancy received acupuncture using sternal and LI4 points. Fourteen of the 20 patients reported marked symptomatic benefit. There was also a significant decrease in the patients' respiratory rates lasting up to 90 minutes post-treatment.

General supportive care

Xia *et al.* of the Institute of Acupuncture of the China Academy of Traditional Chinese Medicine reported on the use of acupuncture in conjunction with radiotherapy or chemotherapy[26]. The patients had lung, esophageal or gastric cancer. Seventy-six patients were randomly assigned to acupuncture with radiotherapy or chemotherapy (38 patients) or radiotherapy or chemotherapy alone (38 patients). The patients were treated to the P6 and ST36 points along with other points chosen on the basis of the patients' illness and symptoms. The authors reported that the acupuncture-treated patients gained weight after treatment, whereas the control group lost weight ($p < 0.001$). The acupuncture patients also had better amelioration of their symptoms and maintained their hemogram and leukocyte levels better.

TAI CHI/QI GONG

Chen and Yeung reviewed all published studies done in China of Qi Gong for cancer patients[27]. They reviewed more than 50 studies, including *in vitro*, *in vivo* and human trials. They found no randomized, blinded studies. Among the published trials there were 21 human trials involving 1883 patients. These reports are summarized below.

At the Meijing Miyun Capital Tumor Hospital, 1648 cancer patients over 8 years were treated with a combination of self-control Qi Gong together with conventional therapies[28]. Data were collected on immune response and the physical health of the patients. The patients reportedly showed 'significant improvement in 32.4%, some effectiveness in 59.2% and only 8.4% reported no effect'[27].

At the Guang Am-Men Hospital 97 patients with advanced cancer received standard therapy plus 2 hours of Qi Gong a day for 3 months. Thirty patients received conventional therapy only. Among the Qi Gong patients 82% regained strength, 63% had improved appetite and 33% had normal defecation. Among the conventionally treated patients, the rates were 10%, 10% and 6%, respectively.

At the Henan Medical University patients with 'cardiac' adenocarcinomas were randomly assigned to four treatment groups: surgery only (48 patients), chemotherapy only with epiallo-pregnanolone (42 patients), Chinese herbal treatment only (46 patients) or Qi Gong plus Chinese herbal treatment (50 patients)[29]. Table 12.11 summarizes the results. The herbs used were not identified. The review stated that the difference in survival between the combined herbal and Qi Gong arm versus the surgery-only arm was statistically significant at $p < 0.01$.

At the Zhejiang Institute of TCM 80 patients with previous treatment with radiation or chemotherapy were randomly assigned to Qi Gong (30 patients), chemotherapy (25 patients) or Qi Gong and chemotherapy (25 patients)[30]. The patients were followed for red and white blood cell counts, serum hemoglobin and T lymphocytes. After 60 days of treatment the Qi Gong group had significantly higher values of the above, and the control groups significantly lower values.

It is difficult to evaluate the results of the above studies for various reasons: the differences in treatment relative to the methods used as standard in Western medicine; the lack of specific control arms, and the problem of possible publication bias from the Chinese literature. Qi Gong as a supportive therapy may have benefits, but there are no definitive data concerning its use as an antineoplastic activity.

CHINESE HERBAL MEDICINE

Hot flushes

Davis *et al.* studied the effects of Chinese medicinal herbs on hot flushes[31]. The trial was not for cancer patients. In this study 78 women with at least 14 hot flushes per week were randomized to a single formulation of 11 Chinese medicinal herbs or placebo. There were 42 patients in the active arm, 39 of whom received any herbal treatment and 28 completed the trial. Of the 36 patients in the placebo arm, 35 received the placebo and 27 completed the trial. The frequency of vasomotor symptoms was reduced in both groups, but to a greater extent in the placebo arm: −15% with the herbs and -31% with placebo ($p = 0.09$).

AYURVEDIC MEDICINE

There is little in the literature on the use of ayurvedic medicine for cancer. Two recent comprehensive reviews of the theoretical basis of cancer and cancer treatment within the ayurvedic framework are by Singh[32] and by Balachandran and Govindarajan[33]. Preclinical studies of the anticancer effects of ayurvedic preparations have also been reported[34].

The only published randomized trial found utilizing ayurvedic medicine is a study of

Table 12.11 Henan Medical University study results (from reference 28)			
	1-year survival	3-year survival	5-year survival
Surgery only	80.1	36.5	20.8
Chemotherapy only	85.7	45.2	25.1
Herbal only	84.5	43.5	26.1
Qi Qong and herbal	86.0	64.0	36.0

preventing morphine-induced constipation[35]. Patients were randomized to Misrakasneham (21 kinds of herbs, castor oil, ghee and milk) or Sofsena (a commercial senna product). Fifty patients starting morphine treatment were randomized to one of the products for 2 weeks. Twenty of the Misrakasneham and 16 of the Sofsena patients completed the trial. Seventeen of the Misrakasneham and 11 of the Sofsena patients maintained satisfactory bowel movements, a non-significant difference.

HOMEOPATHIC MEDICINE

Treatment of radiation effects during breast irradiation

Two trials have been reported of homeopathic preparations to reduce the dermal effects of radiation during breast irradiation. A third, recently published trial utilized a common homeopathic ingredient from a homeopathic pharmaceutical house, calendula, but did not use it in a homeopathic formulation[36].

Balzarini *et al.* reported on a randomized trial of sublingual 3 granules belladona 7cH BID and sublingual 3 granules of X-ray 15 cH versus placebo treatments[37]. The endpoint was an unvalidated measure of 'edema + hyperpigmentation + heat + color'. This was measured weekly for the 6 weeks of radiation therapy and then at 15 days after treatment and 30 days after treatment. The weekly scores were summed and used as one measure, along with the 15-day and 30-day scores. Fifty-one of the sixty-six randomized patients were evaluable. The average scores of the above measure during treatment were 7.4 for treatment and 9.1 for placebo ($p = 0.23$). After radiation the average scores were 2.3 vs. 3.2 ($p = 0.05$). Although the authors claimed statistical significance, they did not state whether this latter measure was an intended endpoint or an *ad-hoc* evaluation.

Schlappack reported on a prospective study of the use of individualized homeopathic treatment for radiation-induced itching of the breast during or after radiation therapy[38]. The measure was a VAS of patient-reported itchiness. Fourteen of the 25 patients had relief of their itching with the first formulation prescribed, and seven of nine responded to a second formulation, with an overall response of 21 of 25 patients.

Oral mucositis

Oberbaum *et al.* reported on a randomized, double-blinded, phase III trial of Traumeel for the prevention of oral mucositis during pediatric bone marrow transplantation[39]. Thirty-two patients, 30 evaluable, were randomized to five-time daily rinses with the Traumeel or placebo (saline). The World Health Organization (WHO) mucositis score and an *ad-hoc* scoring system were the primary measures. The Traumeel patients had significantly less mucositis by area under the curve for total mucositis.

Hot flushes

Thompson and Reilly reported on a prospective study of 45 women with breast cancer suffering estrogen withdrawal symptoms, primarily hot flushes[40]. The intervention was individualized homeopathic treatments. They found a significant improvement in symptom scores and 'effect of daily living' scores with the homeopathic treatments.

Based on this, their group completed a randomized, double-blind, placebo-controlled trial of individualized homeopathic treatment (E. Thompson, personal communication). A single, experienced homeopath saw all of the patients and prescribed an individualized treatment. The prescription was sent to a separate pharmacy and either the prescribed formulation or placebo was sent to the patient. The prescription could be changed at follow-up visits, but the active/

Table 12.12   Clinical trials of alternative medical systems for cancer patients

Intervention	Symptom	Benefit	Level of evidence
Acupuncture or acupressure	Nausea	Positive	I
Auricular acupuncture	Cancer pain (neuropathic)	Positive	I
Acupuncture	Fatigue	Possibly positive	II
Acupuncture	Xerostomia	No clear benefit	I
Acupuncture	Xerostomia	Possible benefit	II
Acupuncture	Hot flushes	No clear benefit	I
Acupuncture	Hot flushes	Possible benefit	II
Acupuncture	Cancer-related breathlessness	Possible benefit	II
Acupuncture with Chinese medicinal herbs	Reduced conventional treatment toxicities	Possible benefit	I
Qi Gong	Reduction in symptoms	Possible benefit	I, II
Chinese Herbal Medicine	Hot flushes (non-cancer patients)	No benefit	I
Ayurvedic herbs	Constipation	Possible benefit, not better than senna	I
Homeopathic formulations	Breast pruritis from radiation therapy	Possible benefit	II
Homeopathic formulations	Breast erythema	Possible benefit	I
Homeopathic formulations	Oral mucositis during bone marrow transplant	Positive benefit	I
Homeopathic formulations	Estrogen withdrawal symptoms	No benefit	I

placebo randomization would not change. The primary outcome was the Measure Yourself Medical Outcome Profile (MYMOP)[41]. Fifty-three patients were randomized. Accrual was stopped early, owing to staffing changes. There was no difference in the primary outcome of the MYMOP score (1.6 at the end of treatment and 1.3 at the 16-week follow-up for the homeopathic group versus 1.5 and 1.2, respectively, for the placebo group). There were no differences in any of the secondary outcomes measured (Table 12.12).

References

1. Roscoe JA, Morrow GR, Hickok JT, et al. The efficacy of acupressure and acustimulation wrist bands for the relief of chemotherapy-induced nausea and vomiting. A University of Rochester Cancer Center Community Clinical Oncology Program multicenter study. J Pain Symptom Manage 2003; 26: 731–42

2. Roscoe JA, Morrow GR, Bushunow P, et al. Acustimulation wristbands for the relief of chemotherapy-induced nausea. Altern Ther Health Med 2002; 8: 56–7, 59–63

3. Shen J, Wenger N, Glaspy J, et al. Electro-acupuncture for control of myeloablative chemotherapy-induced emesis: A randomized controlled trial. J Am Med Assoc 2000; 284: 2755–61

4. Dibble SL, Chapman J, Mack KA, Shih AS. Acupressure for nausea: results of a pilot study. Oncol Nurs Forum 2000; 27: 41–7

5. Dodd MJ. Measuring informational intervention for chemotherapy knowledge and self-care behavior. Res Nurs Health 1984; 7: 43–50

6. Rhodes VA, Watson PM, Johnson MH. Development of reliable and valid measures of nausea and vomiting. Cancer Nurs 1984; 7: 33–41

7. Noga SJ, Tolman AM, Roman JJ, et al. Acupressure as an adjunct to pharmacologic control of nausea, vomiting and retching (N/V) during blood and marrow transplantation (BMT): a randomized, placebo-controlled, algorithm based study. Proceedings of the American Society of Clinical Oncology, 2002; Abstract 1443

8. Pearl ML, Fischer M, McCauley DL, et al. Transcutaneous electrical nerve stimulation as an adjunct for controlling chemotherapy-induced nausea and vomiting in gynecologic oncology patients. Cancer Nurs 1999; 22: 307–11

9. Ozgur Tan M, Sandikci Z, Uygur MC, et al. Combination of transcutaneous electrical nerve stimulation and ondansetron in preventing cisplatin-induced emesis. Urol Int 2001; 67: 54–8

10. Treish I, Shord S, Valgus J, et al. Randomized double-blind study of the Reliefband as an adjunct to standard antiemetics in patients receiving moderately-high to highly emetogenic chemotherapy. Support Care Cancer 2003; 11: 516–21

11. Alimi D, Rubino C, Pichard-Leandri E, et al. Analgesic effect of auricular acupuncture for cancer pain: a randomized, blinded, controlled trial. J Clin Oncol 2003; 21: 4120–6

12. Preiss J, Meisel O. Successful auricular neural therapy in oxaliplatin-induced sensory neuropathy. Proceedings of the American Society of Clinical Oncology, 2003; Abstract 1454

13. Vickers AJ, Straus DJ, Fearon B, Cassileth BR. Acupuncture for postchemotherapy fatigue: a phase II study. J Clin Oncol 2004; 22: 1731–5

14. Johnstone PA, Niemtzow RC, Riffenburgh RH. Acupuncture for xerostomia: clinical update. Cancer 2002; 94: 1151–6

15. Rydholm M, Strang P. Acupuncture for patients in hospital-based home care suffering from xerostomia. J Palliat Care 1999; 15: 20–3

16. List T, Lundeberg T, Lundstrom I, Lindstrom F, Ravald N. The effect of acupuncture in the treatment of patients with primary Sjögren's syndrome. A controlled study. Acta Odontol Scand 1998; 56: 95–9

17. Andersen SW, Machin D. Acupuncture treatment of patients with radiation-induced xerostomia. Oral Oncol 1997; 33: 146–7

18. Blom M, Lundeberg T. Long-term follow-up of patients treated with acupuncture for xerostomia and the influence of additional treatment. Oral Dis 2000; 6: 15–24

19. Wong RK, Jones GW, Sagar SM, et al. A Phase I-II study in the use of acupuncture-like transcutaneous nerve stimulation in the treatment of radiation-induced xerostomia in head-and-neck cancer patients treated with radical radiotherapy. Int J Radiat Oncol Biol Phys 2003; 57: 472–80

20. Blom M, Dawidson I, Fernberg JO, et al. Acupuncture treatment of patients with radiation-induced xerostomia. Eur J Cancer B Oral Oncol 1996; 32B: 182–90. Comment in: Oral Oncol 1997; 33: 146–7

21. Blom M, Kopp S, Lundeberg T. Prognostic value of the pilocarpine test to identify patients who may obtain long-term relief from xerosto-

mia by acupuncture treatment. Arch Otolaryn-gol Head Neck Surg 1999; 125: 561–6

22. Tukmachi E. Treatment of hot flushes in breast cancer patients with acupuncture. Acupuncture Med 2000; 18: 22–7

23. Hammar M, Frisk J, Grimas O, et al. Acupuncture treatment of vasomotor symptoms in men with prostatic carcinoma: a pilot study. J Urol 1999; 161: 853–6

24. Wyon Y, Wijma K, Nedstrand E, Hammar M. A comparison of acupuncture and oral estradiol treatment of vasomotor symptoms in post-menopausal women. Climacteric 2004; 7: 153–64

25. Filshie J, Penn K, Ashley S, Davis CL. Acupuncture for the relief of cancer-related breathlessness. Palliat Med 1996; 10: 145–50

26. Xia YQ, Zhang D, Yang CX, et al. An approach to the effect on tumors of acupuncture in combination with radiotherapy or chemotherapy. J Tradit Chin Med 1986; 6: 23–6

27. Chen K, Yeung R. Exploratory studies of Qigong therapy for cancer in China. Integr Cancer Ther 2002; 1: 345–70

28. Zhang RM. Clinical observation and experimental study of qigong therapy for cancer [in Chinese]. China Qigong Sci 1995; 2: 24–9

29. Fu JZ, Fu SL, Qin JT. Effect of qigong and anticancer body-building herbs on the prognosis of postoperative patients with cardiac adenocarcinoma. Third World Conference on Medical Qigong, Beijing, China, 1996

30. Luo S, Tong T, et al. Effects of vital gate qigong on malignant tumor. First World Conference for Academic Exchange of Medical Qigong, Beijing, China, 1988

31. Davis SR, Briganti EM, Chen RQ, et al. The effects of Chinese medicinal herbs on post-menopausal vasomotor symptoms of Australian women. A randomised controlled trial. Med J Aust 2001; 174: 68–71

32. Singh RH. An assessment of the ayurvedic concept of cancer and a new paradigm of anticancer treatment in Ayurveda. J Altern Complement Med 2002; 8: 609–14

33. Balachandran P, Govindarajan R. Cancer – an ayurvedic perspective. Pharmacol Res 2005; 51: 19–30

34. Smit HF, Woerdenbag HJ, Singh RH, et al. Ayurvedic herbal drugs with possible cytostatic activity. J Ethnopharmacol 1995; 47: 75–84

35. Ramesh PR, Kumar KS, Rajagopal MR, et al. Managing morphine-induced constipation: a controlled comparison of an Ayurvedic formulation and senna. J Pain Symptom Manage 1998; 16: 240–4

36. Pommier P, Gomez F, Sunyach MP, et al. Phase III randomized trial of Calendula officinalis compared with trolamine for the prevention of acute dermatitis during irradiation for breast cancer. J Clin Oncol 2004; 22: 1447–53

37. Balzarini A, Felisi E, Martini A, De Conno F. Efficacy of homeopathic treatment of skin reactions during radiotherapy for breast cancer: a randomised, double-blind clinical trial. Br Homeopath J 2000; 89: 8–12

38. Schlappack O. Homeopathic treatment of radiation-induced itching in breast cancer patients. A prospective observatioonal study. Homeopathy 2004; 93: 210–15

39. Oberbaum M, Yaniv I, Ben-Gal Y, et al. A randomized, controlled clinical trial of the homeopathic medication TRAUMEEL S in the treatment of chemotherapy-induced stomatitis in children undergoing stem cell transplantation. Cancer 2001; 92: 684–90

40. Thompson EA, Reilly D. The homeopathic approach to the treatment of symptoms of oestrogen withdrawal in breast cancer patients. A prospective observational study. Homeopathy 2003; 92: 131–4

41. Paterson C. Measuring outcomes in primary care: a patient generated measure, MYMOP, compared with the SF-36 health survey. Br Med J 1996; 312: 1016–20

13

Modalities – antineoplastic therapy

Antineoplastic therapy includes all types of intervention whose mechanism of action results in the eradication of cancer cells from the body. This will generally include the three major categories of conventional medicine: chemotherapy, radiation therapy and surgery. It is in the arena of antineoplastic therapy that the practitioners of complementary and alternative medicine (CAM), conventional medicine providers and patients experience the greatest misunderstanding and heated debate. Indeed, it is mostly here that the term 'alternative' comes into play as meaning the opposite of evidence-based, scientifically proven, and effective conventional therapy. This conflict is unfortunate on several levels. First, it has placed the patient squarely in the middle – especially patients for whom few effective conventional treatment options are available. Purveyors of alternative medicine continue to provide expensive, sometimes useless and dangerous forms of purported antineoplastic treatment as an option to patients. Conventional providers cannot advise them as to the value of therapies on which they have not received education. Second, the conflict has delayed the implementation of effective preventive and supportive CAM options. These options may indeed improve the

results of conventional antineoplastic therapy through improved tolerance to treatment, or any number of yet to be elucidated biologic mechanisms. Finally, the conflict has delayed important research into modalities that may ultimately prove beneficial to the patient on a number of different levels. All of this is changing rather rapidly, as evidenced by the growth in research dollars targeted for CAM modalities, and the presence of scientific publications such as those reported in this text.

The Office of Cancer Complementary and Alternative Medicine (OCCAM) is a branch of the National Cancer Institute (NCI), which is specifically responsible for CAM research relative to cancer. In an attempt to monitor modalities that have their primary action through measurable tumor response, the NCI Best Case Series (NCI-BCS) was introduced. This has resulted in several active trials of novel antineoplastic alternative approaches. Some examples include the Kelly-Gonzalez approach for the treatment of pancreatic cancer, and the use of antineoplastons in brain tumors. The NCI-BCS begins with inquiries into therapies proposed by users or developers. Case scenarios are submitted followed by rigorous evaluation of pathology, radiographic studies and other diagnostic and treatment aspects of specific cases. Included in this analysis, there must be documented and objective assessment of tumor response, lack of concurrent conventional therapy and documentation that the alternative treatment was delivered. Once all of the data have been reviewed, therapies that appear promising are presented to an advisory panel. If there is sufficient evidence to justify further research, the panel may recommend pursuing the therapy further either as a part of a Practice Outcomes Monitoring and Evaluation System (POMES) or as an implementation of other prospective preclinical or clinical investigations. Over the past 5 years, three therapies have made it through to the phase of further research: a homeopathy approach at a clinic in India for lung cancer; insulin potentiation therapy, which uses insulin with low doses of conventional chemotherapy; and macrobiotic diet therapy. The NCI-BCS system may be expanded in the future to support collaborative projects between conventional researchers and CAM practitioners, in order to accomplish research in a more timely fashion.

This chapter will examine antineoplastic therapy approaches from the CAM world – specifically those therapies whose primary mechanism of action is antineoplastic – defined as killing cancer cells. Interventions that may have an antineoplastic effect through improved immune function or improved tolerance to conventional therapy are included in other sections where appropriate.

13a

Nutrition

Mara Vitolins and Cynthia Thomson

There are certain foods that contain phytonutrients with antineoplastic activity *in vivo* and *in vitro*. Select foods/dietary constituents are being investigated as adjuvant therapy to chemotherapy and radiation, including some foods high in antioxidants (green tea), as well as foods that could modulate phase 1 and II enzymes or drug clearance (cruciferous vegetables), but this work is very preliminary. Please see the Phytochemical chart in 11b for further information.

13b

Mind–body interventions

Linda E. Carlson and Shauna L. Shapiro

ANTINEOPLASTIC CARE

The area of mind–body medicine and antineoplastic care is best illustrated indirectly by the research into psychoneuroimmunology (PNI). PNI research generally measures the effects of psychosocial interventions on indicators that are considered to be potentially important mediators of disease outcomes such as progression and survival, such as natural killer cell numbers. Few studies in the area of PNI have demonstrated direct links between mind–body interventions and disease course, but those few have garnered a great deal of attention and excited the imaginations of a generation of researchers. These studies are included in the section on tertiary prevention. Currently the state of the science is such that it is not possible to state definitive conclusions about the effect of mind–body therapies on cancer progression and survival, although several very provocative studies have been conducted. The types of interventions that appear to hold the most promise in terms of promoting survival are those that include social support and emotional expression, as well as components of stress reduction and/or relaxation. Much more well-controlled research needs to be done in this area

before unequivocal conclusions can be drawn or recommendations made.

Some studies have investigated the effects of psychosocial interventions on intermediary mechanisms such as immune cell counts and function, and stress hormones. Mindfulness-based stress reduction (MBSR) was shown to engender changes in hormone and endocrine profiles of breast and prostate cancer patients towards patterns more characteristic of healthy individuals, suggesting a process of normalization of these systems[1,2]. Another interesting study combining MBSR and dietary changes for men with prostate cancer investigated the effects of the program on prostate-specific antigen (PSA) levels, an indicator of tumor activity. In a pilot study of ten men and their partners, the rate of PSA increase decelerated in eight of the ten men, while three had a decrease in the absolute level of PSA. Doubling time increased from 6.5 months before to 17.7 months after the intervention, indicating a possible slowing of the rate of tumor progression in cases of biochemically recurrent prostate cancer[3].

Other interventions, such as experiential–existential group psychotherapy for breast cancer have also shown changes in immune and hormone profiles. This suggests a trend towards normalization of cortisol levels[4] and less reactivity to stress as a possible consequence of enhanced abilities of emotional expression[5]. The thorny issue of whether these types of change are relevant or important to cancer progression have been addressed recently in a special issue of the journal *Brain, Behavior and Immunity* entitled 'Biological mechanisms of psychosocial effects on disease: implications for cancer control'[6]. The volume was dedicated to addressing issues of possible pathways by which psychosocial factors and interventions could affect the incidence and progression of general and specific cancer-related disease processes. This area of research remains a hotbed of interest and innovation.

In summary, increased attention has been directed towards the possible antineoplastic potential of mind–body interventions, as evidenced by the growing body of literature investigating the impact of a variety of interventions on outcomes such as immune function, stress hormone levels and survival. Further work in this emerging area of interest will hopefully link specific mind–body therapies with particular antineoplastic effects.

References

1. Carlson LE, Speca M, Patel KD, Goodey E. Mindfulness-based stress reduction in relation to quality of life, mood, symptoms of stress and levels of cortisol, dehydroepiandrostrone-sulftate (DHEAS) and melatonin in breast and prostate cancer outpatients. Psychoneuroendocrinology 2004; 29: 448–74

2. Carlson LE, Speca M, Patel KD, Goodey E. Mindfulness-based stress reduction in relation to quality of life, mood, symptoms of stress, and immune parameters in breast and prostate cancer outpatients. Psychosom Med 2003; 65: 571–81

3. Saxe GA, Hebert JR, Carmody JF, et al. Can diet in conjunction with stress reduction affect the rate of increase in prostate specific antigen after biochemical recurrence of prostate cancer? J Urol 2001; 166: 2202–7

4. van der Pompe G, Duivenvoorden HJ, Antoni MH, et al. Effectiveness of a short-term group psychotherapy program on endocrine and immune function in breast cancer patients: An exploratory study. J Psychosom Res 1997; 42: 453–66

5. van der Pompe G, Antoni MH, Duivenvoorden HJ, et al. An exploratory study into the effect of group psychotherapy on cardiovascular and immunoreactivity to acute stress in breast cancer patients. Psychother Psychosom 2001; 70: 307–18

6. Miller AH, ed. Biological mechanisms of psychosocial effects on disease: implications for cancer control. Brain Behav Immun 2003; 17 (Suppl 1): S1–134

13c

Botanicals

Lise Alschuler

NEGATIVE INTERACTIONS OF BOTANICALS

There are examples of herbal and chemotherapeutic drug interactions that may affect the antineoplastic activity of chemotherapy agents. An example of this is an *in vitro* study which demonstrated that berberine, an alkaloid from *Berberis* spp. plants with significant antimicrobial actions, upregulates the multidrug-resistant transporter expression in gastrointestinal cell lines. This effect was specifically confirmed by cells pretreated with berberine that then demonstrated resistance to paclitaxel-induced cytotoxicity[1]. In humans, berberine is extremely poorly absorbed from the lumen of the gastrointestinal tract. Thus, whether this interaction is clinically relevant outside the gastrointestinal tract is difficult to ascertain.

Other potential interactions between curcumin, the major component of *Curcuma longa* (turmeric), and camptothecin, mechlorethamine and doxorubicin (DOX) have important clinical implications. All of these chemotherapeutics induce apoptosis through the generation of reactive oxygen species (ROS) and the activation of the c-Jun NH(2)-terminal kinase (JNK)

pathway. *In vitro* studies suggest that curcumin may interfere with chemotherapeutic-induced ROS and JNK activation. *In vitro* data demonstrated up to 70% inhibition of camptothecin-, mechlorethamine-, and DOX-induced apoptosis of MCF-7, MDA-MB-231, and BT-474 human breast cancer cells[2]. The same investigation used an *in vivo* model of human breast cancer. In this model, dietary supplementation with curcumin resulted in significant inhibition of cyclophosphamide-induced tumor regression. While this interaction remains unobserved in humans, and it is unknown whether sufficient quantities of curcumin could be ingested to produce this interaction, caution is warranted nonetheless.

Genistein, an isoflavone from soy, can have negative results when taken with tamoxifen. At doses of 10 µmol/l or above, genistein inhibits the growth of estrogen-dependent breast cancer cells *in vitro*. However, at lower doses (0.01–1.0 µmol/l) genistein stimulates cell growth and proliferation. The addition of low-dose genistein to tamoxifen-treated cells reversed the inhibitory effects of tamoxifen[3]. Genistein blood levels in humans on a high-soy diet are reported at 0.10 to 6.0 µmol/l. This indicates that it may be very difficult to attain and sustain a concentration of genistein that is high enough to induce tumor inhibition. Thus, genistein may be contraindicated with tamoxifen in breast cancer chemotherapy regimens.

POSITIVE INTERACTIONS OF BOTANICALS

Cisplatin

The antineoplastic activity of cisplatin may be enhanced with co-administration of *Silybum marianum* (milk thistle). In an *in vitro* study, silybin exerted a dose-dependent growth-inhibitory effect on drug-resistant ovarian cancer cells. Additionally, silybin potentiated the cytotoxic effect of cisplatin on these cells[4]. Quercetin, a flavonoid derived from onions and found ubiquitously in plants, amplifies the antiproliferative and proapoptotic effects of cisplatin on lung tumor cell lines *in vitro*[5].

Mitomycin C

Panax ginseng (ginseng) may have synergistic effects with mitomycin C. A treatment group of mice with Ehrlich carcinoma were given 70% methanolic extract of *P. ginseng* orally at varying doses for 10 to 12 days, starting 2 days after tumor implantation. The mice also received intraperitoneal mitomycin C on alternate days for 6 days starting 2 days after tumor implantation. This study found that the *P. ginseng* increased the antitumor activities of mitomycin C and that combined administration of *P. ginseng* and mitomycin C produced significant inhibitory activities compared with those of mitomycin C alone. The study confirmed that the ginseng extract alone had no marked antitumor activity, therefore the authors concluded that ginseng enhanced the antitumor activities of mitomycin C[6].

Doxorubicin and idarubicin

Botanical agents, most notably green tea extracts, have been studied with doxorubicin (DOX) (Adriamycin®). Although there are no human trials, the preliminary *in vitro* and animal *in vivo* data are consistent and indicative of a beneficial relationship between these two agents. DOX is an anthracycline antibiotic widely used against a variety of cancers. The use of DOX can be limited by its side-effects, notably cardiac toxicity. When DOX was administered intraperitoneally to mice with implanted Ehrlich ascites carcinoma, a 25% reduction in tumor weight was observed. When mice ingested green tea during the period of DOX administration, a decrease of 37% in tumor weight was observed. The ingestion of green tea enhanced the DOX tumor inhibition 2.5-fold. The tumors of the green tea-fed mice demonstrated an increase in DOX concentration 1.7-fold compared to the DOX-alone group. Additionally, the DOX concentrations in the heart and liver did not increase with ingestion of green tea; in fact, the DOX contraction in the heart was lower than in the DOX-alone group[7]. These results suggest that the addition of green tea to DOX may intensify the antitumor action of DOX while protecting healthy tissue against DOX-induced toxicity. The enhancing effect of green tea on the antitumor actions of DOX was also demonstrated in a mouse model of M5076 ovarian sarcoma, which exhibits lower sensitivity to DOX than does Ehrlich carcinoma. The injection of DOX alone did not significantly reduce the tumor weight, whereas the combined treatment with oral administration of theanine, a component of green tea, reduced the tumor size by 37% of the control level. Co-administration of green tea (orally administered) with DOX injections also decreased the tumor weight, and the DOX concentration in the tumor increased 1.5-fold ($p < 0.01$). Conversely, the combination of green tea and DOX reduced the DOX concentration in the heart to 75% of that in the

DOX-alone group ($p < 0.01$). The green tea and theanine each decreased the DOX concentration in the liver as well. Green tea, and theanine in particular, appeared to inhibit the efflux of DOX selectively from tumor cells[8]. The co-administration of green tea and of theanine (oral route) with DOX in DOX-resistant mice bearing P388 leukemia cells led to the same effects, namely increased DOX concentration in the tumor, decreased tumor burden and decreased DOX concentration in healthy tissues[9].

Idarubicin (IDA) is a similar type of chemotherapeutic agent. IDA is an anthracycline antibiotic used in the treatment of acute myelocytic leukemia. IDA also exerts significant bone marrow suppression which limits its use. When mice with implanted P388 leukemia cells received oral green tea or oral theanine along with intraperitoneal injections of IDA, the tumor weight decreased by 49%, whereas the IDA-alone group experienced no change in tumor weight ($p < 0.001$). The tumors of the theanine plus IDA group had an IDA concentration 2.0-fold higher than in the IDA-alone group. In addition, theanine reversed the IDA-caused leukocyte depletion and bone marrow cellularity depletion[10]. These reports cumulatively suggest that green tea, and theanine in particular, induce a tumor-selective chemosensitizing effect for DOX and IDA.

Tamoxifen

Several botanical agents have been studied in relation to tamoxifen. Co-treatment with tamoxifen and epigallocatechin gallate (EGCG) from green tea on human PC-9 lung cancer cells induces apoptosis more strongly than does tamoxifen alone or EGCG alone. The enhancement of the inhibitory effect of tamoxifen on MCF-7 breast cancer cells by the addition of EGCG has also been observed[11]. Both agents induce apoptosis and appear to have a synergistic effect in *in vitro* models.

When a standardized extract of American ginseng (*Panax quinquefolius*) was applied to MCF-7 breast cancer cells along with tamoxifen, further suppression of cell proliferation in comparison to either one alone was observed. Components of the ginseng extract were demonstrated to bind to estrogen receptors. Low doses of ginseng had no effect on cell growth, while higher doses significantly decreased cell proliferation. The antiproliferative effect of ginseng was even more pronounced with the addition of tamoxifen[12].

Interleukin-2

Recombinant interleukin-2 (IL-2) is used to stimulate lymphokine-activated killer (LAK) cells in the treatment of leukemias and melanoma. LAK cells are generated from both natural killers (NK) cells and from T cells. The generation of LAK cells is associated with an antitumor effect. Unfortunately, high doses of IL-2 are required to generate LAK cells. High-dose IL-2 therapy is limited by its cardiovascular side-effects, namely: edema, capillary leak syndrome, myocardial infarction and arrhythmias. Co-administration of a non-toxic immunostimulatory agent with the capacity of non-specifically activating all effector pathways would constitute an ideal antineoplastic immunomodulatory approach. When human melanoma cells (A375P and HS294T) were incubated with low-dose IL-2 combined with *Astragalus membranaceus* (astragalus), LAK cell generation and associated tumor-cell killing activity were significantly increased over IL-2 alone. In essence an equivalent level of tumor cell lysis was achieved by a 10-fold lower concentration of IL-2 when astragalus extract was added[13]. This synergism would allow for lower requirements for IL-2 and thus a reduced side-effect profile.

The polysaccharide ginsan, extracted from *Panax ginseng*, has been studied *in vitro* and *in vivo* (rodent) in combination with IL-2.

Leukemia and melanoma cells were incubated with low-dose IL-2 plus ginsan. This combination increased LAK cell activity significantly over cells treated with IL-2 alone. When ginsan was given to a tumor-bearing rat, *in vivo* activation of all effector cells including T cells, NK cells and macrophages occurred. In turn, this caused activation of LAK cells[14]. Although the data on ginseng and on astragalus are preliminary, they do indicate a synergistic effect between astragalus or *P. ginseng* and low-dose IL-2. If this relationship can be proved in humans, it will allow for IL-2 therapy that is better tolerated and equally effective.

Combination chemotherapy

A randomized trial conducted in 1995 of Japanese women with operable breast cancer assessed the impact on prognosis of PSK, a polysaccharide fraction extracted from *Coriolus versicolor,* and levamisole (LMS), an imidazothiazole derivative. In this trial, 227 women with operable breast cancer with vascular invasion in the tumor and/or in metastatic lymph node(s) were randomized to one of three groups. One group received adjuvant chemotherapy for a 23-day course consisting of 5-fluorouracil (5-FU) (100 mg/day, PO), cyclophosphamide (50 mg/day, PO), mitomycin-C (2 mg/day, PO) and prednisolone (5 mg/day, PO) (FEMP); another group received FEMP along with PSK (3 g/day, PO for 28 days); and a third group received FEMP along with LMS (150 mg/day, PO on day 1–3 and day 15–17). All groups received their treatments at 6-month intervals for 5 years. Although this chemotherapy regimen is unusual, the implications are, nonetheless, applicable. Disease-free survival and overall survival rates were compared among the three groups. In disease-free survival or overall survival, there was no significant difference between the three groups. However, the survival curve of the FEMP + PSK group tended to be better than that of the FEMP group (logrank, $p = 0.0706$; generalized Wilcoxon, $p = 0.0739$). At 10 years after tumor resection, the survival rate for the FEMP + PSK group was 81.1%, for the FEMP + LMS group 76.9%, and for FEMP alone group 64.6%. The disease-free survival at this same time point was 74.1% for FEMP + PSK, 70.7% for FEMP + LMS and 64.6% for FEMP alone. The authors concluded that the addition of PSK to this chemotherapy regimen improved the prognosis of the study patients, although this was not statistically significant at $p < 0.05$[15].

Another trial examined the role of PSK on prognosis in patients with operable gastric cancer. In this trial, 262 patients were enrolled. All patients had a histological diagnosis of gastric cancer and underwent curative gastrectomy. Patients were stratified according to the extent of the tumor which is the primary prognostic factor. Patients were randomly assigned to either standard treatment with mitomycin and fluorouracil or standard treatment plus PSK. The mitomycin was given as bolus injections on postoperative days 1 and 7. The standard treatment group then received oral fluorouracil, 150 mg daily for 4 weeks alternated with 4 weeks of rest from treatment. The PSK group received the oral fluorouracil in the same manner for 4 weeks alternated with 4 weeks of oral PSK, 3 g daily. The patients were followed regularly for 5 years. The treatment groups were well balanced in terms of clinical and demographic characteristics. The 5-year disease-free survival rate was 70.7% in the PSK group and 59.4% in the standard treatment group. The reduction in risk was 35% (95% CI 1–58%, $p = 0.047$) without adjustments and 44% (95% CI 13–64%, $p = 0.009$) after adjustment for pTNM stage. The 5-year survival rate was 73% for the PSK group and 60.0% for the standard treatment group. The reduction in risk was 36% (95% CI 1–58%, $p = 0.044$) without adjustments and 44% (95% CI 14–64%, $p = 0.008$) after adjustment for pTNM stage. There were no significant side-effects reported throughout the study. The overall reduction of approximately 20% in recurrence and death rates is a significant finding. The authors of the study noted that PSK induced gene expression for interleukins 1, 6 and 8, as well as for tumor necrosis factor (TNF) and macrophage chemotactic factor. They further surmised that these effects may correct the immunosuppression associated with both the surgery and the subsequent chemotherapy, thus contributing to increased survival[16].

A prospective, randomized, placebo-controlled trial on postoperative patients with stage III gastric cancer was conducted to determine the effects of *Panax ginseng* on immunity and survival in patients receiving 5-FU and cisplatin chemotherapy[17]. After exclusion criteria were applied, 42 patients who had undergone curative gastric resection with D2 lymph node dissection for histologically proven American Joint Committee on Cancer (AJCC) stage III gastric adenocarcinoma were enrolled in this study. The patients were followed postoperatively for 5 years. All patients received monthly 5-FU infusion at 500 mg/m^2 per day, on days 1–5. In addition, bolus cisplatin was given at a dosage of 60 mg/m^2 per day on day 1. The course of chemotherapy was 6 months. Prior to surgery, the patients were randomly assigned additionally to receive *P. ginseng* powder capsules orally at a dosage of 4.5 g/day or sucrose capsules as a placebo throughout the 6-month course of chemotherapy. T-lymphocyte subsets were evaluated preoperatively and at postoperative months 1, 3 and 6. On the basis of clinical examination, ultrasound scanning, abdominal computer tomography and tumor markers evaluation, patients were defined as having tumor recurrence ($n = 19$) or not ($n = 23$) at the 5-year follow-up. No adverse effects were observed in either group. The recurrence rate was greater in the non-ginseng group than in the ginseng group (7/22 versus 13/20, $p < 0.05$). Mean duration of disease free survival was significantly longer in the ginseng group (44.4 ± 13.1 months versus 33.5 ± 17.9 months, $p < 0.05$). The 5-year disease-free survival rate of the ginseng-treated group was 68.2% versus 33.3% in the non-ginseng group. The CD3 and CD4 levels were significantly higher in patients taking the ginseng, which suggests that ginseng may facilitate recovery of immune function during chemotherapy. This, in turn, may help prevent metastatic recurrence. Although this study was small, it is excellent evidence of the survival benefit of *Panax ginseng* root capsules in postoperative gastric cancer patients receiving 5-FU and cisplatin chemotherapy.

The ginsenosides from *Panax ginseng* have also been the subject of two *in vitro* studies on multidrug resistance. One study found that ginsenosides partially reversed multidrug resistance of L5178 mouse lymphoma cells. This study further discovered that the ginsenosides had an overall moderate inhibitory effect on the drug efflux pump[18]. This mechanism of drug resistance is a factor for most chemotherapeutics. The reversal of multidrug resistance by ginsenosides was further clarified in a later *in vitro* study. This study demonstrated that protopanaxatriol gensenosides have a chemosensitizing effect on P-glycoprotein-mediated multidrug-resistant cells by increasing the intracellular accumulation of drugs through a direct interaction with P-glycoprotein[19]. This protein acts as an efflux pump for drugs such as DOX, vincristine, vinblastine, paclitaxel, colchicines, actinomycin D and mitomycin C. These studies suggest that the concurrent use of *P. ginseng* with these chemotherapeutic drugs may delay or reverse chemoresistance.

Botanicals and radiation therapy

Withania somnifera (ashwagandha) has been studied for its radiosensitizing properties. At least five *in vivo* animal studies have confirmed a radiosensitizing effect of ashwagandha. One study studied the effect of intraperitoneal injections of an extract of ashwagandha root powder in mice with implanted sarcoma-180 tumor. The mice received 10 Gy gamma radiation. The mice that received the ashwagandha experienced increased tumor cure, growth delay of partially responding tumors and prolonged survival over radiation-only mice[20]. The radiosensitizing effect of ashwagandha was further characterized. Withaferin A, a steroidal lactone from *Withania somnifera* was injected intraperitoneally into mice with Ehrlich ascites carcinoma. The mice received 7.5 Gy of abdominal gamma radiation. The mice injected with withaferin A also showed an increased life span and tumor-free survival over the mice that received radiation only[21]. The withaferin A appeared to inhibit the repair of radiation damage in tumor cells. In addition to its radiosensitizing effects, withaferin A appears to have antineoplastic actions. This extract has a growth inhibitory effect on Chinese hamster V79 cells. The withaferin A induced a G2/M block *in vitro* at higher doses[22]. This cytotoxic effect may be synergistic with its radiosensitizing effect in prolonging survival time of the tested rodents. While these *in vivo* data are compelling, the applicability to human patients remains unstudied and therefore unknown. The ashwagandha extracts in these studies were injected intraperitoneally. It is unknown how oral dosing of ashwagandha in humans compares to intraperitoneal administration in rodents. In addition, it is unclear whether the radiosensitizing effect is localized to tumor cells only, or whether normal cells in the radiation field would also experience increased radiation effects. If the latter occurred, the concomitant use of ashwagandha could increase radiation therapy-induced side-effects. Nonetheless, the increased tumor response and prolonged survival time of rodents who received ashwagandha extracts along with radiation are encouraging and support the need for human trials.

The addition of EGCG derived from green tea to irradiation increased cell apoptosis in a dose-dependent fashion. This effect was observed in three human cancer cell lines: HeLA (cervical carcinoma), K-562 (chronic myelogenous leukemia), and IM-9 (multiple myeloma). The increased rate of apoptosis correlated with a decrease in proliferation of all three cell lines[23]. The same investigator also looked at the effect of curcumin, from *Curcuma longa*, on these same three cell lines and demonstrated a radiosensitizing effect with increased apoptosis in the curcumin-treated cells[24]. The radiosensitizing effects of curcumin were further demonstrated in the p53 mutant prostate cancer cell line (PC-3)[25]. The mechanisms studied suggest that the genetic effects of curcumin overcome radiation resistance.

The concurrent use of botanicals with chemotherapy and/or radiation therapy is summarized in Table 13.1.

Antineoplastic care with botanicals

The antineoplastic effects of selected botanicals have been demonstrated *in vitro* and *in vivo* animal models. Clinical evidence of significant antineoplastic effects in humans for botanical agents is scarce. The dilemma inherent to initiating these trials lies in the ethical issue of enrolling patients into a trial utilizing unproven botanical therapies at the exclusion of standard conventional therapies. Once a patient's malignancy has progressed through standard treatment options, they become excellent candidates for experimental therapies, but the likelihood of obtaining benefit from these therapies is slim, given the state of the cancerous process. This is particularly true of botanical therapies which tend to exert their effects in a physiological, time-dependent manner. Thus, one is left with the uncomfortable, but necessary, position of extrapolating tentative conclusions about the antineoplastic use of botanicals largely from experimental data.

Table 13.2 summarizes the evidence supporting the antineoplastic effects of botanicals.

Table 13.1   Evidence for co-management with botanicals. Level IV of evidence includes *in vitro* studies, *in vivo* studies and traditional use. Level I of evidence includes level IV and randomized controlled trials

Therapy	Level of evidence IV	Level of evidence I
Multidrug resistance	Panax ginseng	
Taxanes	(-) *Hypericum* spp. (St John's wort) (-) berberine (-) quercetin green tea Panax ginseng soy	
Cisplatin	Coriolus versicolor silybinin	ginger Panax ginseng – gastric CA; Rx cisplatin/5FU
Camptothecin	(-) curcumin	
Doxorubicin	(-) curcumin, green tea	
Mechlorethamine	(-) curcumin	
Cyclophosphamide	Astragalus membranaceous Withania somnifera (ashwagandha)	
Mitomycin-C	Panax ginseng	Coriolus versicolor (PSK) – breast and gastric CA; Rx with 5FU
Interleukin-2	Astragalus membranaceous Panax ginseng	
Radiation therapy	Withania somnifera (ashwagandha) EGCG (derived from Camellia sinensis) Curcumin (derived from Curcuma longa)	

The symbol '(-)' denotes evidence against the use of the therapy. CA, cancer; Rx, the chemotherapeutic agents used in the study; EGCG, epigallocatechin gallate; 5FU, 5-fluorouracil; PSK, a polysaccharide fraction extracted from *Coriolus versicolor*

Table 13.2 Evidence for antineoplastic effects of botanicals

Cancer type	Evidence level IV	Evidence level II	Evidence level I
Breast cancer	curcumin proanthocyanidins (grape seed extract) (-) *Panax ginseng*		
Ovarian cancer	*Panax ginseng* quercetin soy isoflavones		
Prostate cancer		red clover isoflavones green tea	
Colon cancer	PSK (*Coriolus versicolor*) green tea		
Lung cancer	*Panax ginseng*		
Melanoma	curcumin catechin		
Leukemia	*Glycyrrhiza glabra* *Artemesia princeps*		
Renal carcinoma		(-) iscador (*Viscum* spp.)	
Bladder cancer			(-) iscador *Viscum alba*
Sarcoma	*Withania somnifera* green tea (EGCG) *Grifola frondosa* (β1,3-glucan) *Coriolus versicolor* (PSK) *Lentinus edodes* (shiitake mushroom)		

References

1. Lin H, Liu TY, Wu CW, Chi CW. Berberine modulates expression of mdr1 gene product and the responses of digestive tract cancer cells to Paclitaxel. Br J Cancer 1999; 81: 416–22

2. Somasundaram S, Edmund NA, Moore DT, et al. Dietary curcumin inhibits chemotherapy-induced apoptosis in models of human breast cancer. Cancer Res 2002; 62: 3868–75

3. Jones JL, Daley BJ, Enderson BL, et al. Genistein inhibits tamoxifen effects on cell proliferation and cell cycle arrest in T47D breast cancer cells. Am Surg 2002; 68: 575–7; discussion 577–8

4. Scambia G, De Vincenzo R, Ranelletti FO, et al. Antiproliferative effect of silybin on gynaecological malignancies: synergism with cisplatin and doxorubicin. Eur J Cancer 1996; 32A: 877–82

5. Borska S, Gebarowska E, Wysocka T, et al. The effects of quercetin vs cisplatin on proliferation and the apoptotic process in A549 and SW1271

cell lines in in vitro conditions. Folia Morphol (Warsz) 2004; 63: 103–5

6. Kubo M, Tong CN, Matsuda H. Influence of the 70% methanolic extract from red ginseng on the lysosome of tumor cells and on the cytocidal effect of mitomycin C. Planta Med 1992; 58: 424–8

7. Sadzuka Y, Sugiyama T, Hirota S. Modulation of cancer chemotherapy by green tea. Clin Cancer Res 1998; 4: 153–6

8. Sugiyama T, Sadzuka Y. Enhancing effects of green tea components on the antitumor activity of adriamycin against M5076 ovarian sarcoma. Cancer Lett 1998; 133: 19–26

9. Sadzuka Y, Sugiyama T, Sonobe T. Efficacies of tea components on doxorubicin induced antitumor activity and reversal of multidrug resistance. Toxicol Lett 2000; 114: 155–62

10. Sadzuka Y, Sugiyama T, Sonobe T. Improvement of idarubicin induced antitumor activity and bone marrow suppression by theanine, a component of tea. Cancer Lett 2000; 158: 119-24

11. Suganuma M, Okabe S, Kai Y, et al. Synergistic effects of (-)-epigallocatechin gallate with (-)-epicatechin, sulindac, or tamoxifen on cancer-preventive activity in the human lung cancer cell line PC-9. Cancer Res 1999; 59: 44–7

12. Duda RB, Zhong Y, Navas V, et al. American ginseng and breast cancer therapeutic agents synergistically inhibit MCF-7 breast cancer cell growth. J Surg Oncol 1999; 72: 230–9

13. Chu D-T, Lepe-Zuniga J, Wong WL, et al. Fractionated extract of Astragalus membranaceus, a Chinese medicinal herb, potentiates LAK cell cytotoxicity generated by a low dose of recombinant interleukin-2. J Clin Lab Immunol 1988; 26: 183–7

14. Kim K-H, Lee YS, Jung IS, et al. Acidic polysaccharide from Panax ginseng, ginsan, induces Th1 cell and macrophage cytokines and generates LAK cells in synergy with rIL-2. Planta Med 1998; 64: 110–15

15. Iino Y, Yokoe T, Maemura M, et al. Immunochemotherapies versus chemotherapy as adjuvant treatment after curative resection of operable breast cancer. Anticancer Res 1995; 15: 2907–12

16. Nakazato H, Koike A, Saji S, et al. Efficacy of immunochemotherapy as adjuvant treatment after curative resection of gastric cancer. Lancet 1994; 343: 1122–6

17. Suh SO, Kroh M, Kim NR, et al. Effects of red ginseng upon postoperative immunity and survival in patients with stage III gastric cancer. Am J Chin Med 2002; 30: 483–94

18. Molnar J, Szabo D, Pusztai R, et al. Membrane associated antitumor effects of crocine-, ginsenoside- and cannabinoid derivates. Anticancer Res 2000; 20: 861–7

19. Choi CH, Kang G, Min YD. Reversal of P-glycoprotein-mediated multidrug resistance by protopanaxatriol ginsenosides from Korean red ginseng. Planta Med 2003; 69: 235–40

20. Devi PU, Sharada AC, Solomon FE. Antitumor and radiosensitizing effects of Withania somnifera (Ashwagandha) on a transplantable mouse tumor, Sarcoma-180. Indian J Exp Biol 1993; 31: 607–11

21. Sharada AC, Solomon FE, Devi PU, et al. Antitumor and Radiosensitizing effects of withaferin A on mouse Ehrlich ascites carcinoma in vivo. Acta Oncol 1996; 35: 95–100

22. Devi PU, Akagi K, Ostapenko V, et al. Withaferin A: a new radiosensitizer from the Indian medicinal plant Withania somnifera. Int J Radiat Biol 1996; 69: 193–7

23. Baatout S, Jacquet P, Derradji H, et al. Study of the combined effect of X-irradiation and epigallocatechin-gallate (a tea component) on the growth inhibition and induction of apoptosis in human cancer cell lines. Oncol Rep 2004; 12: 159–67

24. Baatout S, Derradji H, Jacquet P, et al. Effect of curcuma on radiation-induced apoptosis in human cancer cells. Int J Oncol 2004; 24: 321–9

25. Chendil D, Ranga S, Meigooni D, et al. Curcumin confers radiosensitizing effect in prostate cancer cell line PC-3. Oncogene 2004; 23: 1599–607

13d

Energy medicine

Suzanne Clewell

ANTINEOPLASTIC CARE

In his book *A Practical Guide to Vibrational Medicine*, Richard Gerber writes that, by harnessing the energies of light, magnetism, pulsed electromagnetic fields, the life energies of plants (captured in flower essences, homeopathic remedies, herbs and essential oils), the environmental energies of Chi and Prana, as well as the healing energy of the life force itself (via healing touch therapies), we are expanding the physician's armamentarium for healing illness with simple, powerful and cost-effective methods[1].

There are thousands of forms of Qi Gong. Most are designed for preventive health care and not for cancer treatment. Although most Qi Gong may bring health benefits, medical Qi Gong is the only form specifically developed for treating and curing disease. Two forms of Qi Gong in China have openly challenged cancer: Guo-Lin new Qi Gong and Chinese Taiji five-element Qi Gong[2].

Guo-Lin New Qi Gong was developed by Guo Lin, a late-stage cancer patient who is said to have recovered from cancer by self Qi Gong practice. There are many reported cases of cancer recovery attributed to practicing Qi Gong, but it is usually used as a supplementary therapy to conventional treatments[3].

In one 8-year study looking at treatment using a modified form of Guo-Lin Qi Gong in 1648 patients with various cancers, 32.4% experienced significant improvement and 59.2% some improvement. Only 8.4% reported no effect. More than 500 of the cancer patients survived 5 years or longer (> 30%)[4].

Zheng Rongrong of Shanghai Qi Gong Academy used Qi Gong combined with Chinese herbs to treat 100 advanced cancer patients. Results showed that comprehensive Qi Gong therapy had effectively prolonged patients' lives. Among the patients treated by Qi Gong therapy, the 1-year survival rate for lung cancer patients was 83%, and the 5-year survival rate for lung cancer patients was 17% (7% in the control group). The 5-year survival rate for colon cancer patients was 23% (12% in the control group). The median survival for liver cancer patients was 22.7 months, compared to 3.5 months in the control group[5].

There have not been many studies on Qi Gong therapy for cancer. However, reported findings have been consistent that cancer patients had more significant improvement (measured by length of life, tumor shrinkage or remission of cancer) when they received Qi Gong therapy partnered with conventional medicine than those groups who received conventional medicine alone[6]. Although the research designs may be somewhat lacking in format, some scientific studies have confirmed the inhibitory effect of external Qi therapy on cancer growth[7]. At the same time, Qi Gong practice is said to increase Qi or the vital energy flow in the body and boost the immune system.

Numerous controlled studies have validated the non-local nature of prayer. Much of this evidence suggests that the individuals sending the prayer or intended healing are able purposefully to affect the physiology of the recipients – even without the receiver being aware that they are the focus of intention[8]. Currently the National Institutes of Health are funding a study on prayer intervention. This 5-year study joins the Johns Hopkins's Center for Health Promotion and Duke's Center for the Study of Religion/Spirituality and Health in an attempt to determine whether spiritual involvement and belief affect immune functioning and cancer prognosis. The population will be Afro-American women recovering from breast cancer surgery[9].

Distant healing has received little attention from mainstream medicine; however, a substantial body of published data supports the possibility of a significant effect. Over 150 formal, controlled studies have been published over the course of the past 40 years, more than two-thirds of which demonstrated significant effects[10].

Although research is demonstrating that spiritual healing/energy medicine works, we still do not know how. In his book *Healing Words: The Power of Prayer and the Practice of Medicine,* Larry Dossey states: 'To acknowledge that we don't know how something works is not a particularly damaging confession in medicine.' (reference 8, p. 277). He goes on to remind us that no one knew how penicillin worked when it was discovered but, had that stopped the process, the introduction of life-saving antibiotics would have been delayed. People who are suffering from pain or infection do not first ask how a therapy works but rather, *does it work?* 'As history shows, full explanations frequently come later. So it may be for prayer and spiritual healing.'[8]

References

1. Gerber R. A Practical Guide to Vibrational Medicine: Energy Healing and Spiritual Transformation. New York: Harper-Collins Publishers, 2000: 404
2. Chen K, He B. Preliminary studies of the effect of qigong therapy on cancer. Presented at Comprehensive Cancer Care 2001: Integrating Alternative and Complementary Therapies, Arlington, VA, October 2001
3. Huang N. The effect of Guo-Lin new Qigong on the lung function micro-circulation in cancer patients. Chin J Somat Sci 1996; 6: 51–4
4. Zang RM. Clinical observation and experimental study of qigong therapy for cancer. [in Chinese]. China Qigong Sci 1995; 2: 24–9
5. Huang GH. A review of scientific research of Qigong anti-cancer therapy. China Qigong Sci 1997; 10: 24–8
6. Cong J, Lu Z. Curative effect on 120 cancer cases treated by Chinese–Western medicine and Qigong therapy. Presented at the 2nd World Conference for Academic Exchange of Medical Qigong, Beijing, China, 1993: 131

7. Chen XL, et al. Double-blind test of emitted Qi on tumor formation of a nasopharyngeal carcinoma cell line in nude mice. Presented at the 2nd World Conference for Academic Exchange of Medical Qigong, Beijing, China, 1993: 105

8. Dossy L. Healing Words: The Power of Prayer and the Practice of Medicine. New York: Harper-Collins, 1997: 61

9. Website: www.dukespiritualityandhealth.org/studies.html#breastcancer

10. Benor DJ. Healing Research, vol 1. Deddington, England: Helix Editions, 1992

14

Tobacco, alcohol and integrative oncology

Dennett Gordon

'There is no chance of beating cancer unless we use both conventional medicine that seeks to cure illness by fixing one's body and unconventional medicine that aims at curtailing the possibility of illness through transforming one's life. It is not possible for a bird to fly on only one wing.' – Joe Pinky

Three sets of facts related to cancer support an aggressive, multipronged attack on tobacco and alcohol consumption. First, and perhaps most significant, is that biological links between tobacco use and many types of cancer are well established in the literature[1–3] and comparable connections between alcohol use and cancer are strongly suggested if not substantiated[4,5]. Certainly this alone would justify making tobacco and alcohol prevention and cessation therapies an integral part of cancer care.

A second set of facts evidences sharp increases in tobacco use during the past several decades[6,7], adding further credence to the necessity of widespread prevention and cessation programs. In fact, experts speculate that medical historians will call the 1900s the 'Tobacco and Cancer Century'[1]. Combine this prediction with the fact that 'a synergistic, multiplicative effect appears to exist between smoking and drinking'[1] and it is easy to see that alcohol consumption is an integral part of the rapidly growing tobacco–cancer tragedy.

Third, salient demographic data punctuate the social, political and moral dimensions of the implication of tobacco and alcohol consumption with cancer, and further underscore the urgent need for prevention and cessation programs that are affordable, effective and accessible to everyone. Studies indicate that worldwide those who are least powerful and most uninformed tend to have the greatest exposure to tobacco and alcohol, thus placing them at the highest risk for cancer and many other diseases[8–10]. This includes young people who have long been targeted by tobacco and alcohol companies because they are often extremely impressionable and innocent of consequences[11,12]. This also includes a disproportionate percentage of minority and low-income groups who can least afford and have the least access to health care but are among the most vulnerable when it comes to tobacco and alcohol products, leading to catastrophic illnesses[8,13]. The lopsided impact of tobacco and alcohol consumption upon the most vulnerable populations in society is arguably not merely the result of poor individual choices, but is also due to inequitable social and institutional forces. The vicious cycle between poverty on the one hand, and smoking and drinking on the other hand, is well documented[14,15]. For many decades, tobacco companies and related interest groups have used their considerable resources to skew public opinion in favor of images and arguments supporting widespread and unrestrained use of their products[1].

All the above reasons support the diffusion of cessation and prevention strategies related to tobacco and alcohol use as widely as possible, as quickly as possible, as cheaply as possible and as early in life as possible. Such strategies could include complementary and alternative therapies as well as conventional therapies, so long as they were efficacious and cost-effective. However, a truly integrative attack on cancer must go beyond these individual approaches to tobacco and alcohol use by also exposing and overturning social, institutional and public policies, and practices that effectively permit and promote such use. After all, one ultimate goal of an integrative approach to oncology is a healthier society and world.

This chapter addresses each of these issues. Emphasis is given to cessation and prevention strategies as adjuncts to mainstream medical care, in that they eliminate or lower the risk of a cause of cancer, reduce the risk of recurrence and improve the chances for actively treated patients. The approaches of complementary and alternative medicine (CAM) are discussed with traditional modalities. In addition to individual approaches, broader-based social and political interventions relating to tobacco and alcohol use are also touched upon.

SCOPE OF THE PROBLEM AND LINK TO CANCER

In the USA, smoking accounts for about 30% of all cancer deaths and 87% of lung cancer deaths[1].

Smokeless tobacco use is unfortunately not a safe substitute for smoking, as oral cancers are many times higher for snuff-dippers compared with non-tobacco users[16]. Regrettably, secondhand smoke, which contains numerous human carcinogens, causes approximately 3000 deaths from lung cancer among non-smokers each year[17].

In contrast to tobacco, alcohol has not been shown to be carcinogenic and far less public attention has been given to the effect of alcohol use on the development of cancer[5]. Possibly as a result of inadequate attention, the actual biological mechanisms affected by alcohol that lead to cancer are still somewhat speculative[4,5]. Nevertheless, the American Cancer Society states that 'alcohol consumption is an established cause of cancers of the mouth, pharynx, larynx, esophagus, liver, and breast.'[6] Although other literature reviews present more conflicted findings in some of these areas, particularly regarding the etiologies of liver and breast cancers, current research is in strong agreement that the use of alcohol plays a causal role in the development of many cancers[4,5]. Moreover, the consumption of alcohol in combination with tobacco increases the risk of cancers of the mouth, larynx, pharynx and esophagus much more significantly than does the independent use of either substance[1,6].

TRENDS AND RISK FACTORS

Both positive and negative trends in tobacco use have been noted during the past few decades. Encouragingly, adult cigarette smoking has declined significantly among most ethnic groups during the past 20 years[6]. However, this decline appears to have leveled off in recent years[6]. Also, while the number of daily smokers decreased in the USA between 1996 and 2001, the number of occasional ('some day') smokers increased during the same period, thus making the prevalence of current smoking relatively stable[18]. In addition, the use of large cigars and cigarillos actually rose during a similar timeframe[6]. The fact that the output of moist snuff increased over 40% during the 1990s is an alarming indication of the substitution of smokeless tobacco products for cigarettes and cigars[19]. These trends do not bode well for the future. It is estimated that the annual deaths attributable to smoking will rise from the current rate of 2.5 million to 12 million by the year 2050[1].

Another disturbing trend is the persistence of social and political constructs underlying alcohol and tobacco consumption. The enduring pattern has been that population groups with the least medical access and the lowest income with which to cope with lifestyle changes due to catastrophic illnesses tend to be among those most severely impacted by tobacco and alcohol factors leading to cancer[16]. The prevalence of major cancer risk factors due to tobacco use is, for example, highest for both men and women living below the poverty line. This group is about three times higher on a percentage basis for African Americans, Hispanics and Native Americans than it is for Caucasian Americans. Similar discrepancies exist for the same socioeconomic groups under age 65 without health-care coverage or any source of regular medical care[8]. Impoverished and near-impoverished groups, a disproportionate share of whom are ethnic minorities, are thus more apt to be at risk for cancer due to tobacco use and less apt to have access to health-care information, reinforcement and treatment.

In addition, cigarette advertising in the USA quadrupled between 1975 and 1997. As mentioned above, a specific target has been young people who are especially impressionable to images portraying the attractiveness of smoking or dipping. Capturing consumers when they are young obviously means that their dependence upon tobacco products will probably be all the more intractable when they reach adulthood, thus ensuring continued sales across their lifespan. Not only does this take a toll on the well-being of individuals, but it also exacts a price

on society as a whole in burdening social services and driving up health-care costs[1].

The tobacco industry has also used its considerable resources to shape public policy by seeking to 'frame the increasing public debate about smoking regulations around rights and liberty rather than health, portray adversaries as extremists, and invest millions of dollars in campaign contributions to the leading political parties.'[1] Such efforts work against an enlightened medicine that promotes health as well as treating illness.

INDIVIDUAL AND SMALL GROUP APPROACHES: CESSATION AND PREVENTION

These unfortunate trends highlight the need for making prevention and cessation programs for tobacco and alcohol users an integral part of oncology. Eliminating a cause of cancer through prevention and reducing the risk of cancer through permanent cessation would have obvious health benefits. Such programs would also have positive economic benefits in reducing the need for costly medical treatments and lowering absenteeism in the workplace[6].

Several effective methods for smoking cessation and abstinence at the level of the individual have been identified (Table 14.1). The Agency for Health Care Policy and Research (AHCPR)

Table 14.1 Categories of effective interventions for smoking cessation and abstinence at the level of the individual
Nicotine replacement
Social support
Skills training and problem-solving education for achieving and maintaining abstinence
Clinician-driven support: four A's – Ask, Advise, Assist and Arrange

has set an approach to smoking cessation stipulating that the 'three particularly effective elements of smoking cessation treatment are (1) nicotine replacement (NRT), (2) social support (clinician-provided encouragement and assistance), and (3) skills training and problem-solving techniques for achieving and maintaining abstinence.'[20] The National Cancer Institute (NCI) recommends the 'four As' for tobacco cessation: *Ask*, *Advise*, *Assist* and *Arrange*[20].

Similar guidelines have been laid down for alcohol curtailment or cessation. The Best Practices Series sponsored by Health Canada and the National Population Health Fund[21], for example, recommends a strategy adaptable to the NCI's 'four As': (1) When *asking* for or recommending cessation, recognize the health of the user, the amount of the use, and the motivations for using; (2) when *advising* the user, normalize the cessation or withdrawal process and address barriers; (3) when *assisting* an individual in withdrawing from alcohol, continue to address barriers and tailor the approach to the individual's needs and situation; and (4) when *arranging* and implementing the withdrawal strategy, focus on reducing harm, developing rapport and mirroring the individual's goals and degree of readiness to stop drinking.

Specific psychosocial interventions for alcohol cessation also parallel the AHCPR's recommendations for tobacco cessation[22]. For example, Australia's National Drug and Alcohol Research Centre (NDARC)[23] advises that the following complementary psychosocial interventions are effective strategies for withdrawal from alcohol: counseling, motivational interviewing, cognitive–behavioral interventions, skills training, behavioral self-management, cognitive restructuring, and self-guided materials (such as reading materials). Roth and Fonagy[24] uncover similar findings in their review of the research on psychotherapy for alcohol dependency and abuse. They further note that alcohol treatment has shifted over the years from long-term residential treatment of 'alcoholics' to briefer therapies with incremental goals that address the context of the drinker. In a more focused meta-analysis of psychosocial treatments for alcohol use disorders, Finney and Moos[25] observe that interpersonally oriented therapies appear more effective with higher-functioning individuals, whereas cognitive–behavioral treatments have better outcomes with more impaired individuals. Finney and Moos also find that empathy from the practitioner seems to have a higher efficacy rate than does confrontation, and that outpatient treatment is about as effective as inpatient treatment for individuals eligible for both[25].

Generally speaking, these recommendations with respect to psychosocial approaches to alcohol withdrawal are reflected in the handbook by Abrams *et al.* of best practices for the treatment of tobacco dependence[26]. It should also be mentioned that Alcoholics Anonymous, the famous 12-step group program dating back to the 1930s, which encourages total abstinence around alcohol use, has been applied to tobacco or nicotine cessation as well[27]. Lundberg and Passik point out a potential problem in withdrawing from both alcohol and tobacco in as much as 'cigarette smoking should not be continued in moderate amounts, whereas moderate alcohol consumption is a part of society's lifestyle in general.'[5] Since the use of alcohol and tobacco often go together, with one triggering the other, it may be difficult to stop smoking while continuing to drink moderately. Also, 'separating "moderate" from "excessive" may be a harder differentiation than an out-and-out recommendation of total abstinence.'[5]

WHAT IS COMPLEMENTARY AND ALTERNATIVE MEDICINE?

A definition of CAM therapies with regards to tobacco and alcohol is difficult, because there is no standard intervention for cessation[1,2]. For the purpose of our discussion, we will maintain the convention that *complementary* therapies complement mainstream medicine and, with increasing data on efficacy, are becoming part of standard conventional medicine[28,29]. Examples of complementary therapies for tobacco cessation include: acupuncture, hypnosis, physical activity, nutrition, mind–body stress reduction, massage and the psychosocial therapies mentioned above. Alternative therapies are promoted as *alternatives* to mainstream treatment. As such, they tend to be more controversial than complementary modalities, as they may delay appropriate conventional medical care[28,29]. An example of an alternative therapy in this context is faith healing or chelation therapy as tobacco or alcohol cessation options.

CAM and conventional modalities directed to the level of the individual that have been used with some success include: nicotine replacement, pharmacotherapy with antidepressants or other agents[6], individual and group counseling and psychosocial interventions, acupuncture and hypnosis (Table 14.2)[30–32]. Successful interventions directed to the societal level include advertising, quit lines, increasing the tax on tobacco products and education[1,2,8]. It is probable that a comprehensive strategy including a broad range of societal and individual approaches would be more successful with a wider array of individuals[1].

Table 14.2 Well-accepted individual methods of tobacco cessation: description and efficacy. From references 30–32

Method	How it works	Success rate
Person-to-person contact	Talking face-to-face with a health-care professional, four or more sessions for 90–300 minutes	About 30% remain smoke-free for at least 5 months; a single 3-minute session results in 14% success rate
Telephone counseling	Counselor calls to the smoker	13% of all smokers in this group quit for at least 5 months
Group therapy	Trained leader meets with a group to discuss techniques and offer support	14% quit rate at the 5-month mark
Individual therapy	Trained therapist coaches the smoker, shares problems and solutions	17% quit rate at the 5-month mark
Zyban (bupropion): requires a doctor's prescription	Helps to ease cravings; method of action not understood	31% success rate
Nicotine gum (nicotine polacrilex): available over the counter	Chewing-gum that releases nicotine, absorbed into bloodstream through the gums	23% success rate
Nicotine skin patch: available over the counter	Nicotine is absorbed through the skin in a steady dose over time	18% success rate
Nicotine nasal spray: requires a doctor's prescription	Nicotine is sprayed into the nose where it is absorbed into the bloodstream	31% success rate

In addition, there are several CAM methods and systems approaches that merit further research. Acupuncture applied to the inner ear has been shown to be potentially helpful with regards to coping with withdrawal symptoms from alcohol, tobacco and other substances. Herbs are commonly used by Chinese medical doctors, often in conjunction with acupuncture. Ayurvedic medicine also employs herbs in the treatment of substance abuse, along with dietary changes and yoga. Biofeedback, which improves control over the autonomic body functions, is also occasionally used in the treatment of substance abuse. A commitment to a 'higher power', the center piece of the 12-step programs for alcohol and nicotine addiction mentioned above, has demonstrated a strong influence on recovery and maintenance of abstinence[33,34].

FOCUS ON THE INDIVIDUAL: COMPREHENSIVE MODEL OF BEHAVIOR CHANGE AND MAINTENANCE

It is easy to see that a variety of approaches to tobacco and alcohol cessation are recommended in the literature. Many of these are meant to be used in combination with each other. Most guidelines appear to advocate a pragmatically eclectic approach lacking in theoretical integration. A welcomed exception to this trend in the literature is the recommendation by several commentators[1,35] – among them Robert Lutz in this volume – that prevention and cessation approaches to tobacco and alcohol use be carried out within the framework of the transtheoretical model of change (TTM) developed by Prochaska and colleagues over the past two decades. It is a research-based, sequential model that synthesizes stages and processes of change within the context of a specific problem. Initially developed to treat the abuse of tobacco, alcohol and other substances[36], TTM has been applied across the field

of health psychology and has shown much promise as a framework for counseling and behavior modification in general[37].

Five stages of change in TTM have emerged through factor analysis or cluster analysis: precontemplation, contemplation, preparation, action and maintenance. Each stage identifies an individual's readiness (motivation) to change. Further elaboration of these stages can be found in Chapter 9. The stages naturally follow in a linear format, so movement between them is straightforward with progression to a successive stage depending on the completion of the tasks that define the prior stage. However, the possibility of a stage regression or a repetition of a series of stages at a more advanced level is also possible. A 'Stages of Change Questionnaire' is available to help ensure an accurate assessment of the client's stage of readiness and the tasks to be completed[37].

Each stage of change is identified with a unique subset of ten psychotherapeutic processes which have also been gleaned through statistical analyses. These processes are 'the ways in which individuals attempt to change with or without therapy.'[38] They include consciousness raising, self-re-evaluation, self-liberation, counterconditioning, stimulus control, reinforcement management, helping relationships, dramatic relief, environmental re-evaluation, and social liberation. A 'Processes of Change Questionnaire' may be used to assess which method or process of change is needed by an individual to complete a task associated with that individual's stage of readiness[37] (Table 14.3).

In addition to stages and processes of change, Prochaska's research has further isolated what he calls five levels of change. A level of change is the particular context of the problem to be addressed. There are five such levels in TTM: symptom/situational problems; maladaptive cognitions, current interpersonal conflicts; family systems conflicts, and intrapersonal conflicts[37] (Table 14.4).

Table 14.3 Ways in which individuals attempt to change according to the transtheoretical mode of change

Consciousness raising

Self re-evaluation

Counterconditioning

Stimulus control

Reinforcement management

Helping relationships

Dramatic relief

Environmental re-evaluation

Social liberation

Table 14.4 Five levels of change – context of the problem to be addressed

Symptom/situational problems

Maladaptive cognitions

Current interpersonal conflicts

Family systems conflicts

Intrapersonal conflicts

Thus, the level of change situates the identified problem in a life context, which helps clarify an individual's stage of readiness to change with respect to that problem. Knowing the level of change also helps identify the processes or interventions that are needed to help the individual work towards a higher stage of readiness. For example, treatment of the problem of tobacco or alcohol consumption is approachable in several ways depending on the current context of the consumption. The problem may be relatively isolated (symptom/situational level), tied to emotional difficulties (intrapersonal level), reinforced by irrational justifications (maladaptive cognitive level), compensation for spousal or family stress (interpersonal level or family system level), or the result of peer pressure (symptom/situational

level). A knowledge of the level of the problem – whether it is associated with cognitive, emotional, or interpersonal issues – informs the assessment of the stage of readiness and the appropriate processes of change.

In summary, TTM integrates a variety of perspectives and techniques under a single theoretical umbrella that is easily understandable and generalizable. Originally developed to treat substance usage, it has been shown to be particularly effective in the treatment of tobacco and alcohol consumption. Its effectiveness appears to be due to the fact that it focuses not only on the usage *per se*, but also on the motivation and situational context of the user.

SOCIAL, POLITICAL, AND INSTITUTIONAL APPROACHES: REFRAMING THE NATIONAL AND INTERNATIONAL AGENDA

Several effective methods for smoking cessation and abstinence on the societal level have been identified (Table 14.5). On community and governmental levels, a prominent goal of tobacco and alcohol curtailment programs is to change social norms regarding consumption, marking a societal shift toward viewing tobacco and alcohol prevention as a public health, cultural and macroeconomic issue[39,40]. The American Cancer Society reports the National Institutes of Health estimates of health costs for cancer in 2003 to be 'at $189.5 billion: $64.2 billion for direct medical costs (total of all health expenditures); $16.3 billion for indirect morbidity costs (costs of lost productivity due to illness); and $109 billion for indirect mortality costs (cost of productivity due to premature death)'[6]. The effects of cancer on mental health are unfortunately less agreed upon and, hence, less well defined[41,42]. Nevertheless, the consensus among policy makers tends to be that, regardless of how they are valued, the human suffering and accompanying economic burden wrought by tobacco- and alcohol-related disease and premature death is highly significant and deserving of immediate attention[39–42].

Substantial cultural shifts typically accompany a change in social norms and economic conditions. Much has been written on the complex interaction of economic, social and cultural factors influencing health, particularly in light of the increased cancer incidence and mortality among those living below the poverty line[1]. A national study by the American Cancer Society in 1986[43] concluded that 'the primary cause of disparities in cancer between African Americans and whites is poverty'[6]. In 1991, the director of the US National Cancer Institute expressed the same view more poignantly: 'Poverty is a carcinogen.'[44] In 2003, several reports, including one by the prestigious Institute of Medicine (IOM), describe similar findings in more detail[14]. The consensus is that socioeconomic status affects numerous factors, including high-risk characteristics (such as tobacco and alcohol consumption), as well as poor access to prevention, early detection, diagnosis, medical treatment, palliative care and post-treatment quality-of-life supports. Cultural barriers, such as language, beliefs, values and traditions, were also noted to be inhibitors of cancer care. In more economically advantaged regions, cultural changes are also enacted when public policy moves from a laissez faire attitude built around individual liberty and the free market system, toward a philosophy that emphasizes community and governmental promotion of public health and well-being. This change in social norms is tied to notions of individual rights embedded in the social contract rather than to individual constraints due to the social condition of poverty. Across the world stage, changes in social norms affecting tobacco and alcohol consumption require a multifaceted approach that varies from region to region depending on relevant political barriers, governmental organizations, and population needs[14,39,40,44]. In the *The Economics of Tobacco*[41], the World Bank outlined

such a strategy of addressing specific factors and structural problems related to tobacco use. The following excerpt provides a good summary of their recommendations regarding governmental interventions:

> *Where governments decide to take strong action to curb the tobacco epidemic, a multipronged strategy should be adopted. Its aims should be to deter children from smoking, to protect nonsmokers, and to provide all smokers with information about health effects of tobacco. The strategy, tailored to individual country needs, would include: (1) raising taxes [particularly on the retail price of cigarettes]; (2) publishing and disseminating research results on the health effects of tobacco…; (3) widening access to nicotine replacement and other cessation therapies[41].*

The same report proposed several kinds of global strategy as complements or alternatives to governmental actions.

> *International organizations such as the United Nations agencies should review their existing programs and policies to ensure that tobacco control is given due prominence; they should sponsor research into the causes, consequences, and costs of smoking, and cost-effectiveness of interventions at the local level; and they should address tobacco control issues that cross borders, including working with the WHO's [World Health Organization] proposed Framework Convention for Tobacco Control. Key areas for action include facilitating international agreements on smuggling control, discussions on tax harmonization to reduce the incentives for smuggling, and bans on advertising and promotion involving the global communications media[41].*

These cost-effective interventions to reduce tobacco use at the level of society are presented in Table 14.5.

Table 14.5   Effective interventions at the societal level. From reference 45

Interventions	Beneficiaries/target group	Process indicators
Higher taxes on cigarettes and other tobacco products	Smokers, potential smokers (especially youth)	Price of cigarettes, tax as percentage of final sale price
Bans/restrictions on smoking in public and work places: schools, health facilities, public transport, restaurants, cinemas, etc.	Non-smokers protected from second-hand smoke	Smoke-free public spaces and places
Comprehensive bans on advertising and promotion of all tobacco products, logos and brand names	Smokers and potential smokers (especially youth) Societal attitudes to smoking	Laws, regulations, extent to which respected/enforced
Better consumer information: education, counter advertising, media coverage, research findings	Smokers and potential smokers Societal norms and attitudes to smoking	Knowledge of health risks, attitudes to smoking
Large, direct warning labels on cigarette boxes and other tobacco products	Smokers	Perecentage of box surface covered by label, message, color/font specifications
Help for smokers who wish to quit, including increased access to nicotine replacement therapy (NRT) and other cessation therapies, quit lines, etc.	Smokers	Number of ex-smokers

The evidence indicates that the greatest effectiveness is achieved when interventions are implemented together. There is no silver bullet! Price increases have been shown to be the most effective deterrent (particularly among youth), which has a positive effect on the economy by giving individuals and households increased discretionary income. However, a negative side-effect of a decrease in demand for tobacco products is the temporary net job loss due to decreases in tobacco farming, manufacturing and distribution. Another potentially negative effect of reducing demand for tobacco output is that poor consumers who find it too difficult to quit and continue to consume tobacco will be hurt by rising prices resulting from falling demand. Thus, compensating them in other product areas, such as basic foods, and targeting those groups with aggressive cessation programs might be advisable.

Measures to reduce the supply of tobacco (e.g. prohibition, youth access restrictions, crop substitutions and trade restrictions) are typically ineffective with the exception of controls on smuggling.

Similar plans have been proposed regarding alcohol consumption, although they are fewer and far less detailed in terms of their political constructions[10,23]. This may be a sign of the paucity of public attention paid to drinking compared with that which is now given to smoking and dipping[5]. As mentioned, alcohol is an established cause of cancer and when combined with tobacco has been shown to increase the risk of many cancers[1,6]. Alcohol has an established relation to poverty and a substantial negative social impact, particularly on the young and in the Third World[8–10]. Given these facts, it stands to reason that alcohol prevention and cessation deserves a comparable national and global agenda.

By eliminating or greatly reducing individual factors and structural problems in society that are driving up tobacco and alcohol consumption, the average human life will be likely to lengthen and improve in quality. This benefit extends not only to individuals, but also to their relationships and ultimately to society as a whole. As people gain support and insight about how to transcend unhealthy dependencies on substances such as tobacco and alcohol, they have an opportunity to change the compulsive ways in which they relate to themselves and each other, and through that to transform their world.

SUMMARY AND CONCLUSION

Tobacco and alcohol, either alone or in combination with each other, pose significant risk factors related to several different forms of cancer. The causal agents pertain to lifestyle and, in the case of tobacco and possibly alcohol, are also associated with biological mechanisms. Social, economic and political contexts have been shown to facilitate consumption as well. These facts militate strongly in favor of cessation and prevention programs that are affordable, effective and widely accessible. These programs must be geared toward both individuals and societies. As a practical matter, the fact that tobacco abstinence is typically encouraged whereas moderate alcohol consumption is a pervasive social norm, may pose a further challenge when treating people who use both in combination. Readiness to change, and all of its associated components, must be assessed continually in order to provide optimal care to the individual and assist in comprehensive behavior change.

The political and socioeconomic factors underlying the diffusion of tobacco and alcohol products call for community, national, and even international programs of action. The eradication of cancer, particularly as it relates to tobacco and alcohol consumption, poses a daunting task for clinicians, researchers, patient advocates, health-care administrators, politicians, and other opinion leaders. It requires a network extending across linguistic, cultural and political boundaries, and an alliance among people who may have specific disagreements with each other but who nevertheless share a common purpose. A lone intervention between individuals, as necessary as it might be, lights a single flame that may soon die when exposed to its surrounding environs, but a global agenda of activities could ignite a bonfire with the potential to significantly lower tobacco- and alcohol-related morbidity and mortality worldwide.

References

1. Koh HK, Kannler C, Geller AC. Cancer prevention: Preventing tobacco-related cancers. In Devita VT, et al., eds. Cancer: Principles and Practices of Oncology, 6th edn. Philadelphia: Lippincott Williams &Wilkins, 2001: 549–60

2. Hecht SS. Tobacco smoke carcinogens and lung cancer. J Natl Cancer Inst 1999; 91; 1194

3. Doll R, Peto R. The Causes of Cancer. New York: Oxford University Press, 1981

4. Bagnardi V, Blangiardo M, La Vecchia C, Corrao G. A meta-analysis of alcohol drinking and cancer risk. Br J Cancer 2001; 85: 1700–5

5. Lundberg JC, Passik SD. Alcohol and cancer. In: Holland J, ed. Psycho-oncology. New York: Oxford University Press, 1998; 45–8

6. American Cancer Society. Cancer Facts and Figures 2004. Atlanta, GA: American Cancer Society, 2004

7. National Center for Health Statistics. Health, United States, 2002, with chartbook on trends in the health of Americans. Hyattsville, MD: Public Health Service, 2002

8. Singh G, Miller B, Hankey BF, Edwards BK. Area socioeconomic variations in US cancer incidence, mortality, stage, treatment, and survival 1975–1999. NCI Cancer Surveillance Monograph Series. Number 4. Bethesda, MD: National Cancer Institute; 2003. NIH Publications No. 03-5417. http://seer.cancer.gov/publications/ses

9. Jones-Webb R, Snowden L, Herd D, et al. Alcohol-related problems among black, Hispanic, and white men: the contribution of neighborhood poverty. J Stud Alcohol 1997; 58: 539–45

10. Mosher J. Alcohol and poverty: analyzing the link between alcohol-related problems and social policy. In: Samuels SE, Smith MD, eds. Improving the Health of the Poor. Menlo Park, CA: The Henry J. Kaiser Family Foundation, 1992: 97–121

11. Centers for Disease Control and Prevention. Youth tobacco surveillance – United States, 2000. CDC Sur Summaries. Morbid Mortal Weekly Rep 2001; 50: SS–4

12. Centers for Disease Control and Prevention. School health policies and programs study 2000, state level summaries, health education. Atlanta, GA: Centers for Disease Control and Prevention (online). Available at: http://www.cdc.gov/nccdphp/dash/shpps/summaries/health_ed/index.htm

13. Ries LAG, Eisner MP, Kosary CL, et al., eds. SEER Cancer Statistics Review, 1975–2002. Bethesda, MD: National Cancer Institute. http://seer.cancer.gov/scr/1975_2002/, based on November 2004 SEER data submission, posted to the SEER website 2005

14. Institute of Medicine. Unequal Treatment: Confronting Racial and Ethnic Disparities in Health Care. Washington, DC: National Academy Press, 2003

15. Freeman HP. Commentary on meaning of race in science and society. Cancer Epidemiol Biomarkers Prev 2003; 12: 232S–236S

16. US Department of Health and Human Services. The Health Consequences of Using Smokeless Tobacco: A Report of the Advisory Committee to the Surgeon General. Atlanta, GA: US Department of Health and Human Services, National Institutes of Health, National Cancer Institute, 1986

17. US Environmental Protection Agency. Respiratory Health Effects of Passive Smoking: Lung Cancer and Other Disorders. EPA/600/6-90/006F. Washington, DC: US Environmental Protection Agency, 1992

18. Centers for Disease Control and Prevention. Prevalence of current cigarette smoking among adults and changes in prevalence of current and some day smoking. United States, 1996–2001. Morbid Mortal Weekly Rep 2003; 52: 303–7

19. US Department of Agriculture. Tobacco Situation and Outlook Report. Washington, DC: US Department of Agriculture, Market and Trade Economics Division, Economics Research Service, 2002

20. Agency for Health Care Policy and Research, Smoking Cessation Clinical Practice Guideline Panel and Staff. Smoking cessation clinical practice guidelines. JAMA 1996; 275: 1270

21. Seeking Solutions. Best Practices: Alcohol and other substances use withdrawal. Vancouver, BC: Health Canada and the National Population Health Fund, 2004. www.agingincanada.ca

22. Myrick H, Anton R. Treatment of alcohol withdrawal. Alcohol Health Res 1998; 22: 38–43

23. Shand F, Gates J, Fawcett J, Mattick R. Guidelines for the Treatment of Alcohol Problems. Canberra: National Drug and Alcohol Research Centre, 2003

24. Roth A., Fonagy P. What Works for Whom? A Critical Review of Psychotherapy Research. New York: Guilford Press, 1996

25. Finney JW, Moos RH. Psychosocial treatments for alcohol use disorders. In: Nathan PE, Gorman JM, eds. A Guide to Treatments that Work. New York: Oxford University Press, 1998: 156–66

26. Abrams DB, Niaura R, Brown RA, et al. The Tobacco Dependence Treatment Handbook: A

Guide to Best Practices. New York: Guilford Press, 2003

27. Yoder B. The Recovery Resource Book: The Best Available Information on Addictions and Co-dependence. New York: Simon & Schuster, 1990

28. Deng G, Cassileth BR, Yeung KS. Complementary therapies for cancer-related symptoms. J Support Oncol 2004; 2: 419–26

29. Richardson MA, Sanders T, Palmer JL. Complementary/alternative medicine use in a comprehensive cancer center and the implications for oncology. J Clin Oncol 2000; 18: 2505–14

30. Ullman K, Quit smoking now. Intouch, January 2002

31. Fiore MC, Bailey WC, Cohen SJ, et al. Treating tobacco use and dependence. Rockville, MD: US Department of Health and Human Services, 2000

32. Springfield Publishing. Nursing 99 Drug Handbook. Springfield, IL: Springfield Publishing, 1999

33. Fugh-Berman A. Alternative Medicine: What Works. Baltimore, MD: Williams & Wilkins, 1997

34. Pelletier KR. The Best Alternative Medicine: What Works? What Does Not? New York: Simon & Schuster, 2000

35. DiClemente CC, Prochaska JO, Fairhurst SK, et al. The process of smoking cessation: An analysis of precontemplation, contemplation, and preparation stages of change. J Consult Clin Psychol 1991; 59: 295–304

36. Prochaska JO, DiClemente CC, Norcross JC. In search of how people change. Applications to addictive behaviors. Am Psychol 1992; 47: 1102

37. Prochaska JO, DiClemente CC. The transtheoretical approach. In: Norcross JC, Goldfried MR, eds. Handbook of Psychotherapy Integration. New York: Basic Books, 1992: 300–34

38. Petrocelli JV. Processes and Stages of Change: Counseling with the Transtheoretical model of change. J Counsel Dev 2002; 80: 22–30

39. Brundtland G. Framework Convention on Tobacco Control. Geneva, Switzerland: World Health Organization, May 2000. http://www.who.int/tobacco/fctc/text/en/fctc_en.pdf

40. World Health Organization. Tobacco Free Initiative. Geneva, Switzerland: World Health Organization, 2004

41. US Department of Health and Human Services. The Health Consequences of Smoking: Cancer. A report of the Surgeon General. DHHS Pub. No. (PHS)82-50179. Rockville, MD: US Department of Health and Human Services, Public Health Service, Office of Smoking and Health, 1982

42. US Department of Health and Human Services. The Health Consequences of Smoking: Cancer and Chronic Lung Disease in the Workplace. A report of the surgeon general. DHHS Pub. No. (PHS)85-50207. Washington, DC: US Department of Health and Human Services, Public Health Service, Office of Smoking and Health, 1985

43. American Cancer Society. Special Report on Cancer in the Economically Disadvantaged. Atlanta, GA: American Cancer Society, 1986

44. Broder S. Progress and challenges in the National Cancer Program. In: Burgge J, Curran T, Harlow E, McCormick F, eds. Origins of Human Cancer: A Comprehensive Review. Plainview, NY: Cold Spring Harbor Laboratory Press, 1991: 27-33

45. The World Bank Group. Tobacco Control. Geneva, Switzerland: World Bank Group, 2004

15

Specific malignancies

(a) Breast cancer

Matthew P. Mumber

Breast cancer is the most common female malignancy in the Western world. In women aged 40–55, it is the leading cause of cancer-related death in the USA. There has been a slight decrease in the rates of breast cancer mortality over the past several years, probably as a result of improvements in early detection and conventional therapies, especially new agents used for systemic chemotherapy. This decreased risk of death has been accompanied by an increased incidence of pre-invasive lesions, namely ductal carcinoma *in situ* (DCIS), largely the result of increased ability to find this disease early through appropriate screening mammography[1].

RISK FACTORS

Rates of development of breast cancer increase with increasing age. A female baby born today has a 1 in 8 chance of developing breast cancer within her lifetime, according to statistics from the National Cancer Institute. Major risk factors for breast cancer are listed in Table 15.1. Epidemiologic studies show a wide variation of breast cancer incidence in different cultures – specifically a near ten-fold increased risk in Western versus Asian countries. Interestingly, this difference in risk is changed if a woman migrates to the West from Asia – i.e. her risk of breast cancer matches that of women born in the Western world. This points to possible modifiable risk factors such as nutrition, lifestyle and environmental exposures.

Scientists are defining family-related risk factors through the identification of specific genes, such as *BRCA1* and *BRCA2*. These genes were identified by following families in which a heritable breast cancer syndrome was suspected, owing to multiple cases through many generations. Unfortunately, only 10–15% of breast cancer cases appear to be genetically linked, and there is still significant debate as to how to manage patients with these gene mutations[2,3].

The Gail model quantifies a woman's breast cancer risk prospectively, based on many of the above factors, and can be used to estimate the relative risk for individual patients interested in primary and secondary prevention[4].

SCREENING AND EARLY DETECTION

The two general modalities for screening and early detection include mammography and breast self-examination, although the latter has been debated because of some conflicting research findings. New applications of existing technologies (such as magnetic resonance imaging (MRI) of the breast) hold promise for screening, especially in high-risk populations[4].

DIAGNOSIS

Diagnosis of breast cancer is usually made by breast biopsy, often guided by radiographic techniques using mammography and ultrasound.

Table 15.1   Risk factors for breast cancer

Risk factor	Relative risk
Irradiation of breast	Over 20 (age 10–20 years) 15.0 (age 20–30 years) 1.0 (age older than 50)
Family history of breast cancer	1.4–2.8 (one first-degree relative) 4.2–6.8 (two first-degree relatives)
Biopsied breast disease	1.5–2.0 (hyperplasia) 3.0-5.0 (atypia)
Age at first birth	1.8 (35 years or older) 1.0–1.9 (nulliparous) 0.8 (20 or younger)
Last menstrual period after age 55	1.5–2.0
First menstrual period before age 12	1.2–1.3
Oral contraceptives	1.5 (use before first birth) 1.0 (use)
Prior breast cancer	0.5–1% added risk per year
Postmenopausal estrogen replacement	1.1–2.0
Alcohol use	1.4 (one drink per day) 1.7 (two drinks per day) 2.0 (three drinks per day)
Obesity	1.2
High-fat diet	1.2
History of breast feeding	0.8
Oophorectomy	0.5
Prolonged exposure to pesticides	?
Chlorinated solvents	?
Polychlorinated biphenyls (PCBs)	?
BRCA1 mutation positive	36–85% lifetime risk – tends to occur at an early age

Examples of relative risk factor: 1.0 = no added risk; 0.5 = 50% normal risk; 2.0 = twice normal risk

Table 15.2	Examples of advances in conventional therapies and improved patient tolerence	

Conventional therapy	Advance	Patient impact
Surgery	sentinel lymph node mapping	lessens need for complete axillary dissection in selected patients
Chemotherapy	improved antiemetic regimens less toxic gene-based agents	improved nausea control improved efficacy and tolerance
Radiation therapy	improved treatment planning	less early and delayed normal tissue toxicity (lung, heart)

CONVENTIONAL THERAPY

Conventional treatment of breast cancer is generally guided by patient factors, disease stage and tumor characteristics. Surgery, chemotherapy and radiation therapy all play significant roles of variable intensity depending upon these factors. The general trend is toward maintaining the cosmetic form and function of the breast and surrounding tissues, while decreasing the morbidity of conventional treatment options. Table 15.2 illustrates some significant advances in conventional therapies, and the impact on patient tolerance. The text in these specific malignancy sections does not include an exhaustive review of all modalities, and some of the information presented in the tables was presented in earlier sections. Levels of evidence are listed below.

The following sections will focus on modalities mentioned throughout this text with regards to prevention, supportive care, and antineoplastic uses. Table 15.3 presents a list of modalities, their benefit and level of evidence for use. Please also note that therapies which have some potential for dangerous interactions with conventional therapies are denoted with an asterisk, owing to these potential safety issues.

- Level one – well-designed randomized controlled clinical trial(s);

- Level two – prospective and retrospective non-randomized clinical trials and analyses;

- Level three – opinions of expert committees, best-case series;

- Level four – preclinical *in vitro* and *in vivo* studies, and traditional uses.

Physical activity

Robert B. Lutz

PRIMARY PREVENTION

After colon cancer, breast cancer is the most well-studied for its relationship to physical activity. Although the relationship appears to be less robust than that seen with colon cancer, nonetheless data support a protective role for physical activity, with an approximate 20–30% overall decrease seen for women, irrespective of their life-stage[1]. Data from a case–control study suggest that physical activity during puberty may be especially important in decreasing a woman's lifetime risk[2]. This finding is consistent with the presumed biologic mechanisms for the protective role of physical activity in breast cancer. Exercise during puberty may delay the age of menarche as well as affecting the development of breast tissue (e.g. density of tissue). It is probable, however, that the protective role of physical activity varies across a woman's lifespan as a function of hormonal variability and other related factors. Therefore, physical activity throughout life is probably just as important as exercise at a specific point. A dose–response relationship exists, with the majority of studies suggesting lower risks with higher levels of activity, the recommendation being leisure time moderate to vigorous physical activity of at least 4 hours per week.

TERTIARY PREVENTION

Of interest is a single small study in which self-reported exercise suggested increased survival[3]. This finding has recently been supported by data from the Nurses' Health Study. Women who were diagnosed with breast cancer after enroll-ment were followed for up to 16 years (1986–2002) or until their deaths. Almost 2300 women reported being physically active after diagnosis, with 230 deaths from breast cancer identified. Women who were physically active for 1–3 hours per week had a relative risk (RR) of 0.81 (95% CI 0.59–1.13); those who were active for 3–5 hours per week had a RR of 0.46 (95% CI 0.26–0.82); for 5–8 hours per week, a RR of 0.58 (95% CI 0.38–0.90); and for > 8 hours per week, a RR of 0.71 (95% CI 0.46–1.09). The *p* value for a linear trend was 0.05. Walking was the primary activity performed[4].

SUPPORTIVE CARE

In contrast to other cancers, more research has looked at the role of physical activity and exercise in survivors of breast cancer. These studies have looked at individuals both during, as well as after, treatment. Although using a variety of methodologies and exercise protocols (supervised vs. unsupervised; aerobic and/or resistance training; prescribed exercise), the research strongly supports a positive role for physical activity in addressing a number of physical and quality of life issues. These include objective measures, such as exercise capacity, body weight and composition, flexibility, fatigue, measures of immune function and nausea. Additionally, subjective measures, such as symptoms of depression and/or anxiety, mood, self-esteem, functional and physical well-being, overall quality of life and satisfaction with life, have been positively affected[5] (Table 15.3).

Table 15.3	Benefits of interventions in breast cancer	

Modality/intervention	Benefit	Level of evidence
Primary prevention		
Physical activity		
Mild, moderate	lower relative risk (RR)	II, III, IV
Nutrition		
Diet		
plant based	lower RR	II, III, IV
fiber	lower RR	III, IV
individual foods		
soy	possible lower RR	conflicting II, III, IV
green tea	possible lower RR	II, III, IV
flax seed	possible lower RR	IV
fish oil	possible lower RR	II, III, IV
individual phytochemicals	possible lower RR	conflicting II, IV
Supplementation		
multivitamins	possible lower RR	conflicting II, III, IV
Obesity		
BMI in normal range	lower RR	II, III, IV
Mind–body		
yoga	possible psychneuroimmunologic	none
hypnosis	benefit	
meditation		
support groups		
Botanicals		
Curcumin	lower RR	IV
Energy medicine	unknown	none
Alternative systems	unknown	none
Spirituality	social support protective, religiosity protective, marriage protective	II
Tobacco cessation	lower RR	II, III, IV
Environment		
Pesticide exposure	possible lower RR	IV
Secondary prevention		
Physical activity		
Mild	lower RR	III
Moderate		
Nutrition		
Diet		
plant based	lower RR	III
fiber	unknown	III
individual foods		
soy		
high concentration	possible lower RR	II, IV
low concentration	possible higher RR	II, IV

Continued

413

Table 15.3 *Continued*

Modality/intervention	Benefit	Level of evidence
Nutrition		
Diet		
flax seed	possible lower RR	II, IV
fish oil	possible lower RR	II, IV
green tea	possible lower RR	II, IV
individual phytochemicals	possible lower RR	IV
Supplementation		
multivitamins	possible lower RR	II, IV
Obesity		
BMI in normal range	Possibly lower RR	II, III, IV
Mind–body		
yoga	possible psychneuroimmunologic	none
hypnosis	effect	
meditation		
support groups		
Botanicals	phytoestrogenic effect? positive or negative effect	IV
Energy medicine	unknown	none
Alternative systems	unknown	none
Spirituality	unknown	none
family support	possible lower RR	II
Tobacco cessation	lower RR	II, III
Tertiary prevention		
Physical activity		
Mild	possible lower RR	II, III, IV
Moderate	possible lower RR	II, III, IV
Nutrition		
Diet		
plant based	possible lower RR	III
fiber	possible lower RR	III
individual foods		
soy		
high concentration	possible lower RR	III, IV
low concentration	possible higher RR	III, IV
flax seed		
lignan component	possible higher RR	III, IV
omega-three component	possible lower RR	III, IV
green tea	possible lower RR	II, III, IV
fish oil	possible lower RR	II, III, IV
individual phytochemicals	possible lower RR	II, III, IV
Supplementation		
CoQ10	possible lower RR	II, III, IV

Continued

Table 15.3 *Continued*

Modality/intervention	Benefit	Level of evidence
Tertiary prevention		
Obesity		
BMI in normal range	possibly lower RR	II, III, IV
Mind–body		
yoga	possible lower RR	II, III
support groups	improved survival	conflicting I, II, III
Botanicals	improved recovery from conventional therapy (Ashwagandha, Astragalus)	IV
Energy medicine	unknown	none
Alternative systems	unknown	none
Spirituality	support group participation (improved survival)	conflicting levels I, II, II
Tobacco cessation	lower RR	II, III, IV
Supportive care during treatment		
Physical activity		
Mild	improved fatigue, quality of life (QOL)	II, III
Moderate		
Nutrition		
Diet		
individual foods		
soy*	decreased hot flushes	conflicting level II, III
individual phytochemicals*	improved tolerance of conventional therapy	conflicting III, IV
CoQ10*	possible cardiac protection	IV
Supplementation	improved tolerance of conventional therapies	IV
multivitamins*		
Mind–body		
yoga	improved QOL, sleep, anxiety	II, III
hypnosis	improved anxiety	II, III
meditation	improved anxiety, sleep	II, III
support groups	improved QOL	I, II, III
Manual therapy		
massage and manual lymphatic drainage	improved lymphedema	I, II, III
Botanicals		
black cohosh*	improved hot flushes	conflicting level I, II, III
*Panax ginseng**	improved fatigue	II, III
calendula cream	improved skin reaction to radiation	II, III, IV
Energy medicine	improved fatigue	II, III
biofield techniques	improved QOL	

Continued

Table 15.3 *Continued*

Modality/intervention	Benefit	Level of evidence
Supportive care during treatment		
Alternative systems	acupuncture nausea prevention	I, II, III
Spirituality	social support improved anxiety, QOL	I, II, III
Following treatment		
Physical activity		
Mild	improved fatigue	II, III
Moderate	improved depression	II, III
	improved sleep	II, III
	improved QOL	II, III
Nutrition		
CoQ10	improved fatigue	II, III
Mind–body		
yoga	improved sleep, QOL, anxiety	II, III
hypnosis	symptom control	II, III
meditation	improved QOL, pain, immune parameters	I, II, III
support groups		
Manual therapy		
massage	decreased lymphedema	I, II, III
strain–counterstrain therapy	improved musculoskeletal complaints	III
Botanicals		
Panax ginseng*	improved fatigue	II, III
black cohosh*	improved hot flushes	II, III
calendula ointment	improved skin recovery following radiation	I, II, III, IV
Energy medicine		
biofield techniques	improved QOL	II, III
Alternative systems	acupuncture for fatigue	II
Spirituality	improved QOL	II, III
Antineoplastic therapy		
Nutrition		
Diet		
plant based	none	none
fiber	none	none
specific diets (macrobiotic, Gerson)	cell kill	conflicting III, IV
individual foods		
green tea	cell kill	IV
soy	cell kill	IV
grape seed extract (proantho-cyanidin)	cell kill	IV
curcumin	cytostatic	IV

Continued

Table 15.3 *Continued*

Modality/intervention	Benefit	Level of evidence
Following treatment		
Nutrition		
Diet		
individual phytochemicals	improved cell kill	IV
individual vitamins (A, C, E, selenium)	cell kill	IV
Supplementation	none	none
Obesity	none	none
Mind–body		
yoga	none	none
hypnosis	none	none
meditation	none	none
support groups	improved overall survival	conflicting level I, II, III
Manual therapy		
massage	none	none
chiropractic		
strain–counterstrain		
Botanicals		
*Panax ginseng**	estrogen-like activity – AVOID	IV
flax lignans*		
red clover*		
iscador	anti-tumor efficacy	conflicting II, III, IV
Energy medicine	none	none
Alternative systems		
Chinese herbs	cell kill	IV
Spirituality	increased cell kill	IV
prayer	improved overall survival	II

BMI, body mass index; QOL, quality of life

Nutrition

Cynthia Thomson and Mara Vitolins

Considerable controversy surrounds the discussions regarding the dietary pattern associated with a reduced risk of breast cancer. A number of studies, but not all, advise a diet that is low in fat, high in fruits and vegetables and with limited or no alcohol consumption reduces the risk of breast cancer[1–5]. In 1997, the American Institute for Cancer Research/World Cancer Research Fund panel report concluded that there is 'probable' evidence that a diet rich in fruits and vegetables, carotenoids and fiber reduces the risk of breast cancer[6]. Additionally, they indicated that it is also 'probable' that alcohol and obesity increase the risk[6].

The macronutrient (carbohydrate, fat, protein) distribution associated with breast cancer risk has been vigorously debated over the past 20 years and the role of dietary fat in breast cancer prevention has been particularly controversial. Pooled results of large, prospective studies investigating fat and breast cancer have not found significant associations between total fat or specific types of fat and breast cancer risk[7,8]. After 8 years of follow-up, data reported from the Nurses' Health Study revealed no association between total fat consumption and breast cancer risk. However, there was a significant association between the highest quintile of animal fat consumption and breast cancer risk among premenopausal women[9]. Red meat and high-fat dairy products were identified as the major contributors to total animal fat in this cohort[9]. Although most studies of macronutrient distribution have focused on fat, few studies have investigated the optimal amount of protein and carbohydrate for breast cancer prevention with conflicting results[10–12]. It is important to note that many studies have not distinguished between animal protein and plant protein or specific types of carbohydrate (simple versus complex). This area of research continues to unfold and dietary intervention studies such as the diet modification arm of the Women's Health Initiative Trial will hopefully provide additional insight concerning this complex area of nutrition and cancer research.

Mind–body interventions

Linda E. Carlson and Shauna L. Shapiro

Mind–body supportive care was generally summarized in Chapter 12c, and much of the data reviewed applies to breast cancer patients. In terms of tertiary prevention, a significant example of supportive therapy and tertiary prevention for breast cancer patients includes the landmark psychosocial intervention study for women with metastatic breast cancer in which supportive/expressive group therapy was utilized[1]. Findings demonstrated that the year-long weekly psychosocial intervention enhanced patients' psychosocial functioning and reduced pain as compared to a standard care treatment control group, *and increased survival time by an average of*

18 months. However, a large replication trail failed to find a survival advantage for the group therapy[2]. There is debate as to whether this intervention affects survival rates, and a recent meta-analysis of this and ten other trials was inconclusive[3].

Other interventions such as experiential–existential group psychotherapy and mindfulness-based stress reduction for breast cancer have also shown changes in immune and hormone profiles, again suggesting a trend towards normalization of cortisol levels and less reactivity to stress as a consequence of enhanced emotional expression abilities[4–6].

Botanicals

Lise Alschuler

CHEMOPREVENTION OF BREAST CARCINOGENESIS

There are several herbs that have demonstrated chemoprevention effects in the development of breast cancer. Some of the most controversial, yet compelling, chemopreventive botanical agents are soy isoflavones. Soy-derived isoflavones have a multitude of effects, the summative impact of which may modulate the risk of breast carcinoma.

Soy isoflavones, namely genistein and diazdein, have been shown to increase serum levels of sex hormone binding globulin (SHBG), which, in turn, decreases the bioavailability of free estrogen. This action may explain the results of clinical studies that have documented reductions in estrogen levels. Additionally, soy isoflavones favor the 2-hydroxylation metabolic pathway of estrogen over the 17-hydroxylation pathway[1]. The metabolites of 2-hydroxylation exert a much weaker proliferative effect on breast cells than do the 17-hydroxylation metabolites. In a prospective, double-blind, randomized controlled trial, 68 premenopausal, omnivorous women between the ages of 25 and 55 years were enrolled. The experimental group consumed 40 mg genistein a day for 12 weeks. The mean menstrual cycle length increased by 3.52 days in the experimental group compared to a mean decrease of 0.06 days in the placebo group ($p = 0.04$). The experimental group had their mean follicular phase increase by 1.46 days compared with a mean increase of 0.14 days for participants on placebo ($p = 0.08$). The lengthened follicular phase and longer menstrual cycle shortens the luteal phase. Breast cells proliferate 2–3 times more rapidly during the luteal phase than during the follicular phase; thus, over time,

a shortened luteal phase may decrease the overall breast carcinoma risk[2]. It is of note that the amount of genistein used in this study, namely 40 mg, reflects the amount of soy isoflavones in a traditional diet in Asia (40–80 mg daily), where the incidence of breast cancer (and prostate cancer) is among the lowest in the world. A typical Western diet contains approximately 1 mg of isoflavones per day. Thus, the relevance and practical implications of this study in a Western population are questionable. Nonetheless, a population-based case–control study of breast cancer prior to the age of 50 in southern Germany demonstrated a significant reduction of breast cancer risk in both the highest and the lowest intake quartiles of diadzein and genistein. The OR (95% CI) for breast cancer risk was 0.62 (0.4–0.95) for the highest quartile and 0.47 (0.29–0.74) for the lowest quartile. This protective effect was only evident in hormone-receptor positive tumors. This study indicates that low levels of soy isoflavones may, in fact, confer protective benefits on premenpausal women[3].

Experimental data regarding soy isoflavones have both clarified and confused the role of these isoflavones in breast cancer prevention. A recent study by Zhou *et al.* demonstrated that genistein inhibited the growth of estrogen-dependent MCF-7 breast tumors *in vivo*[4]. This effect was postulated to be due to inhibition of tumor angiogenesis, reduction of estrogen receptor (ER)-α protein levels in MCF-7 tumors, and via modulation of the insulin-like growth factor (IGF)-I signaling pathway (IGF-I normally stimulates the proliferation of MCF-7 cells). On the other hand, Maggiolini *et al.* demonstrated that, at relatively low concentrations (at or below

1 μmol/l), genistein was a full agonist for ERα and ERβ and stimulated the proliferation of ER-dependent breast cancer cells[5]. Po *et al.* also demonstrated a proliferative effect on MCF-7 cells by low concentrations of genistein[6]. Both groups also demonstrated that 10 μmol/l and higher concentrations of genistein exerted cytotoxic effects on MCF-7 cells in an ER-independent fashion. The cytotoxic effects are proposed to be the result of inhibition of both tyrosine kinases and topoisomerase II. This high concentration of genistein corresponds to serum concentrations achieved in humans with a soy-rich and soy-supplemented diet. A typical Japanese diet, known to be soy-rich, produces phytoestrogen concentrations above 5 μmol/l in adults. Thus, it appears from these studies that exposure to phytoestrogens levels below 1 μmol/l may produce estrogenic effects, and upon long-term exposure, may promote breast cancer development and progression. Conversely, a diet rich in soy and supplemented with soy isoflavones may prevent breast cancer development. A 2004 study comparing soy flour, soy molasses, Novasoy and a mixture of isoflavones and genistein on MCF-7 (ER+) breast cancer cells in mice produced fascinating results. Soy flour-fed mice experienced stable tumors. Tumors in the mice fed soy molasses, Novasoy, mixed isoflavones or genistein alone grew in size. All groups received genistein aglycone equivalent products. Collectively, these results suggest that minimally processed soy flour may have chemopreventative effects, while processed soy foods and soy ingredients may actually stimulate tumor growth[7].

The cytotoxic effects of genistein have been further elaborated. Genistein, at 50 μmol/l and 100 μmol/l, up-regulated heat shock protein mRNA and down-regulated mRNA expression of ER-α and serum response factor (SRF)[8]. SRF is an important transcription factor that mediates the action of growth factors and the non-genomic actions of estrogen. Thus, the inhibitory effect of genistein on MCF-7 cells may involve the down-regulation of the ER at both the transcriptional and the post-transcriptional levels. Genistein may also inhibit the response of MCF-7 cells to growth factors by decreasing tyrosine kinase activities as well as decreasing the expression of downstream tyrosine kinase-responsive transcription factors, such as SRF. Genistein causes cell-cycle arrest in the G_0–G_1 and G_2–M phases by down-regulating the cell-cycle regulator gene, p21[9]. Decreased p21 sensitizes MDA-MB-231 malignant breast cells to genistein-mediated apoptosis. Genistein has also been demonstrated to induce DNA strand breakage by inhibiting topoisomerase II[10]. This breakage is generally lethal to the cell. It is of note that a subfraction of damaged cells can survive with permanent genetic alterations. If these alterations involve oncogenes, tumor suppressor genes or transcription factors, these genetic alterations may initiate carcinogenesis. It appears that, even at a molecular level, the overall effect of genistein is confusing.

Despite the compelling epidemiologic evidence, until the molecular effects of genistein are more clearly elucidated, soy should be thought of cautiously with regards to breast cancer chemoprevention.

A less controversial botanical agent that is chemopreventive for breast cancer is green tea. Green tea has been studied for its secondary and tertiary chemoprevention effects. Nakachi *et al.* determined that consumption of over five cups of green tea daily lowered the recurrence rate of stage I and II breast cancer and induced a longer disease-free period[11]. In this prospective cohort study, 472 Japanese women with histologically confirmed invasive breast carcinomas (stages I, II and III) were assessed for axillary lymph node metastases and progesterone and ER expression at the time of partial or total mastectomy and axillary dissection. In addition, these women were followed for 7 years with regards to recurrence in relation to green tea consumption. This study found that the premenopausal women who drank more than 5 cups of green tea daily had a lower mean number of metastasized lymph nodes. Subsequent to surgery, among the women with stage I and II breast cancer, drinkers of more than 5 cups daily of green tea experienced a 16.7% recurrence rate, while consumers of less than 4 cups per day experienced a 24.3% recurrence rate ($p < 0.05$). In addition, the drinkers of over 5 cups per day of green tea had a longer disease-free period (by 3.6 years) than did the green tea drinkers of fewer than 4 cups each day. The investigators adjusted for lifestyle factors inclusive of dietary intake of selected foods, cigarette smoking, alcohol use, frequency of pregnancy, child birth and abortion, body mass index and age. The mean consumption of green tea among those consuming more than 5 cups per day was estimated to be 8 cups. Stage III breast cancer patients did not show response to the green tea consumption, with 54% of the patients experiencing recurrence within 4 years. The lack of effect from green tea in this group is possibly the result of the fact that stage III cancer involves more accumulated genetic changes and that estrogen dependence is lost from stage II to stage III.

Inoue *et al.* also looked at the impact of regular green tea consumption on the risk of breast cancer recurrence[12]. This study began in 1990 with the collection of lifestyle information from 1160 new surgical cases of invasive breast cancer in female patients at a Japanese cancer center. These women were monitored for recurrence and daily green tea consumption over a 9-year period. The average age was 51.5 years. During 5264 person-years of follow-up (average 4.5 years per subject), 133 subjects (12%) experienced recurrence. A 31% decrease in risk of recurrence, as measured by hazard ratio (HR), adjusted for stage, was observed with consumption of 3 or more daily cups of green tea (HR = 0.69). This risk reduction was particularly statistically significant in stage I patients with a 57% decrease in risk. The risk reduction was present, but less significant, in stage II and not present among more advanced stages.

A recent study of primary breast cancer risk reduction from green tea consumption was published in 2003[13]. This was a 3-year population-based, case-controlled study of 501 Chinese, Japanese and Filipino women with an initial diagnosis of breast cancer, living in Los Angeles County. The control group consisted of 594 women without a diagnosis of breast cancer. Information on lifestyle habits during the year prior to the diagnosis was collected in addition to information about green tea consumption. Drinkers of at least 85.7 ml of green tea, (this represents approximately 2.85 oz or less than 1 cup) showed a significantly reduced risk of breast cancer (40–50% reduction in breast cancer risk), with a statistically significant trend of decreasing risk with increasing amount of green tea intake (intake of over 209.4 ml (this represents one cup of tea) conferred the greatest risk reduction) compared to non-drinkers of green tea. Interestingly, this study observed a protective effect on breast cancer risk from soy consumption that was most pronounced in non-drinkers of green tea. Conversely, the benefit of green tea was primarily observed among subjects who were low soy consumers. The significance of this observation is unknown.

Of the many herbs that have been investigated for their chemoprevention actions in breast carcinogenesis, there are several that are promising, but still in need of further research. Grape juice has demonstrated anticarcinogenic actions in several cancer cell types. Both *in vitro* and *in vivo* studies have demonstrated significant aromatase inihibition in an aromatase-transfected MCF-7 cell line with resultant 70% reduction in tumor size in mice[14]. The aromatase inhibition from grape juice appears to be the result of several active components. Aromatase inhibition is a particularly desirable chemoprevention strategy in postmenopausal women given the important role that tumor aromatase plays in the autocrine and paracrine stimulation of tumor growth.

Flax seed oil may also have chemoprevention actions. Rats with already established mammary tumors were fed flax seed oil or corn oil. The flax oil-supplemented rats experienced a decreased mammary tumor volume and fewer new mammary tumors than rats who received corn oil alone[15]. This effect was correlated with the omega-3 fatty acids, in particular the α-linolenic acid in flax seed oil.

Curcumin, derived from *Curcuma longa*, has anticarcinogenic activity in animals. These activities include a chemoprevention action on diethylstilbestrol (DES)-induced tumor promotion of rat mammary glands initiated with radiation. After a year of supplemental curcumin feeding, DES-fed rats demonstrated a 28.0% incidence of mammary tumors as opposed to a 84.6% incidence in the DES-fed control group[16]. This reduction of incidence was postulated to be due to interference by curcumin with DES-dependent promotion, possibly the result of lipid peroxidation inhibition by curcumin. In addition, curcumin-fed rats had higher concentrations of n-3 polyunsaturated fatty acids, which may prevent tumorigenesis via various anti-inflammatory mechanisms.

Glycyrrhiza uralensis has also been demonstrated to inhibit cell proliferation in human breast cancer cells (MCF-7) in a dose- and time-dependent manner. *Glycyrrhiza* extracts up-regulate proapoptotic protein in the Bax family[17]. Finally, flavonoids quercetin and naringenin act as estradiol mimetics on ER-α transcriptional activity. However, they impair the activation of rapid signaling pathways, thus decoupling ER-α signal transduction. This could explain the antiproliferative effect of these flavonoids in estrogen-related cancers[18].

and epigallocatechin gallate (EGCG) from green tea on human PC-9 lung cancer cells induces apoptosis more strongly than tamoxifen alone or EGCG alone. The enhancement of the inhibitory effect of tamoxifen on MCF-7 breast cancer cells by the addition of EGCG has also been observed[19]. Both agents induce apoptosis and appear to have a synergistic effect in *in vitro* models.

When a standardized extract of American ginseng (*Panax quinquefolius*) was applied to MCF-7 breast cancer cells along with tamoxifen, further suppression of cell proliferation in comparison to either one alone was observed. Components of the ginseng extract were demonstrated to bind to estrogen receptors. Low doses of ginseng had no effect on cell growth, while higher doses significantly decreased cell proliferation. The antiproliferative effect of ginseng was even more pronounced with the addition of tamoxifen[20]. The opposite effect has been observed with genistein, an isoflavone from soy, and tamoxifen. At doses of 10 μmol/l or above, genistein inhibited the growth of estrogen-dependent breast cancer cells *in vitro*. However, at lower doses (0.01–1.0 μmol/l) genistein stimulated cell growth and proliferation. Furthermore, the addition of low-dose genistein to tamoxifen-treated cells reversed the inhibitory effects of tamoxifen[21]. Genistein blood levels in humans on a high-soy diet are reported at 0.10–6.0 μmol/l. This indicates that it may be very difficult to attain and sustain a concentration of genistein that is high enough to induce tumor inhibition. Thus, genistein may be contraindicated with tamoxifen in breast cancer chemotherapy regimens.

Tamoxifen

Several botanical agents have been studied in relation to tamoxifen. Co-treatment with tamoxifen

ANTINEOPLASTIC THERAPY

Several herbs have suggestive antineoplastic effects against breast cancer. Curcumin extracted from *Curcuma longa* (turmeric) inhibited the proliferation of MCF-7 human breast cancer cells *in vitro*[22]. This inhibition occurred in a dose-dependent manner. Curcumin exerts a cytostatic effect at the G_2/M stage. This effect may be the result of inhibition of protein kinase C, which is involved in signal transduction and regulation of cellular proliferation.

A proanthocyanidin extract from grape seed exerted cytotoxic effects on MCF-7 breast cancer cells[23]. The cytotoxic effect was concentration- and time-dependent. This cytotoxic effect was not observed when the proanthocyanidin extract was applied to normal human gastric mucosal cells and normal human J774A.1 macrophages. In fact, the growth and viability of these cells was enhanced. Proanthocyanidins are a group of polyphenolic bioflavonoids found in fruits and vegetables. Proanthocyanidins have been shown to inhibit DNA topoisomerase II and to modulate protein kinase C which may explain its cytoxic effect on MCF-7 cells.

In contrast, ginsenoside Rg1 derived from *Panax notoginseng* demonstrated estrogen-like activity on MCF-7 cells *in vitro*[24]. Rg1 is one of the most abundant ginsenosides in ginseng. This study merits cautious use of ginseng in estrogen-dependent cancers.

Energy medicine

Suzanne Clewell

The patient with breast cancer presents with a myriad of symptoms that may be discovered, in future research, to be very amenable to energy medicine.

Chemotherapy-induced acute vomiting occurs in approximately 15% of women treated for breast cancer despite the use of 5-HT$_3$ antagonists. More than one-third of women receiving chemotherapy for breast cancer will experience delayed chemotherapy-induced vomiting[1]. It is hypothesized that the use of energy medicine while administering chemotherapy may assist the drugs to work optimally, with reduced side-effects.

The often-experienced skin reactions associated with radiation therapy to the breast are also an area of great concern for the patient as well as the physician and clinic staff. Practitioners of energy medicine believe that subtle energy can be used to increase the healing vibration of the patient to speed healing and reduce pain. There is evidence that points to the benefits of energy medicine in the treatment of burns[2]. The National Center for Complementary and Alternative Medicine (NCCAM) is currently recruiting patients for a study looking at distant healing in wound healing, psychological functioning and physiological symptoms after surgery for breast reconstruction[3].

Lymphedema occurs in patients with various types of cancer, but it is probably most common in the patient with breast cancer. Secondary lymphedema may occur in the breast cancer patient who has had removal of or injury (radiation therapy) to the axillary lymph nodes. In addition to compression garments and patient teaching, treatment of lymphedema often includes massage therapy. Many massage therapists incorporate energy medicine in some form into the massage session feeling that the combination may be more beneficial than massage alone. The hypothesis is that energy medicine will allow for the best outcome to occur for that individual. The assumption is that the increased flow of energy would assist in the optimal flow of lymph, with resulting reduction of edema.

Fatigue, often described by the patient as overwhelming, is a common complaint. Fatigue often continues to present a problem for many months after treatment and is an important factor when considering the patient's quality of life. A study entitled *Healing Touch and the Quality of Life in Women Receiving Radiation Treatment for Cancer* was conducted by the staff at Barnes-Jewish Hospital in St Louis along with the School of Social Service at St Louis University[4]. The study population consisted of 62 women who were receiving radiation treatment for newly diagnosed gynecologic or breast cancer. The randomization was to receive either Healing Touch or mock treatment, along with standard care. All were blinded to their group assignment. The primary outcome measure was health-related quality of life as assessed by using the SF-36 tool, which measures nine health-related areas such as pain, general mental health, vitality and limitations in social activities due to physical or emotional problems. Scores ranged from 0 to 100 with higher scores associated with better functioning. The overall average score at baseline was 53. After intervention the Healing Touch group had an average score of 63.3 while the mock-treatment group scored an average of 54.3.

According to the researchers, the Healing Touch group scored higher in all nine areas of the assessment of quality of life. It was found that the Healing Touch group showed statistically significant improvements in pain, vitality and physical functioning[4].

Research in the area of the specific symptoms experienced by breast cancer patients is scarce.

This is an area that could benefit immensely from additional data.

References

Breast cancer

1. Leibel S, Phillips T. Textbook of Radiation Oncology. Philadelphia: WB Saunders, 1998: 1013–46
2. Perez C, Brady L, Halperin EC, Schmidt-Ull-rich RK. Principles and Practice of Radiation Oncology. Philadelphia: Lippincott, Williams and Wilkins, 2004: 1315–1553
3. LowDog T, Micozzi M. Womens Health in Complementary and Integrative Medicine. St Louis, MO: Elsevier, 2005
4. DeVita VJ, Hellman S, Rosenberg S. Cancer Principles and Practice of Oncology. 5th edn. Philadelphia: Lippincott-Raven, 1997: 1541–1616

Physical activity

1. Thune I, Furberg A-S. Physical activity and cancer risk: dose–response and cancer, all sites and site-specific. Med Sci Sports Exerc 2001; 33 (Suppl): S530–S550
2. Marcus PM, Newman B, Moorman PG, et al. Physical activity at age 12 and adult breast cancer risk (United States). Cancer Causes Control 1999; 10: 293–302
3. Cunningham AJ, Edmonds CVI, Jenkins BP, et al. A randomized controlled trial of the effects of group psychological therapy on survival in women with metastatic breast cancer. Psycho-oncology 1998; 7: 508–17
4. Holmes MD, Chen WY, Feskanich D, et al. Physical activitiy and survival after breast cancer diagnosis. J Am Med Assoc 2005; 293: 2479–86

5. Courneya KS. Exercise in cancer survivors: an overview of research. Med Sci Sports Exerc 2003; 35: 1846–52

Nutrition

1. Hunter DJ, Spiegelman D, Adami HO, et al. Non-dietary factors as risk factors for breast cancer, and as effect modifiers of the association of fat intake and risk of breast cancer. Cancer Causes Control 1997; 8: 49–56
2. Smith-Warner SA, Spiegelman D, Yaun SS, et al. Alcohol and breast cancer in women: a pooled analysis of cohort studies. J Am Med Assoc 1998; 279: 535–40
3. Willett WC, Hunter DJ, Stampfer MJ, et al. Dietary fat and fiber in relation to risk of breast cancer. An 8-year follow-up. J Am Med Assoc 1992; 268: 2037–44
4. Terry P, Suzuki R, Hu FB, Wolk A. A prospective study of major dietary patterns and the risk of breast cancer. Cancer Epidemiol Biomarkers Prev 2001; 10: 1281–5
5. Block G, Patterson B, Subar A. Fruit, vegetables, and cancer prevention: a review of the epidemiological evidence. Nutr Cancer 1992; 18: 1–29
6. World Cancer Research Fund Panel. Food, Nutrition and the Prevention of Cancer: a Global Perspective. Washington, DC: American Institute for Cancer Research, 1997
7. Hunter DJ, Spiegelman D, Adami HO, et al. Cohort studies of fat intake and the risk of breast cancer—a pooled analysis. N Engl J Med 1996; 334: 356–61

8. Smith-Warner SA, Spiegelman D, Yaun SS, et al. Intake of fruits and vegetables and risk of breast cancer: a pooled analysis of cohort studies. J Am Med Assoc 2001; 285: 769–76

9. Cho E, Spiegelman D, Hunter DJ, et al. Premenopausal fat intake and risk of breast cancer. J Natl Cancer Inst 2003; 95: 1079–85

10. Toniolo P, Riboli E, Shore RE, Pasternack BS. Consumption of meat, animal products, protein, and fat and risk of breast cancer: a prospective cohort study in New York. Epidemiology 1994; 5: 391–7

11. Toniolo P, Riboli E, Protta F, et al. Calorie-providing nutrients and risk of breast cancer. J Natl Cancer Inst 1989; 81: 278–86

12. Sieri S, Krogh V, Muti P, et al. Fat and protein intake and subsequent breast cancer risk in postmenopausal women. Nutr Cancer 2002; 42: 10–17

Mind–body interventions

1. Spiegel D, Bloom JR, Draemer HC, Gottheil E. Effect of psychosocial treatment on survival of patients with breast cancer. Lancet 1989; 2: 888–91

2. Goodwin PJ, Leszcz M, Ennis M, et al. The effect of group psychosocial support on survival in metastatic breast cancer. N Engl J Med 2001; 345: 1719–26

3. Smedslund G, Ringdal GI. Meta-analysis of the effects of psychosocial interventions on survival time in cancer patients. J Psychosom Res 2004; 57: 123–31

4. van der Pompe G, Duivenvoorden HJ, Antoni MH, et al. Effectiveness of a short-term group psychotherapy program on endocrine and immune function in breast cancer patients: an exploratory study. J Psychosom Res 1997; 42: 453–66

5. Carlson LE, Speca M, Patel KD, Goodey E. Mindfulness-based stress reduction in relation to quality of life, mood, symptoms of stress and levels of cortisol, dehydroepiand-osterone-sulfate (DHEAS) and melatonin in breast and prostate cancer outpatients. Psychoneuroendocrinology 2004; 29: 448–74

6. Carlson LE, Speca M, Patel KD, Goodey E. Mindfulness-based stress reduction in relation to quality of life, mood, symptoms of stress, and immune parameters in breast and prostate cancer outpatients. Psychosom Med 2003; 65: 571–81

Botanicals

1. Lu L, Anderson KE, Grady J, Nagamani M. Effects of soya consumption for one month on steroid hormones in premenopausal women: implications for breast cancer risk reduction. Cancer Epidemiol Biomarkers Prev 1996; 5: 63–70

2. Kumar NB, Cantor A, Allen K, et al. The specific role of isoflavones on estrogen metabolism in premenopausal women. Cancer 2002; 94: 1166–74

3. Linseisen J, Piller R, Hermann S, et al. Dietary phytoestrogen intake and premenopausal breast cancer risk in a German case-control study. Int J Cancer 2004; 110: 284–90

4. Zhou JR, Vu L, Mai Z, Balckburn GL. Combined inhibition of estrogen-dependent human breast carcinoma by soy and tea bioactive components in mice. Int J Cancer 2004; 108: 8–14

5. Maggiolini M, Bonofiglio D, Marsico S, et al. Estrogen receptor alpha mediates the proliferative but not the cytotoxic dose-dependent effects of two major phytoestrogens on human breast cancer cells. Mol Pharmacol 2001; 60: 595–602

6. Po LS, Chen ZY, Tsang DS, Leung LK. Baicalein and genistein display differential actions on estrogen receptor (ER) transactivation and apoptosis in MCF-7 cells. Cancer Lett 2002; 187: 33–40

7. Allred CD, Allred KF, Ju YH, et al. Soy processing influences growth of estrogen-dependent breast cancer tumors in mice. Carcinogenesis 2004; 25: 1649–57

8. Chen WF, Huang MH, Tzang CH, et al. Inhibitory actions of genistein in human breast cancer (MCF-7) cells. Biochim Biophys Acta 2003; 1638: 187–96

9. Upadhyay S, Neburi M, Chinni SR, et al. Differential sensitivity of normal and malignant breast epithelial cells to genistein is partly mediated by p21(WAF1). Clin Cancer Res 2001; 7: 1782–9

10. Constantinou AI, Lantvit D, Hawthorne M, et al. Chemopreventive effects of soy protein and

purified soy isoflavones on DMBA-induced mammary tumors in female Sprague–Dawley rats. Nutr Cancer 2001; 41: 75–81

11. Nakachi K, Suemasu K, Suga K, et al. Influence of drinking green tea on breast cancer malignancy among Japanese patients. Jpn J Cancer Res 1998; 89: 254–61

12. Inoue M, Tajima K, Mizutani M, et al. Regular consumption of green tea and the risk of breast cancer recurrence: follow-up study from the Hospital-based Epidemiologic Research Program at Aichi Cancer Center (HERPACC), Japan. Cancer Lett 2001; 167: 175–82

13. Wu AH, Yu MC, Tseng CC, et al. Green tea and risk of breast cancer in Asian Americans. Int J Cancer 2003; 106: 574–9

14. Chen S, Sun X-Z, Kao Y-C, et al. Suppression of breast cancer cell growth with grape juice. Pharm Biol 1998; 36 (Suppl): 53–61

15. Thompson L, Rickard SE, Orcheson L, Seidl M. Flaxseed and its lignan and oil components reduce mammary tumor growth at a late stage of carcinogenesis. Carcinogenesis 1996; 17: 1373–6

16. Inano H, Onoda M, Inafuku N, et al. Chemoprevention by curcumin during the promotion stage of tumorigenesis of mammary gland in rats irradiated with γ-rays. Carcinogenesis 1999; 20: 1011–18

17. Jo EH, Hong HD, Ahn NC, et al. Modulations of the Bcl-2/Bax family were involved in the chemopreventive effects of licorice root (Glycyrrhiza uralensis Fisch) in MCF-7 human breast cancer cell. J Agric Food Chem 2004; 52: 1715–19

18. Virgili F, Acconcia F, Ambra R, et al. Nutritional flavonoids modulate estrogen receptor alpha signaling. IUBMB Life 2004; 56: 145–51

19. Suganuma M, Okabe S, Kai Y, et al. Synergistic effects of (-)-epigallocatechin gallate with (-)-epicatechin, sulindac, or tamoxifen on cancer-preventive activity in the human lung cancer cell line PC-9. Cancer Res 1999; 59: 44–7

20. Duda RB, Zhong Y, Navas V, et al. American ginseng and breast cancer therapeutic agents synergistically inhibit MCF-7 breast cancer cell growth. J Surg Oncol 1999; 72: 230–9

21. Jones JL, Daley BJ, Enderson BL, et al. Genistein inhibits tamoxifen effects on cell proliferation and cell cycle arrest in T47D breast cancer cells. Am Surg 2002; 68: 575–7; discussion 577–8

22. Simon, A, Allais DP, Duroux JL, et al. Inhibitory effect of curcuminoids on MCF-7 cell proliferation and structure–activity relationships. Cancer Lett 1998; 129: 111–16

23. Ye X, Krohn RL, Liu W, et al. The cytotoxic effects of a novel IH636 grape seed proanthocyanidin extract on cultured human cancer cells. Mol Cell Biochem 1999; 196: 99–108

24. Chan RY, Chen WF, Dong A, et al. Estrogen-like activity of ginsenoside Rg1 derived from Panax notoginseng. J Clin Endocrinol Metab 2002; 87: 3691–5

Energy medicine

1. Dibble SL, Casey K, Nussey B, et al. Chemotherapy-induced vomiting in women treated for breast cancer. Oncol Nurs Forum 2004; 31: 1

2. Wirth DP. The effect of non-contact Therapeutic Touch on the healing of full-thickness dermal wounds. Subtle Energies 1990; 1(1): 1–20

3. www.clinicaltrials.gov

4. Cook CA, Guerrerio JF, Slater VE. Healing Touch and quality of life in women receiving radiation treatment for cancer. Altern Ther Health Med 2004; 10: 34–40

15

Specific malignancies

(b) Prostate cancer

Matthew P. Mumber

Prostate cancer is the most common malignancy affecting American men and also the most controversial with regards to diagnosis, treatment options and efficacy of therapy. The incidence of prostate cancer more than doubled in the late 1980s and early 1990s following the introduction of the prostate-specific antigen (PSA) blood level as an effective screening tool. The incidence has slowly declined since then. The overall survival has also increased substantially with this rise in incidence – perhaps as a result of stage migration – picking up disease earlier than was possible prior to the advent of PSA testing. There remain no firm data that early detection reduces disease morbidity and mortality. However, it does appear that disease caught at an earlier stage is curable using currently available therapies, while there is no cure for metastatic disease. Watchful waiting is a viable treatment option for patients with early-stage, low-risk disease and multiple medical problems, owing to the indolent natural history of low-risk disease. There are also significant implications for the cost of health care with regards to early detection and treatment options[1].

RISK FACTORS

The cause of prostate cancer is not known. The disease is most common in older men, with the average age being 72 at diagnosis. The number of men diagnosed at an earlier age is expected to increase with routine screening. Epidemiologic studies show a wide variation of prostate cancer incidence. There is over a ten-fold increase in prostate cancer mortality in Scandanavian versus Asian countries. Within a single country, incidence can vary, as in the two-fold relative risk for African American men relative to Whites living in the USA. Similar to breast cancer, the risk of prostate cancer for a man who migrates from Asia to a country with higher incidence rates will change to match the risk level of the new country. This points to possible modifiable risk factors such as nutrition, lifestyle and environmental exposures. Smoking has been associated with an increased incidence of the disease, and with more aggressive disease. A positive family history is also an important risk factor. Table 16.4 shows potential likely and less likely risk factors relative to the gathered data concerning each factor[1,2].

Table 15.4 Potential risk factors for prostate cancer

Likely risk factors	Less likely risk factors
Age	Sexual behavior (multiple partners, sexually transmitted diseases)
Race (Black versus White)	Vasectomy
Ethnicity	Benign prostatic hyperplasia (BPH)
Diet (fat intake, specific foods)	
Family history	
Hormonal factors (serum testosterone)	
Tobacco use	
Histologic precursors (prostate intraepithelial neoplasia)	

SCREENING AND EARLY DETECTION

There is considerable controversy that surrounds the use of early detection capabilities for prostate cancer. The general methods for screening include serum PSA and digital rectal examination (DRE). The American Cancer Society recommends that men 50 years of age and older with a life expectancy of at least 10 years undergo annual DRE and a serum PSA determination in order to identify prostate cancer at its earliest possible stage. There are several different iterations of PSA that may also prove to be prognostic with regards to improving the diagnostic accuracy of the test. These include the PSA velocity, free/total PSA ratio and PSA density. PSA velocity accounts for the change in PSA over time, while the latter two measures attempt to factor in the differential effect of benign prostatic hyperplasia to cancerous tissue[3].

DIAGNOSIS

Prostate cancer is diagnosed by needle biopsy performed under ultrasound guidance. The extent of biopsy and the areas addressed have been debated in recent years, with a trend toward a larger number of biopsies directed toward the peripheral zones of the gland[3].

CONVENTIONAL THERAPY

There is no consensus as to the best form of treatment for prostate cancer at any stage of disease, mainly owing to the wide variability in disease aggressiveness, patient-related factors and treatment risks and benefits. Generally a patient's disease can be separated into three risk levels – low, intermediate and high – based on serum PSA level, Gleason's score and DRE stage; the number of positive biopsies may also come into play prognostically. Options for treatment include watchful waiting, radiation therapy, surgery and hormonal therapy. Conventional approaches have improved with regards to limiting patient morbidity, as shown in Table 15.5.

The following sections will focus on modalities mentioned throughout this text with regards to prevention, supportive care and antineoplastic uses. The text in these specific malignancy sections does not include an exhaustive review of all modalities, and some of the information

Table 15.5 Approaches to therapy for prostate cancer

Conventional therapy	Advance	Patient impact
Surgery	nerve-sparing prostatectomy	improved postoperative potency rates
Radiation therapy	intensity-modulated radiation and image-guided tretament	lowered morbidity and improved disease control

presented in the tables was presented in earlier sections. Tables will present a list of modalities, their benefit, and level of evidence for use. Levels of evidence are as follows:

- Level one: well-designed randomized controlled clinical trial(s);

- Level two: prospective and retrospective non-randomized clinical trials and analyses;

- Level three: opinions of expert committees, best-case series;

- Level four: preclinical *in vitro* and *in vivo* studies, and traditional uses.

Physical activity

Robert B. Lutz

PREVENTION

Although there are a number of studies that have looked at the relationship between physical activity and risk of prostate cancer, the findings have been inconsistent. Approximately half of the reported studies from around the world reported decreased risks of 10–70% (average risk reduction of 10–30%) for prostate cancer with physical activity, with men who expended at least 1000 kcal per week and up to 3000 kcal per week demonstrating the greatest risk reductions[1].

Initial data from the Harvard Alumni Health Study suggested that men who expended more than 4000 kcal per week had lower incidence rates of prostate cancer than those individuals who expended < 1000 kcal per week. These findings were most marked in men in their seventies[2]. Follow-up data did not support this finding, however[3].

Overall, the inconsistency of findings and the difference in research methodology challenge recommending physical activity for prostate cancer prevention. The discrepancies may be explained by many of the previously mentioned unknowns that plague this field of inquiry. The significant lag time between cancer initiation and presentation affects the detection of latent disease and may be affected by recall bias, as individuals may be unable to remember their previous physical activity patterns accurately. Additionally, screening for prostate cancer has changed over the past few decades with the advent of prostate-specific antigen (PSA) testing. Individuals who are more health conscious may create a selection bias by seeking testing more often and be identified earlier, thereby affecting the results of population studies. The lack of intervention trials prevents many of these unknowns from being answered.

SUPPORTIVE CARE

In a follow-up report of a small trial of survivors of prostate cancer (n = 12) who participated in a 20-week supervised exercise program followed by a self-monitored program, participants reported no significant changes in quality of life indices (activities of daily living, perceived fitness, pain rating), but did note improvement in vigor. Non-statistically significant improvements were made in both aerobic conditioning and strength. The researchers explained the lack of improvement in quality of life bt the fact that these individuals reported a very good quality of life prior to entrance into the study[4].

Table 15.6   Benefits of interventions in prostate cancer

Modality/intervention	Benefit	Level of evidence
Primary prevention		
Physical activity Mild Moderate	Positive benefit	II, III
Nutrition Diet		
plant based	possible positive	II, III
fiber	unknown	
individual foods		
soy	possible positive	II, IV
garlic	possible positive	II, IV
omega three fats from fish, walnuts, flax (also lignans)	possible positive	II, IV
tomato-sauce based dishes	possible positive	II, IV
individual phytochemicals		
vitamin E	possible positive	II, IV
selenium	possible positive	II, IV
Supplementation	possible positive	II, IV
Obesity	possible positive	II, IV
Mind–body		
yoga	unknown	
hypnosis	unknown	
meditation	unknown	
support groups	unknown	
Manual therapy		
massage	unknown	
chiropractic		
strain–counterstrain		
Botanicals		
green tea	possible positive	II, IV
milk thistle	possible positive	IV
Scutellaria baicalensis	possible positive	IV
Energy medicine	unknown	
Alternative systems	unknown	
Spirituality	unknown	
Tobacco cessation	positive	II, III, IV
Secondary prevention		
Physical activity Mild Moderate	unknown	

Continued

Table 15.6 *Continued*

Modality/intervention	Benefit	Level of evidence
Secondary prevention		
Nutrition		
Diet		
plant based	possible positive	IV
fiber	unknown	
individual foods		
soy	possible positive	IV
garlic	possible positive	IV
omega threes	possible positive	IV
tomato-based products	possible positive	IV
individual phytochemicals		
vitamin E	possible positive	IV
selenium	possible positive	IV
Supplementation	possible positive	IV
Obesity	possible positive	IV
Mind–body		
yoga	unknown	
hypnosis		
meditation		
support groups		
Manual therapy		
massage	unknown	
chiropractic		
strain–counterstrain		
Botanicals		
green tea	possible positive	IV
milk thistle	possible positive	IV
Scutellaria baicalensis	possible positive	IV
Energy medicine	unknown	
Alternative systems	unknown	
Spirituality	unknown	
Tobacco cessation	possible positive	III, IV
Tertiary prevention		
Physical activity	possible positive	III
Mild		
Moderate		
Nutrition		
Diet		
plant based	possible positive	IV
fiber	unknown	

Continued

Table 15.6 *Continued*

Modality/intervention	Benefit	Level of evidence
Tertiary prevention		
Nutrition		
Diet		
individual foods		
soy	possible positive	II, IV
garlic	possible positive	II, IV
omega threes	possible positive	II, IV
tomato-based products	possible positive	II, IV
flax lignans	possible positive	II, IV
individual phytochemicals	possible positive	IV
vitamin E	possible positive	IV
selenium	possible positive	IV
Supplementation		
Obesity	possible positive	II, IV
Mind–body		
yoga	unknown	
hypnosis		
meditation		
support groups		
Manual therapy		
massage	unknown	
chiropractic		
strain–counterstrain		
Botanicals		
green tea	possible positive	IV
milk thistle	possible positive	IV
Scutellaria baicalensis	possible positive	IV
Energy medicine	unknown	
Alternative systems	unknown	
Spirituality	unknown	
Tobacco cessation	positive	II, III, IV
Supportive care		
Physical activity	improved vigor, no change in quality of	II
Mild	life (QOL)	
Moderate		
Nutrition		
Diet		
plant based	unknown	
fiber	unknown	
individual foods		
soy	positive effect of hot flushes	II
garlic	unknown	

Continued

Table 15.6 *Continued*

Modality/intervention	Benefit	Level of evidence
Supportive care		
Nutrition		
Diet		
individual foods		
omega threes	unknown	
tomato-based products	unknown	
individual phytochemicals		
vitamin E	unknown	
selenium	unknown	
Supplementation	unknown	
Obesity	unknown	
Mind–body		
yoga	improved QOL and symptom	II, III, IV
hypnosis	control – decreased anxiety and	
meditation	depression	
support groups		
Manual therapy		
massage	improved musculoskeletal	II, III
chiropractic	symptoms, lowered anxiety	
strain–counterstrain		
Botanicals		
green tea	improved fatigue	II
Energy medicine	improved QOL	II
Alternative systems	unknown	
Spirituality	improved QOL	II
Tobacco cessation	general health and well-being	II, III, IV
Antineoplastic care		
Physical activity	unknown	
Mild		
Moderate		
Nutrition		
Diet		
plant based	unknown	
fiber	unknown	
individual foods		
soy	possible positive	IV
garlic	possible positive	IV
omega threes	unknown	
tomato-based products	possible positive	IV
flax lignans	possible positive	II, IV

Continued

Table 15.6 *Continued*

Modality/intervention	Benefit	Level of evidence
Antineoplastic care		
Nutrition		
Diet		
individual phytochemicals	possible positive	IV
vitamin E	possible positive	IV
selenium	unknown	
Supplementation		
Obesity	possible positive (losing weight)	II
Mind–body		
yoga	possible positive	II
hypnosis		
meditation		
support groups		
Manual therapy		
massage	unknown	
chiropractic		
strain–counterstrain		
Botanicals		
green tea	possible positive	IV, negative level II trial in hormone refractory
red clover	possible positive	II, IV
Energy medicine	unknown	
Alternative systems	unknown	
Spirituality	unknown	
Tobacco cessation	unknown	

Nutrition

Mara Vitolins and Cynthia Thomson

A significant amount of data exists concerning prostate cancer and certain foods and phyto-chemicals. This includes data concerning foods such as green tea, tomato-based products, garlic, soy and foods containing omega-3 fats such as salmon, sardines and walnuts. Phytochemicals such as lycopene, vitamin E and selenium have also been researched (see Table 11.5). The large SELECT trial is specifically examining the effects of vitamin E and selenium in a randomized fashion.

Mind–body interventions

Linda E. Carlson and Shauna L. Shapiro

A recent pilot study examined the effect of dietary change combined with a mindfulness-based stress reduction (MBSR) intervention, including yoga, in prostate cancer patients. Preliminary results show a lowering of levels of prostate-specific antigen[1]. A larger randomized study is currently under way. Another study of patients with breast or prostate cancer found that MBSR practice resulted not only in improved sleep and quality of life, but also in reductions in cortisol levels and enhancement of some measures of immune function[2,3].

Botanicals

Lise Alschuler

CHEMOPREVENTION OF PROSTATE CARCINOGENESIS

Prostate cancer is an ideal candidate for chemoprevention given the typical age of onset of this disease. Even small delays in the neoplastic process could have significant impact on the incidence of this disease. However, the evidence for plant-based chemoprevention is largely experimental. There are several promising agents, but it is important to keep in mind that these agents lack conclusive evidence. Soy is a potential chemopreventive agent in the development of prostate cancer. Of the major isoflavones in soy, daidzein is most extensively metabolized by intestinal microflora. This metabolism converts daidzein into 4-hydroxyequol, or equol. Equol is more potent than daidzein or genistein in terms of its antioxidant index, antiproliferative actions and its binding affinity for estrogen receptor (ER)-β in prostatic cells. At experimental levels that correlate with prostatic concentrations of equol obtained from men living in Asian countries who consume soy as part of their normal diet, equol arrests prostate cancer cell lines in the G_0/G_1 phase of the cell cycle[1]. Of interest is the finding that, upon consuming soy, Asian men convert diadzein to equol more effectively than do their North American and European counterparts. This is postulated to be the result of differing intestinal microflora, the composition of which is heavily influenced by dietary factors. Asian men consume fewer meat products and more vegetable foods than do European or North American men, leading to different populations of intestinal microflora. This is relevant to the chemoprevention properties of soy, because experimental data suggest that men consuming a typical Western diet may not benefit from the potential chemoprevention effects of soy without radically altering their dietary habits towards that of the Asian-type diet. This was recently confirmed in a double-blinded, parallel-arm randomized clinical trial. Male subjects aged 50–80 years in apparent good health were randomized to consume either a soy protein drink providing 83 mg/day of isoflavones or a similar drink with the isoflavones removed. Eighty-one out of 128 subjects were analyzed at study completion. There were no changes in the values of prostate-specific antigen (PSA). In fact, men who consumed the isoflavones-containing drink experienced a 0.5% greater increase in PSA level than did the isoflavones-negative group[2]. These results were further confirmed in an open-label pilot study of 62 men aged 61–89 years (mean age 73.6 years) with histologically proven prostate carcinoma. The men either had had radical prostatectomy, radiotherapy, both prostatectomy and radiotherapy, or were in off-cycle during hormonal treatment or in active surveillance. The study required the men to consume an encapsulated genistein-rich extract from soy on a daily basis. The primary endpoint of 50% reduction in PSA from the start of the trial was only seen in one man in the active surveillance group. An additional seven men in the active surveillance group had reduced PSA levels by less than 50%. These results were not attributable to the genistein[3]. From these trials, the clinical impact of soy consumption on the prevention of prostate carcinoma remains dubious. Certainly the quantity of isoflavones, the source of isoflavones, the required length of time of consumption, the efficiency of gastrointestinal metabolism of isoflavones and the hormonal status of the cancer are all factors which need to be elucidated in order to gain more understanding of the chemoprevention potential of soy isoflavones in prostate cancer.

Another promising chemopreventive agent for prostate cancer is green tea. Epidemiological studies suggest a chemopreventive effect of tea against prostate cancer in humans[4]. The experimental administration of epigallocatechin gallate (EGCG) from green tea to androgen-dependent and androgen-independent human prostate cancer cells (LNCaP, DU145 and PC-3 cells) results in apoptosis. Additionally, green tea-fed rats evidenced increased tumor-free and overall survival rates over controls. EGCG causes cell arrest in the G_0/G_1 phase of the cell cycle. This arrest is independent of p53 status. Additionally, EGCG inhibits proteasome, which results in tumor-growth arrest. EGCG also represses at least nine genes, including protein kinase C, which are involved with protein signaling leading to inhibition of cell progression. Finally, EGCG inhibits 5α-reductase, thus inhibiting the conversion of testosterone to its activated form, dihydrotestosterone, resulting in decreased hyperplasia[5].

Scutellaria baicalensis is a herb used extensively in Chinese herbalism. *S. baicalensis* was one of the herbs in an herbal product known as PC-SPES. PC-SPES included seven herbs and was efficacious as an antineoplastic agent in prostate carcinoma, as demonstrated by *in vitro* experiments, animal experiments and limited clinical trials. However, PC-SPES was recalled by the Food and Drug Administration (FDA) owing to the discovery of warfarin, diethylstilbestrol and indomethacin in the product. The efficacy of this product has led to research on the herbs it contained in an effort to identify active components. Of the herbs in the product, *S. baicalensis* displayed antineoplastic activities similar to those of PC-SPES and greater than any of the other herbs in the formula[6]. In fact, *S. baicalensis* had even greater potency in suppressing PSA than did PC-SPES. *S. baicalensis* contains several flavonoids, of which baicalin and its metabolite,

baicalein, appear to have the strongest ability to exert anticarcinogenic activity. These flavonoids possess anti-inflammatory, antibacterial, antiproliferative and lipoxygenase-inhibitory activities, some or all of which may explain its possible chemopreventive properties.

Ganoderma lucidum (reishi mushroom) may be of benefit in the chemoprevention of prostate cancer. An *in vitro* experiment demonstrated the ability of a reishi extract to down-regulate the expression of NF-κB-regulated urokinase plasminogen activator (uPA) and the uPA receptor. This action resulted in suppression of cell migration of invasive prostate cancer cells. In addition, by down-regulating NF-κB, Bcl-2 and Bcl-xl were down-regulated which, in turn, induced apoptosis. In addition, the reishi extract inhibited cell proliferation in a dose-dependent manner by down-regulation of expression of cyclin B and cdc-2 and up-regulation of p21 expression in PC-3 cells[7].

A final botanical agent that is worthy of attention as a potential chemopreventive agent for prostate carcinogenesis is silymarin, derived from *Silybum marianum* (milk thistle). Silymarin is a flavonoid antioxidant which experimentally inhibited human prostate carcinoma DU145 cells[8]. The anticarcinogenic effects are likely to involve impairment of cell signaling pathways and induction of cyclin-dependent kinase inhibitors with resultant G_1 cell-cycle arrest. While these data are preliminary, there is a possibility that silymarin may exert significant chemopreventive effects against human prostate cancer.

ANTINEOPLASTIC EFFECTS

Preliminary human trial data are suggestive of an antineoplastic effect of red clover-derived isoflavones in prostate cancer. A non-randomized, non-blinded trial with historically matched controls examined the effect of an acute exposure to a dietary supplement of isoflavones prior to radical prostatectomy[9]. Thirty-eight patients with non-metastatic prostate cancer and a Gleason score of ≥ 5 were recruited to the study. Prior to surgery, 20 patients consumed 160 mg of red clover-derived isoflavones consisting of genistein, diadzein, formononetin and biochanin A in tablet form for a median time of 20 days (range of 7–54 days). Biopsy specimens from the removed prostate tissue revealed a significantly higher rate of apoptosis in the isoflavone group than in the control group ($p = 0.0018$), specifically in the regions of low- to moderate-grade cancer (Gleason grades 1–3). No adverse effects related to treatment were observed.

A Phase II trial of green tea in the treatment of patients with androgen-independent metastatic prostate carcinoma failed to demonstrate significant antineoplastic activity[10]. Forty-two men with asymptomatic, biopsy-proven and clinically evidenced androgen independent prostate cancer were eligible for the study. All patients were prescribed green tea at a dose of 6 g/day orally in six divided doses. The tea was administered as a pulverized green tea powder that was mixed into water. Patients were evaluated every month for 4 months; however, the median time on the trial was only 1 month. Toleration of the green tea was good, with no toxicity in 31% of the patients. Other patients experienced nausea, emesis, insomnia, fatigue, diarrhea, abdominal pain or confusion. Compliance was generally good. Among the 42 patients, one patient manifested a 50% decrease in PSA level from baseline (229 ng/dl to 105 ng/dl). This decrease was not sustained beyond 2 months. No patient manifested a tumor response on radiographic assessment or physical examination. The overall response rate was 2% (95% CI 1–14%). This response rate was below the hypothesized level of 5% attributable to mere chance. This study indicates that green tea may not exert antineoplastic effects in hormone-refractory prostate cancer. However, the length of time of exposure to the green tea may not have been long enough and the extract may not have contained sufficient amounts of EGCG to uncover a benefit. These concerns are relevant in light of the fact that the epidemiologic benefits of green tea in prostate cancer prevention suggest that long-term exposure may be necessary. Additionally, *in vitro* data indicate that the antineoplastic effects of green tea are derived from individual catechins with varying intensity. Namely, apoptosis of DU145 cells is induced mostly by epigallocatechin, followed by epigallocatchein-3-gallate then epicatechin-3-gallate, and finally epicatechin[11]. Thus, an extract that contains high amounts of epigallocatechin would be expected to yield more favorable clinical results.

Promising *in vitro* data demonstrated the ability of silybinin (derived from *Silymarin marianum*) to inhibit telomerase activity and to down-regulate PSA in LNCaP prostate cancer cell lines[12]. These results suggest a possible therapeutic role for silybinin as an antiproliferative agent in prostate cancer.

Energy medicine

Suzanne Clewell

The National Center for Complementary and Alternative Medicine (NCCAM) has recently proposed a new study to determine whether Reiki energy healing affects progression and anxiety in patients newly diagnosed with prostate cancer. It is scheduled for completion in September 2005[1].

Several clinical situations exist in which prostate cancer patients could hypothetically benefit from energy medicine approaches. These areas deserve further study. For example, hormone therapy (androgen deprivation therapy) for the treatment of prostate cancer often produces unnerving symptoms for the patient. Impotence, incontinence, loss of libido, hot flushes, osteoporosis and gynecomastia may need to be addressed in the form of diverse modalities combined with energy medicine to assist in providing relief to the patient. For the patient receiving hormonal therapy these symptoms should disappear when the hormones are discontinued. However, for the patient on long-term therapy or for the patient who has had an orchiectomy, these symptoms may persist. Once attuned to Reiki, a patient could provide needed healing and symptom relief to himself any time a need arose.

Fortunately, with the state-of-the-art intensity-modulated radiation therapy (IMRT) technology used in radiation therapy today we are seeing fewer bowel-related side-effects in the treatment of prostate cancer. If patients do experience diarrhea, increased urinary urge, fatigue, rectal burning or pain, energy medicine can be useful in promoting relaxation, which may tend to calm the bowel and reduce symptoms. Energy can be passed to reduce anxiety in the patient having a prostate seed implant procedure as well as reducing postoperative side-effects.

References

Prostate cancer

1. DeVita VJ, Hellman S, Rosenberg S. Cancer Principles and Practice of Oncology, 5th edn. Philadelphia: Lippincott-Raven, 1997: 1322–85
2. Leibel S, Phillips T. Textbook of Radiation Oncology. Philadelphia: WB Saunders, 1998: 741–84
3. Perez C, Brady L, Halperin EC, Schmidt-Ullrich RK. Principles and Practice of Radiation Oncology. Philadelphia: Lippincott, Williams and Wilkins, 2004: 1692–62

Physical activity

1. Thune I, Furberg A-S. Physical activity and cancer risk: dose–response and cancer, all sites and site-specific. Med Sci Sports Exerc 2001; 33 (Suppl): S530–S550
2. Lee I-M, Paffenbarger RS, Hsieh CC. Physical activity and risk of prostatic cancer among college alumni. Am J Epidemiol 1992; 135: 169–79
3. Lee I-M, Sesso HD, Paffenbarger RS. A prospective cohort study of physical activity and body

size in relation to prostate cancer risk, United States. Cancer Causes Control 2001; 12: 187–93

4. Durak EP, Lilly PC, Hackworth JL. Physical and psychosocial responses to exercise in cancer patients: a two year follow-up survey with prostate, leukemia, and general carcinoma. J Exerc Physiol online 1999; 2(1)

Mind–body interventions

1. Saxe GA, Hebert JR, Carmody JF, et al. Can diet in conjunction with stress reduction affect the rate of increase in prostate specific antigen after biochemical recurrence of prostate cancer? J Urol 2001; 166: 2202–7

2. Carlson LE, Speca M, Patel KD, Goodey E. Mindfulness-based stress reduction in relation to quality of life, mood, symptoms of stress and levels of cortisol, dehydroepiandrostrone-sulfate (DHEAS) and melatonin in breast and prostate cancer outpatients. Psychoneuroendocrinology 2004; 29: 448–74

3. Carlson LE, Speca M, Patel KD, Goodey E. Mindfulness-based stress reduction in relation to quality of life, mood, symptoms of stress, and immune parameters in breast and prostate cancer outpatients. Psychosom Med 2003; 65: 571–81

Botanicals

1. Hedlund TE, Johannes WU, Miller GJ. Soy isoflavonoid equol modulates the growth of benign and malignant prostatic epithelial cells in vitro. Prostate 2003; 54: 68–78

2. Adams KF, Chen C, Newton KM, et al. Soy isoflavones do not modulate prostate-specific antigen concentrations in older men in a randomized controlled trial. Cancer Epidemiol Biomarkers Prev 2004; 13: 644–8

3. deVere White RW, Hackman RM, Soares SE, et al. Effects of a genistein-rich extract on PSA levels in men with a history of prostate cancer. Urology 2004; 63: 259–63

4. Jain MG, Hislop GT, Howwe GR, et al. Alcohol and other beverage use and prostate cancer risk among Canadian men. Int J Cancer 1998; 78: 707–11

5. Adhami VM, Ahmad N, Mukhtar H. Molecular targets for green tea in prostate cancer prevention. J Nutr 2003; 133 (Suppl 7): 2417S–2424S

6. Hsieh TC, Lu X, Chea J, Wu JM. Prevention and management of prostate cancer using PC-SPES: a scientific perspective. J Nutr 2002; 132 (Suppl 11): 3513S–3517S

7. Jiang J, Slivova V, Valachovicova T, et al. Ganoderma lucidum inhibits proliferation and induces apoptosis in human prostate cancer cells PC-3. Int J Oncol 2004; 24: 1093–9

8. Zi X, Grasso AW, Kung HJ, Agarwal R. A flavonoid antioxidant, silymarin, inhibits activation of erbB1 signaling and induces cyclin-dependent kinase inhibitors, G1 arrest, and anti-carcinogenic effects in human prostate carcinoma DU145 cells. Cancer Res 1998; 58: 1920–9

9. Jarred RA, Keikha M, Dowling C, et al. Induction of apoptosis in low to moderate-grade human prostate carcinoma by red clover-derived dietary isoflavones. Cancer Epidemiol Biomarkers Prev 2002; 11: 1689–96

10. Jatoi A, Ellison N, Burch PA, et al. A phase II trial of green tea in the treatment of patients with androgen independent metastatic prostate carcinoma. Cancer 2003; 97: 1442–6

11. Chung LY, Cheung TC, Kong SK, et al. Induction of apoptosis by green tea catechins in human prostate cancer DU145 cells. Life Sci 2001; 68: 1207–14

12. Thelen P, Wuttke W, Jarry H, et al. Inhibition of telomerase activity and secretion of prostate specific antigen by silibinin in prostate cancer cells. J Urol 2004; 171: 1934–8

Energy medicine

1. Reiki Healing in Prostate Cancer, sponsored by NCCAM, www.ClinicalTrials.gov

15

Specific malignancies

(c) Lung cancer

Matthew P. Mumber

Lung cancer is the leading cause of death in the USA for both men and women, and is among the most commonly occurring malignancies in the world, with an incidence that is increasing. In the USA, only about 15% of patients who are diagnosed with lung cancer survive for 5 years. It is expected that, with changes in smoking rates and lower-tar cigarettes, the incidence of lung cancer may decrease[1,2].

RISK FACTORS

Tobacco is the most important cause of lung cancer, and its incidence increases with exposure. There is a relative risk of dying from lung cancer of approximately 13:1 for smokers versus non-smokers; those who smoke more than 1.5 packs per day (30 cigarettes) have an increased risk of 22:1. Lower-tar and filtered cigarettes carry less risk and the 40–50% of smokers who quit may have a five- to eight-fold risk reduction. The risk of developing a second lung cancer once one has already developed is about 2% per year. Other carcinogens such as radon and asbestos can also increase risk. The presence of increased risk from a genetic predisposition is unknown[1,2].

SCREENING AND EARLY DETECTION

Routine chest X-rays and sputum samples have been analyzed in the past as methods for screening and early detection of lung cancer in high-risk individuals (smokers and those with second-hand tobacco exposure). Unfortunately, these have not proved effective. There are some encouraging data that high-speed spiral computed tomography (CT) scans might detect earlier cancers, although this process is costly and also detects many benign lesions. Current trials are under way investigating CT scanning as a screening tool[1].

DIAGNOSIS

The diagnosis of lung cancer is usually made through bronchoscopy or CT-guided biopsy. Often, a surgical procedure such as

Table 15.7   Advances in conventional tools in lung cancer

Conventional tool	Advance	Patient impact
Positron emission tomography (PET scan)	improved staging accuracy	can eliminate morbidity of unnecessary procedures in advanced disease; can better define patients who have early-stage disease
Combined chemotherapy and radiation	concurrent delivery	improved overall survival in selected patients
Ethyol (amifostine)	radiation protectant	lower rates of lung and esophagus damage
Chemotherapy	biologic agents (e.g. Iressa)	lower toxicity and improve disease response (in small number who do respond)

mediastinoscopy can be used further to define areas of concern.

CONVENTIONAL THERAPY

Lung cancer is generally treated with surgery, radiation and chemotherapy, the uses of which vary depending upon the stage of disease. Surgery is used for early-stage lesions, while combination radiation and chemotherapy treatments are often used in patients with locally advanced disease. Despite modest improvements for patients with both early and advanced disease offered by adjuvant chemotherapy or by the combination of all three conventional options, the results for lung cancer treatment remain poor, owing to a high rate of development of distant metastases[1]. Some modest improvements in conventional therapy are listed in Table 15.7.

The following sections will focus on modalities mentioned throughout this text with regards to prevention, supportive care and antineoplastic uses. The text in these specific malignancy sections does not include an exhaustive review of all modalities, and some of the information presented in the tables was presented in earlier sections. Tables will present a list of modalities, their benefit and level of evidence for use. Levels of evidence are listed below:

- Level one: well-designed randomized controlled clinical trial(s);

- Level two: prospective and retrospective non-randomized clinical trials and analyses;

- Level three: opinions of expert committees, best-case series;

- Level four: preclinical *in vitro* and *in vivo* studies, and traditional uses.

Physical activity

Robert B. Lutz

PREVENTION

There are few research studies that have looked at physical activity and risk of lung cancer. It is difficult in many of these studies completely to adjust for tobacco usage, and comparisons of smokers versus non-smokers is likewise difficult, owing to the low incidence of lung cancer in this latter group. Overall, however, there does appear to be a preventive role, with an average risk reduction of 30–40% noted for both leisure-time physical activity as well as occupational physical activity[1]. An inverse dose–response relationship is evident, suggesting that 4 hours per week of moderate to vigorous leisure-time physical activity is required to impart benefit[2]. In the Harvard Alumni Health Study, an inverse graded dose–response relationship was noted between physical activity and lung cancer. Men who expended ≥ 3000 kcal per week in overall physical activity pursuits demonstrated a 39% reduction in risk as compared to men who expended < 1000 kcal per week, the equivalent of about 2.5 hours per week of moderate-intensity activity[3].

SUPPORTIVE CARE

No available studies addressing quality of life in survivors of lung cancer are available. To a degree, this may be attributable to the overall poor prognosis that still exists for lung cancer. Additionally, the rates of physical activity in smokers tend to be less than in non-smokers and it would be unlikely that non-active individuals would become active after diagnosis and treatment. Nonetheless, the overall benefits of physical activity are well identified, to include significant benefits in relieving symptoms of depression and improving mood[4]. The current public health guidelines are potentially achievable for individuals with lung cancer, based upon their debility and functional capacity. Beginning simple activities, such as walking, with gradual increases as tolerated, would be beneficial.

Table 15.8 Benefits of interventions in lung cancer		
Modality/intervention	*Benefit*	*Level of evidence*
Primary prevention		
Physical activity		
Mild		
Moderate	possible positive	II
Nutrition		
Diet		
plant based	possible positive	II
fiber	unknown	
individual foods		
carrots	possible positive	II
individual phytochemicals		
synthetic β-carotene alone in smokers	negative	I, II
Supplementation	possible positive	II, IV
Low glycemic index	possible positive	II, IV
Obesity	unknown	
Mind–body		
yoga	unknown	
hypnosis		
meditation		
support groups		
Manual therapy		
massage	unknown	
chiropractic		
strain–counterstrain		
Botanicals		
green tea	possible positive	IV
Energy medicine	unknown	
Alternative systems	unknown	
Spirituality	unknown	
Tobacco cessation	positive	II, III, IV
Secondary prevention		
Physical activity		
Mild	unknown	
Moderate		
Nutrition		
Diet		
plant based	unknown	
fiber		
individual foods		

Continued

Table 15.8 *Continued*

Modality/intervention	Benefit	Level of evidence
Secondary prevention		
Nutrition		
Diet		
individual phytochemicals		
β-carotene alone in smokers	negative (increased risk)	I
Supplementation		
Obesity	unknown	
Mind–body		
yoga	unknown	
hypnosis		
meditation		
support groups		
Manual therapy		
massage	unknown	
chiropractic		
strain–counterstrain		
Botanicals		
green tea	possible positive	II, IV
Energy medicine	unknown	
Alternative systems	unknown	
Spirituality	unknown	
Tobacco cessation	positive	II, III, IV
Tertiary prevention		
Physical activity		
Mild		
Moderate	unknown	
Nutrition		
Diet		
plant based	unknown	
fiber		
individual foods		
individual phytochemicals		
Supplementation		
Obesity	unknown	
Mind–body		
yoga	unknown	
hypnosis		
meditation		
support groups		

Continued

Table 15.8 *Continued*

Modality/intervention	Benefit	Level of evidence
Tertiary prevention		
Manual therapy massage chiropractic strain–counterstrain	unknown	
Botanicals green tea	possible positive	IV
Energy medicine	unknown	
Alternative systems	unknown	
Spirituality	unknown	
Tobacco cessation	positive	II, III, IV
Supportive care		
Physical activity Mild Moderate	Possible improved quality of life (QOL), symptom control	II

Nutrition
Diet
  plant based
  fiber
  individual foods
  individual phytochemicals
Supplementation
	unknown	

Obesity	unknown	
Mind–body yoga hypnosis meditation support groups	improved QOL and symptom control, decreased anxiety and depression	II
Manual therapy massage chiropractic strain–counterstrain	improved symptom control	II
Botanicals green tea	improved fatigue	II
Energy medicine	improved QOL and symptom control	II
Alternative systems	unknown	
Spirituality	unknown	
Tobacco cessation	improved pulmonary function	II

Continued

Table 15.8 *Continued*

Modality/intervention	Benefit	Level of evidence
Antineoplastic care		
Physical activity Mild Moderate	unknown	

Nutrition
Diet
   plant based
   fiber
   individual foods
   individual phytochemicals
Supplementation
	unknown	

Obesity	unknown	

Mind–body
   yoga
   hypnosis
   meditation
   support groups
	unknown	

Manual therapy
   massage
   chiropractic
   strain–counterstrain
	unknown	

Botanicals
   Panax ginseng
   Curcumin
	possible positive
	possible positive
		IV
		IV

Energy medicine	unknown	
Alternative systems	unknown	
Spirituality	unknown	
Tobacco cessation	unknown	

Nutrition

Mara Vitolins and Cynthia Thomson

Very little research has been conducted evaluating dietary intake and lung cancer. One study conducted by De Stefani *et al.*[1] examined whether sugar consumption modified lung cancer risk. This case–control study involved 463 cases with lung cancer and 465 hospitalized controls. After adjustment for potential confounders (tobacco smoking and total energy, total fat, vitamin C and α-carotene intakes) an increased risk for sugar-rich foods, total sucrose intake, sucrose/dietary fiber ratio and glycemic index for lung cancer was reported (odds ratio for highest category of total sucrose intake: 1.55, 95% CI 0.99–2.44). The joint effect of pack-years, total fat intake, and sucrose intake was associated with an increased risk of 28.3 (95% CI 13.4–59.7) for high values of the three variables. Additional studies are needed to elucidate the role of sugar intake and lung cancer risk.

Mind–body interventions

Linda E. Carlson and Shauna L. Shapiro

Support group participation may be beneficial in lung cancer with regards to quality of life and symptom control, as is relaxation/imagery and hypnosis for dealing with dyspnea and pain, and for end-of-life issues.[1]

Botanicals

Lise Alschuler

CHEMOPREVENTION OF LUNG CANCER

There is fairly good evidence to support a chemo-preventive effect of green tea in reducing the risk of developing lung cancer. Two population-based cohort studies have demonstrated this effect. One study identified 649 incident cases of primary lung cancer diagnosed among women 35–69 years of age, living in Shanghai, China. A control group of 675 women from the general population were frequency-matched to the age distribution of the subject group. All participants were questioned regarding the type and amount of tea consumed annually over the past 5 years. Among non-smoking women, consumption of green tea was associated with a reduced risk of lung cancer (OR 0.65; 95% CI 0.45–0.93) and the risks decreased with increasing consumption. There was no association among women who smoked[1].

Another population case-control study conducted in Okinawa, Japan on 333 cases and 666 age-, sex- and residence-matched controls led to similar conclusions. The greater the intake of Japanese green tea, the smaller the risk, particularly in women. The risk decreased in proportion to the amount of tea consumed daily, with over 10 cups daily conferring the greatest benefit (OR 0.38; 95% CI 0.12–1.18) and 1–4 cups conferring the least, but still significant, benefit (OR 0.77; 95% CI 0.28–2.13) over non-drinkers.

The risk reduction was detected mainly in squamous cell carcinoma[2]. Epigallocatechin gallate (EGCG), epigallocatechin (EGC) and epicatechin-3-gallate (ECG) have been shown to inhibit cell growth of human lung cancer cells (PC-9 cell line) via the induction of apoptosis[3]. The induction of apoptosis may be mediated by the ability of EGCG to produce H_2O_2 which mediates apoptosis in cultured lung cells[4].

Curcumin, from *Curcuma longa*, has been shown to induce apoptosis in human lung cancer cell lines A549 and H1299 in a concentration-dependent manner. A549 is p53 proficient and H1299 is a p53 null mutant. Curcumin resulted in p53-independent apoptosis in both cell lines[5].

ANTINEOPLASTIC THERAPY

Panax ginseng may prove to be of value as an antineoplastic agent for pulmonary adenocarcinoma. An *in vitro* study examined the antitumor activity of a ginseng saponin metabolite, 20-*O*-β-D-glucopyranosyl-20(*S*)-protopanaxadiol (IH-901) against pulmonary adenocarcinoma cells resistant to cisplatin[6]. The mean concentration required to inhibit the proliferation of the cells by 50% was 20.3 µmol/l for IH-901 and 60.8 µmol/l for cisplatin. This suggests that IH-901 could be used for the treatment of cisplatin-resistant pulmonary cancer.

Energy medicine

Suzanne Clewell

Side-effects from conventional treatments for lung cancer are always dependent upon the individual but, if/when they arise, energy medicine may have some effectiveness in reducing or eliminating them.

Energy healing may be an effective tool for smoking cessation, and deserves further research. Unfortunately, as we are aware, the majority of cases of lung cancer are directly related to tobacco use. A great number of patients that we see in our facility are not able or willing to stop smoking, even after receiving a diagnosis of lung cancer. If there is a desire to quit, energy medicine may be able to provide the inner strength needed to succeed by allowing the growth and change necessary for healing in our lives.

References

Lung cancer

1. DeVita VJ, Hellman S, Rosenberg S. Cancer Principles and Practice of Oncology, 5th edn. Philadelphia: Lippincott-Raven, 1997: 841–950
2. Leibel S, Phillips T. Textbook of Radiation Oncology. Philadelphia: WB Saunders, 1998: 567–600

Physical activity

1. Friedenreich CM. Physical activity and cancer prevention: from observational to intervention research. Cancer Epidemiol Biomarkers Prev 2001; 10: 287–301
2. Thune I, Furberg A-S. Physical activity and cancer risk: dose–response and cancer, all sites and site-specific. Med Sci Sports Exerc 2001; 33 (Suppl 6): S530–S550
3. Lee I-M, Sesso HD, Paffenbarger RS. Physical activity and risk of lung cancer. Int J Epidemiol 1999; 28: 620–5
4. US Department of Health and Human Services. Physical Activity and Health: A Report of the Surgeon General. Atlanta, GA, US Department of Health and Human Services, Centers for Disease Control and Prevention, National Center for Chronic Disease Prevention and Health Promotion, 1996

Nutrition

1. De Stefani E, Deneo-Pellegrini H, Mendilaharsu M, et al. Dietary sugar and lung cancer: a case–control study in Uruguay. Nutr Cancer 1998; 31: 132–7

Mind–body interventions

1. Newell SA, Sanson-Fisher RW, Savolainen NJ. Systematic review of psychological therapies for cancer patients: overview and recommendations for future research. J Natl Cancer Inst 2002; 94: 558–84

Botanicals

1. Zhong L, Goldberg M, Gao Y-T, et al. A population-based case-control study of lung cancer and green tea consumption among women liv-

ing in Shanghai, China. Epidemiology 2001; 12: 695–700

2. Ohno Y, Wakai K, Genka K, et al. Tea consumption and lung cancer risk: a case-control study in Okinawa, Japan. Jpn J Cancer Res 1995; 86: 1027–34

3. Suganuma M, Okabe S, Sueoka N, et al. Green tea and cancer chemoprevention. Mutat Res 1999; 428: 339–44

4. Yang GY, Liao J, Kim K, et al. Inhibition of growth and induction of apoptosis in human cancer cell lines by tea polyphenols. Carcinogenesis 1998; 19: 611–16

5. Radhakrishna Pillai G, Srivastava AS, Hassanein TI, et al. Induction of apoptosis in human lung cancer cells by curcumin. Cancer Lett 2004; 208: 163–70

6. Lee S-J, Sung H, Lee SJ, et al. Antitumor activity of a novel ginseng saponin metabolite in human pulmonary adenocarcinoma cells resistant to cisplatin. Cancer Lett 1999; 144: 39–43

15

Specific malignancies

(d) Colorectal cancer

Matthew P. Mumber

Colorectal cancer ranks third and second in frequency in men and women, respectively. It is the fourth leading cause of cancer mortality, because it has a better prognosis than more common cancers. The incidences of colon cancer vary ten-fold with a higher incidence in Western countries relative to Asia. Japan is an interesting example of a country in which low incidences have increased significantly – this increase is felt to be due to dietary and environmental exposures imposed upon a background of genetic susceptibility. An individual who migrates from an area with a low incidence to an area with a higher incidence will increase their individual risk accordingly. The overall incidence of colon cancer has continued to decrease since the 1980s, as have cancer mortality rates. These decreases are felt to be due to changes in the use of endoscopic polypectomy, dietary factors, energy intake, physical activity, serum cholesterol, cigarette smoking and obesity[1].

RISK FACTORS

A variety of risk factors exist for colon cancer. The main cause of colon cancer on a cellular level is a genetic change in the epithelial cells of the colonic mucosa. Several factors can initiate the process of carcinogenesis, and these are listed in Table 15.9. Table 15.10 lists factors that affect relative risk. Criteria have been developed to differentiate patients with familial polyposis syndromes – who have a near 100% risk of developing colon cancer – from patients with hereditary non-polyposis colon cancer (HNPCC) in whom the risk can increase to 57–80% by age 60, from patients who only have first degree relatives with colon cancer, in whom the relative risk is much lower. These are called the Amsterdam II criteria[1,2].

Table 15.9   Initiators for colon carcinogenesis
Lack of detoxification enzymes in the gut
Presence of fecal mutagens
Meat intake, especially fried red meat
Lack of calcium, vitamin D and folate from a multivitamin
Increased bile acids associated with a high-fat diet
Increased fecal pH

15.10	Risk factors for colon cancer

Hereditary polyposis syndromes

Family history of non-polyposis-related colon cancer

Increased age

Inflammatory bowel disease

High dietary animal fat

Alcohol and tobacco intake

Low-fiber diet

Low physical activity

Obesity, high-energy intake

DIAGNOSIS

Diagnosis is generally made by either the workup of a symptomatic patient or through the screening of asymptomatic patients. Symptomatic patients are generally worked up more aggressively with a minimum of total colonic examination through endoscopic and radiologic means, whereas asymptomatic patients are generally diagnosed through the use of screening examinations, such as flexible sigmoidosopy.

SCREENING AND EARLY DETECTION

Screening for asymptomatic individuals with normal risk should begin at age 50 and include digital rectal examination with fecal occult blood testing and flexible sigmoidoscopy every 5 years[1]. Patients in higher-risk groups, such as those with an HNPCC family history, should have earlier onset of screening and more frequent and thorough colonic examinations. Recommendations for this group include colonoscopy every 1–3 years, beginning at age 25 for those with known HNPCC mutations. Screening is not an effective management tool for the population with known familial adenomatous polyposis syndromes, and total colectomy should be considered[1].

CONVENTIONAL THERAPY

Conventional therapy options include surgery, radiation therapy and chemotherapy, the degree of which varies depending upon the location (colon versus rectum) and stage of disease. Advances in conventional therapy options that may lower morbidity are listed in Table 15.11. New chemotherapy drugs have significantly improved overall patient survival.

The following sections will focus on modalities mentioned throughout this text with regards to prevention, supportive care and antineoplastic uses. The text in these specific malignancy sections does not include an exhaustive review of all modalities, and some of the information presented in the tables was presented in earlier sections. Tables will present a list of modalities, their

Table 15.11	Advances in conventional therapy options for colorectal cancer

New chemotherapy drugs	
irinotecan, oxaloplatin	improved survival
Xeloda ™	oral chemotherapy agent, improved convenience
Avastin™ and Erbitux™ (biologic agents)	improved survival and tolerance
Improvements in surgical techniques	improved tolerance
Radiation therapy: technical improvements	improved tolerance, decreased late reactions

benefit and level of evidence for use. Levels of evidence are listed below.

- Level one: well-designed randomized controlled clinical trial(s);

- Level two: prospective and retrospective non-randomized clinical trials and analyses;

- Level three: opinions of expert committees, best-case series;

- Level four: preclinical *in vitro* and *in vivo* studies, and traditional uses.

Physical activity

Robert B. Lutz

PRIMARY PREVENTION

Cancer of the colon provides the most available research for the preventive role of physical activity, with at least 50 studies identified[1]. The data are generally consistent in demonstrating an inverse relationship between physical activity and cancer incidence, with an average risk reduction of 40–50% noted[2]. These findings have been identified for both men and women. This benefit appears to be present for both leisure-time physical activity as well as occupational physical activity; a dose–response relationship is most evident for leisure-time physical activity, however. Men and women expending more than 1000 kcal/week in vigorous activity during at least three specific periods in their lives have been noted to have a 40% decrease in risk of colon cancer[3]. There is a suggestion that lifelong physical activity may be more beneficial in prevention[4]. Data from the two large epidemiologic studies – the Harvard Alumni Health Study[4] and the Nurses' Health Study[5] – suggest that 30–60 minutes per day of moderate to vigorous physical activity is preventive for colon cancer.

SECONDARY PREVENTION

Whereas the majority of data on physical activity are drawn from epidemiologic studies, the APPEAL Study (A Program Promoting Exercise and an Active Lifestyle) is one of the few intervention studies currently available in cancer research. It is a randomized controlled clinical trial enrolling physically inactive men and women between the ages of 40 and 75 and is oversampling individuals with a history of adenomatous polyps. It is testing the effects of a 1-year moderate- to vigorous-intensity exercise program on a number of physiological endpoints (e.g. cell proliferation, apoptosis, levels of insulin-like growth factor I). Data from this intervention trial may provide researchers with the opportunity of determining the specific attributes of exercise that may most affect cancer outcomes relevant to cause and prevention[6].

SUPPORTIVE CARE

There is a single study that has examined quality of life for individuals who have survived colorectal cancer[7]. Individuals who had been diagnosed with colorectal cancer within 4 years of the study and received adjuvant therapies were surveyed to assess their exercise behavior (prediagnosis, treatment, post-treatment), quality of life and overall satisfaction with life. Findings indicated that an individual's functional quality of life significantly affected their satisfaction with life; exercise levels decreased from pre-diagnosis to post-treatment; and those individuals who were previously active but did not resume activity post-treatment experienced the lowest quality of life.

CONCLUSIONS

The research to date in colon cancer strongly supports a preventive role for physical activity. Recommendations of 30–60 minutes of moderate- to vigorous-intensity activity per day performed over an individual's lifetime appear to incur the most benefit. Survivors of colon cancer should be encouraged to be physically active, respectful of their limits and with the understanding that they may not achieve levels of activity previously experienced before diagnosis.

RECTAL CANCER

Prevention and supportive care

The data are inconsistent for rectal cancer, but generally support no association between physical activity and rectal cancer risk. Rectal gastrointestinal transit time is not affected in a similar fashion to that seen in the colon, the presumed mechanism by which physical activity imparts its protective role. As mentioned for colon cancer, a single study looking at quality of life did not differentiate between colon and rectal cancers. Findings supported the beneficial role for physical activity in positively affecting the functional quality of life of cancer survivors[7].

Table 15.12   Benefits of interventions in colorectal cancer

Modality/intervention	Benefit	Level of evidence
Primary prevention		
Physical activity		
Mild	positive	II, III
Moderate		
Nutrition		
Diet		
plant based	possible positive	II, III, IV
fiber	possible positive	II, III, IV
individual foods		
cruciferous vegetables	possible positive	II, III, IV
individual phytochemicals	positive	II, IV
folate, calcium, selenium	possible positive	II, IV
Supplementation		
multivitamins	possible positive	II
Obesity	positive	II, III, IV
Mind–body		
yoga	possibly positive (if considered as a	II
hypnosis	form of exercise)	
meditation	unknown	
support groups 'psychotherapy' – individual and/or group		
Manual therapy		
massage	unknown	
chiropractic		
strain–counterstrain		
Botanicals		
green tea	possible positive	IV
Energy medicine	unknown	
Alternative systems	unknown	

Continued

Table 15.12 *Continued*

Modality/intervention	Benefit	Level of evidence
Primary prevention		
Spirituality	unknown	
Tobacco cessation	positive	II, III, IV
Secondary prevention		
Physical activity Mild Moderate	possible positive	II, III, IV
Nutrition Diet		
plant based	possible positive	II, III, IV
fiber	possible positive	II, III, IV
individual foods		
ginger	possible positive	IV
curcumin	possible positive	IV
individual phytochemicals		
folate	positive	II, IV
calcium	possible positive	II, IV
Supplementation		
multivitamins	possible positive	II, IV
Obesity	possible positive	II, III, IV

Mind–body
  yoga
  hypnosis
  meditation
  support groups
	unknown	

Manual therapy
  massage
  chiropractic
  strain–counterstrain
	unknown	

Botanicals green tea	possible positive	IV
Energy medicine	unknown	
Alternative systems	unknown	
Spirituality	unknown	
Tobacco cessation	positive	II, III, IV
Tertiary prevention		
Physical activity Mild Moderate	possible positive	II, III, IV

Continued

Table 15.12 *Continued*

Modality/intervention	Benefit	Level of evidence
Tertiary prevention		
Nutrition		
Diet		
plant based	possible positive	III, IV
fiber	possible positive	III, IV
individual foods		
ginger	possible positive	IV
curcumin	possible positive	IV
individual phytochemicals		
folate	possible positive	III, IV
calcium	possible positive	III, IV
Supplementation		
multivitamins	possible positive	IV
Obesity	possible positive	II, III, IV
Mind–body		
yoga	unknown	
hypnosis		
meditation		
support groups		
Manual therapy		
massage	unknown	
chiropractic		
strain–counterstrain		
Botanicals		
green tea	possible positive	IV
Energy medicine	unknown	
Alternative systems	unknown	
Spirituality	unknown	
Tobacco cessation	positive	II, III, IV
Supportive care		
Physical activity		
Mild	positive effect on quality of life (QOL),	II, III
Moderate	symptom control	
Nutrition		
Diet		
plant based	unknown	
fiber	unknown	
individual foods	unknown	
individual phytochemicals	unknown	
Supplementation	unknown	
Obesity	unknown	

Continued

Table 15.12 *Continued*

Modality/intervention	Benefit	Level of evidence
Supportive care		
Mind–body		
yoga	improved QOL and symptom control,	II
hypnosis	decreased anxiety and depression	II
meditation		II
support groups		II
Manual therapy		
massage	improved symptom control	II
chiropractic		
strain–counterstrain		
Botanicals		
green tea	symptom control (see chart in supportive care section)	II
Energy medicine	improved QOL and symptom control	II
Alternative systems	improved nausea, pain	II
Spirituality	improved symptom control	II
Tobacco cessation	unknown	II
Antineoplastic care		
Physical activity		
Mild		
Moderate	unknown	
Nutrition		
Diet		
plant based	unknown	
fiber	unknown	
individual foods		
ginger	possible positive	IV
curcumin	possible positive	IV
individual phytochemicals	unknown	
Supplementation	unknown	
Obesity	unknown	
Mind–body		
yoga	unknown	
hypnosis		
meditation		
support groups		
Manual therapy		
massage	unknown	
chiropractic		
strain–counterstrain		

Continued

Table 15.12 *Continued*

Modality/intervention	Benefit	Level of evidence
Antineoplastic care		
Botanicals		
green tea	possible positive	IV
PSK from *Coriolus versicolor*	possible positive	IV
Energy medicine	unknown	
Alternative systems	unknown	
Spirituality	unknown	
Tobacco cessation	unknown	

PSK, polysaccharide K

Nutrition

Mara Vitolins and Cynthia Thomson

DIETARY FIBER AND CANCER

In recent years much attention has been focused on the possible protective role of fiber in the prevention of cancer of the colon and rectum. Historically, this concept stemmed from the observations that the incidence of colon cancer was lower among Africans, who consumed a diet high in insoluble fiber, than among African-Americans, who consumed diets low in fiber[1]. However, once again, other dietary factors cannot be ignored. Consuming high amounts of dietary fiber requires a person to eat a great deal of fruits, vegetables, grains, beans and other unrefined foods. Typically, this means that a person has less room to eat high fat meats and highly refined foods.

Fiber consumed as part of a healthy diet stimulates colon muscle activity and supports beneficial microflora activity[2,3]. Dietary fiber (water insoluble) provides bulk that decreases the transit time through the colon and reduces the risk of constipation[2,3]. The quantity of dietary fiber also affects bile salt metabolism and fecal bulk, all of which may be involved in colon cancer[3,4]. This provides biologic plausibility to the hypothesis that a high-fiber diet would be associated with a lower incidence of colorectal cancers. Fiber can also favorably affect the balance of steroid hormones by lowering levels of the precursor molecule cholesterol, impacting levels of sex hormones including estrogen and testosterone[5].

Bonithon-Kopp *et al.* provide study evidence that fiber supplements might actually have a detrimental effect on colon health, suggesting that fiber should be consumed as part of a healthy diet rather than in the form of a fiber supplement[6].

Additional information regarding fiber intake can be found in Chapter 11b.

Mind–body interventions

Linda E. Carlson and Shauna L. Shapiro

Although research has not focused specifically on colorectal cancer, there is good support for interventions such as meditation, yoga, supportive group therapy and individual psychotherapy and hypnosis as being beneficial for supportive care, in terms of decreasing symptoms of anxiety and depression, and improving overall quality of life for a variety of cancer patients[1,2].

Botanicals

Lise Alschuler

In vivo data suggest an antimetastatic effect of PSK, a protein-bound polysaccharide obtained from culture mycelia of *Coriolus versicolor*, on mouse colon cancer. The oral administration of PSK significantly reduced the development of liver metastasis and prolonged the survival of the host mice[1]. PSK was found to interfere with many steps of metastasis including detachment, intravasation, intravascular migration and attachment to vessels, extravasation, migration, proliferation and tumor angiogenesis. In addition, PSK enhanced T cell-mediated immunity. The pharmacokinetics of oral PSK has been demonstrated in rats and rabbits[2]. The plasma half-life is between 4.2 and 5.9 hours, with complete disappearance after 72 hours. After oral absorption, PSK concentrates in secretory organs, adrenal glands, thyroid gland, pancreas, liver and bone marrow. The majority of PSK is excreted via the lungs, with minor amounts excreted in the urine and feces.

An *in vitro* study examined the antineoplastic activity of green tea in several human colon carcinoma cell lines. (-)-Epigallocatechin-3-gallate (EGCG) was shown to inhibit topoisomerase I, but not topoisomerase II in several human carcinoma cell lines[3]. Topoisomerase I and II activities are higher in colon tumors and in various colon carcinoma cell lines compared to normal tissue. This study suggests that there may be potential benefit from combining green tea, or EGCG, with antitumor agents that also inhibit topoisomerase in order to reduce the dose of the antitumor agent and its associated side-effects.

CHEMOPREVENTION OF COLON CANCER

Green tea offers promise as a chemopreventive agent for colon cancer. However, it appears not to be chemopreventive against the development of gastric cancer. Catechin, a flavonoid derived from green tea, inhibits colonic aberrant crypt formation in rats[4]. A phase I/II study of human volunteers demonstrated that a single dose of 1.2 g of standardized green tea powder, which was equivalent to 2–3 cups of brewed tea, resulted in significant levels of tea polyphenols in plasma, urine and rectal biopsy samples. Additionally, the half-life for each EGCG and epicatechin (EC) was approximately 4 hours. The rectal biopsies also revealed decreased mucosal concentrations of prostaglandin E_2 at 4 and 8 hours after tea administration, which indicated tissue response to the tea[5]. There are no chemopreventive clinical trials to date, leaving the clinical significance of these preliminary data undetermined.

Energy medicine

Suzanne Clewell

Side-effects of chemotherapy in cancers of the gastrointestinal system will, of course, vary with the individual patient and conventional therapies used. Some of the commonly seen side-effects are diarrhea, mouth sores, lowering of blood cell counts, changes to the nails and skin, and sometimes nausea and vomiting or hair thinning. Along with the appropriate medications that have been found to be effective for the symptoms mentioned, energy medicine may hypothetically be used to enhance their effect and possibly allow for lower and fewer doses to be required.

References

Colorectal cancer

1. DeVita VJ, Hellman S, Rosenberg S. Cancer Principles and Practice of Oncology, 5th edn. Philadelphia: Lippincott-Raven, 1997: 1134–233
2. Perez C, Brady L, Halperin EC, Schmidt-Ullrich RK. Principles and Practice of Radiation Oncology. Philadelphia: Lippincott, Williams and Wilkins, 2004: 1607–29

Physical activity

1. Lee I-M. Physical activity and cancer prevention – data from epidemiologic studies. Med Sci Sports Exerc 2003; 35: 1823–7
2. Friedenreich CM. Physical activity and cancer prevention: from observational to intervention research. Cancer Epidemiol Biomarkers Prev 2001; 10: 287–301
3. Slattery ML, Potter J, Caan B, et al. Energy balance and colon cancer – beyond physical activity. Cancer Res 1997; 57: 75–80
4. Lee I-M, Paffenbarger RS Jr, Hsieh C. Physical activity and risk of developing colorectal cancer among college alumni. J Natl Cancer Inst 1991; 83: 1324–9

5. Martinez ME, Giovannucci E, Spiegelman D, et al. Leisure-time physical activity, body size, and colon cancer in women: Nurses' Health Study Research Group. J Natl Cancer Inst 1997; 89: 948–55
6. McTiernan A. Intervention studies in exercise and cancer prevention. Med Sci Sports Exerc 2003; 35: 1841–5
7. Courneya KS, Friedenreich CM. Relationship between exercise pattern across the cancer experience and current quality of life in colorectal cancer survivors. J Altern Complement Med 1997; 3: 215–26

Nutrition

1. Levy RD, Segal I, Hassan H, Saadia R. Stool weight and faecal pH in two South African populations with a dissimilar colon cancer risk. S Afr J Surg 1994; 32: 127–8
2. Slavin J. Why whole grains are protective: biological mechanisms. 1994; 32: 127–8
3. Jenkins DJ, Kendall CW, Popovich DG, et al. Effect of a very-high-fiber vegetable, fruit, and nut diet on serum lipids and colonic function. Metabolism 2001; 50: 494–503
4. Blackwood AD, Salter J, Dettmar PW, Chaplin MF. Dietary fibre, physicochemical properties

and their relationship to health. J R Soc Health 2000; 120: 242–7

5. Adlercreutz H. Western diet and Western diseases: some hormonal and biochemical mechanisms and associations. Scand J Clin Lab Invest 1990; 201 (Suppl): 3–23

6. Bonithon-Kopp C, Kronborg O, Giacosa A, et al. Calcium and fibre supplementation in prevention of colorectal adenoma recurrence: a randomised intervention trial. European Cancer Prevention Organisation Study Group. Lancet 2000; 356: 1300–6

Mind–body interventions

1. Newell SA, Sanson-Fisher RW, Savolainen NJ. Systematic review of psychological therapies for cancer patients: overview and recommendations for future research. J Natl Cancer Inst 2002; 94: 558–84

2. Speca M, Carlson LE, Goodey E, Angen M. A randomized, wait-list controlled clinical trial: the effect of a mindfulness meditation-based stress reduction program on mood and symptoms of stress in cancer outpatients. Psychosom Med 2000; 62: 613–22

Botanicals

1. Kobayashi H, Matsunaga K, Oguchi Y. Antimetastatic effects of PSK (Krestin), a protein-bound polysaccharide obtained from basidiomycetes: an overview. Cancer Epidemiol Biomarkers Prev 1995; 4: 275–81

2. Ikuzawa M, et al. Fate and distribution of an antitumor protein-bound polysaccharide PSK (Krestin). Int J Immunopharmac 1988; 10: 415–23

3. Berger SJ, et al. Green tea constituent (–)-epigallocatechin-3-gallate inhibits topoisomerase I activity in human colon carcinoma cells. Biochem Biophys Res Commun 2001; 288: 101–5

4. Franke AA, et al. Inhibition of colonic aberrant crypt formation by the dietary flavonoids (+)-catechin and hesperidin. Adv Exp Med Biol 2002; 505: 123–33

5. August DA, et al. Ingestion of green tea rapidly decreases prostaglandin E2 levels in rectal mucosa in humans. Cancer Epidemiol Biomarkers Prev 1999; 8: 709–13

15

Specific malignancies

(e) Skin cancer

Matthew P. Mumber

Skin cancer is the most common malignancy in the USA, and can be divided into melanomatous and non-melanomatous varieties. The non-melanomatous varieties are very common, and include basal cell (65% of total) and squamous cell cancers (30% of total). Melanomas are much less common, and more potentially life-threatening, owing to their tendency to spread and relative unresposiveness to conventional therapeutic options. Over the past decade, the incidence of skin cancer, and melanoma particularly, has increased greater than any other cancer except lung cancer in women[1].

RISK FACTORS

Risk factors for all types of skin cancer include sun exposure, and especially sunburn and blistering at a young age in light-skinned individuals. Skin trauma, chronic irritation, smoking, chemical exposure, genetic syndromes and immunosuppression also increase the relative risk[2].

SCREENING AND EARLY DETECTION

Patients at high risk should be screened for unusual changes in skin lesions and moles on a consistent basis. Moles should be watched for changes in color, size and appearance.

DIAGNOSIS

Diagnosis is usually made by skin biopsy through incisional or excisional biopsy.

CONVENTIONAL THERAPY

Surgery and radiation therapy are the most commonly used conventional therapies for all types of skin cancer. Advanced and metastatic melanomatous and non-melanomatous skin cancers can be treated with chemotherapy, but the results have been disappointing[1].

The following sections will focus on modalities mentioned throughout this text with regards to prevention, supportive care and antineoplastic uses. The text in these specific malignancy sections does not include an exhaustive review of all modalities, and some of the information presented in the tables was presented in earlier sections. Tables will present a list of modalities, their benefit, and level of evidence for use. Levels of evidence are listed below.

• Level one: well-designed randomized controlled clinical trial(s);

• Level two: prospective and retrospective non-randomized clinical trials and analyses;

• Level three: opinions of expert committees, best-case series;

• Level four: preclinical *in vitro* and *in vivo* studies, and traditional uses.

Physical activity

Robert B. Lutz

An inverse relationship has been seen in melanoma for men and women exercising 5–7 days per week (OR 0.7); however, no mechanism is readily apparent for this finding[1]. One hypothesis is immune mediation, as melanoma is known to be an immune-responsive cancer type.

Table 15.13 Benefits of interventions in skin cancer		
Modality/intervention	*Benefit*	*Level of evidence*
Primary prevention		
Physical activity		
Mild		
Moderate	positive	II
Nutrition		
Diet		
plant based	unknown	
fiber	unknown	
individual foods	unknown	
individual phytochemicals		
selenium	possible positive	II, IV
Supplementation		
multivitamins	possible positive	II, IV
Obesity	unknown	
Mind–body		
yoga	unknown	
hypnosis		
meditation		
support groups		
Manual therapy		
massage	unknown	
chiropractic		
strain–counterstrain		
Botanicals		
green tea	possible positive	II, IV
silymarin	possible positive	IV
resveratrol	possible positive	IV
Energy medicine	unknown	
Alternative systems	unknown	
Spirituality	unknown	
Tobacco cessation	positive	II, III, IV
		Continued

Table 15.13 *Continued*

Modality/intervention	Benefit	Level of evidence
Secondary prevention		
Physical activity		
Mild		
Moderate	unknown	
Nutrition		
Diet		
plant based	unknown	
fiber	unknown	
individual foods		
individual phytochemicals		
selenium	possible positive	II, IV
Supplementation		
multivitamins	possible positive	II, IV
Obesity	unknown	
Mind–body		
yoga	unknown	
hypnosis		
meditation		
support groups		
Manual therapy		
massage	unknown	
chiropractic		
strain–counterstrain		
Botanicals		
Energy medicine	unknown	
Alternative systems	unknown	
Spirituality	unknown	
Tobacco cessation	positive	II, III, IV
Tertiary prevention		
Physical activity		
Mild		
Moderate	unknown	
Nutrition		
Diet		
plant based	unknown	
fiber	unknown	
individual foods	unknown	
individual phytochemicals		
selenium	possible positive	II

Continued

Table 15.13 *Continued*

Modality/intervention	Benefit	Level of evidence
Tertiary prevention		
Nutrition		
Supplementation		
multivitamins	possible positive	II
Obesity	unknown	
Mind–body		
yoga	unknown	
hypnosis	unknown	
meditation	unknown	
support groups	possible positive (melanoma)	I
Manual therapy		
massage		
chiropractic	unknown	
strain–counterstrain		
Botanicals		
Energy medicine	unknown	
Alternative systems	unknown	
Spirituality	unknown	
Tobacco cessation	positive	II, III, IV
Supportive care		
Physical activity		
Mild	improved quality of life (QOL) and	II, III
Moderate	symptom control	
Nutrition		
Diet		
plant based		
fiber	unknown	
individual foods		
individual phytochemicals		
Supplementation		
Obesity	unknown	
Mind–body		
yoga		
hypnosis	improved quality of life (QOL) and	II, III
meditation	symptom control	
support groups		
Manual therapy		
massage		
chiropractic	improved symptom control	II, III
strain–counterstrain		

Continued

Table 15.13 *Continued*

Modality/intervention	Benefit	Level of evidence
Supportive care		
Botanicals	see supportive care chart	II, IV
Energy medicine	improved QOL and symptom control	II, IV
Alternative systems	improved QOL and symptom control	II, III, IV
Spirituality	improved QOL and symptom control	II
Tobacco cessation	unknown	
Antineoplastic care		
Physical activity Mild Moderate	unknown	

Nutrition
Diet
  plant based
  fiber
  individual foods
  flax lignan
  individual phytochemicals
Supplementation
	
	unknown
	
	possible positive (melanoma)
		
		IV

Obesity	unknown	

Mind–body
  yoga
  hypnosis
  meditation
  support groups
	
	unknown	

Manual therapy
  massage
  chiropractic
  strain–counterstrain
	
	unknown	

Botanicals
  green tea
  curcumin and catechin
	
	possible positive
	possible positive (melanoma)
		
		IV
		IV

Antineoplastic care		
Energy medicine	unknown	
Alternative systems	unknown	
Spirituality	unknown	
Tobacco cessation	unknown	

Nutrition

Cynthia Thomson and Mara Vitolins

Studies conducted utilizing animal models have reported that orally administered fractions of tea inhibited skin cancers and other tumors induced by carcinogens and ultraviolet light[1,2], and that caffeinated teas were more protective than decaffeinated teas[1]. Caffeine or tea alone also has been found to have an inhibitory effect on ultraviolet light-induced tumorigenesis, and adding caffeine to decaffeinated teas has been shown to restore their inhibitory effect[2].

Whether or not individuals should consume caffeine to prevent skin cancer is still under investigation.

Mind–body interventions

Linda E. Carlson and Shauna L. Shapiro

Fawzy *et al.* showed a survival advantage in patients with melanoma who participated in a 6-week psychoeducational intervention, which was associated with increases in natural killer cell function as well as 5–6-year survival[1,2]. The intervention consisted of group support, relaxation exercises, coping skills training and education. Interestingly, the survival advantage was weaker, but was still upheld at the 10-year follow-up[3]. At the 10-year follow-up, the survival advantage only held for women (who had a better prognosis than the men), and those who had shallower tumor depth at the time of diagnosis.

This seemed to indicate that those patients with the worst medical prognosis benefited less over the longer term from the intervention.

It is also well known that interferon and interleukin treatments for melanoma are often associated with increased levels of depression, thought to be due to the pro-inflammatory effects of these cytokines in the brain. It thus becomes even more important to offer supportive care in the form of individual counseling or prophylactic antidepressant therapy for patients undergoing this arduous treatment.

Botanicals

Lise Alschuler

CHEMOPREVENTION OF SKIN CANCER

There are no human population studies or intervention trials on botanical agents as chemopreventives against the development of skin cancers. However, there are two botanicals that show promise based on experimental data. Silybum, a flavonoid in *Silymarin marianum* (milk thistle), inhibited skin tumor promotion in human epidermoid carcinoma cells A431 and in mice. Epidermal growth factor receptor (EGFR) is a recognized mediator of tumor promotion. EGFR mediates tyrosine phosphorylation, thus stimulating signal transduction-induced cell growth and proliferation. EGFR is activated in skin cells exposed to ultraviolet B radiation and oxidative stress. Treatment of A431 cells that overexpressed EGFR with silymarin resulted in a significant inhibition of both ligand-induced activation of EGFR and tyrosine phosphorylation. Cells treated with silymarin showed a significant G_2–M arrest in cell-cycle progression and a highly significant inhibition of DNA synthesis and cell growth in a dose-dependent manner[1].

Another antioxidant compound that had chemopreventive actions in mouse skin tumorigenesis is resveratrol. Resveratrol is a phytoalexin that is generated in response to fungal infection in species such as *Vitis vinifera* (grape).

As a result, resveratrol is found in relatively high quantities in grape skins and red wines. Resveratrol significantly inhibits oxidative stress via inhibition of arachindonic acid metabolites catalyzed by both cyclo-oxygenase (COX)-1 and COX-2. Resveratrol also inhibits the expression of certain genes such as *c-fos* and *TGF-β1*. These mechanisms result in decreased tumorigenesis in mouse skin tumors induced by chemical carcinogens[2]. While these experimental data indicate a chemopreventive effect of both silymarin and resveratrol, human trials are needed to ascertain the significance of these results.

MELANOMA

The inhibitory effects of curcumin and catechin on lung metastasis induced by B16F-10 melanoma cells were studied in mice. Curcumin and catechin each significantly ($p < 0.001$) inhibited lung tumor formation (89.3% and 82.2%, respectively) and increased survival (143.9% and 80.8%, respectively) of the mice. In addition, in an *in vitro* model, curcumin and catechin significantly inhibited the invasion of the melanoma cells across a collagen matrix. The ability of curcumin and catechin to inhibit the invasion of B16F-10 melanoma cells appeared to be due to inhibition of metalloproteinases[3].

Energy medicine

Suzanne Clewell

The side-effects of skin cancer treatment will differ depending upon the pathology.

Less aggressive cancers are easily removed by curettage and electrodesiccation; others by freezing with liquid nitrogen, or with the use of laser therapy. Surgery is used when appropriate for cancers that may be larger or of greater concern. Skin grafts may sometimes be necessary if a large amount of tissue was removed. Radiation is often used to treat those skin cancers that are difficult to manage with surgery, and in some cases topical chemotherapy may be prescribed.

The effects of various energy healing modalities on the healing of wounds has been inconclusive so far. Further study is required for definitive answers. However, owing to the low risk/benefit ratio of energy medicine, it would not be unreasonable to direct energy to the specific site for healing.

References

Skin cancer

1. DeVita VJ, Hellman S, Rosenberg S. Cancer Principles and Practice of Oncology, 5th edn. Philadelphia: Lippincott-Raven, 1997: 1879–934
2. Leibel S, Phillips T. Textbook of Radiation Oncology. Philadelphia: WB Saunders, 1998: 1165–82

Physical activity

1. Shors AR, Solomon C, McTiernan A, et al. Melanoma risk in relation to height, weight, and exercise (United States). Cancer Causes Control 2001; 12: 599–606

Nutrition

1. Wang ZY, Huang MT, Lou Y-R, et al. Inhibitory effects of black tea, green tea, decaffeinated black tea, and decaffeinated green tea on ultraviolet B light-induced skin carcinogenesis in 7,12-dimethylbenz(a)anthracene-initiated SKH-1 mice. Cancer Res 1994; 54: 3428–35
2. Huang M-T, Xie J-G, Wang ZY, et al. Effects of tea, decaffinated tea, and caffine on UVB light-induced complete carcinogenesis in SKH-1 mice: demonstration of caffeine as a biologically important constituent of tea. Cancer Res 1997; 57: 2623–9

Mind–body interventions

1. Fawzy FI, Fawzy NW, Hyun CS, et al. Malignant melanoma. Effects of an early structured psychiatric intervention, coping, and affective state on recurrence and survival 6 years later. Arch Gen Psychiatry 1993; 50: 681–9
2. Fawzy FI, Kemeny ME, Fawzy NW, et al. A structured psychiatric intervention for cancer patients. II. Changes over time in immunological measures. Arch Gen Psychiatry 1990; 47: 729–35
3. Fawzy FI, Canada AL, Fawzy NW. Malignant melanoma: effects of a brief, structured psychiatric intervention on survival and recurrence at

10-year follow-up. Arch Gen Psychiatry 2003; 60: 100–3

Botanicals

1. Ahmad N, Javed S, Agarwal R. Skin cancer chemopreventive effects of a flavonoid antioxidant silymarin are mediated via impairment of receptor tyrosine kinase signaling and perturbation in cell cycle progression. Biochem Biophys Res Commun 1998; 248: 294–301

2. Jang M, Pezzuto JM. Resveratrol blocks eicosanoid production and chemically-induced cellular transformation: implications for cancer chemoprevention. Pharm Biol 1998; 36: 28–34

3. Menon LG, Kuttan R, Kuttan G. Anti-metastatic activity of curcumin and catechin. Cancer Lett 1999; 141: 159–65

15f

Other cancers

Matthew P. Mumber

There has been significant research regarding several of the modalities covered in this text and less common malignancies. This chapter will cover some selected highlights concerning these other malignancies and various applications investigated. It is important to realize that, with regards to cancer prevention and antineoplastic therapy, all malignancies are not alike. Indeed, every specific malignancy has its own set of conventional treatment options, which varies widely among different cancers and stages of disease. What works in one cancer, may not work in another. This requires that specific malignancies be studied separately, especially when antineoplastic action is the goal of therapy[1–3].

Following each discussion point a level of data and possible effect are noted. The level of evidence is the same as that used throughout the text.

Physical activity

Robert B. Lutz

PREVENTION

In general, there are fewer epidemiologic studies looking at causes of other than the leading cancers (colon, lung, breast, prostate). Likewise, results are often inconsistent, combining to provide difficulty in determining a protective role for physical activity and cancer, although for some types an association does appear to exist. Therefore, any positive findings must be viewed as preliminary, pending further research.

For example, the available research has suggested an average risk reduction of 30–40% for endometrial cancer with physical activity[1–3]. As reported at the American Association of Cancer Research in March 2004, women in China who reported lifetime activity (exercise, walking and cycling for errands, housework) were found to have approximately 33% lower rates of endometrial cancer[4] (level II data, possible positive effect).

In a pooled analysis of data from the Health Professional's Follow-up Study and the Nurses' Health Study, an inverse relationship was identified for moderate physical activity and pancreatic cancer (multivariable RR of 55%), while total physical activity was inversely related to risk in overweight individuals (pooled multivariable RR of 0.59)[5] (level II data, possible positive effect).

In a case–control study of women with papillary thyroid cancer, the risk of thyroid cancer was reduced among women who reported regular leisure-time physical activity during the 2 years preceding diagnosis compared to women who did not report exercise during that period (OR = 0.76). Similarly, women who reported exercising regularly between ages 12–21 demonstrated a similar protective effect (OR 0.83)[6] (level II data, possible positive effect).

However, risk has varied for ovarian cancer (RR 0.3–1.1) in case–control studies[7], and in a longitudinal cohort study comparing less active women with moderately active and very-active women, relative risks of 1.4–2.1, respectively, were identified[8]. Overall, however, no risk can be concluded[1] (level II data – possible negative effect of increasing intensity).

No consistent association has been identified in non-Hodgkin's lymphoma overall or in diffuse or follicular lymphoma[9], or in stomach, renal or bladder cancers[10,11] (level II data – no effect).

Botanicals

Lise Alschuler

OVARIAN CANCER

Antineoplastic therapy

Ginsenoside Rh2, isolated from *Panax ginseng*, has been found to inhibit the growth of human ovarian cells in nude mice[1]. The Rh2 was administered to the mice orally for 70 days. After 70 days, the tumor growth in nude mice was significantly inhibited compared to that in a cisplatin-treated group as well as a control group. There were no toxic effects observed in any of the mice. This study is in apparent contradiction to the estrogen-like stimulatory activity of another component of ginseng, Rg1, on estrogen-dependent cells (MCF-7 cells). The complete effect of ginseng on human cancers is hard to predict from these experimental studies on isolated constituents of ginseng. It is thus difficult to know how to utilize these preliminary data in a clinical context (level IV data – possible tumoricidal effect).

Quercetin, a bioflavonoid found in high concentrations in onions, has been demonstrated *in vitro* to interfere with signal transduction pathways in ovarian epithelial cancer cells[2]. Quercetin inhibits protein kinase and thus may reduce ovarian tumor cell growth, survival and progression. Quercetin is a promising antineoplastic herbally derived agent (level IV data – possible tumoricidal effect).

Adding to the debate regarding the effect of soy-derived genistein and daidzein isoflavones on estrogen-dependent cancers is an *in vitro* study that demonstrated a reduction of ovarian cell proliferation from these isoflavones[3]. Genistein and diadzein independently significantly reduced the growth of Caov-3 and NIH:OVCAR-3

ovarian cancer cell lines at dietarily relevant concentrations (10^{-8}–10^{-10} mol/l). The addition of ICI-182780, an estrogen antagonist, blocked these inhibitory effects, suggesting an estrogen receptor-dependent mechanism (level IV – possible tumoricidal effect). However, these results are contraindicated by a more recent *in vitro* study that demonstrated that genistein and daidzein enhanced proliferation of estrogen-sensitive breast cancer MCF-7 cells[4]. This study elucidated a pathway of tumor initiation and cell proliferation by isoflavones involving DNA oxidative damage, and estrogen receptor binding (proliferation). These results are probably transferable to other estrogen-dependent cancers such as those of the ovary. Until further *in vivo* and clinical investigation clarifies the impact of soy isoflavones on estrogen-dependent cancers, their therapeutic role in ovarian cancer is questionable.

LEUKEMIA

Antineoplastic therapy

Glycyrrhizin and its diastereoisomers, active constituents of *Glycyrrhiza glabra* (licorice), were studied *in vitro* against human chronic myeloid leukemic cells. The glycyrrhizin triterpenoids demonstrated approximately 50% inhibition compared to 100% inhibition by daunorubicin[5]. These data are preliminary and future trials are needed to verify this effect in humans. Another approach to treatment of leukemia lies in the use of agents that induce terminal differentiation. This approach is attractive in that it is associated with less morbidity than that produced by cytotoxic drugs. Yosmogin is a sesquiterpene lactone isolated from *Artemisia princeps*. The effect of yosmogin was studied on human promyelocytic leukemia HL-60 cells. Yosmogin by itself was a weak inducer of differentiation. However, when yosmogin was applied to the cells with either 1,25-dihydroxyvitamin D_3 or all-*trans*-retinoic acid, yosmogin strongly enhanced 1,25-dihyrdoxyvitamin D_3 and all-*trans*-retinoic acid-induced differentiation in a concentration-dependent manner[6]. These results suggest a synergism between these substances and a potential role as an adjuvant treatment for chronic leukemias (level IV – possible cell killing effect).

Another promising botanical agent for leukemia is green tea. In an *in vitro* experiment, EGCG, from green tea (*Camellia sinensis*), inhibited tyrosine kinase. This caused a significant increase in apoptosis and cell death in chronic lymphocytic leukemia cells. In addition, epigallocatechin gallate (EGCG) suppressed vascular endothelial growth factor (VEGF)-R1 and VEGF-R2 phosphorylation. This latter effect interrupted the VEGF survival signals in CLL cells, resulting in caspase activation and subsequent cell death[7]. This effect has also been demonstrated for baicalein, derived from *Scutellaria baicalensis*, in human promyelocytic leukemia (HL-60) cells *in vitro*. Baicalein induced apoptosis via promotion of caspase-3 activity[8] (level IV – possible cell killing effect).

PANCREATIC CANCER

EGCG, derived from green tea, caused growth suppression of human pancreatic cells (PANC-1, MIA PaCa-2, BxPC-3) *in vitro*[9]. This suppression was dose-dependent. In addition, EGCG caused a significant suppression of invasiveness into Matrigel™ basement membrane matrix. Quercetin, a flavonoidal compound, has been shown to block the epidermal growth factor

receptor-signaling pathway in MiaPaCa-2 human pancreatic cells[10]. This disruption resulted in significant growth inhibition of these cells and the induction of apoptosis. To date, there are no human trials to confirm the *in vitro* effects of EGCG or quercetin (level IV – possible cell killing).

RENAL CARCINOMA AND BLADDER CANCER

Antineoplastic

In a phase II trial of 14 patients (eight men and six women) with renal adenocarcinoma stage IV and clearly measurable lung metastases, the subjects were treated with subcutaneous injections of Iscador (extract of mistletoe, *Viscum* spp.)[11]. The subjects received injections every other day in escalating doses over 3 weeks followed by maintenance therapy for up to 2 years. All patients died with a median survival of 330 days. The median time to progression was 108 days. Eleven of the 14 patients received additional palliative treatment. The Iscador therapy failed to produce significant improvements in time to progession, survival, laboratory measures or quality of life. This study does not support the use of Iscador for stage IV renal adenocarcinoma, despite popular belief and practice (level II – no effect).

A randomized phase II trial studied the impact of subcutaneous application of mistletoe lectin in 45 patients with pTa G1-2 superficial bladder cancer. The patients were randomized after complete resection to the control arm or to receive 1 ml of mistletoe lectin subcutaneously twice a week for 3 months, followed by a therapy-free 3 months before a second cycle was started. Both groups were similar with regard to the total number of tumors and recurrences at the time of resection. After a follow-up of 18 months, cystoscopic data revealed 30 recurrences in the control group and 31 recurrences in the treatment group with no difference in time to recurrence. There were three cases of progression in each group and there were nine patients in each group who remained without evidence of disease. This study failed to demonstrate any benefit associated with mistletoe therapy in preventing bladder cancer recurrence[12] (level I/II – no effect).

SARCOMA

Antineoplastic therapy

The antitumor effect of *Withania somnifera* (ashwagandha) was demonstrated against mouse tumor, Sarcoma 180[13]. Ashwagandha extract was injected into mice with transplanted sarcoma tumor. Daily doses of the extract to a maximum cumulative dose of 15 g/kg were given. A dose of 750 mg/kg for 15 days resulted in significant reductions in tumor volume doubling time and overall regression (level IV – possible cell killing).

Green tea extracts have also been studied in sarcoma models. Treatment of human chondrosarcoma cells (HTB-94) with EGCG significantly ($p < 0.05$) reduced the viability of these cells and this correlated with the induction of apoptosis[14]. This induction of apoptosis was demonstrated to be mediated through the activation of caspase proteases. Furthermore, EGCG has been shown to bind to, and to inhibit, gelatinases and metalloproteinases. These enzymes are typically overexpressed in cancer and also during the process of angiogenesis. These enzymes are critical for dissolving through basement membrane barriers during the metastatic process. Gelatinases are thus considered necessary for tumor invasion and for angiogenesis. Human fibrosarcoma cells incubated with EGCG solution demonstrated significantly inhibited invasion. Inhibition of tumor cell invasion by at least 50% occurred with concentrations of EGCG similar to those in the plasma of moderate (2–4 cups daily) tea drinkers (0.1–0.3 µmol/l)[15]. This inhibition is thought to be the result of EGCG inhibition of gelatinases and metalloproteinases (level IV – possible cell killing).

Mushroom extracts have been studied in various sarcoma models. Intraperitoneal administration of β-1,3-glucan and β-1,6-glucan obtained from *Grifola frondosa* to mice with fibrosarcoma resulted in enhanced cytotoxic activity and interleukin (IL)-1 productivity by macrophages and T cells. These activities were, in turn, associated with significant reduction in tumor size[16]. This same effect was demonstrated against sarcoma 180 tumors in mice with intraperitoneal injection of polysaccharide peptides (PSP) from *Coriolus versicolor*. The significant reduction in tumor growth was attributed to the immunomodulating effects of the PSP[17]. Antitumor effects of orally administered *Lentinus edodes* (shiitake mushroom) were demonstrated in a mouse sarcoma model. In the shiitake-fed mice, the macrophage production of superoxide anion increased 2–2.3 times, and the cytotoxic activities of natural killer (NK) cells and cytotoxic T cells increased 1.9 times and 1.4 times, respectively, compared to control animals[18]. Although the research on mushroom extracts in sarcoma models is preliminary, the results from the studies are consistent with one another. This is suggestive of a predictive antitumor effect via immunomodulation (level IV – cell killing).

GASTRIC CANCER

Prevention

In contrast with the favorable data trends regarding the chemoprevention properties of green tea against colon carcinogenesis and oral leukoplakia, there appears to be no chemoprevention of gastric cancer. In a population-based, prospective cohort study in Japan, 26 311 volunteers completed a self-administered questionnaire that included questions about the frequency of consumption of green tea. During 199 748 person-years of follow-up (over a period of 8 years), Cox regression estimated the relative risk of gastric cancer according to consumption of green tea and found no association. The study controlled for co-variables[19] (level II – no effect).

In contrast to this study, an epidemiologic study of soy products and death from gastric carcinoma concluded that soy intake may reduce the risk of death from stomach cancer[20]. This study was also conducted in Japan and followed 30 304 participants for over 7 years. During this time 121 deaths from stomach cancer occurred. In men, the highest tertile of soy intake was inversely associated with death from stomach cancer after controlling for co-variates (hazard ratio 0.49; 95% CI 0.22–1.13). This same trend was observed in women; however, the association was of marginal significance. This association was the strongest for non-fermented soy products. Genistein has been previously shown to increase apoptosis, and to decrease proliferation and angiogenesis of gastric carcinomas (Level II – possible positive effect).

Antineoplastic therapy

A trial examined the role of PSK on prognosis in patients with operable gastric cancer. In this trial, 262 patients were enrolled. All patients had a histologic diagnosis of gastric cancer and underwent curative gastrectomy. Patients were stratified according to the extent of the tumor which is the primary prognostic factor. Patients were randomly assigned to either standard treatment with mitomycin and fluorouracil or standard treatment plus PSK. The mitomycin was given as bolus injections on postoperative days 1 and 7. The standard treatment group then received oral fluorouracil, 150 mg daily for 4 weeks alternated

with 4 weeks of rest from treatment. The PSK group received the oral fluorouracil in the same manner for 4 weeks alternated with 4 weeks of oral PSK, 3 g daily. The patients were followed regularly for 5 years. The treatment groups were well balanced in terms of clinical and demographic characteristics. The 5-year disease-free survival rate was 70.7% in the PSK group and 59.4% in the standard treatment group. The reduction in risk was 35% (95% CI 1–58%, $p = 0.047$) without adjustments and 44% (95% CI 13–64%, $p = 0.009$) after adjustment for pTNM stage. The 5-year survival rate was 73% for the PSK group and 60.0% for the standard treatment group. The reduction in risk was 36% (95% CI 1–58%, $p = 0.044$) without adjustments and 44% (95% CI 14–64%, $p = 0.008$) after adjustment for pTNM stage. There were no significant side-effects reported throughout the study. The overall reduction of approximately 20% in recurrence and death rates is a significant finding. The authors of the study noted that PSK induced gene expression for interleukins 1, 6 and 8, as well as for tumor necrosis factor (TNF) and macrophage chemotactic factor. They further surmised that these effects may correct the immuno-suppression associated with both the surgery and the subsequent chemotherapy, thus contributing to increased survival[21] (level I – positive effect).

A prospective, randomized, placebo-controlled trial on postoperative patients with stage III gastric cancer was conducted to determine the effects of *Panax ginseng* on immunity and survival in patients receiving 5-fluorouracil (5-FU) and cisplatin chemotherapy[22]. After exclusion criteria were applied, 42 patients who had undergone curative gastric resection with D2 lymph node dissection for histologically proven AJCC stage III gastric adenocarcinoma were enrolled in this study.

The patients were followed postoperatively for 5 years. All patients received monthly 5-FU infusion at 500 mg/m² per day, on days 1–5. In addition, bolus cisplatin was given at a dosage of

60 mg/m^2 per day on day 1. The course of chemotherapy was 6 months. Prior to surgery, the patients were randomly assigned additionally to receive *P. ginseng* powder capsules orally at a dosage of 4.5 g/day or sucrose capsules as a placebo throughout the 6-month course of chemotherapy. T-lymphocyte subsets were evaluated preoperatively and at postoperative months 1, 3 and 6. On the basis of clinical and ultrasound examination, abdominal computed tomography and tumor markers, patients were defined as having tumor recurrence ($n = 19$) or not ($n = 23$) at the 5-year follow-up. No adverse effects were observed in either group.

The recurrence rate was greater in the nonginseng group than in the ginseng group (7/22 versus 13/20, $p < 0.05$). Mean duration of disease free survival was significantly longer in the ginseng group (44.4 ± 13.1 months versus 33.5 ± 17.9 months, $p < 0.05$). The 5-year disease-free survival rate of the ginseng-treated group was 68.2% versus 33.3% in the nonginseng group. The CD3 and CD4 levels were significantly higher in patients taking the ginseng, which suggests that ginseng may facilitate recovery of immune function during chemotherapy. This, in turn, may help prevent metastatic recurrence. Although this study was small, it is excellent evidence of the survival benefit of *Panax ginseng* root capsules in postoperative gastric cancer patients receiving 5-FU and cisplatin chemotherapy (level I – positive effect).

HEAD AND NECK CANCER

Secondary prevention

There is compelling evidence for a chemopreventive effect of green tea on the development of oral cancers. A randomized, placebo-controlled 6-month trial of 59 male and female subjects was conducted in a dental hospital in China. All subjects had diagnosed oral leukoplakia. Of the subjects, 46 were smokers. Twenty non-smoking dental patients without oral leukoplakia were chosen as a healthy control group. Subjects in the tea-treated group took 8 capsules of green tea extract, which was equivalent to 3 g of tea daily, and painted mixed tea in glycerin on their leukoplakial lesions three times daily. After 6 months of intervention, partial regression of the lesions was observed in 37.9% of the tea-treated group, and in only 10% of the placebo group ($p < 0.05$). Partial regression was defined as 30% or more reduction in the size of a lesion or the sum of sizes of multiple lesions. In addition, after 6 months of intervention, the micronuclei formation in exfoliated oral cells, previously elevated over that in healthy subjects, was significantly reduced in the tea-treated group[23]. EGCG has been demonstrated to arrest human leukoplakia cell lines in G_1 phase[24] (level II – positive effect).

Energy medicine

Suzanne Clewell

All of the situations that are proposed below for the use of energy medicine are hypothetical, and based on level IV data, or traditional use.

GENITOURINARY: BLADDER, KIDNEY

Surgical treatment of bladder cancer may consist of a transurethral resection of the bladder (TURB) for early-stage cancer, cystectomy for more advanced or recurrent cancers and, if the bladder is removed, an ostomy or urostomy. Potential side-effects related to surgery include: pain, bleeding, infection, incontinence and possible impotency. Altered body image is a genuine concern related to the bag the patient must now wear to collect urine. Symptoms related to radiation of the bladder may include redness of the skin and bladder irritation with the need to pass urine frequently during the period of treatment. Chemotherapy for bladder cancer may cause nausea and vomiting, loss of appetite, sores in the mouth, loss of hair, anemia, fatigue, easy bruising and increased chance of infection.

All of these symptoms may hypothetically be addressed by using energy medicine. Remembering that a cure may or may not be the outcome, healing or reduction in symptoms may be experienced by the recipient sometimes far beyond expectations.

People with kidney cancer may present with symptoms related to surgery, radiation therapy and/or immunotherapy. Symptom prevention with energy modalities would include decreased anxiety, pain relief and reduction of the often-severe side-effects associated with immunotherapy. The side-effects from interleukin-2 may include hypotension, excess fluid in the lungs, kidney damage, bleeding, heart-related symptoms, chills and fever.

Patients will usually be hospitalized during treatment and would benefit from energy medicine during that time. The energy received by the patient can hypothetically do no harm to him/her and may assist the success of the therapy by boosting the inner resources of the patient.

AERODIGESTIVE TRACT: HEAD AND NECK, ESOPHAGUS, GASTRIC, LUNG

The symptoms associated with the treatment of cancers in the head and neck region are usually some of the most difficult for a patient to endure. Symptoms vary with the exact area receiving radiation.

Depending upon the condition of a patient's dentition, teeth may be extracted. This not only makes eating difficult but also is a huge body-image concern for some. Food loses its taste and the patient loses his/her appetite. Eventually swallowing, one of the most basic bodily functions related to survival, is made difficult or impossible. Head and neck cancer patients will often have a gastric tube inserted for tube feedings. This can be a source of such anxiety that patients refuse even to look at the area of insertion, much less keep it clean or use it correctly. Skin irritation during radiation is an ongoing concern. Mucositis is commonly observed in these patients and may be brought on by decreased immunity related to chemotherapy treatment, directly related to the chemotherapy drug, or perhaps caused by the radiation therapy.

Energy medicine has been shown to reduce anxiety, increase immune function and facilitate healing. It may help to clear the thought processes so that the patient is better able to assimilate all the information being presented to him. Energy medicine hypothetically optimizes healing when combined with the conventional treatments for these symptoms.

There is a great amount of patient teaching necessary, especially when a person has cancer in this area, and this is an opportune time for the health-care provider to be able to send healing energy through the state of being present. There are numerous appointments to be made and dates to remember, and all of this is extremely anxiety producing. Energy healing may be given to this person through a reassuring arm around the shoulder or holding his/her hand as well as simply through the human-to-human connection that is made when we are truly present with that person. Many times I have seen distinct change in the attitude of a patient within a period of a few minutes after initiating a brief flow of energy. Patients who were in near-panic states often begin to relax and even be joking and laughing as they leave the office.

Esophageal cancer treatments vary depending upon the extent of the disease and the general health of the patient. Treatment is often aggressive and causes multiple symptoms. Radiation to this area will cause a painful sore throat, skin irritation and fatigue. Chemotherapy may also produce fatigue as well as nausea and decreased blood counts. Energy medicine may be an appropriate and effective modality for reduction of these symptoms.

One of the most memorable experiences I have had as a nurse using Reiki in the workplace was with a patient with esophageal cancer. This man was receiving high-dose Brach therapy (HDR). This involved the insertion of a catheter into the esophagus for the purpose of delivering a dose of radiation directly to the cancer. He arrived in our facility from the hospital in some

distress as he had copious amounts of mucus and saliva which needed to be suctioned constantly or he would panic… feeling as if he could not breathe. The computed tomography (CT) scan was performed as soon as he arrived but he would then have to wait on the stretcher (trundle bed) until the medical physicist, radiation oncologist and dosimetry specialist worked on his plan of treatment, at which time he would be taken into the treatment room to receive radiation. He required continuous suctioning as he gagged with a frightened look in his eyes. At one point I had about 2 minutes before he would need to be suctioned again. I took this time to center myself and place both hands upon him. I felt energy, 'electricity', coming into me from the earth into my feet and flowing up through me to a power above. I perceived a warmth, a connection, and just asked that whatever healing was most appropriate for this man would manifest. Almost immediately this man clearly said 'I'd like to take you home with me', meaning that whatever I was doing felt good to him. This was amazing to me, because he had not been able to utter one word since he arrived that day. I said a few words of comfort to him while continuing to pass energy and within a minute he was asleep. He rested comfortably for the next hour and a half. He was taken into the treatment room and tolerated his radiation well. As he was being taken out of the building to go back to the hospital he waved good-bye to me and said, 'see you later'. This man who was drowning in his secretions one minute suddenly could sleep comfortably and did not need suctioning for the entire hour and a half that he remained in our facility. I attribute the majority of this experience to his receiving energy medicine.

The standard of care in the patient diagnosed with gastric cancer is surgery to remove the cancer and lymph nodes in the area of the stomach, wait an appropriate time for healing from the surgery, then treat with radiation and chemotherapy. Surgery can be extensive, so management of pain is a priority. There is the potential for numerous digestive system side-effects (dumping syndrome, etc.) related to loss of the stomach. The individual who is able to self-treat with healing energy has a great advantage in that he/she is able to provide this healing to him/herself at any time necessary. The food eaten may receive healing energy also and thus, it is thought, help with digestion.

GASTROINTESTINAL: COLORECTAL, ANAL, PANCREATIC

Cancer of the pancreas is an especially devastating cancer for all concerned, owing to its reputation for being not only difficult to treat but also seldom curable and often very painful. Quality of life issues may arise when offering treatment such as surgery or chemotherapy.

Probably one of the most appropriate times to offer energy modalities is when the patient may not have many other options to consider. Naturally this concept would need to be approached with the utmost sensitivity. After a patient has had time to assimilate the medical information that has been offered, the subject of energy medicine could be introduced as a method of calming anxieties and relaxing the body and spirit. It may also be explained to the patient that if the body is relaxed it allows medications (narcotics, antiemetics, etc.) to work more effectively. It is of the utmost importance that the person receiving the energy understands the differences between healing and curing, and that expectations are realistic.

CENTRAL NERVOUS SYSTEM

Symptoms related to cancer of the central nervous system depend upon the location of the tumor. Spinal cord tumors may cause paralysis, pain and numerous other symptoms. Tumors of the brain may provoke seizures, nausea, profound weakness, balance problems, vision problems, pain, headache and personality changes.

As humans our being or essence is felt to be intertwined with our personality. This perception makes changes in personality very difficult for loved ones to accept in the patient with brain cancer. Small changes may be easily dealt with, but major changes in personality disrupt the entire family. Patients may become angry, they have lost personal power. The loss of driving privileges is often very difficult to accept, because it signifies their loss of freedom. Family decisions are no longer trusted to this person.

Biofield modalities are appropriate to assist the patient and those who care for him/her. Energy medicine may hypothetically help both the patient and the family to be more accepting of each other and to maintain a greater sense of calm and ease tension. This healing energy will go to wherever in the body or into whatever situation it is most needed.

There is a current study by the National Center for Complementary and Alternative Medicine (NCCAM) to assess whether distant healing effects survival time and loss of function for patients with glioblastoma. This is a double-blind randomized controlled clinical trial of 'distant healing intentionality'. The study findings will provide a basis for developing a larger, definitive trial[1].

References

Other cancers

1. DeVita VJ, Hellman S, Rosenberg S. Cancer Principles and Practice of Oncology, 5th edn. Philadelphia: Lippincott-Raven, 1997
2. Perez C, Brady L, Halperin EC, Schmidt-Ullrich RK. Principles and Practice of Radiation Oncology. Philadelphia: Lippincott, Williams and Wilkins, 2004
3. Leibel S, Phillips T. Textbook of Radiation Oncology. Philadelphia: WB Saunders, 1998

Physical activity

1. Friedenreich CM. Physical activity and cancer prevention: from observational to intervention research. Cancer Epidemiol Biomarkers Prev 2001; 10: 287–301
2. Shu XO, Hatch MC, Zheng W, et al. Physical activity and risk of endometrial cancer. Epidemiology 1993; 4: 342–9
3. Levi R, La Vecchia C, Negri E, et al. Selected physical activities and the risk of endometrial cancer. Br J Cancer 1993; 67: 846–51
4. Available at: http://www.cbsnews.com/stories/2004/03/30/health/main609379.shtm (Accessed 30 March 2004)
5. Michaud DS, Giovannucci E, Willet WC, et al. Physical activity, obesity, height, and the risk of pancreatic cancer. JAMA 2001; 286: 921–99
6. Rossing MA, Remler R, Voigt LF, et al. Recreational physical activity and risk of papillary thyroid cancer (United States). Cancer Causes Control 2001; 12: 881–5
7. Zheng W, Shu XO, McLaughlin JK, et al. Occupational physical activity and the incidence of cancer of the breast, corpus uteri and ovary in Shanghai. Cancer 1993; 71: 3620–4
8. Mink, PJ, Folsom AR, Sellers TA, et al. Physical activity, waist-to-hip ratio, and other risk factors for ovarian cancer: a follow-up study of older women. Epidemiology 1996; 7: 38–45
9. Cerhan JR, Janney CA, Vachon CM, et al. Anthropometric characteristics, physical activity, and risk of non-Hodgkin's lymphoma subtypes and B-cell chronic lymphocytic leukemia: a prospective study. Am J Epidemiol 2002; 156: 527–35
10. McTiernan A, Ulrich C, Slate S, Potter J. Physical activity and cancer etiology: associations and mechanisms. Cancer Causes Control 1998; 9: 487–509
11. Thune I, Furberg A-S. Physical activity and cancer risk: dose-response and cancer, all sites and site-specific. Med Sci Sports Exerc 2001; 33 (Suppl): S530–S550

Botanicals

1. Tode T, Kikuchi Y, Kita T, et al. Inhibitory effects by oral administration of ginsenoside Rh2 on the growth of human ovarian cancer cells in nude mice. J Cancer Res Clin Oncol 1993; 120: 24–6
2. Nicosia SV, Bai W, Cheng JO, et al. Oncogenic pathways implicated in ovarian epithelial cancer. Hematol Oncol Clin North Am 2003; 17: 927–43
3. Chen X, Anderson JJ. Isoflavones inhibit proliferation of ovarian cancer cells in vitro via an estrogen receptor-dependent pathway. Nutr Cancer 2001; 41: 165–71
4. Murata M, Midorikawa K, Koh M, et al. Genistein and daidzein induce cell proliferation and their metabolites cause oxidative DNA damage in relation to isoflavone-induced cancer of estrogen-sensitive organs. Biochemistry 2004; 43: 2569–77
5. Malagoli M, et al. Effect of glycyrrhizin and its diastereoisomers on the growth of human tumour cells: preliminary findings. Phytother Res 1998; 12: S95–S97
6. Kim SH, Kim TS. Synergistic induction of 1,25-dihydroxyvitamin D(3)- and all-trans-retinoic acid-induced differentiation of HL-60 leukemia cells by yomogin, a sesquiterpene lactone from Artemisia princeps. Planta Med 2002; 68: 886–90
7. Lee YK, Bone ND, Stege AK, et al. VEGF receptor phosphorylation status and apoptosis is

modulated by a green tea component, epigallo-catechin-3-gallate (EGCG) in B cell chronic lymphocytic leukemia. Blood 2004; 104: 788–94

8. Li YC, Tyan YS, Kuo HM, et al. Baicalein induced in vitro apoptosis undergo caspases activity in human promyelocytic leukemia HL-60 cells. Food Chem Toxicol 2004; 42: 37–43

9. Takada M, Nakamura Y, Koizumi T, et al. Suppression of human pancreatic carcinoma cell growth and invasion by epigallocatechin-3-gallate. Pancreas 2002; 25: 45–8

10. Lee LT, Huang YT, Huang JJ, et al. Blockade of the epidermal growth factor receptor tyrosine kinase activity by quercetin and luteolin leads to growth inhibition and apoptosis of pancreatic tumor cells. Anticancer Res 2002; 22: 1615–27

11. Kjaer M. Misteltoe (Iscador) therapy in stage IV renal adenocarcinoma. A phase II study in patients with measurable lung metastases. Acta Oncol 1989; 28: 489–94

12. Goebell PJ, Otto T, Suhr J, Rubben H. Evaluation of an unconventional treatment modality with mistletoe lectin to prevent recurrence of superficial bladder cancer: a randomized phase II trial. J Urol 2002; 168: 72–5

13. Devi PU, Sharada AC, Solomon FE, Kamath MS. In vivo growth inhibitory effect of Withania somnifera (Ashwagandha) on a transplantable mouse tumor, Sarcoma 180. Ind J Exp Biol 1992; 30: 169–72

14. Islam S, Islam N, Kermode T, et al. Involvement of caspase-3 in epigallocatechin-3-gallate-mediated apoptosis of human chondrosarcoma cells. Biochem Biophys Res Commun 2000; 270: 793–7

15. Garbisa S, Sartor L, Biggins S, et al. Tumor gelatinases and invasion inhibited by the green tea flavanol epigallocatechin-3-gallate. Cancer 2001; 91: 822–32

16. Takeyama T, Suzuki I, Ohno N, et al. Host-mediated antitumor effect of grifolan NMF-5N, a polysaccharide obtained from Grifola frondosa. J Pharmacobiol Dyn 1987; 10: 644–51

17. Dong Y, Kwan CY, Chen ZN, Yang MM. Antitumor effects of a refined polysaccharide peptide fraction isolated from Coriolus versicolor: in vitro and in vivo studies. Res Commun Mol Pathol Pharmacol 1996; 92: 140–8

18. Nanba H. Kuroda H. Antitumor mechanisms of orally administered shiitake fruit bodies. Chem Pharm Bull (Tokyo) 1987; 35: 2459–64

19. Tsubono Y, Nishino Y, Komatsu S, et al. Green tea and the risk of gastric cancer in Japan. N Engl J Med 2001; 344: 632–6

20. Nagata C, et al. A prospective cohort study of soy product intake and stomach cancer death. Br J Cancer 2002; 87: 31–6

21. Nakazato H, Takatsuka N, Kawakami N, Shimizu H. Efficacy of immunochemotherapy as adjuvant treatment after curative resection of gastric cancer. Lancet 1994; 343: 1122–6

22. Suh SO, Kroh M, Kim NR, et al. Effects of red ginseng upon postoperative immunity and survival in patients with stage III gastric cancer. Am J Chin Med 2002; 30: 483–94

23. Li N, Sun Z, Han C, Chen J. The chemopreventive effects of tea on human oral precancerous mucosa lesions. Proc Soc Exp Biol Med 1999; 220: 218–24

24. Khafif A, Chantz SP, Chou TC, et al. Quantitation of chemopreventive synergism between (-)-epigallocatechin-3-gallate and curcumin in normal, premalignant and malignant human oral epithelial cells. Carcinogenesis 1998; 19: 419–24

Energy medicine

1. Efficacy of Distant Healing in Glioblastoma Treatment, sponsored by NCCAM, www.ClinicalTrials.gov. Estimated completion date late 2004

15g

Palliative and end-of-life care

Matthew P. Mumber

Palliative and end-of-life care are increasingly becoming models for an integrative approach to oncology that focuses on the mental, emotional, physical and spiritual needs of patients, families and providers. The Institute of Medicine defines palliative care as that which 'seeks to prevent, relieve or soothe the symptoms of disease or disorder without effecting a cure… in this broad sense [it] is not restricted to those who are dying or those enrolled in hospice programs… it attends closely to the emotional, spiritual and practical needs and goals of patients and those close to them'[1].

Palliative care should not only be used in the end-of-life situation, it should be used as a routine part of cancer care[2,3]. Palliative and end-of-life care are a part of a continuum that can exist for all involved in the process of serving patients with chronic diseases that have exhausted active treatment options. In this setting, there exists a fine balance of what may seem to be competing principles and therapeutic goals, as depicted in Table 15.14.

This realm of treatment is currently much closer to an integrative approach than conventional biomedicine, owing to the fact that 'curing' is no longer an option, and therefore a focus on 'healing' can take priority[4]. Complementary and alternative modalities are also being considered as a part of palliative care and end-of-life processes. Studies show that patients are more satisfied with hospice services when complementary care is used, and that about 60% of hospices use complementary therapies.[5–14]

Table 15.14 Issues to balance in palliative and end-of-life care

First do no harm	Do good
Truth telling in prognosis	Preserving hope
Relief of pain and suffering	Maintenance of quality of life
Physician and caregiver empathy and involvement	Physician and caregiver self-care
Significant change, loss of defined roles, loss of meaning	Transcendence and transformation

Working with a significant population of patients in the palliative and end-of-life setting can be overwhelming for oncology providers. Historically, in medical training, very little emphasis was placed on the needs of palliative care patients[1,15]. The result of this process has been to disconnect with the preferences of the majority of the population and the reality of interventions provided[1], as depicted in Table 15.15.

In his book *The Palliative Response*, Bailey offers a practical framework to address suffering as it occurs on physical, social, emotional and spiritual levels[16]. These considerations are outlined in Table 15.16.

The following sections list some complementary and alternative medicine (CAM) and conventional approaches that add value to palliative and end-of-life care as supportive care options. This list includes issues from Bailey's descriptions of various forms of suffering at the end of life, and offers possible therapeutic options, with appropriate levels of evidence. An excellent general source of information is the End of Life Nursing Education Consortium[17].

Level of evidence is defined as follows:

- Level one – well-designed randomized controlled clinical trial(s);

- Level two – prospective and retrospective non-randomized clinical trials and analyses;

- Level three – opinions of expert committees, best-case series;

- Level four – preclinical *in vitro* and *in vivo* studies, and traditional uses.

PHYSICAL SUFFERING

Pain and distress

- Intentional sedation is a treatment goal that differs from physician-assisted suicide[16];

- Subcutaneous therapy offers a lower morbidity option to intravenous therapy, and includes specific procedures[16];

- Mind–body interventions such as yoga, meditation, support groups, self-hypnosis, creative art therapy, music therapy, relaxation/imagery[7,14] (level II);

- Gentle massage, energy medicine[6,18] (level II);

- Auricular acupuncture may be helpful[19] (level II).

Anorexia

- Dexamethasone is an inexpensive and efficacious method to help with appetite enhancement, relative to more expensive drugs such as Megace and Marinol[16];

- Omega-three fat supplementation[20] (conflicting level I);

- Physical activity as tolerated[21] (level II).

Fatigue

- Fatigue can respond to simple interventions such as physical therapy, reframing of goals and getting up out of bed[16];

- Mind–body therapies – yoga, meditation (level II);

- Physical activity[22] (level II);

- Healing Touch and massage[23] (level I).

Constipation

- Fruits and vegetables, fluids (level II);

- Physical activity as tolerated (level II);

- Abdominal massage[24] (level II);

- Herbal laxatives such as *Cascara sagrada* (senna) (level IV).

Table 15.15   Patient preferences and reality in palliative and end-of-life care

Preferences	Reality
90% would prefer to die at home	15% die at home
Adequate pain control	Pain control inadequate
Patients would like to talk about spiritual, emotional issues	Infrequent dialog about spiritual, emotional issues

Table 15.16   Key elements in palliative care

Type of suffering	Specific examples
Physical	Pain and distress, anorexia, fatigue, constipation, dyspnea, insomnia, nausea and vomiting, feeding by mouth, hydration, opioid side-effects, debility, symptom prevention, advance planning
Emotional	Depression, anxiety, delirium, loneliness, grief and bereavement
Social	Limited income, lack of insurance, inadequate housing, social isolation, caregiver fatigue
Spiritual	Loss of hope, loss of relations with faith community, search for meaning

Dyspnea

- Dyspnea can often be relieved by the use of a fan or air conditioner[16];

- Acupuncture[14] (level II);

- Muscle relaxation with breath retraining[14] (level II).

Insomnia

- Insomnia can respond to changing rituals – exercise earlier in day, using relaxation techniques, restricting use of bed for sleep[16];

- Yoga, relaxation techniques, guided imagery, hypnosis[25,26] (level II);

- *Matricaria recutita* (chamomile tea), *Valeriana officinalis* (valerian), *Lavendula officinalis* (lavender) pillows (levels II–IV).

Nausea and vomiting

- Nausea has many causes, including fear and anxiety, constipation, medications and vertigo[16];

- Acupressure, acupuncture, electroacupuncture[14] (levels I, II, III);

- Mind–body relaxation techniques[14,26] (level II).

Feeding by mouth

- Continuing feeding and hydrating by mouth, even in small quantities, offers similar length of survival for most patients, and allows for less morbidity than feeding tubes or intravenous feeding[16];

- Feeding tubes can serve as an effective bridge to resuming oral intake for some patients, e.g.

esophageal and head and neck cancer patients undergoing radiation[16].

Opioid side-effects

- An equianalgesic chart should be on hand for conversion of pain medication doses; when medication type is changed, one can often reduce the equianalgesic dose by up to 25% and provide similar pain relief with less toxicity[16].

Symptom prevention

- While all ethical principles are important, working with the patient and family toward 'doing good' or beneficience will often achieve the other principles, such as 'do no harm'[16].

Advance planning

- The physician should not delegate sharing bad news. Bad news is best shared at a scheduled appointment with the entire family, and the physician should stop frequently to assess understanding and show empathy[16,27].

EMOTIONAL SUFFERING

Depression

- Mind–body therapies[26] (levels I and II);
- Physical activity[28] (level II).

Anxiety

- Mind–body therapies[10,29] (level II);
- Physical activity[30] (level II);
- Creative arts/music[7,9–11,31] (level II);
- *Valeriana officinalis* (valerian) (level IV).

Loneliness, grief and bereavement, social isolation

- Support groups[14] (level II).

CAREGIVER FATIGUE

Self-care for the provider dealing with palliative care includes the R&Rs: Recuperation with rest and sleep, Restoration with good nutrition, Relaxation with regular vacations, Recreation in the form of hobbies, Rejuvenation with regular exercise, self-Referral if concerned about your health (physically and emotionally), fostering Relationships with family, friends and colleagues on personal and professional levels, and by finding and being a mentor, finding methods for Reflection on personal, religious or philosophical issues. All of this can help one to develop a sense of the transcendent[16,32,33].

SEARCH FOR MEANING

- Five things that everyone needs to say at life's end: forgive me; I forgive you; thank you; I love you; good bye[16];

- It is appropriate for physicians to share in a patient's wondering about unanswerable questions[16];

- Transcendence at life's end is a state of meaning and hope that provides connection with family and others across life-changing events and across even death itself. Physicians can help to support this process through an open and honest dialog concerning spiritual issues and by supporting each individual patient and family's unique process[16];

- Mind–body therapies[14] (level II);

- Residential retreats and support groups[33] (level II).

For a listing of Hospice programs around the country that use various CAM approaches in palliative care, see Chapter 12f.

CURRENT RESEARCH

REST trial: Reducing End of Life Symptoms with Touch – determines whether massage therapy is effective in reducing pain and distress and improving quality of life among cancer patients at life's end. Expected completion: October 2005 (see NCCAM website).

END-OF-LIFE RESOURCES

Advanced Directives: A Selected Bibliography – includes living wills, guardianships, durable powers of attorney and health proxies. Includes a comprehensive bibliography with a small section on ethnic, cultures and nations. State University of NY, Buffalo Health Sciences Library (ublib.buffalo.edu)

Approaching Death: Improving Care at the End of Life – published by the Institute of Medicine, Committee on Care at the End of Life.

Partnership for Caring: America's Voices for the Dying – national non-profit organization that partners individuals and organizations to improve how people die in our society. (www.partnershipforcaring.org)

End of Life Physician Education Resource Center (EPERC) – supported by the Robert Wood Johnson Foundation and located at the Medical College of Wisconsin. The EPERC is a central repository for educational materials and information about end of life issues. (www.eperc.mcw.edu/)

End-of-Life Nursing Education Consortium (ELNEC) Project – a comprehensive, national education program to improve end-of-life care by nurses, and is funded by a major grant from The Robert Wood Johnson Foundation. Primary project goals are to develop a core of expert nursing educators and to co-ordinate national nursing education efforts in end-of-life care. www.aacn.nche.edu/ELNEC/index.htm)

Education on Palliative and End Of Life Care – Oncology (EPEC-O) – organization sponsored by the American Society of Clinical Oncology in order to educate physicians concerning end-of-life care. (www.epeconline.net)

American Hospice Foundation
www.americanhospice.org

Hospice Foundation of America
www.hospicefoundation.org

National Hospice and Palliative Care Organization (NHPCO)
www.nhpco.org

Palliative care

The Cochrane Pain, Palliative Care and Supportive Care Collaborative Review Group – systematic reviews of randomized controlled trials of interventions concerned with pain and palliative care. (www.jr2.ox.ac.uk/Cochrane/)

The Center to Advance Palliative Care – a national initiative supported by the Robert Wood Johnson Foundation and Mount Sinai School of Medicine. The mission of the Center to Advance Palliative Care is to increase the availability of quality palliative care services in hospitals and other health-care settings for people with life-threatening illnesses, their families and caregivers by providing technical support and resources. (www.capcmssm.org)

Palliative Care Leadership Center – helps hospitals develop palliative care programs. (www.capc.org/pclc)

References

1. Approaching death: improving care at the end of life – a report of the Institute of Medicine. Health Serv Res 1998; 33: 1–3

2. Stacey B, Martin K, Underwood R. A continuum of palliative care services: reflections on an Australian model of care. J Palliat Care 1997; 13: 45–9

3. Yurk R, Morgan D, Franey S, et al. Understanding the continuum of palliative care for patients and their caregivers. J Pain Symptom Manage 2002; 24: 459–70

4. Choi YS, Billings JA. Changing perspectives on palliative care. Oncology (Huntingt) 2002; 16: 515–22

5. Byass R. Auditing complementary therapies in palliative care: the experience of the day-care massage service at Mount Edgcumbe Hospice. Complement Ther Nurs Midwifery 1999; 5: 51–60

6. Fellowes D, Barnes K, Wilkinson S. Aromatherapy and massage for symptom relief in patients with cancer. Cochrane Database Syst Rev 2004: CD002287

7. Lewis CR, de Vedia A, Reuer B, et al. Integrating complementary and alternative medicine (CAM) into standard hospice and palliative care. Am J Hosp Palliat Care 2003; 20: 221–8

8. Wright LD. Complementary and alternative medicine for hospice and palliative care. Am J Hosp Palliat Care 2004; 21: 327–30

9. Brenner ZR, Krenzer ME. Using complementary and alternative therapies to promote comfort at end of life. Crit Care Nurs Clin North Am 2003; 15: 355–62

10. Zappa SB, Cassileth BR. Complementary approaches to palliative oncological care. J Nurs Care Qual 2003; 18: 22–6

11. Demmer C. A survey of complementary therapy services provided by hospices. J Palliat Med 2004; 7: 510–16

12. Demmer C, Sauer J. Assessing complementary therapy services in a hospice program. Am J Hosp Palliat Care 2002; 19: 306–14

13. Penson J. Complementary therapies: making a difference in palliative care. Complement Ther Nurs Midwifery 1998; 4: 77–81

14. Pan CX, Morrison RS, Ness J, et al. Complementary and alternative medicine in the management of pain, dyspnea, and nausea and vomiting near the end of life. A systematic review. J Pain Symptom Manage 2000; 20: 374–87

15. Burge FI, Latimer EJ. Palliative care in medical education at McMaster University. J Palliat Care 1989; 5: 16–20

16. Bailey FA. The Palliative Response. Birmingham, AL: Menasha Ridge Press, 2003

17. Sherman DW, Matzo ML, Coyne P, et al. Teaching symptom management in end-of-life care: the didactic content and teaching strategies based on the end-of-life nursing education curriculum. J Nurs Staff Dev 2004; 20: 103–15

18. Post-White J, Kinney ME, Savik K, et al. Therapeutic massage and healing touch improve symptoms in cancer. Integr Cancer Ther 2003; 2: 332–44

19. Alimi D, Rubino C, Pichard-Leandri E, et al. Analgesic effect of auricular acupuncture for cancer pain: a randomized, blinded, controlled trial. J Clin Oncol 2003; 21: 4120–6

20. Jho DH, Cole SM, Lee EM, Espat NJ. Role of omega-3 fatty acid supplementation in inflammation and malignancy. Integr Cancer Ther 2004; 3: 98–111

21. Zinna EM, Yarasheski KE. Exercise treatment to counteract protein wasting of chronic diseases. Curr Opin Clin Nutr Metab Care 2003; 6: 87–93

22. Schneider CM, Dennehy CA, Roozeboom M, Carter SD. A model program: exercise intervention for cancer rehabilitation. Integr Cancer Ther 2002; 1: 76–82

23. Post-White J, Kinney ME, Savik K, et al. Therapeutic massage and healing touch improve symptoms in cancer. Integr Cancer Ther 2003; 2: 332–44

24. Preece J. Introducing abdominal massage in palliative care for the relief of constipation. Complement Ther Nurs Midwifery 2002; 8: 101–5

25. Douglas DB. Hypnosis: useful, neglected, available. Am J Hosp Palliat Care 1999; 16: 665–70

26. Wolsko PM, Eisenberg DM, Davis RB, Phillips RS. Use of mind–body medical therapies. J Gen Intern Med 2004; 19: 43–50

27. DiBartola LM. Listening to patients and responding with care: a model for teaching communication skills. Jt Comm J Qual Improv 2001; 27: 315–23

28. Keats MR, Courneya KS, Danielsen S, Whitsett SF. Leisure-time physical activity and psychosocial well-being in adolescents after cancer diagnosis. J Pediatr Oncol Nurs 1999; 16: 180–8

29. Wolsko PM, Eisenberg DM, Davis RB, Phillips RS. Use of mind–body medical therapies. J Gen Intern Med 2004; 19: 43–50

30. Mackey KM, Sparling JW. Experiences of older women with cancer receiving hospice care: significance for physical therapy. Phys Ther 2000 May; 80: 459–68

31. Deng G, Cassileth BR, Yeung KS. Complementary therapies for cancer-related symptoms. J Support Oncol 2004; 2: 419–26

32. Baumrucker SJ. Palliative care, burnout, and the pursuit of happiness. Am J Hosp Palliat Care 2002; 19: 154–6

33. Feldman MK. Time out. Physician sabbaticals can provide relief from burnout, a chance to learn new skills, and time for introspection. Minn Med 1999; 82: 23–4

Index

academic medical center setting 83–6

access to treatments 103

acupuncture 248, 249

  guideline for eligibility 116

  placebo effect and 30

  supportive care 367–71

    breathlessness 371

    fatigue 369–70

    nausea 367–9

    pain 369

    side-effect management 370–1

adjuvant therapy 178

Agency for Health Care Policy and Research (AHCPR), levels of evidence 19–20, 21

alcohol consumption 397–8

  abuse, burnout and 63

  behavior change and maintenance model 402–3

  CAM therapies 400–2

  cessation and prevention 399–400

  national and international approaches 403–6

  scope of problem 398

  trends and risk factors 398–9

Alexian Brothers Hospital Network model 50

Alitus Integrative Health & Wellness, Vernon Hills, IL 96–7

aloe vera 335–6

α-linolenic acid (ALA) 265–6

alternative medicine 78, 243–53

  definition 4

  supportive care 367–74

  see also ayurvedic medicine; complementary and alternative medicine (CAM); homeopathy; traditional Chinese medicine (TCM)

American Cancer Society (AMS), nutritional guidelines 263–6

animal therapy 355–6

anorexia 496

antineoplastic therapy 11–12, 377–8

  botanicals 388–90

    bladder cancer 486–7

    breast cancer 423–4

    gastric cancer 488–9

    leukemia 485–6

    lung cancer 454

    ovarian cancer 485

    prostate cancer 441–2

    renal carcinoma 486

    sarcoma 487

  energy medicine 393–4

  mind–body interventions 381–2

  nutrition 379

antioxidants 178–9

supportive care 310–13
anxiety management 498
    energy medicine 342–3, 348
    environment 343
apoptosis 179
appetite enhancement 313–14
    palliative/end-of-life care 496
arginine supplementation 311–13
art 344–5
ashwagandha (*Withania somnifera*) 334, 335
    radiation therapy and 387–8
    sarcoma therapy 487
astragalus (*Astragalus membranaceus*) 334, 335
    interleukin-2 interaction 385
aura 206, 217
ayurvedic medicine 249–51
    diagnosis 250
    pathogenesis 249–50
    supportive care 372–3
    treatment of disease 250
        cancer 250–1

bad news sharing 498
Balint groups 71
beneficence 8
berberine 383
best case series 20
biofield 217
    see also energy medicine
black cohosh (*Cimicifuga racemosa*) 331
bladder cancer 486–7, 490
body composition 174
body fat distribution 258
body mass index (BMI) 179
    see also obesity
body weight management *see* weight management
botanicals 191–5, 485–9
    antineoplastic therapy 388–90
        bladder cancer 486–7
        breast cancer 423–4
        gastric cancer 488–9
        leukemia 485–6
        lung cancer 454

ovarian cancer 485
prostate cancer 441–2
renal carcinoma 486
sarcoma 487
cancer prevention 287–92
    breast cancer 420–3
    colorectal cancer 468
    garlic 287–8
    gastric cancer 487–8
    green tea 288–90
    head and neck cancer 489
    lung cancer 454
    milk thistle 290–1
    prostate cancer 440–1
    recommendations 291–2
    skin cancer 479
    soy 291
drug interactions 33, 192–3, 331–2, 333, 383–4
    positive interactions 384–8, 389, 423
glossary of terms 194
pancreatic cancer and 486
radiation therapy and 387–8
research 191–4
    current trials 193–4
resources 194–5
supportive care 331–7
    chemotherapy-related symptom management 334–5
    immunosuppression 333–4
    nausea/vomiting 332–3
    radiation therapy side-effects 335–6
    recommendations 336–7
    side-effect management 331–2
    see also herbal treatments; *specific botanicals*
brain cancer 492
breast cancer 409–26
    benefits of interventions 413–17
    botanicals and 420–4
    conventional therapy 411
    diagnosis 410
    energy medicine 425–6
    mind–body interventions 419
    nutrition and 418

physical activity and 412
risk factors 409, 410
screening and early detection 409–10
breathlessness, acupuncture benefits 371
burnout
costs of 63–4
drug and alcohol abuse 63
relationships 63–4
suicide 63
factors 62–3
in oncology 61–2
medical training and 62
patient care issues 62
risk of 61
business assessment 121–38
costs 122–4
reasons for service provision 121–2
reimbursement 122–3
analysis 124–5
CAM and 127–34
CPT® codes 125–7
service users 122

C-reactive protein (CRP) 314
Calendula officinalis 336
California Hematology Oncology Medical
Group, Los Angeles and Torrance, CA
86–7
calories 179
restriction benefits 258
Camellia sinensis see green tea
Cancell/Entelev 23
cancer 179
incidence 123
prevention *see* preventive care
see also specific forms of cancer
Cancer Treatment Centers of America, Zion, IL
and Tulsa, OK 90–2
Canyon Ranch, Tucson, AZ 98
carbohydrate 179
carcinogen 179
carcinogenesis 179
cardiovascular fitness 174
caregiver fatigue 498

Carolinas Integrative Health, Charlotte, NC
93–4
case series 20
catechins 266
protective effect 289–90, 468
see also green tea
Cell Theory 244
Center for Frontier Medicine in Biofield Science 216
Center for Integrated Healing, Vancouver,
Canada 89–90
Center for Integrative Medicine and Healing
Therapies, Largo, FL 94–5
central nervous system cancer 492
chakra system 206–8, 217
chemoprevention 194, 287
garlic 287–8
green tea 288–90
see also preventive care
chemotherapy
positive interactions with botanicals 384–7,
423
combination chemotherapy 386–7
side-effect management 331–2, 334–5,
349–51
acupuncture 367–9
cisplatin 334–5
cyclophosphamide 335
energy medicine 341–6, 469
immunosuppression 333–4
myelosuppression 350–1
nausea and vomiting 332–3, 367–9
toxin elimination 357
Chi 204, 217, 245
see also energy medicine
Chi Kung 209
see also energy medicine
Children's Hospitals and Clinics, Minneapolis,
MN 92–3
chiropractic therapy 197–8, 199
reimbursement 136
see also manual therapies
cisplatin
activity enhancement 384

side-effect management 334–5
'clinic without walls' model 81, 95–6
clinical decision making *see* decision making
clinical guidelines *see* guidelines
clinical trials 23–5
    non-randomized controlled clinical trials 20
    phase I trials 24
    phase II trials 24–5
    phase III trials 25
    phase IV trials 25
    randomized controlled clinical trials 20,
        25–31
        nocebo effect 31
        placebo effect 26–31
cognitive–behavioral therapy (CBT) 187,
    281–2, 323
color therapy 343–4
colorectal cancer 457–69
    benefits of interventions 461–5
    botanicals and 468
    conventional therapy 458–9
    diagnosis 458
    energy medicine 469, 492
    mind–body interventions 467
    nutrition and 466
    physical activity and 460–1
    risk factors 457, 458
    screening and early detection 458
community environment 360–1
compassion 9
complementary and alternative medicine
    (CAM) 3–4, 17–18, 78
    classifications 18–19
    education *see* physician training
    guidelines 114–15
    legal issues 101–2
        failure to inform about CAM options 112
        referrals 112–13
        relevant law 102–4
    placebo effect and 30–1
    'push and pull' factors 5
    reimbursement and 127–34, 135–6
    safety considerations 32–4
    tobacco and alcohol cessation 400–2

    users 122
complementary medicine 4, 78
connection 354–5
    animal/pet therapy 355–6
    nature therapy 356
consent form 116–17
Consortium of Academic Health Centers for
    Integrative Medicine (CAHCIM) 44,
    52–3
constipation 496
consultation-based integrative medicine 80–1,
    83–90, 93–4
contaminants, herbal products 32–3
    hypothetical clinical trial 104–5
continuing medical education (CME) 45–50
    CAM and cancer and 47–50
        continuing CAM education 50–4
            Alexian Brothers Hospital Network model
                50
            resources 51–2
            starting a program 51
        improvements in options 47
        obstacles to 46–7
conventional medicine 4, 243–4
Coriolus versicolor 334, 335
    colorectal cancer and 468
    positive drug interactions 386–7
    sarcoma and 487
costs 122–4
creative therapies 187
    supportive care 324–5
curcumin
    antineoplastic effect 423–4
    drug interactions 383
    protective effect 423, 454
    radiosensitizing effect 388
curing, versus healing 9
Current Procedure Terminology (CPT®) codes
    125–6
    category I codes 126
    category II codes 127
    category III codes 127
    getting a CPT code added 126–7
cyclophosphamide side-effect management 335

Dana-Farber Cancer Institute Zakim Center, Boston, MA 83–5, 131
decision making 34–7, 145–63
    decision trees 146–63
    guidelines 145–6
    individual clinical situation 35
    level of evidence and CAM 35–6
    therapy type and goal 34–5
deep tissue massage 199
delay in treatment, liability for 113–14
depression 282, 498
    energy medicine and 342–3, 348
diet 177, 263–9
    guidelines for cancer prevention 263–6
    history 179
    palliative care 314–15
        food as comfort 315
        hydration 315
    protective effect of plant-based diet 266–9
        dietary fiber 267–8, 466
        evidence 266–7
        phytochemicals 268–9
        vegetable and fruit intake 267
    supportive care 313–14
        appetite enhancement 313–14
        maintaining visceral protein stores 314
        meal replacements/supplements 313
    see also nutrition
dietary 24-hour recall 179
dietary fiber 179–80
    colorectal cancer and 466
    protective effect 267–8, 466
dietary records 179
Dietary Supplement Health and Education Act, 1994 (DSHEA) 103, 192
dietary supplements
    reimbursement 132
    supportive care 310–13
        assessment of supplement use 311
        glutamine and arginine 311–13
        meal replacements 313
distant healing 209
    current trial 214–15
    see also energy medicine

docosahexanoic acid (DHA) 264
doctor–patient relationship 360
Doctoring to Heal 72
doxorubicin (DOX), green tea interaction 384–5
drug abuse, burnout and 63
drug interactions 33, 192–3, 331–2, 333, 383–4
    positive interactions 384–8, 389, 423
dyspnea 497

eicosapentaenoic acid (EPA) 264
electromagnetic field 208, 211–12
    see also energy medicine
end-of-life care 361–3, 495–9
    caregiver fatigue 498
    current research 499
    emotional suffering 498
    physical suffering 496–8
    resources 499
    search for meaning 498–9
energy 217
energy medicine 203–19, 490–2
    antineoplastic care 393–4
    bladder cancer 490
    breast cancer 425–6
    cancer prevention 295–9
        recommendations 296–7, 299
    CNS cancer 492
    colorectal cancer 469, 492
    definition 203–4
    end-of-life care 361–3
    environmental 357–61
        community environment 360–1
        doctor–patient relationship 360
        energetic environment 357–8
        family environment 359–60
        natural environment 358–9
    esophageal cancer 491
    gastric cancer 491–2
    glossary of terms 217–18
    head and neck cancers 490–1
    lung cancer 455
    modalities 204, 205

pancreatic cancer 492
prostate cancer 443
renal cancer 490
research 212–17
   current questions 213–14
   current trials 214–17
resources 218–19
skin cancer 480
treatment-related symptom management
   346–51
   depression/anxiety 348
   fatigue 346–7
   sexuality 349
   sleep changes 348–9
   weight gain/loss 347–8
treatment-related symptom prevention
   341–6
   color and light therapy 343–4
   depression/anxiety 342–3
   environment 343
   pain relief 341–2
vitality enhancement 351–7
   animal/pet therapy 355–6
   connection 354–5
   hope 353
   meaning 353–4
   nature therapy 356
   spirituality 356–7
   toxin elimination 357
environment
   anxiety and 343
   community environment 360–1
   doctor–patient relationship 360
   energetic environment 357–8
   family environment 359–60
   natural environment 358–9
epidermal growth factor receptor (EGFR) 479
epigallocatechin gallate (EGCG) 385, 388
   breast cancer protection 423
   colorectal cancer and 468
   leukemia and 486
   pancreatic cancer and 486
   prostate cancer protection 441
   sarcoma and 487

esophageal cancer 491
exercise 173
   see also physical activity
exercise testing 173
Exploratory Program Grant for Frontier Medicine 216

faith 238
   see also spirituality
family members 352
   family environment 359–60
Family Practice Center of Integrative Health
   and Healing, Burlington, Ontario 94
fat 179
   saturated 180
   trans 180
fat distribution 258
fatigue
   acupuncture benefits 369–70
   breast cancer patients 425
   caregiver fatigue 498
   energy medicine 346–7
   palliative/end-of-life care 496
   physical activity benefits 303–4
feeding by mouth 497–8
Feng Shui 343
fiber, dietary 179–80
   colorectal cancer and 466
   protective effect 267–8, 466
fibrosarcoma 487
Finding Meaning in Medicine® 72
fish oils, protective effect 264
fitness center setting 81, 96–7
flax seed, protective effect 265–6, 423
food frequency questionnaires 180
free radicals, physical activity and 258–9
fruit intake, protective effect 267
   see also diet; nutrition
functional foods 180

Ganoderma lucidum 441
garlic, preventive effect 287–8
gastric cancer 487–9, 491–2
   antineoplastic therapy 488–9

prevention 487–8
genistein, tamoxifen interaction 383–4, 423
  see also soy
ginger, anti-emetic action 332–3
ginseng
  breast cancer and 423, 424
  gastric cancer and 488–9
  lung cancer and 454
  ovarian cancer and 485
  positive drug interactions 387
    interleukin-2 385–6
    mitomycin C 384
    tamoxifen 385, 423
glucose, physical activity effect 258
glutamine supplementation 311–13
glycemic index 180
Glycyrrhiza 423, 485–6
grape juice, protective effect 422
grape seed, antineoplastic effect 424
green tea 22–3, 266
  antineoplastic effect 442, 486, 487
  doxorubicin/idarubicin interaction 384–5
  preventive effects 288–90
    breast cancer 421–2
    colorectal cancer 468
    lung cancer 454
    oral cancers 489
    prostate cancer 441
Grifola frondosa 487
group therapeutic procedures 137–8
guided imagery *see* imagery
guidelines 10, 12, 114–15
  decision making 145–6
  nutritional guidelines 263–6
guiding principles of medicine 6–10
Gwinnett Health System, Lawrenceville, GA
  97–8

harmlessness 8
head and neck cancer 489, 490–1
healing
  focus on 9, 204
  sacredness of 236–8
  spirituality and 71

Healing Touch 209, 299, 341
  breast cancer patients 425–6
  current trial 215–16
  see also energy medicine
health insurance 122–5
  CPT® codes 125–6
    getting a CPT code added 126–7
  see also reimbursement
Health Insurance Portability and Accountability
  Act (HIPPA) 125
health resort setting 81, 98
health-care fraud 103–4
health-care provider wellness *see* provider wellness
health-related physical fitness 173–4
herbal treatments
  contaminants 32–3
    hypothetical clinical trial 104–5
  herb–drug interactions 33, 192–3, 331–2,
    333, 383–4
    positive interactions 384–8, 389, 423
  in Traditional Chinese Medicine 248
    hot flushes 372
  reimbursement 132
  see also botanicals
heterocyclic amines (HCA) 274–5
holistic approach 244–5
homeopathy 251–3
  cancer and 252–3
  placebo effect and 30
  supportive care 373–4
    hot flushes 373–4
    oral mucositis 373
    radiation therapy side-effects 373
hope 239, 353
  see also spirituality
hospital-based integrative care 83, 90–2
  pediatric 92–3
hot flushes 331
  acupuncture benefits 370–1
  Chinese herbal medicine 372
  homeopathic medicine 373–4
hydration, in palliative care 315
Hypericum perforatum see St John's wort

hypnosis 187
    supportive care 319–20
    see also mind–body interventions
hypothesis-driven research 21–3

idarubicin (IDA), green tea interaction 385
imagery 187, 320
    supportive care 320
    see also mind–body interventions
immune function
    enhancement 273–4
    physical activity effects 257
immunosuppression 333–4
informed CAM-trained clinician model 82
informed clinician model 82
informed consent form 116–17
informed networking clinician model 82, 87–8
insoluble fiber 179, 268
insomnia 497
insulin
    control of 269–72
    physical activity effect 258
insulin-like growth factor 269–72
    physical activity effect 258
Integrative Internal Medicine Clinic, San Diego,
    CA 95–6
integrative medicine (IM) 3–4, 78
    consultation-based integrative medicine
        80–1, 83–90, 93–4
    definition 78, 102
    expanded domain 6, 7
    hospital-based 83, 90–2
        pediatric 92–3
    in academic medical center 83–6
    in fitness center 81, 96–7
    in spa or health resort 81, 98
    integrative primary care 81, 94–5, 96–7
    legal issues 101–19
        clinical cases 104–12
        law relevant to integrative care 102–4
        liability for delay 113–14
        referrals 112–13
        resources 117–19
    models 80–3, 84

    positive and negative attributes 6
    virtual integrative medicine services 81,
        97–8
    see also integrative oncology
integrative medicine (IM) centres 78–80
    examples 83–98
    models of integrative care 80–3, 84
integrative oncology (IO) 3, 78
    decision making 34–7, 145–63
        decision trees 146–63
        guidelines 145–6
        individual clinical situation 35
        level of evidence and CAM 35–6
        therapy type and goal 34–5
    definition 4
    functional aspects 10–13
        Precautionary Principle 12–13
        preventive, supportive and antineoplastic
            care 11–12
        translation versus transformation 10–11
    principles of 7–10
    reasons for 5–6
    service establishment *see* business assessment
    see also integrative medicine (IM)
interdisciplinary integrative group practice
    82–3, 89–90, 93–4
International Society for the Study of Subtle
    Energies and Energy Medicine (ISSSEEM)
    203
isoflavones 264–5, 291
    breast cancer prevention 420–1
    ovarian cancer and 485
    prostate cancer prevention 440–2

joint mobilization 137

Kemper classification of CAM therapies 18–19
kidney cancer 486, 490

legal issues 101–19
    clinical cases 104–12
    law relevant to integrative care 102–4
    liability for delay 113–14
    referrals 112–13

resources 117–19
Lentinus edodes 487
leukemia 485–6
levels of evidence 19–21
licensure 102
light therapy 343–4
lignans 265–6
lung cancer 445–57
   benefits of interventions 448–51
   botanicals and 454
   conventional therapy 446
   diagnosis 445–6
   energy medicine 455
   mind–body interventions 453
   nutrition and 452
   physical activity and 447
   risk factors 445
   screening and early detection 445
lymphedema 425

macronutrient 180
magnet therapy 210
   see also energy medicine
malpractice 102–3
   liability 105–9
managed care plans 125
manual therapies 137, 197–200
   current research 198–9
   glossary of terms 199
   resources 199–200
   supportive care 339
   see also chiropractic therapy; massage therapy;
     osteopathy
massage therapy 137, 197–8, 209–10
   lymphedema 425
   reimbursement 131
   supportive care 339, 341
   see also manual therapies
meaning 353–4
   search for 229–32, 498–9
Medicaid program 124–5
medical culture 64–5
Medical Knowledge Self-Assessment Program
   (MKSAP) 47

medical school 44
Medicare reimbursement 122–3, 124, 126,
   127, 133
   CAM services 131–3, 135–6
meditation 187
   supportive care 321–2
   see also mind–body interventions
melanoma 471
   botanicals and 479
   mind–body interventions 478
   physical activity and 473
Memorial Sloan-Kettering Cancer Center, New
   York 130, 131
menopausal symptoms
   acupuncture benefits 370–1
   see also hot flushes
MET (metabolic equivalent) 174–5
micronutrients 180
   protective effects 272–3
     immune enhancement 273–4
   supportive care 310–13
milk thistle 335
   cisplatin interaction 384
   protective effect 290–1, 441
   skin cancer protection 479
mind–body interventions 183–8
   antineoplastic therapy 381–2
   breast cancer 419
   cancer prevention 281–3, 419
   colorectal cancer 467
   definition 183–4, 187
   glossary of terms 187–8
   lung cancer 453
   prostate cancer 439
   reimbursement 132
   research 184–7
     current questions 185
     current trials 185–6
   resources 188
   skin cancer 478
   supportive care 319–27, 419
     creative therapies 324–5
     hypnosis 319–20
     imagery/relaxation 320

meditation 321–2
  psychotherapy 323–4
  yoga 322–3
mindfulness-based cognitive therapy (MBCT)
  282
mindfulness-based stress reduction (MBSR)
  282, 283
  antineoplastic care 381
  prostate cancer 439
  supportive care 321–2
mistletoe (*Viscum*) 486–7
mitomycin C, ginseng synergistic effect 384
moxibustion 248, 249
multidisciplinary integrative group practice 82,
  86–7, 94–5, 96–7
musculoskeletal fitness 174
music therapy 299, 342, 345–6
myelosuppression 350–1

National Cancer Institute (NCI), ranking of
  levels of evidence 19–21
National Center for Complementary and Alternative Medicine (NCCAM)
  CAM fellowship education 45
  classification scheme 18
  definition of integrative medicine 102
natural environment 358–9
nature therapy 356
nausea 332–3, 350–1, 497
  acupuncture benefits 367–9
neck cancer 489, 490–1
negligence 102–3, 105
neuromuscular therapy 199
nocebo effect 31
non-randomized controlled clinical trials 20
nutrition 177–80
  antineoplastic therapy 379
  breast cancer risk and 418
  cancer prevention 263–76
    dietary fiber 267–8, 466
    food preparation 274–5
    guidelines 263–6
    immune enhancement 273–5
    insulin control 269–72

micronutrients 272–3
  phytochemicals 268–9, 270–2
  plant-based diet 266–9
  recommendations 275–6
  weight control 269
colorectal cancer and 466
counseling, reimbursement 131–2, 135
glossary of terms 178–80
lung cancer and 452
prostate cancer and 438
research 177–8
  current questions 178
  current trials 178
skin cancer and 477
supportive care 307–15
  antioxidant/micronutrient supplements
    310–13
  unintentional weight loss 307–10
  weight management 307
see also botanicals

obesity 258, 269
  weight control 269
occupational activity 173
opioid side-effects 498
oral cancers 489
oral mucositis 373, 490
osteopathy 197–8, 199
  see also manual therapies
outcomes
  ranking of 20
  uncertainty of 8–9
ovarian cancer 485
Oxford Health Plans 128, 129
oxidative damage, physical activity and 258–9

pain relief
  acupuncture 369
  energy medicine 341–2
  palliative/end-of-life care 496
palliative care 314, 495–9
  caregiver fatigue 498
  current research 499
  emotional suffering 498

energy medicine 361–3
  nutrition therapy 314–15
    food as comfort 315
    hydration 315
  physical suffering 496–8
  resources 499
  search for meaning 498–9
Panax see ginseng
pancreatic cancer 486, 492
PC-SPES 23
  contaminants 32–3
pediatric integrative oncology 92–3
personal emotion work 71
pet therapy 355–6
physical activity 171–5, 347–8
  cancer prevention 257–60, 484
    breast cancer 412
    colorectal cancer 460
    lung cancer 447
    mechanisms of preventive effect 257–9
    prostate cancer 432
    recommendations 259–60
  definition 173
  glossary of terms 173–5
  research 172–3
    current questions 172
  resources 175
  skin cancer and 473
  supportive care 303–5, 412, 432, 447, 460
    colorectal cancer 460
    recommendations 304–5
physical fitness 173
  health-related 173–4
physical therapy 137
physician training 43–54
  CAM associate fellowship program 45
  medical school 44
  residency and fellowship 44–5
  resources 51–4
  specialized CAM fellowship programs 45
  see also continuing medical education (CME)
physician wellness *see* provider wellness
Physician's Information and Education Resource (PIER) 47

phytochemicals 180, 194, 270–2
  protective effect 268–9
phytotherapy 194
placebo effect 26–31, 349
  as confounding factor in clinical research 28–30
  CAM and 30–1
Place...of wellness, MD Anderson Cancer Center, Houston, TX 85–6
Polarity Therapy 210
  see also energy medicine
prayer
  antineoplastic care 394
  current trial 216–17
  see also energy medicine
pre-clinical trials 22–3
Precautionary Principle 12–13
presence 346
preventive care 11–12, 255
  botanicals 287–91
    breast cancer 420–3
    colorectal cancer 468
    garlic 287–8
    gastric cancer 487–8
    green tea 288–90
    head and neck cancer 489
    lung cancer 454
    milk thistle 290–1
    prostate cancer 440–1
    recommendations 291–2
    skin cancer 479
    soy 291
  breast cancer 412, 419, 420–3
  colorectal cancer 460, 461, 468
  energy medicine 295–9
    recommendations 296–7, 299
  gastric cancer 487–8
  lung cancer 447, 454
  mind–body clinical interventions 281–3, 419
  nutrition 263–76
    food preparation 274–5
    guidelines 263–6
    immune enhancement 273–5

insulin control 269–72
micronutrients 272–3
plant-based diet 266–9
recommendations 275–6
weight control 269
physical activity 257–60, 484
breast cancer 412
colorectal cancer 460
lung cancer 447
mechanisms of preventive effect 257–9
prostate cancer 432
recommendations 259–60
prostate cancer 432, 440–1
reimbursement 132–3
skin cancer 479
professional satisfaction 59–60
prostate cancer 429–43
benefits of interventions 433–7
botanicals and 440–3
conventional therapy 430–1
diagnosis 430
energy medicine 443
mind–body interventions 439
nutrition and 438
physical activity and 432
risk factors 429–30
screening and early detection 430
protein 180
provider wellness 57–74
burnout 61–2
costs of 63–4
factors 62–3
medical training and 62
patient care issues 62
risk of 61
challenge of 65–6
connecting with other providers 72–3
residential retreat programs 72–3
connecting with self 67–8
integrative approach to self-care 58
medical culture role 64–5
narrative approach 68–9
personal emotion work 71
professional satisfaction 59–60

provider as patient 60–1
psychosocial support 71
self-care deficit 60
spirituality 69–71
healing and 71
religious practices 69
spiritual self-inquiry 70–1
transformation of 'sick care' into health care 66–7
wellness practices 68
working with the impossible 66
Prudential Insurance 128, 129
PSK polysaccharide 335, 386, 468, 488
psychoneuroimmunology (PNI) 282
antineoplastic care 381
psychosocial services
reimbursement 132
support for providers 71
psychotherapy 323–4

Qi 245
Qi Gong 209, 213, 299
antineoplastic care 393–4
chemotherapy side-effect management 350
supportive care 371–2
quercetin 485, 486

radiation therapy
botanicals and 387–8
side-effect management 335–6
homeopathy 373
salivary dysfunction 370
randomized controlled clinical trials 20, 25–31
nocebo effect 31
placebo effect and 26–31
rectal cancer 461
see also colorectal cancer
reductionist approach 244
referrals to CAM therapists, legal aspects 112–13
Regional Radiation Oncology Center, Rome, GA 87–8
Reiki 208–9
anxiety management 343

current trial 215
    end-of-life care 361–2
    pain management 341–2
    vitality enhancement 351
    see also energy medicine
reimbursement 103, 122–3
    analysis 124–5
    CAM and 127–34, 135–6
    CPT® codes 125–6
        getting a CPT code added 126–7
    dietary supplements 132
    herbal therapies 132
    massage therapy 131
    mind–body (stress reduction) 132
    non-conventional providers 133, 136
    nutritional counseling 131–2, 135
    preventive medicine 132–3
    psychosocial services 132
relationship-centred care 58
relationships
    doctor–patient relationship 360
    importance of 354–5
    see also connection
Relative Value Units (RVU) 125–6
relaxation 187–8
    supportive care 320
    see also mind–body interventions
religion 69, 222
    see also spirituality
renal cancer 486, 490
research design 19–23
    hypothesis-driven research 21–3
    levels of evidence 19–21
    see also clinical trials
residential retreat programs 72–3
resting energy expenditure (REE) 180
resveratrol 479
risk–benefit analysis 36

safety considerations 32–4
St John's wort
    drug interactions 33, 332
    placebo effect and 26–8
salivary dysfunction, radiation-induced 370

sarcoma 487
saturated fat 180
scanning 217
Schwartz Center Rounds 72
scope of practice 102
Scutellaria baicalensis 441
seasonal affective disorder (SAD) 344
self-care
    deficit 60
    integrative approach 58
    see also provider wellness
service among equals 9
service establishment *see* business assessment
sexuality problems 349
shiatsu 199
shiitake mushroom 487
side-effect management 331–2, 334–5, 349–51
    energy medicine 341–6, 469
    immunosuppression 333–4
    myelosuppression 350–1
    nausea and vomiting 332–3
        acupuncture 367–9
    opioid side-effects 498
Silybum marianum (milk thistle) 335
    cisplatin interaction 384
    protective effect 290–1, 441
    skin cancer protection 479
skin cancer 471–80
    benefits of interactions 473–6
    botanicals and 479
    conventional therapy 471–2
    diagnosis 471
    energy medicine 480
    mind–body interventions 478
    nutrition and 477
    physical activity and 473
    risk factors 471
    screening and early detection 471
sleep disturbances 497
    deprivation 64
    energy medicine 348–9
smoking *see* tobacco use
soluble fiber 179–80, 268
soy, protective effect 264–5, 291

breast cancer 420–1
gastric cancer 488
ovarian cancer and 485
prostate cancer 440–1
spa setting 81
spirituality 69, 221–40
  connectedness 233–6
  definitions 221–3
  faith, hope and trust 238–9
  from doing to being 232–3
  loss of control 226–9
  provider wellness and 69–71
    healing and 71
    religious practices 69
    spiritual self-inquiry 70–1
  research 223
  sacredness of healing 236–8
  search for meaning 229–32
  spiritual assessment 223, 224
  vitality enhancement 356–7
  'why' questions 223–6
'stages of change' model 165–8
  action 166
  contemplation 166
  counseling patients 166
    assessment 167
    evaluation and reformulation 168
    implementation 167
    planning 167
    target identification 167
  maintenance 166
  pre-contemplation 166
  preparation 166
standardized extract 194
steroid sex hormones, physical activity effects 257–8
  females 258
  males 257–8
stomach cancer see gastric cancer
stress reduction, reimbursement 132
subtle energy 218
sugar intake, lung cancer and 452
suicide, burnout and 63
supportive care 11, 301

acupuncture 367–71
  breathlessness 371
  fatigue 369
  nausea 367–9
  pain 369
  side-effect management 370–1
ayurvedic medicine 372–3
botanicals 331–7
  chemotherapy-related symptom management 334–5
  immunosuppression 333–4
  nausea/vomiting 332–3
  radiation therapy side-effects 335–6
  recommendations 336–7
  side-effect management 331–2
breast cancer 412, 419
Chinese herbal medicine 372
colorectal cancer 460, 461
energy medicine 341–63
  treatment-related symptom management 346–51
  treatment-related symptom prevention 341–6
  vitality enhancement 351–7
homeopathy 373–4
lung cancer 447
manual therapies 339
mind–body interventions 319–27, 419
  creative therapies 324–5
  hypnosis 319–20
  imagery/relaxation 320
  meditation 321–2
  psychotherapy 323–4
  yoga 322–3
nutrition 307–15
  antioxidant/micronutrient supplements 310–13
  dietary intervention 313–15
  unintentional weight loss 307–10
  weight management 307
physical activity 303–5, 412, 432, 447, 460
  recommendations 304–5
prostate cancer 432
Qi Gong 371–2

supportive–expressive therapy 281, 282
systems approach 34

Tai Chi 209, 371–2
  see also energy medicine
tamoxifen
  activity enhancement 385, 423
  hot flush induction *see* hot flushes
tea 266
  skin cancer protection 477
  see also green tea
team approach 6
Therapeutic Touch 209, 299, 341
  end-of-life care 361
  myelosuppression and 350
  see also energy medicine
third-party reimbursement 103
  see also reimbursement
tiredness *see* fatigue
tobacco use 397–8
  behavior change and maintenance model
    402–3
  CAM therapies 400–2
  cessation and prevention 399–400
  lung cancer and 445
  national and international approaches 403–6
  scope of problem 398
  trends and risk factors 398–9
toxin elimination 357
Traditional Chinese Medicine (TCM) 245–9
  disease 246–9
    cancer 248–9
    diagnosis 247–8
    pathogenesis 246–7
    treatment 248
  physiology 245–6
trans fat 180
transformation 10
  'sick care' into health care 66–7
  versus translation 10–11
translation 10
  versus transformation 10–11
transtheoretical model of change (TTM)
  402–3

trust 238–9
  see also spirituality
type C personality 281

Uncaria tomentosa (cat's claw) 334

vegetable intake, protective effect 267
virtual integrative medicine services 81, 97–8
visceral protein stores 314
vitality enhancement 351–7
  animal/pet therapy 355–6
  connection 354–5
  family 352
  hope 353–4
  nature therapy 356
  physician 351–2
  spirituality 356–7
vitamins *see* micronutrients
vocational activity 173
vomiting 332–3, 350, 497
  acupuncture benefits 367–9
  breast cancer patients 425

waist circumference 180
weight management 269, 307
  energy medicine 347–8
  unintentional weight loss 307–10, 347–8
wellness 58–9
  see also provider wellness
Western medicine 243–5
Withania somnifera (ashwagandha) 334, 335
  radiation therapy and 387–8
  sarcoma therapy 487

Yin and Yang 210, 246
yoga 188
  supportive care 322–3
  see also mind–body interventions
yosmogin 486

Zakim Center for Integrated Therapies, Dana-
  Farber Cancer Institute, Boston, MA
  83–5, 131